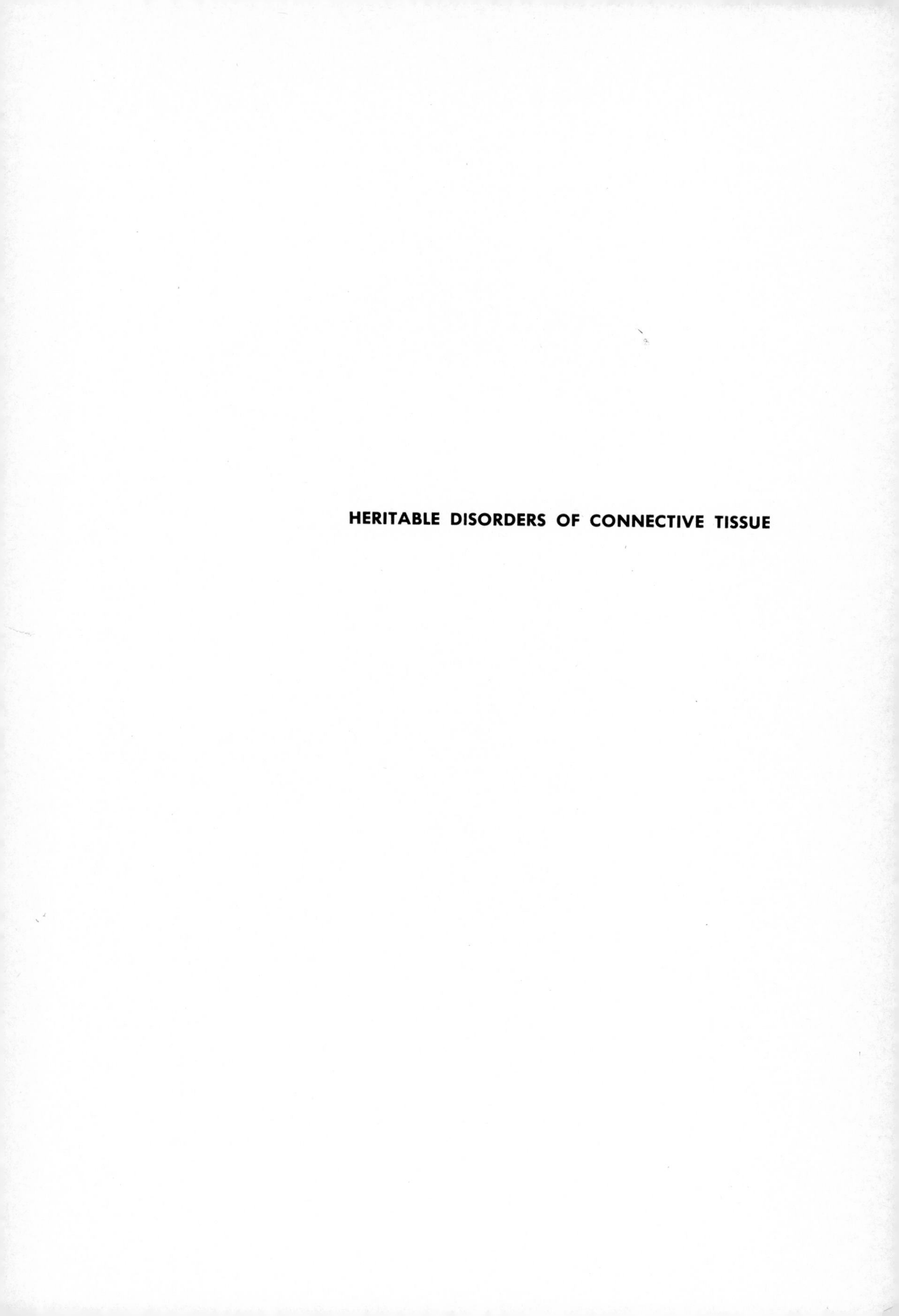

HERITABLE DISORDERS OF CONNECTIVE TISSUE

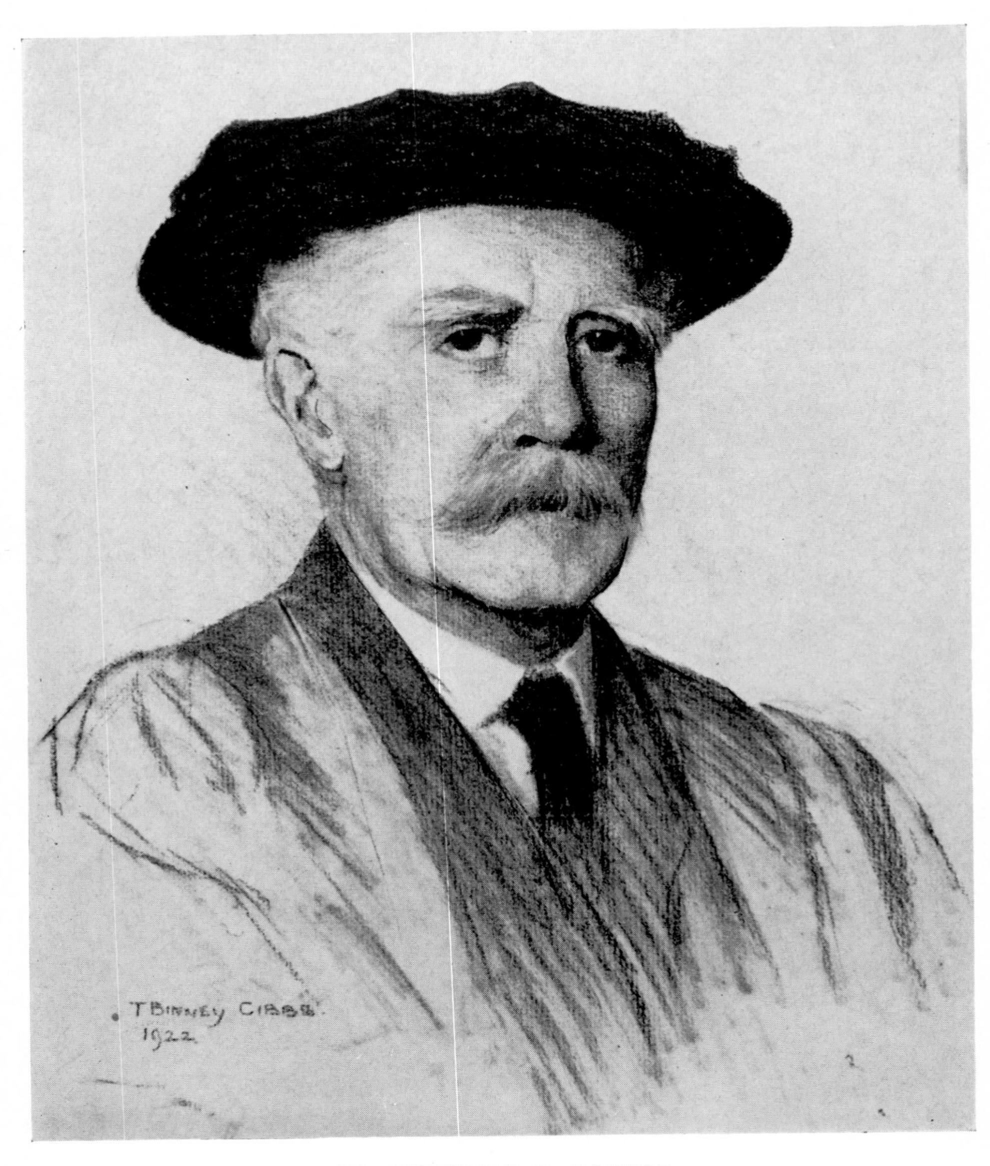

SIR ARCHIBALD E. GARROD

Author of Inborn Errors of Metabolism (1909, 1923) and Successor to Osler as Regius Professor of Medicine at Oxford

(From a previously unpublished crayon drawing made in 1922. Reproduced here through the kindness of Sir Archibald's daughter, Miss Dorothy A. E. Garrod.)

Heritable disorders of connective tissue

VICTOR A. McKUSICK, M.D.

Professor of Medicine, The Johns Hopkins University School of Medicine; Physician, The Johns Hopkins Hospital, Baltimore

THIRD EDITION

With 190 illustrations and two in color

The C. V. Mosby Company

Saint Louis 1966

Third edition

Previous editions copyrighted 1956, 1960
Printed in the United States of America
Library of Congress Catalog Card Number 65-28046
Distributed in Great Britain by Henry Kimpton, London

Dedicated
to the memory of

SIR ARCHIBALD E. GARROD (1857-1936)

and

to all who believe, as he did, that the clinical investigation of hereditary disorders can shed light on normal developmental and biochemical mechanisms

Preface

It has been ten years since some of this material was first published as a series of articles in the *Journal of Chronic Diseases.* The continued interest in the heritable disorders of connective tissue and their continued importance to clinical medicine and the biology of connective tissue are notable. In the interval, understanding of these diseases from both the clinical and the biologic points of view has increased appreciably. The collagen molecule has become more familiar in its physicochemical details, although it has far to go to match that paragon of protein molecules—hemoglobin. Characterization of the nature and metabolism of mucopolysaccharides has also advanced.

In connection with the Marfan syndrome, surgical treatment of the aortic complications is entirely a development of the last decade. An exciting discovery is that an inborn error of metabolism (homocystinuria) is responsible for a clinical picture which, because of ectopia lentis and vascular disease, simulates the Marfan syndrome. The vascular complications of the Ehlers-Danlos syndrome have become better appreciated. The existence of a recessive form of osteogenesis imperfecta now seems more likely. Evidence for involvement primarily of the elastic fiber in pseudoxanthoma elasticum has forced revision of the view held ten years ago. Furthermore, the recessive inheritance and histopathologic features, as well as the experience with homocystinuria, suggest that an inborn error of metabolism should be sought. The example of homocystinuria also suggests that alkaptonuria deserves classification as a heritable disorder of connective tissue.

Nosology has advanced farthest in this field in the mucopolysaccharidoses. Whereas in 1955 the nature of gargoylism as a mucopolysaccharidosis was recognized on histochemical grounds and two genetic forms, the autosomal recessive and the X-linked, were distinguished, characterization of the mucopolysacchariduria and identification of at least four other distinct varieties are developments of the last decade.

It is especially the generalist—the *general practitioner* and the *internist* and *pediatrician* without particular subspecialization—to whom the problems related to the several syndromes discussed here are of importance and to whom this book is addressed. He is in the best position to size up the total situation in the individual patient and with reference to the family background, with which he is most likely to have firsthand familarity. He can best evaluate what may be excessive loose-jointedness and "ganglingness" or mild pectus excavatum, pigeon breast, kyphoscoliosis, and flat feet. In the light of the general manifestations and the family background he can best appraise the significance of internal medical manifestations, which may be integral parts of a generalized syndrome.

Asboe-Hansen* has made the following cogent comment:

> Connective tissue connects the numerous branches of medical science. Without connective tissue, medicine would come to pieces, even non-viable pieces, just like the cells of the human body.

The ubiquity of connective tissue is responsible for its unifying influence on medicine, referred to in the statement quoted above. Furthermore, its ubiquity is responsible for the fact that concern with the problems of generalized and hereditary disorders of connective tissue extends also to many divisions of medical science and practice.

The *ophthalmologist* sees grave changes in the eyes in pseudoxanthoma elasticum, in the Marfan syndrome, and in homocystinuria and sees less serious, yet significant, alterations in osteogenesis imperfecta, the Ehlers-Danlos syndrome, and the mucopolysaccharidoses.

The *otologist* sees the patients with the Hurler syndrome, those with osteogenesis imperfecta, and rarely those with the Marfan syndrome.

The *orthopedist* is concerned with the cases of osteogenesis imperfecta, the Ehlers-Danlos syndrome, the Hurler syndrome, and sometimes the Marfan syndrome. Patients with fibrodysplasia ossificans progressiva are frequently seen by him.

The *general surgeon* repairs the hernias of the patient with the Marfan syndrome, the Ehlers-Danlos syndrome, osteogenesis imperfecta, or the Hurler syndrome.

The *hematologist* is consulted for the bruisability in the Ehlers-Danlos syndrome, for the tendency to multiple hemorrhages in patients with pseudoxanthoma elasticum, and for the multiple venous and arterial thromboses in homocystinuria.

The *gastroenterologist* is likely to encounter a case of pseudoxanthoma elasticum if he treats a sizable group of patients with gastrointestinal hemorrhage.

Increasingly the *cardiologist* is finding the Marfan syndrome of greater importance among the "causes" of aortic regurgitation and of dissecting aneurysm of the aorta than he had previously realized. In the Hurler syndrome the cardiac involvement may bring the patient to medical attention and is frequently the cause of death at an early age. Among cases of *peripheral vascular disease,* pseudoxanthoma elasticum or homocystinuria occasionally figures as a predominant etiologic factor.

Aside from the cardiovascular manifestations, the *chest physician* will be interested in the occurrence of cystic disease of the lung in the Marfan syndrome and of rupture of the lung with pneumothorax or mediastinal emphysema in the Marfan syndrome and in the Ehlers-Danlos syndrome.

The *dermatologist* treats patients with pseudoxanthoma elasticum and the Ehlers-Danlos syndrome.

Even the *plastic surgeon* is called in to provide cosmetic relief for the unsightly changes in the skin of the neck in pseudoxanthoma elasticum.

---

*Asboe-Hansen, G., editor: Connective tissue in health and disease, Copenhagen, 1954, Ejnar Munksgaards Forlag.

The *dentist* sees abnormalities, especially in osteogenesis imperfecta and the Hurler syndrome.

The *rheumatologist,* interested in connective tissues in general, is likely to see in these heritable disorders of connective tissue, derangements in purer culture and more easily analyzed form than in the acquired disorders of connective tissue such as the arthritides. Specifically, the rheumatologist may be consulted for the repeated hydrarthroses which may accompany the loose-jointedness of the Ehlers-Danlos syndrome, for the stiff joints of the mucopolysaccharidoses, and for the arthritis of alkaptonuria.

The *endocrinologist* is frequently consulted by the parents of a child with the Marfan syndrome or the Hurler syndrome and by the patient with osteogenesis imperfecta or fibrodysplasia ossificans progressiva, the incorrect supposition being that an endocrinopathy is present.

By reason of their hereditary nature, all these conditions are of interest to the *medical geneticist.*

The *pathologist,* of course, must be familiar with them, and the *radiologist* will find in every one of these syndromes diagnostic features which can be revealed by his rays.

Obviously, one objective of this book and of the clinical investigations on which it is based is a synthesis of the scattered information about several conditions which have in common the facts that they are (1) generalized disorders of connective tissue and (2) heritable, even if not inherited in the individual instance. To my knowledge, only Bauer and Bode have previously attempted such a synthesis.*

A second objective has been to see what justification could be found for a favorite, although (witness the following quotation from Harvey as well as the dedication) far from original, notion of mine: that clinical investigation of pathologic states is as legitimate a method as any other for studying biology. Specifically, the hereditary syndromes are tools for study of the normal situation—in this case for the elucidation of connective tissue. When he compares his methods as biologic tools with the electron microscope, analytical chemistry, tissue culture, and others, the clinician tends to get an inferiority complex. I will leave it to the reader to judge whether the clinical researches, which are reported here but which are in only small part my own, demonstrate that the clinician can take his place with the so-called "pure scientists" in the group now trying to fit together the varishaped pieces of the intricate jigsaw puzzle that is connective tissue.

> Nature is nowhere accustomed more openly to display her secret mysteries than in cases where she shows traces of her workings apart from the beaten path; nor is there any better way to advance the proper practice of medicine than to give our minds to the discovery of the usual law of Nature by careful investigation of cases of rarer forms of disease. For it has been found, in almost all things, that what they contain of useful or applicable nature is hardly perceived unless we are deprived of them, or they become deranged in some way.†

Victor A. McKusick
The Johns Hopkins Hospital

*Bauer, K. H., and Bode, W.: Erbpathologie der Stützgewebe beim Menschen. In Handbuch der Erbbiologie, vol. 3, Berlin, 1940, Julius Springer.

†From letter written by William Harvey in 1657, six weeks before his death. Quoted by Garrod, Sir Archibald: The lessons of rare maladies, Lancet 1:1055, 1928.

Acknowledgments

The original investigations referred to in this book were supported in part by a grant from the Daland Fund of the American Philosophical Society Held at Philadelphia for Promoting Useful Knowledge and in part by grants-in-aid from the National Institutes of Health, Public Health Service.

The late Dr. Joseph Earle Moore encouraged these studies, by wise suggestions improved their published form, and in general made this book possible.

To the late Dr. Richard H. Follis, Jr., I owe the largest debt of conceptual nature; his concept of osteogenesis imperfecta as a generalized unitary defect of connective tissue probably catalyzed my own thinking along these lines.

I am grateful for the patient work of Mrs. Mary von Heimburg, Mrs. Nelle Garrett, Mrs. Geneva Roberts, Miss Eugenia Morgan, and Mrs. Ruth Kimmerer in the typing and other work associated with preparation of the manuscipt.

It would be impossible to name all the individuals who have assisted in accumulating the data presented. Nor can I list all the persons whose thoughts have influenced mine during the course of analyzing these disorders.

To my fellow members of the Galton-Garrod Society, founded at the Johns Hopkins University a few years ago by several of us who share an interest in human genetics, I am indebted for the pleasure and profit of many stimulating exchanges of ideas. Among others, Dr. Barton Childs, Dr. Bentley Glass, and Dr. Abraham Lilienfeld have been especially helpful to me.

The course in biophysical and biochemical cytology conducted by Professor F. O. Schmitt, Dr. Jerome Gross, and colleagues at the Massachusetts Institute of Technology, June, 1955, was of great assistance in the preparation of the brief survey of the biology of normal connective tissue.

In the study of the Marfan syndrome my studies were assisted by the contemporaneous studies of ectopia lentis by Dr. Howard A. Naquin of the Wilmer Ophthalmological Institute. Dr. Russell S. Fisher permitted me to examine the files of the Medical Examiners Office of the City of Baltimore for cases of dissecting aneurysm of the aorta in young persons. Dr. Robert A. Robinson called my attention to the experiments which are the basis for my tentative theory of the pathogenesis of dolichostenomelia and arachnodactyly in the Marfan syndrome. The editors and publishers of *American Journal of Human Genetics, Bulletin of The Johns Hopkins Hospital, Circulation, Bulletin of the New York Academy of Medicine, Medicine,* and *Annals of Internal Medicine* kindly permitted reuse of illustrative material.

Dr. William S. McLaughlin, urologist, of Hanover, New Hampshire, provided the data on the disease of the urinary tract in the patient with the Ehlers-Danlos syndrome pictured in Fig. 5-4.

In the study of osteogenesis imperfecta, Dr. George O. Eaton, chief of staff at the Children's Hospital School, permitted me to use the resources of that institution. Further kinships were identified through the cooperation of the staff of the Kernan Hospital for Crippled Children.

Dr. Stanton L. Eversole, Jr., reviewed the pathologic material in the cases of pseudoxanthoma elasticum and of the Ehlers-Danlos syndrome.

The interest and experience of James B. Sidbury, Jr., in the Hurler syndrome were of great assistance during that phase of the study. Dr. Harry Butler and other members of the staff of the Rosewood State Training School, Ownings Mills, Maryland, cooperated with me in the study of the patients at that institution.

In recent years several of my research fellows have contributed importantly in the study of several of the heritable disorders of connective tissue. Deserving particular mention are Roswell Eldridge, Richard M. Goodman, W. Bryan Hanley, R. Neil Schimke, and David Wise. Dr. A. E. Maumenee and several members of his staff in the Wilmer Ophthalmological Institute, particularly Drs. James P. Gills, Jr., Morton F. Goldberg, David Paton, and Gunter K. von Noorden, have contributed in many ways to the study of these disorders of connective tissue, almost all of which seem to have ocular manifestations. Other associates I would acknowledge—even at the risk of omitting others of the many who have contributed—are Drs. Ronald A. Bergman (Department of Anatomy), Michael A. Naughton (Department of Biophysics), Robert A. Milch (Department of Orthopedic Surgery), and Ernest W. Smith (Department of Medicine).

Conversations with Dr. Karl Meyer of Columbia University have been stimulating and informative. Dr. David Kaplan, Downstate Medical Center, Brooklyn, New York, contributed significantly in the biochemical study of the mucopolysaccharidoses.

The late Dr. Ernst Oppenheimer, in preparing the German translation of the first edition, made several worthwhile suggestions which were incorporated in this edition.

I am indebted to Professor Charles E. Dent, London, for directing my attention specifically to the simulation of the Marfan syndrome by homocystinuria. Dr. R. Neil Schimke was mainly responsible for a survey of cases of ectopia lentis and/or presumed Marfan syndrome in which over twenty families with homocystinuria were ascertained. We are indebted to a large number of ophthalmologists and other physicians who gave us access to patients for homocystinuria screening. Drs. A. D. Pollack and Thomas Huang studied pathologic material from patients with homocystinuria. Drs. Leonard Laster and S. Harvey Mudd, of the National Institutes of Health, did enzyme and other studies in the homocystinuric patients ascertained in the screening program.

Dr. Robert A. Milch gave valuable assistance in preparation of the chapter on alkaptonuria and has been a constant source of stimulation and insight.

The late Mrs. Hermina Grimm Bird and Miss Sheila Manning were of great assistance in bibliographic research.

To the many others who directly or indirectly contributed to this book I extend my grateful appreciation. Essential to the successful pursuit of a study which is partly retrospective such as this and which concerns disorders of relatively infrequent occurrence are the careful recording of information by many individuals over a long period of time and its careful preservation in the archives of our hospitals and other institutions. I am deeply grateful for the contributions of many members of the staff of The Johns Hopkins Hospital over a period of many years.

Contents

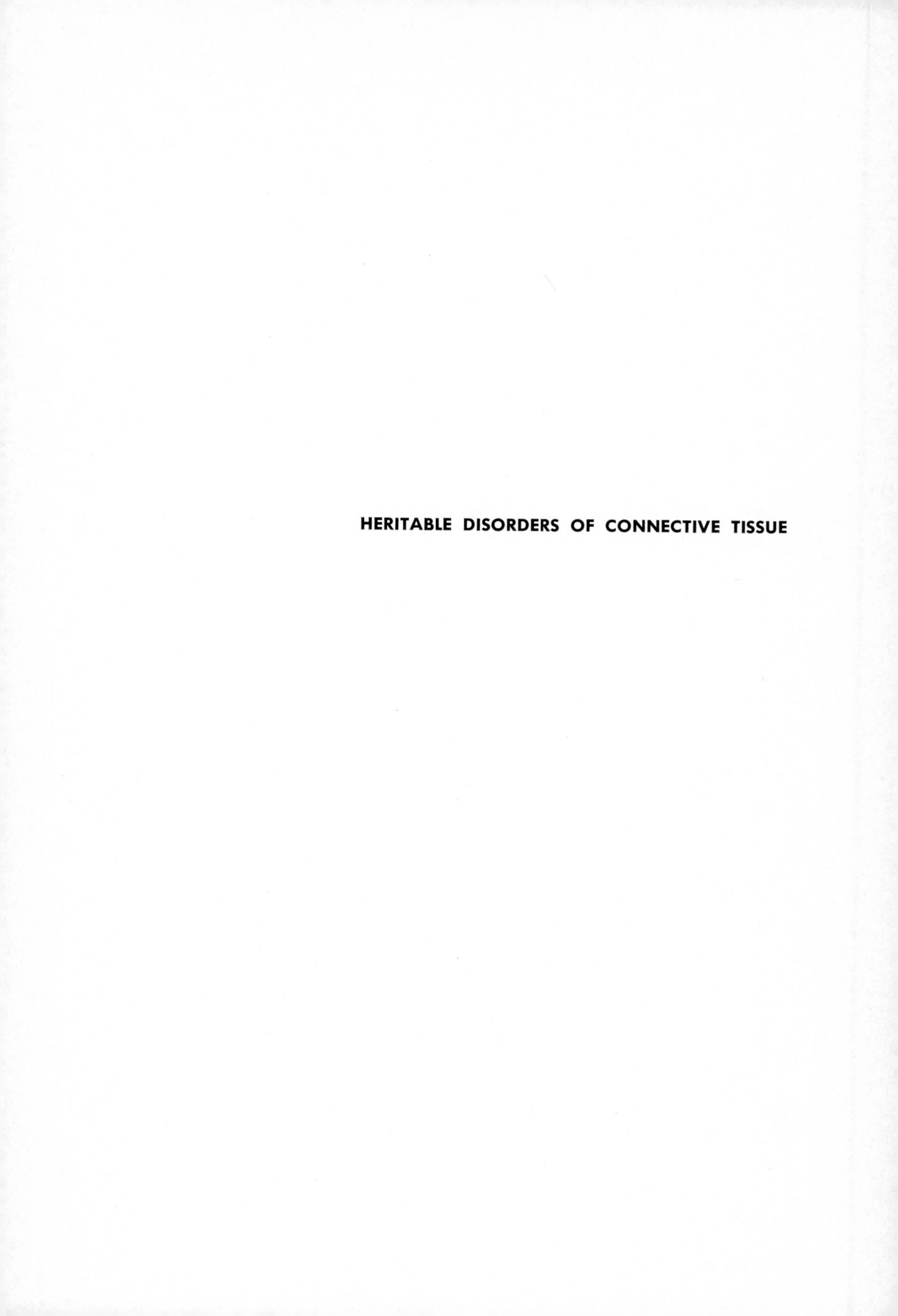

HERITABLE DISORDERS OF CONNECTIVE TISSUE

1

The clinical behavior of hereditary syndromes

We must analyse, and seek to interpret partnerships in disease.
*—Jonathan Hutchinson**

Because of the light they shed on normal mechanisms, many of the inherited ailments of man have importance far out of proportion to their numerical significance. Such is the case, at least potentially, with the hereditary disorders of connective tissue. This consideration, together with the increasing recognition of internal medical ramifications of these diseases, prompted this survey.

Terms

The disorders discussed here present clinically as combinations of clinical manifestations, or syndromes.† (The manifestations in each of the principal heritable disorders of connective tissue are outlined in Table 1.) Meaning literally a "running together," the term syndrome is legitimately applied to any consistent combination of two or more clinical manifestations. The term has no necessary etiologic connotations; specifically a syndrome need not be gene-determined. In the minds of many, *syndrome* and *disease* are distinguishable terms, the latter referring to a specific etiopathogenetic entity and the former to a combination of manifestations that may have diverse causes. In this discussion, however, *syndrome* will be used in a specific sense—to signify a distinct etiopathologic entity, the diverse manifestations of which result from a single primary cause.

The use of the term syndrome in the specific sense need not, and should not, becloud the issue of genetic heterogeneity. Cases that might legitimately be called instances of the Hurler syndrome by satisfying the main criteria described by Hurler are now known to be examples of a distinct entity and are assigned a

*From Hutchinson, Jonathan: Arch. Surg. **4**:361, 1893.

†It has been claimed[13] that the correct pronunciation of this word is "syndrŏmē," not "syndroam."

Table 1. Heritable disorders of connective tissue—a synopsis of symptoms*

Disorders	*Skin*	*Joints*	*Eye*	*Bone*	*Cardiovascular system*	*Fascia*	*Inheritance*	*Fundamental defect*
Marfan syndrome	Striae distensae	Hyperextensibility	*Ectopia lentis*, suspensory ligament of lens	Excessive length of long bones: *dolichostenomelia* (long, thin extremities)	Aortic media, *aneurysm*	Hernia	Autosomal dominant	Defect of elastic tissue? of collagen?
Homocystinuria	Malar flush		*Ectopia lentis*	*Dolichostenomelia*	*Arterial and venous thromboses*		Autosomal recessive	Defect in cystathionine synthetase
Ehlers-Danlos syndrome	*Fragility; hyperelasticity*	*Hyperextensibility*	Ectopia lentis; microhemorrhages of retina		Rupture of aorta and large arteries	Eventration of diaphragm; hernia	Autosomal dominant	Defect in formation of collagen wickerwork?
Osteogenesis imperfecta	Thin; abnormal scar formation	Hyperextensibility	Sclera, thinning of: *blue sclerotics*	*Brittle bones;* otosclerosis *(deafness)*		Hernia	Autosomal dominant	Defect of collagen?
Alkaptonuria	*Ochronotic pigmentation*	*Arthritis*	*Ochronotic pigmentation*		Valvular sclerosis; accelerated arteriosclerosis?		Autosomal recessive	Defect of homogentisic acid oxidase
Pseudoxanthoma elasticum	*Dystrophy* in wear-and-tear areas		Bruch's membrane, crazing of: *angioid streaks*		Peripheral arteries, medial sclerosis of; *hemorrhages*		Autosomal recessive	Degeneration of elastic fibers
Hurler syndrome (prototype mucopolysaccharidosis)	Roughening; nodular thickening; hirsutism	*Limitation of mobility*	*Clouding of cornea*	Dwarfism; *dysostosis multiplex*	Intimal deposits in coronary arteries; valvular lesions	Hernia	Autosomal recessive	Qualitative and/or quantitative defect in formation of mucopolysaccharide

*Italicized items indicate predominant manifestations in the case of each syndrome.

different name. Some patients who show features of the Marfan syndrome have a distinct inborn error of metabolism, homocystinuria. Such cases are called by the more specific designation, leaving "the Marfan syndrome" as a label for those cases which thus far seem to represent a large homogeneous residual group, of which the precise basic defect is not yet known.

The term *heritable* was selected for the title of this book (rather than inherited or hereditary) to convey the sense that in a given individual the gene and/or the disease, although transmissible to offspring, may not have been inherited but rather may have arisen by mutation. The terms *inherited, genetic, hereditary,* and *familial* are essentially synonymous with *heritable* but have particular shades of meaning. Mongolism is a genetic disorder, since it results from a change in the genetic material. It is also heritable but is usually not inherited from a parent. *Familial* is a loose term that can refer to concentration of a given trait in families for reasons other than genetic ones.

Congenital and *hereditary* (and cognate terms of the latter, listed above) are not synonymous. Congenital means simply "present at birth"; it has no etiologic connotations. A disorder may be congenital and not hereditary, or, conversely, may be hereditary and not congenital. Thalidomide embryopathy is congenital but not hereditary. Pseudoxanthoma elasticum is hereditary but not congenital.

Abiotrophy is a term suggested in the early years of this century by Gowers[5] for neurologic disorders in which a particular tissue or cell class is capable of function for only a limited time because of an innate weakness. Friedreich's ataxia and Huntington's chorea are examples. The abiotrophies are not congenital although they are hereditary. The changes in the aorta in the Marfan syndrome; in the skin, eye, and blood vessels in pseudoxanthoma elasticum; and in the joints in alkaptonuria are of abiotrophic nature. Abiotrophy, as a term, means no more than the late onset of degenerative changes. In using the term one should not deceive himself that he understands the nature of the basic defect.

Pleiotropic (meaning loosely "many effects") is a term applied to those single genes which are responsible for multiple manifestations. Although the gene may have many phenotypic effects, the primary action of the gene is unitary. *Polyphenic* is a useful term synonymous with pleiotropic.

Pedigree patterns

Each of the disorders for main discussion is determined by a single mutant gene in either single (heterozygous) state, e.g. the dominant conditions, or in double (homozygous) state, e.g. the recessive conditions. Some are determined by genes on an autosome, i.e. are autosomal, and at least one by a gene on the X chromosome; that is, the disorder is sex-linked or, more precisely, X-linked.

Rare monomeric genetic disorders such as these show characteristic pedigree patterns depending on whether the disorder is autosomal dominant, autosomal recessive, or X-linked recessive.

For rare *autosomal dominant traits,** the affected person is almost always heterozygous and is likely to be married to an unaffected person. Since the af-

---

*Because of the experience with sickle cell anemia (a homozygous state) and sickle cell trait (the corresponding heterozygous state), the word *trait* tends to suggest to clinicians the heterozygous carrier state of any recessive disorder. The geneticist, however, uses the term synonymously with *character* or *characteristic,* to refer to any phenotype.

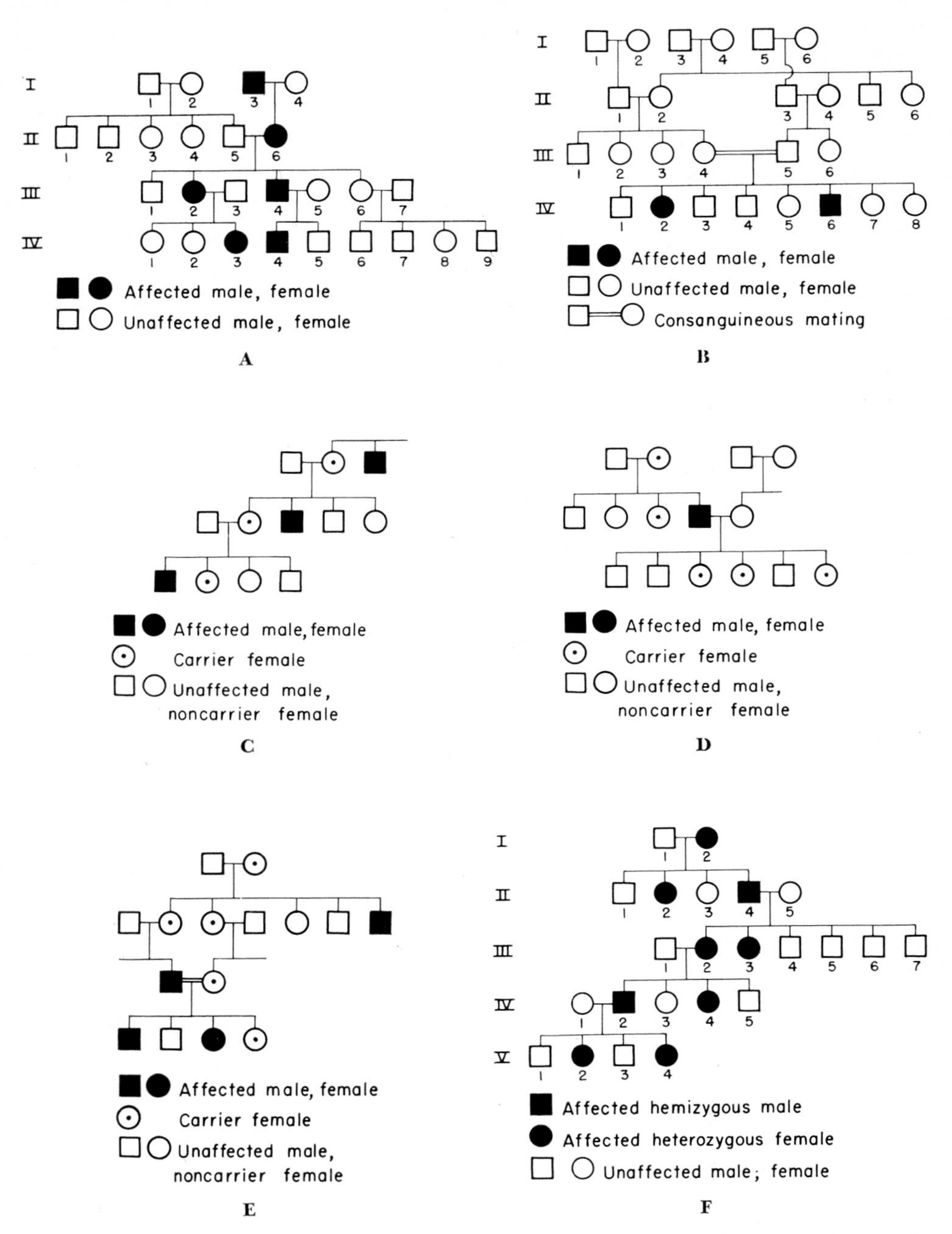

Fig. 1-1. Idealized pedigree pattern. **A,** The pattern of a rare autosomal dominant disorder. **B,** The pattern of a rare autosomal recessive disorder. **C, D,** and **E,** The pattern of an X-linked recessive disorder. In **D** the fact that all daughters of an affected male are carriers and all sons are normal is indicated. In **E** the offspring of the mating of an affected male with a carrier female are represented. The affected son is not an exception to the rule of "no male-to-male transmission," since the gene came from the carrier mother. **F,** The pattern of an X-linked dominant trait. Although the families with affected mother suggest autosomal dominant inheritance, all daughters of affected males are affected and all sons of affected males are normal.

fected person is equally likely to give the "normal" chromosome as to give the homologous chromosome carrying the mutant gene to a particular child, the chance of an offspring's being affected is 50%. Furthermore, since the mutant gene is carried by one of the nonsex chromosomes, both males and females are affected and can transmit it to both their sons and their daughters. (See Fig. 1-1*A*.)

As a generalization, dominant traits are less severe than recessive ones. In part, an evolutionary or selective reason for this observation can be offered. A dominant lethal, i.e. a dominant mutation that determines a grave disorder precluding reproduction, will promptly disappear. On the other hand, a recessive mutation, even if in homozygous state it prevents reproduction, can gain wide dissemination in heterozygous carriers.

A biochemical explanation is also possible for the greater severity of recessive traits. One might expect a greater derangement when both genes specifying a particular protein, let us say an enzyme, are of mutant type than if only one is mutant.

Although, like most generalizations, this one is not always true, dominantly inherited traits tend to be structural anomalies, such as brachydactyly, whereas recessively inherited traits tend to be inborn errors of metabolism, i.e. enzyme defects. The distinction is well illustrated by the two types of hereditary methemoglobinemia. All have cyanosis as the phenotypic characteristic. Some cases are due to a defect in an enzyme of the red blood cell; this type is inherited as an autosomal recessive. Others have an aberrant amino acid sequence of hemoglobin; this type is inherited as an autosomal dominant.

Among the children of two individuals who are both heterozygous for a dominantly inherited trait, the genotypic expectations are precisely those described by Mendel: one fourth homozygous, affected; two fourths heterozygous, affected; and one fourth homozygous, normal. The homozygous state of few dominant traits has been observed. In some disorders that are relatively mild in the heterozygous individual, the homozygous state is lethal. Probably few traits are completely dominant, that is, have the same phenotype in heterozygotes and homozygotes.

Another characteristic of dominant traits is wide variability in severity, or "expressivity" (p. 12). Sometimes the expressivity is so much reduced that the presence of the gene cannot be recognized, at least by methods currently available. When this is the case, the trait or the gene is said to be "nonpenetrant." Sometimes in pedigrees of families with a dominant trait, so-called "skipped generations" occur. In the "skipped" individual, expressivity is so low that the presence of the gene is not recognizable. Closer study of persons who clearly transmitted the trait from grandparent to grandchild sometimes shows mild but definite manifestations.

Another phenomenon based largely on the wide variability of dominant traits is "anticipation": the given hereditary disorder manifests itself earlier, is more severe, and leads to earlier death in each successive generation or at least in one generation than in the one just preceding it. This has been purported for myotonic dystrophy. It is clear, however, that anticipation is the result of biases of ascertainment. Obviously, the affected persons in generation I who have children are those at the milder end of a bell-shaped distribution curve for severity. On the other hand, *their* affected children, in generation II, are likely to cover more nearly the whole range of severity. On the average, then, generation II is likely to be more severely affected than generation I by any gauge, such as age of onset, degree of incapacitation, or age at death. Another source of bias leading to the artefactual phenomenon of anticipation is the following: the parent-child sets used in the calculations are often selected through the children who, the more severely they are affected, are the more likely to come to attention. *Anticipation has no genuine biologic basis.*

Autosomal recessive disorders (Fig. 1-1*B*) likewise occur with equal frequency in males and in females. When the condition is rare, almost all the affected individuals have normal parents, but both are heterozygotes. *Autosomal recessive inheritance is inheritance from both parents.* Since related individuals are more likely to be heterozygous for the same mutant gene, consanguineous matings, of first cousins for example, have a higher probability of producing offspring affected by a recessive disorder. Viewed in another way, a greater proportion of the parental matings in families affected by recessive traits are likely to be consanguineous than is true generally. The rarer the recessive condition is, the higher is the proportion of consanguineous parental matings. For the more frequent autosomal recessive disorders (cystic fibrosis of the pancreas may be an example), there is little or no more consanguinity among the parents than expected by chance. In the case of a very rare recessive disorder, the occurrence of parental consanguinity may be the first clue to the fact that the trait is genetic.

Among the offspring of two heterozygous parents, one fourth of males and females are expected to be homozygous and affected. However, in human genetics, sibships with both parents heterozygous are generally ascertained only through the occurrence in them of at least one affected member. Since there is usually no way to recognize those matings of two appropriately heterozygous parents who are so fortunate as to escape having affected children, a collection of sibships containing at least one affected child is a biased sample. In the ascertained families, more than the expected one fourth are affected. Methods for correcting for the "bias of ascertainment" have been developed.

If an individual affected by a recessive trait marries a heterozygous carrier of the same recessive gene, one half of the offspring, on the average, will be affected, and a pedigree pattern superficially resembling that of a dominant trait results. Previously, it was thought that two genetic forms of alkaptonuria (Chapter 7) exist—one inherited as an autosomal recessive and one as an autosomal dominant. However, closer investigation revealed that the apparently dominant form was the same disease as the clearly recessive one. Because of inbreeding, homozygous affected individuals frequently mated with heterozygous carriers, and a quasidominant pedigree pattern resulted.

As originally defined by Mendel* and as used most accurately, the terms

---

*In 1866, Mendel wrote, "Henceforth . . . those characters which are transmitted entire, or almost unchanged in the hybridization, and therefore in themselves constitute the characters of the hybrid, are termed the *dominant,* and those which become latent in the process *recessive*" [italics mine]. Recall that Mendel was hybridizing pure lines, which were either homozygous dominant or homozygous recessive at any given locus. The hybrid, or F_1, generation was heterozygous. If the word *heterozygote* is substituted for *hybrid* the definition is precisely the one currently used. The terms refer to characters, not genes. That part of the definition saying "almost unchanged in the hybridization" allows for phenotypic differences in the dominant character in the homozygote as compared with the heterozygote.

dominant and *recessive* refer to the character, trait, or phenotype—not to the gene. (For convenience, the geneticist often speaks of a "recessive gene" or a "dominant gene," especially in population genetics. But this is merely a variety of shorthand; he says "recessive gene," for example, to avoid saying "a gene that produces particular phenotypic effects only when present in homozygous state.")

Confusion arises if one fails to remember that dominance and recessivity are attributes of the phenotype, not of the gene. Of two related characters, one may be dominant and the other recessive, depending on the acuteness of the methods for defining phenotype. An illustration: the phenotype sickle cell anemia is recessive, since the homozygous state of the gene is required. Sickling, however, is a dominant phenotype, since the gene in heterozygous state is expressed. By electrophoresis of the blood of heterozygotes, both hemoglobin S and hemoglobin A are demonstrated, so at this level of study the phenotypes are codominant.

X-linked inheritance

Like autosomal traits, those which are determined by genes on the X chromosome may be either dominant or recessive. At least the female with 2 X chromosomes may be either heterozygous or homozygous for a given mutant gene, and in the female the trait can demonstrate either recessive or dominant behavior. But the male with a single X chromosome can have only one genetic constitution—the hemizygous; and, regardless of the behavior of the gene in the female, whether recessive or dominant, it is always expressed in the male.

The critical characteristic of X-linked inheritance, both dominant and recessive, is the *absence of male-to-male, i.e. father-to-son, transmission.* This is a necessary result of the fact that the X chromosome of the male is transmitted to none of his sons although it passes to each daughter.

The pedigree pattern of an autosomal dominant trait tends to be a vertical one, with the trait passed from generation to generation. That of an autosomal recessive trait tends to be a horizontal one, with affected persons confined to a single generation. The pedigree pattern of a rare *X-linked recessive character* (Fig. 1-1*C*) tends to be an oblique one, since the affection is one almost exclusively of males and is transmitted to the sons of their normal carrier sisters. Bateson likened this pattern to the knight's move in chess. Often, tracing of X-linked recessive characters through many generations is difficult because the patronymic of affected persons usually changes with each generation.

Among the children of a male affected by an X-linked recessive trait (Fig. 1-1*D*), all sons are unaffected and all daughters are carriers, provided that the mother is not affected and is not a heterozygous carrier. Father-to-son transmission of X-linked traits cannot occur.

If an affected male marries a carrier female—and for rare conditions this is more likely to occur in a consanguineous marriage, as shown in Fig. 1-1*E*—half the daughters will be homozygous and affected and the others will be carriers. Half the sons are expected to be affected. This is not a true exception to the rule of no male-to-male transmission, because the mutant gene came from the carrier mother.

In some instances it is impossible by pedigree pattern alone to distinguish between an X-linked recessive and an autosomal dominant male-limited trait. In both modes of inheritance, the trait occurs only in males and is transmitted by females who do not show it. Prime examples are the testicular feminization syndrome[8] and the Reifenstein syndrome,[2] both of which are forms of familial male pseudohermaphroditism resulting apparently from a defect in testicular hormonogenesis. Testes must be present for the disorder to be expressed. The female cannot show the disorder even if she possesses the appropriate genotype. The main way to distinguish X-linked recessive and autosomal dominant inheritance is by the findings in the progeny of affected males. If X-linked, the trait will be transmitted to none of his sons by an affected male. The progeny test is not available in the genetic analysis of the two examples cited because affected males are sterile. The test is also not available in X-linked recessive conditions which, although not affecting the reproductive capacity directly, are of such a nature that affected males do not survive to reproduce. The X-linked mucopolysaccharidosis, the Hunter syndrome, is such a condition (Chapter 9). Formally, from pedigree pattern alone, either X-linked recessive or autosomal dominant male-limited inheritance is possible. Favoring X-linked inheritance are the facts (1) that there is no plausible reason that the disorder should not be expressed in the female and (2) that this appears to be an enzyme disorder which in the overwhelming proportion occurs only in homozygous persons or in the hemizygous male.

In *X-linked dominant inheritance* (Fig. 1-1*F*), both females and males are affected, and both males and females transmit the disorder to their offspring, just as in autosomal dominant inheritance. Superficially, the pedigree patterns in the two types of inheritance are similar, but there is a critical difference. In X-linked dominant inheritance, although the affected female transmits the trait to half her sons and half her daughters, the affected male transmits it to *none* of his sons and to *all* of his daughters. One of the best-studied X-linked dominant traits is vitamin D-resistant rickets, or hypophosphatemic rickets. The skeletal defect alone gives a pedigree pattern that tends to be inconclusive. However, when hypophosphatemia is used as the trait for analysis, the inheritance becomes clear. *All* the daughters and *none* of the sons of affected males are affected.

Conventions for the construction of pedigree charts are illustrated by the idealized examples, shown in Fig. 1, of the several modes of inheritance. Squares are used for males and circles for females, rather than the symbols ♂ and ♀, which are more generally used by British writers. Solidly "blacked-in" symbols indicate affected individuals and an arrow indicates the propositus (—a), or proband, the affected person who first brings the kindred to the attention of the medical geneticist.

The genetic basis of syndromes

Some congenital syndromes are nongenetic in etiology, e.g. the thalidomide syndrome and the rubella syndrome. The Marfan syndrome and Down's syndrome (mongolism) are examples of syndromes resulting from a change in the genetic material. Formally, at least four types of genetic change producing syndromes are recognized.

1. Probably the largest number of recognized genetic syndromes result from mutation in a single structural gene. The manifold features of the syndrome result from the fact that the primary gene product, enzyme or nonenzymic protein, has a rather wide role in the body's economy. All the conditions discussed

here seem to fall into this class. Since search for a unitary defect is based on the premise of a one-gene–one-syndrome relationship, it is well to examine the evidence that one gene is primarily responsible for all manifestations and that, for example, two or more closely linked genes are not involved.

(a) It is unlikely that several genes would undergo mutation simultaneously to reproduce these syndromes again and again with such exactitude.

(b) Linkage is the location of genes on the same chromosome. Crossing-over tends to separate even closely linked genes so that with the passage of generations, a larger number of generations if the linkage is close, no particular association of the characters determined by the linked genes is observed in a given individual. *Genetic linkage produces no permanent association of characters.* It is true that for closely neighboring genes the rate of crossing-over is so low that the relatively few human generations available for study may, in any one kindred, be inadequate to demonstrate separation of the components of a given syndrome. However, in the population at large, the situation is as stated by Snyder[11]:

> The occurrence of genetic linkage between the genes for two traits does not change the association for these traits in the population from what it would be if they are not linked. Stated conversely, a correlation between two traits in a free-breeding population does not indicate genetic linkage between the genes for these traits.*

Monogenic determination is given strong support when one component of a dominantly inherited syndrome is present in a grandparent and grandchild and absent in the intervening generation. The failure to appear in the parent could be accounted for by crossing-over, but reappearance in the next generation would be inexplicable.

(c) The most telling argument for a single-gene mechanism for syndromes comes from the possibility of relating all manifestations of a syndrome to a single basic disturbance. In the mouse, in *Drosophila,* and in other species, including man, unitary defects have been demonstrated as the basis of hereditary syndromes. In some instances definition of the basic defect has been carried to the level of the molecule. Sickle cell anemia, which has manifold clinical features constituting a syndrome, represents an instance where definition of the basic defect has met with outstanding success. Elucidation of the basic defect at a more superficial level can still provide strong support for the one-gene–one-syndrome hypothesis. Grüneberg[6] has constructed convincing "pedigrees of causes" for complex single-gene syndromes of the mouse. In osteogenesis imperfecta, although the nature of the defect of connective tissue (probably collagen) is not known at the molecular level, no one would now seriously doubt that the bone fragility, blue sclerotics, and deafness are the result of one and the same defect of connective tissue.

It is true that in the present state of our ignorance it is impossible, in the case of some syndromes, to relate all components to a unitary biochemical anomaly. For example, in the syndrome of polyposis of the small intestine and melanin spots of the buccal mucosa, lips, and digits,[7] there

*From Snyder, L. H.: Principles of gene distribution in human populations, Yale J. Biol. Med. 19:817, 1947.

is no obvious common denominator. Even in such a situation, however, the other arguments listed above make a single-gene mechanism likely.

2. Although genetic linkage is an unlikely explanation for relatively frequent genetic syndromes that have arisen on many separate occasions, some specific populations might have many cases of an unusual syndrome produced by mutation in 2 or more closely linked genes that have not yet become separated by the mechanism of crossing-over. No convincing example in man is known.

3. The operon mechanism is a special case of linkage, since by definition an operon consists of 2 or more closely linked structure genes. Mutation in an operator gene that controls the function of the stucture genes comprising the operon could produce a syndrome. Again, no fully established example is at hand. The most plausible example is provided by the hemoglobin genes. The genes determining the structure of beta polypeptide chains of hemoglobin A and of delta polypeptide chains of hemoglobin A_2 are apparently adjacent and, together with an operator gene that "turns them off and on," may constitute an operon. Mutation in the operator gene may be responsible for a condition called "high fetal hemoglobin," or "hereditary persistence of fetal hemoglobin." The features of this condition, which may be considered a syndrome, are high fetal hemoglobin, low or absent hemoglobin A, and low or absent hemoglobin A_2. (The operon theory is not yet fully established.[12])

4. Chromosomal aberrations can result in syndromes, and a number of examples have been provided by the explosive development of the field of human cytogenetics since 1959. The aberration may consist of abnormalities of chromosome number or abnormalities of chromosome structure or both. The Turner syndrome (XO sex chromosome constitution) results from a deficiency of one sex chromosome. The Klinefelter syndrome (XXY sex chromosome constitution) results from an excess (by one) of sex chromosomes. The Down syndrome (mongolism) results from an excess of an autosome, namely chromosome 21, which is present in triplicate. Deletions, translocations, inversions, insertions, duplications, and isochromosomes are some of the structural abnormalities of chromosomes that can result in syndromes.

As stated earlier, the term syndrome will be used in a specific sense in this book. Medical genetics forces one to think in terms of a specific gene producing a specific disease. (In his scholarly *Nosography*[4] Knut Faber, a Copenhagen professor of medicine, assigned to Gregor Mendel a significant role in the definition of specific disease entities.) One occasionally hears statements such as "That is one of those congenital-familial affairs with which anything can occur." It should not be necessary to emphasize the direct corollary of the single-gene proposition: the clinical picture in each of these syndromes is as clear-cut and specific (with, of course, the clinical variability discussed below) as the clinical picture produced by a pathogenic microorganism. In many respects, hereditary disease differs from infectious disease only in that the etiologic agent is a mutant gene operating from within rather than a bacterium invading from without. The virologists have rather long been aware of the basic analogies between their field and that of the geneticist.[8]

The concept of the specific nature of given entities is not inconsistent with the existence of considerable variability in each. Learning clinical medicine is, to a large extent, a matter of learning the clinical variability in individual disease entities. Medical genetics is no exception.

Mutation, equilibrium, and sporadic cases

All monomeric genetic disorders arose by genetic mutation at some time in recently or more remotely past generations. A proportion of cases of dominant disorders and of X-linked recessive disorders owe their abnormality to a mutation that occurred in the germ cells of one or the other parent. These are sporadic or nonfamilial cases. The more severe the particular dominant or X-linked trait and the more drastically it interferes with reproduction of the affected persons as a group, the higher is the proportion of cases that are new mutants. This follows directly from an assumption of genetic equilibrium. If no mutation occurred and the affected individuals reproduced less often than the average of the population, then the disorder would disappear. If, on the other hand, mutation continued—even at a low frequency—and the reproductive fitness of affected persons were not reduced, the condition would become very frequent. Genetic equilibrium can be compared to a bucket of water from which water (the genes) may be lost through a hole at the bottom (negative selection), but other genes are added from a tap at the top (mutation). At equilibrium, the loss and gain of genes balance each other.

Considerations of equilibrium and the proportion of cases that are sporadic and nonfamilial, having arisen by new mutation, are illustrated by Duchenne's pseudohypertrophic muscular dystrophy, the Hunter type of mucopolysaccharidosis (Chapter 9), and by other X-linked recessive conditions in which few if any affected males reproduce. One third of cases owe their disease to mutation affecting the X chromosome that the mother gave the affected son. In two thirds the mutation occurred in a generation earlier than the mother's, and other affected males may be identified in the family.

When one encounters a "sporadic" case (i.e. an isolated instance, with parents and all other relatives of the subject normal) of a disorder that is generally considered to be heritable or that may be heritable, the following possibilities must be considered.

1. As outlined above, the case in question may be the result of new mutation. This is possible when the condition is dominant or X-linked recessive.
2. The affected individual may have a recessive gene in homozygous state. If the parents are consanguineous, this possibility is strengthened.
3. Although no certain example can be cited in man, it is theoretically possible that the disorder requires the existence of two complementary but independently inherited dominant genes. Neither gene alone can produce abnormality. In such a case, the patient demonstrating a "sporadic case" would have derived one dominant gene from each parent.
4. Possibly the trait is in fact dominant, but the parent who is heterozygous has the disorder in such subtle form that it defies detection.
5. Theoretically, somatic mutation can account for sporadic cases, especially when the anomaly is localized. The genetic change would need to occur in the zygote or in the embryo at a rather early stage.
6. Severely affected sporadic cases could result from a chromosomal aberration.

7. The sporadic case may represent a phenocopy. Goldschmidt introduced the term *phenocopy* to signify the situation when an environment factor produces the same clinical disorder, the same phenotype, that occurs as a genetic derangement. As indicated on p. 282, ochronosis closely similar to that of alkaptonuria was produced by the prolonged use of carbolic acid dressings on chronic cutaneous ulcers.

Genotype, phenotype, expressivity, and penetrance

Although some of these terms have already been used, specific definition and discussion are warranted. The *genotype* is the genetic constitution of the individual, with regard either to a specific genetic locus or to the whole genome. The *phenotype* is the character or trait or the composite of characters that is capable of being observed by one means or another but may be many steps removed from the genotype. The distinction may be compared to that between character and reputation. Genotype and character are what one really is; phenotype and reputation are what one appears to be. (The *karyotype* is the chromosomal constitution of the individual. In normal man there are 46 chromosomes: 2A + XY and 2A + XX, for males and females, respectively.)

Expressivity is the term that has been applied to the variability in phenotype produced by a given genotype and is equivalent to the grade of severity in clinical medicine. *Penetrance* is an all-or-none affair, contingent on whether the methods for studying phenotype do or do not permit identification of the specific genotype in the individual. In a group of persons with the same genotype there

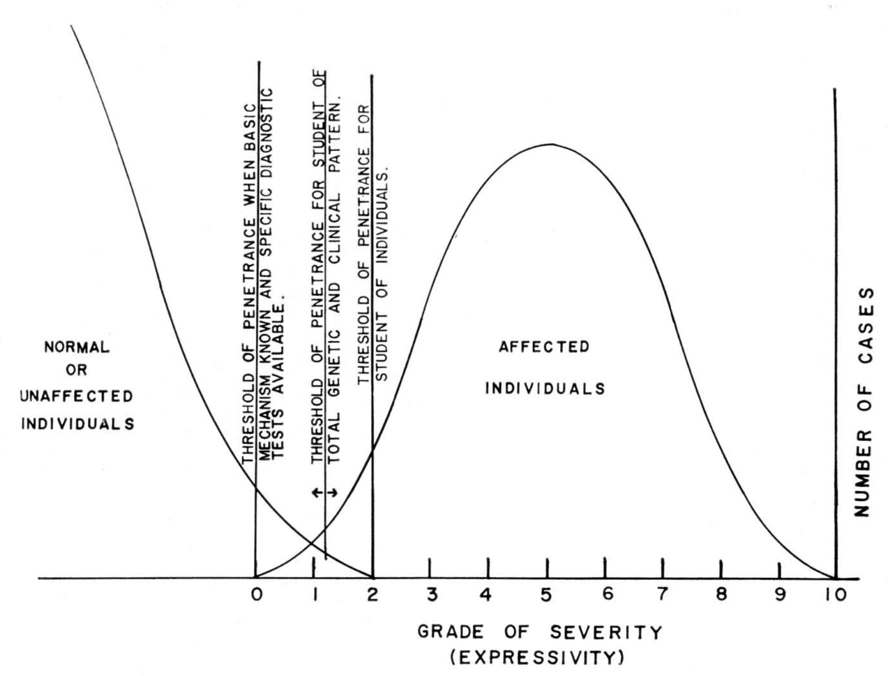

Fig. 1-2. The interrelationship of penetrance and expressivity in hereditary syndromes. (See text.) (Inspired by Dr. H. Bentley Glass.)

may be some with manifestations so mild that they do not deviate sufficiently from certain members of the "normal" group to be recognized as affected. These cases, the instances of incomplete penetrance, or *forme fruste,* correspond to the subclinical cases of infectious diseases. The familiar bell-shaped Gaussian curve probably accurately describes the distribution of cases as to severity (expressivity). (See Fig. 1-2.) The three vertical lines of the diagram indicate various thresholds of penetrance. These lines cross the distribution curve on the side constituted by cases of lesser grades of severity. At this end also the curve is overlapped by the normal distribution curve. The majority of recognizable cases are of intermediate severity; there are some very severe cases and some very mild ones. Those affected individuals in the zone of overlap have mild manifestations which, because of their occurrence as "normal variations" in a small proportion of the normal population, cannot be recognized as abnormal when the individual is studied. For the student of the individual, then, the threshold of penetrance is at the point of overlap of the two curves. A certain number of additional cases can be recognized by the student of the total genetic and clinical picture, by one who investigates the entire family in detail. (There are risks, of course, that some unaffected individuals will be incorrectly classified as affected.) It seems probable that when the basic defect in each of these syn-

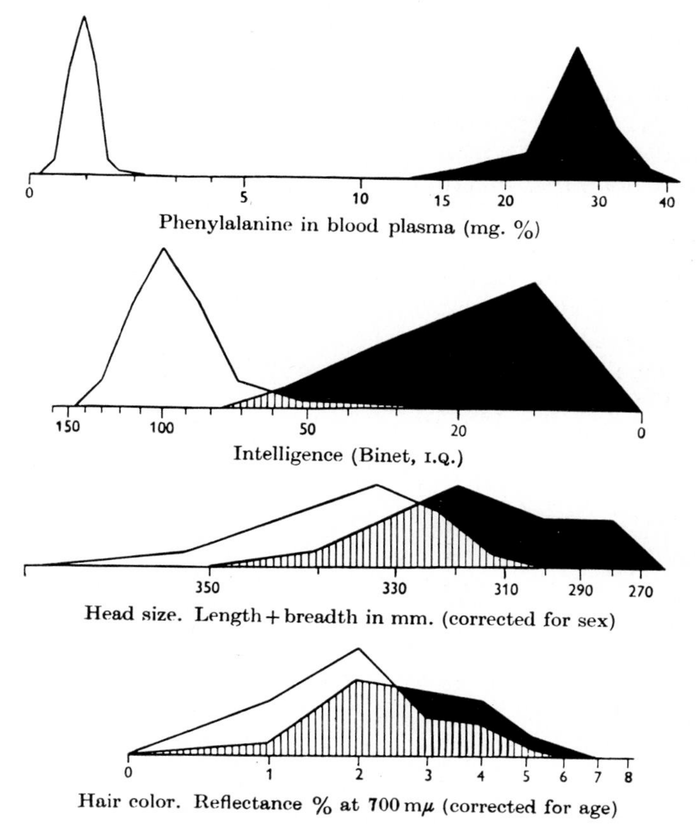

Fig. 1-3. The dependence of penetrance on the phenotype selected for study. (See text.) (From Penrose, L. S.: Ann. Eugen. **16:**134, 1951.)

dromes is known, and when a specific method for demonstrating the defect becomes available, all cases of each syndrome will be identifiable. At this point the threshold of penetrance will be moved back to the limit; and penetrance, an artificial concept at the best, will no longer have significance for these syndromes.

In the case of the multifaceted syndromes of the type discussed in this book, each component may have partially independent behavior so far as penetrance and expressivity are concerned. For example, in the case of the Marfan syndrome, any one of the three major components (ocular, aortic, skeletal) may be present with little or no involvement in the other two areas.

Variations in expressivity and differences of penetrance, depending on what phenotype is analyzed, are well illustrated by phenylketonuria, as pointed out by Penrose.[10] (See Fig. 1-3.) If hair color or head size is taken as the phenotype for study, differentiation of affected from unaffected is poor. Intelligence is a better discriminant. The level of phenylalanine in the blood—a phenotype closely related to the basic defect, which involves the enzymatic conversion of phenylalanine to tyrosine—is by far the best discriminant.

Principles of inborn errors of metabolism

The disorder of connective tissue in alkaptonuria was adequately recognized, characterized, and analyzed from the standpoint of mechanism only after the nature of the disorder as an inborn error of metabolism had been established. Homocystinuria is a second clear example of a heritable disorder of connective tissue owing to an inborn error of metabolism. Both of these conditions are autosomal recessive; and, as stated earlier, this mode of inheritance should always alert one to the possibility of an inborn error of metabolism, i.e. an enzyme defect, whereas dominant inheritance is more suggestive of a structural abnormality in a nonenzymic protein. For example, the dominant inheritance of the Marfan syndrome, Ehlers-Danlos syndrome, and osteogenesis imperfecta suggests an alteration of structure of a connective tissue protein, whereas the recessive inheritance of pseudoxanthoma elasticum and the several mucopolysaccharidoses urges search for an enzyme defect.

Garrod, whose portrait appears as the frontispiece and especially appropriately so with the inclusion of two inborn errors of metabolism, directed thinking along lines of chains of metabolic reactions and blocks at specific points as a result of mutation in the gene controlling a particular enzymatic step. (As Beadle[1] pointed out in his Nobel lecture, the one-gene–one-enzyme hypothesis was implicit in Garrod's work and conclusions.)

As schematized in Fig. 1-4, there are at least three mechanisms by which a genetic enzyme block can result in the phenotypic features of an inborn error of metabolism. (1) Excess substance may accumulate proximal to the block. The connective tissue features of alkaptonuria have this basis. (2) Lack of the product of the chain of reactions may lead to the phenotypic features. Albinism, the several forms of congenital adrenal hyperplasia, and genetic defects in thyroid hormonogenesis leading to familial goiter are examples. (3) The production, through an alternative pathway, of products that normally are of minor quantitative importance may be responsible for some or all of the phenotypic features. Phenylketonuria is a case in point; some of the urinary excretory products are produced through an alternate metabolic pathway.

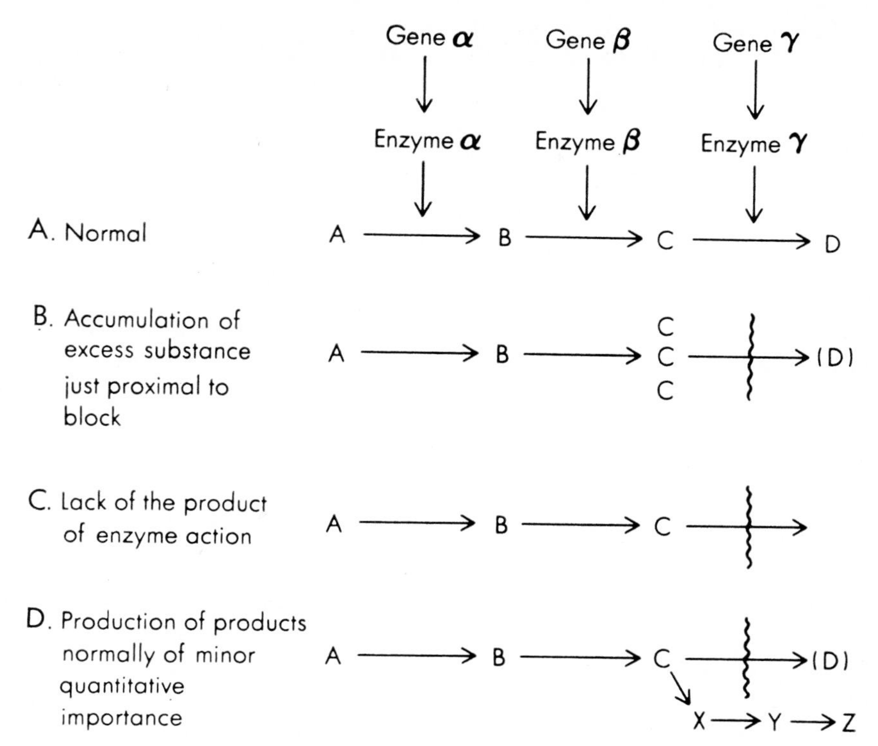

Fig. 1-4. Chains of metabolic reactions and the effects of enzyme blocks.

Defects in active transport systems

Several hereditary syndromes have been shown to be the result of a gene-determined defect in an active transport system. Cystinuria, not to be confused with homocystinuria (Chapter 4), is an example. The defect concerns transport of cystine and related amino acids (lysine, ornithine, and arginine) across the renal tubule cells. The plasma level of cystine and the other three amino acids is normal or low. By contrast the aminoaciduria of inborn errors of metabolism such as homocystinuria is of the overflow type; the plasma level of the amino acid that accumulates proximal to a Garrodian block in intermediary metabolism is elevated or, if there is no renal threshold for the substance, unaltered.

The molecular basis of inherited disease

It is beyond the scope of this presentation to discuss in full the important information on (1) the chemical nature of the gene (DNA, deoxyribonucleic acid) and the manner in which genetic information is encoded therein; (2) the role of RNA (ribonucleic acid) in conveying the genetic code from the chromosome in the nucleus to the ribosomes, sites of protein synthesis in the cytoplasm; and (3) the various mechanisms by which gene action is controlled during development and differentiation.

It is relevant to mention briefly, however, the following facts:

1. The primary product of gene action is a protein.
2. The function of the gene is to specify the sequence of amino acids in a

given protein (or polypeptide chain, because some proteins are made up of more than one polypeptide chain, each determined by a different gene).

3. The series of purine and pyrimidine bases in DNA are the "letters" which in various combinations of three spell the code words (or codons), each specific for a particular amino acid.
4. The codons in the gene are colinear, i.e. in the same linear sequence, with the amino acids in the protein specified by that gene.
5. The protein specified by a given gene may be an enzyme, and mutation may result either in the formation of an enzyme with deficient enzymatic activity or in the failure of any enzyme at all to be formed. In either case, a disorder may result which, if the enzyme involved is concerned in intermediary metabolism, will be classed as an inborn error of metabolism.
6. On the other hand, the protein specified by the gene and formed on the cytoplasmic ribosomes may be a nonenzymic protein. Hemoglobin is an extensively studied example; collagen may be another. (The genetic control of protein synthesis is schematized in Fig. 1-5.)

It was earlier indicated that recessively inherited disorders tend to be inborn errors of metabolism and dominantly inherited disorders have been found, when the molecular defect is known, to be the result of a change in the structure (i.e. amino acid sequence) of a nonenzymic protein. This is perhaps not surprising. Because of a margin of safety with which the organism is blessed, the effects of an enzyme deficiency are likely to be evident only in the homozygote, i.e. when there is none at all of the particular enzyme or when all of the enzyme is of the defective mutant type. On the other hand, when the gene-determined change

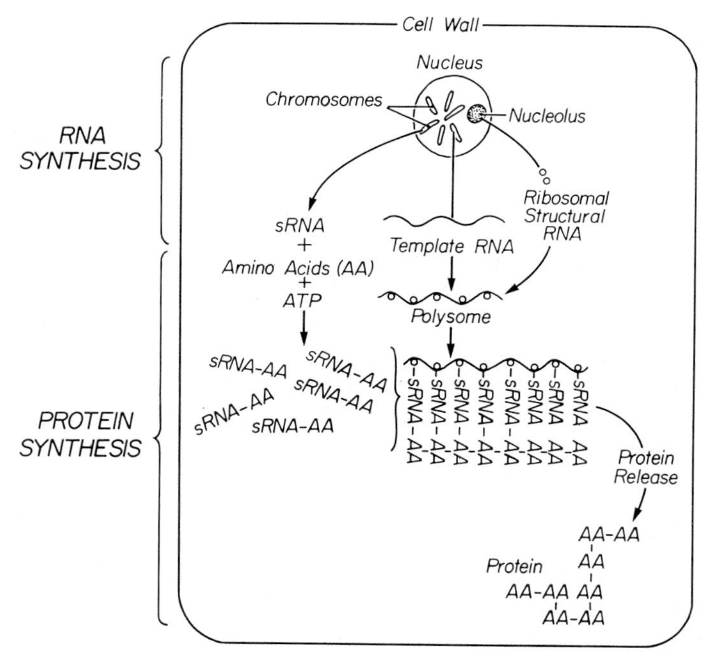

Fig. 1-5. The genetic control of protein synthesis. (Courtesy Dr. J. D. Wilson, Dallas, Texas.)

involves a nonenzymic protein, such as a structural protein like collagen, the resulting change in the physical properties of the protein may be evident in the phenotype even though only part of the total protein is atypical or abnormal, as is the case in the heterozygote.

The above considerations are important as guides to study of the basic defect in each of the heritable disorders of connective tissue. In the dominant disorders—Marfan syndrome, Ehlers-Danlos syndrome, and osteogenesis imperfecta—change in a structural protein should be sought. In the recessive disorders, homocystinuria and alkaptonuria, an enzymatic defect has already been identified; and such should also be sought in pseudoxanthoma elasticum, a recessive. The several mucopolysaccharidoses, all recessives, are probably the result of a defect in one or another enzyme involved in the synthesis of mucopolysaccharides.

Heterogeneity of genetic disease

It has happened so often in medical genetics as to be considered the rule, that—when subjected to penetrating scrutiny—a condition which appears at first to be homogeneous is found in fact to comprise two or more separate and distinct entities. Examples are albinism, the thalassemias, the glycogen storage diseases, intestinal polyposis, and elliptocytosis.

Heterogeneity of genetic disease is a corollary of the axiom that the phenotype is not a necessary indication of the genotype. Several different genotypes can lead to the same phenotype. This is to be expected, since many steps, each separately gene-controlled, go into the determination of most phenotypes, and mutation at any of several different steps can lead to the same end effect. The situation has been compared to stalling of a car, which can have many causes even though the end result or phenotype is identical. "Genetic mimic," or "genocopy," is the term given to a genetic condition that is phenotypically similar or identical to another but has a different genetic basis. (As stated earlier, "phenocopy" is the designation given to a phenotype that is similar or identical to a genetically determined one but is determined by exogenous factors.)

Separate entities are discerned (1) by subtle phenotypic differences, (2) by genetic differences, (3) by biochemical differences, or (4) by physiologic differences. Each of these approaches is illustrated below.

The presence or absence of corneal dystrophy is a feature distinguishing two forms of gargoylism, the autosomal recessive type described by Hurler and the X-linked recessive form described by Hunter (Chapter 9). The association of soft tissue and osseous tumors distinguishes the colonic polyposis of the Gardner syndrome from familial polyposis of the colon.

The genetic means of distinguishing separate genetic entities include demonstration of different modes of inheritance or different linkage relationships and the study of offspring produced by the marriage of two persons with a recessively inherited disorder. Spastic paraplegia, retinitis pigmentosa, and Charcot-Marie-Tooth peroneal muscular atrophy are three disorders that are inherited as autosomal dominant in some families, as autosomal recessive in others, and as X-linked recessive in yet others. Usually, in conditions with these three forms of inheritance, the autosomal recessive form is clinically most severe, the dominant form least severe, and the X-linked recessive form intermediate in severity.

Two distinct forms of elliptocytosis (ovalocytosis), both inherited as dominants, have been distinguished on the basis of linkage relationships, although no definite phenotypic differences are discernible. Linkage studies[9] indicate that one form is determined by a gene at a locus which is on the same pair of chromosomes as the locus occupied by the Rh blood group genes, whereas a second form of elliptocytosis is determined by a gene at some position far removed from the Rh locus.

In many instances, congenital deafness (deafmutism) can be shown to be inherited as a simple autosomal recessive. Assortative (i.e. nonrandom) mating is often practiced by deafmutes; deaf persons marry other deaf persons much more often than would occur on a random basis. All children of two deaf persons, each from a family with a recessive pattern of inheritance, are deaf if the two parents are homozygous at the same locus. Families fulfilling this expectation have been observed. However, in other families the two parents, both affected by phenotypically identical and recessively inherited deafness, have all normal children. The explanation is that the deaf parents are homozygous at different loci and suffer from genetically distinct forms of deafness.

Observations are available on the marriage of two individuals, both of whom appear to be identically affected by albinism. In the case of one such mating, all four children were normally pigmented. When the parents were examined closely it was concluded that the father may in fact suffer from albinoidism, a condition of pigment dilution but not absence, easily confused with albinism.

Biochemical means of differentiating phenotypically similar genetic entities are illustrated by the nonspherocytic hemolytic anemias and by certain of the mucopolysaccharidoses (Chapter 9).

The physiologic method for differentiating phenotypically similar genetic diseases is nicely demonstrated by hemophilia. Prior to about 1950 all sex-linked hemophilia was assumed to be one and the same disease, although the possibility of multiple allelism had been suggested to explain the occurrence of clinically mild and clinically severe forms. It was then discovered that the blood from some hemophilic subjects would correct the clotting defect in others. The correctability was mutual. The explanation is that the location of the defect in the chain of clotting reactions is different and bloods from two hemophilic persons complement each other, each providing an essential clotting factor missing in the other. Thus, hemophilia A (classic hemophilia) and hemophilia B (Christmas disease) were distinguished. Although both are determined by genes on the X chromosome, the genes are known to be on different parts of the chromosome; linkage studies indicate that the hemophilia A gene is fairly close to the color blindness locus, the glucose-6-phosphate dehydrogenase locus, and the Xg blood group locus, whereas the Christmas disease gene is far removed from these loci. Thus, evidence from genetic linkage corroborates the evidence from physiologic studies.

Detection of heterozygous carriers

The detection of heterozygous carriers of recessive traits, either autosomal or X-linked, has practical importance in genetic counselling. It also has scientific importance in the establishment of mode of inheritance; for example, discovery of a partial defect such as an intermediate level of enzyme activity in both parents of affected persons, or in the mother only, is strong support for autosomal recessive or for X-linked recessive inheritance, respectively. Furthermore, the findings in heterozygotes for X-linked traits have special genetic interest in connection with the Lyon hypothesis.

Methods for detecting heterozygotes consist mainly of (1) demonstration of an intermediate deficiency of a gene product, such as an enzyme, and (2) demonstration of less than normal functioning when a particular metabolic step is placed under stress by a so-called loading test, or tolerance test. In a number of recessively inherited inborn errors of metabolism in which the specific defective enzyme has been identified, partial deficiency of that enzyme has been demonstrated in parents. Homocystinuria (Chapter 4) is a case in point. In phenylketonuria, loading tests that use orally administered phenylalanine demonstrate increases in blood levels persisting for a longer time than usual.

Females heterozygous for X-linked recessive traits are likely to show directly or indirectly a reduced level of the particular gene product. Reduced red cell glucose-6-phosphate dehydrogenase (G6PD) activity in primaquine sensitivity or favism and reduced antihemophilic factor in hemophilia A are examples. In addition the considerations of the Lyon hypothesis dictate that if the phenotype is observable at the cellular level heterozygotes for X-linked traits are found to be a mosaic of cells with the same defect as in cells of the hemizygous affected male and cells that are perfectly "normal."

The Lyon hypothesis, or one-active-X principle, suggests that early in the embryologic development of the normal XX female, probably between the time of implantation (seventh to eighth day) and the sixteenth day after fertilization, a "decision" is made in each and every cell as to which X chromosome, that derived from the father or that from the mother, will be the genetically active X chromosome in that particular cell. The other X chromosome becomes essentially inactive genetically and becomes the Barr body, or sex chromatin. It is a further part of the Lyon hypothesis that the decision made in a given anlage cell is abided by in all descendants of that cell.

The consequences of the Lyon hypothesis are several. As stated earlier, the heterozygous female is a mosaic of mutant and wild-type cells. The female has no more genetically active X chromosomes than does the hemizygous male. Since the number of pertinent anlage cells, e.g. those destined to produce the antihemophilic factor, is small at the "time of decision," the proportion of cells having the mutant X chromosome as the active one will vary statistically around 50%, according to a binomial distribution. It is possible, therefore, for a heterozygote to have a majority of mutant X chromosomes active and as a result to be clinically affected—the so-called manifesting heterozygote. Such a situation has been observed in G6PD deficiency and in hemophilia. Heterozygosity is proved, in such instances, by the presence of both normal and affected sons.

Mosaicism in heterozygotes has been demonstrated for several X-linked recessive traits in man. For example, the female who is heterozygous for X-linked ocular albinism shows a mosaic pigmentary pattern of the fundus oculi. The female heterozygous for G6PD deficiency has two classes of erythrocytes, deficient and normal. In the X-linked disorder of mucopolysaccharide metabolism, the Hunter syndrome (Chapter 9), two classes of connective tissue cells can be demonstrated in the heterozygous female.

Complex genetic predisposition

Many disorders have a tendency to run in families, but unlike those conditions with which we are concerned in this book, the pattern of familial occurrence does not suggest simple Mendelian inheritance. Whenever one undertakes to survey the role of genetic factors in the diseases of a given system, it is found that the entities tend to fall into two categories: (1) the relatively uncommon simply inherited one and (2) the common conditions in which genetic factors seem to play some role but environment factors are also involved, often in a complex manner. Rheumatoid arthritis, rheumatic fever, systemic lupus erythematosus, and scleroderma (systemic sclerosis) are generally considered "connective tissue diseases," although it can be argued that they are diseases *in* but not *of* connective tissue. In each of these, some evidence for familial aggregation is available.

The questions which the geneticist considers are different in the two categories of disease. In the rare simply inherited disorders he is interested in gene frequency, mode of inheritance, nature of the basic defect, mechanism of the phenotypic features, mutation rate, selection factors, and so forth. In the more common conditions of multifactorial causation, in which genetic factors—themselves multiple (polygenic)—may play a role, the questions are likely to be: "How important is the genotype in determining the occurrence of the disease?" and "If important, by what mechanism does the genetic constitution contribute to the development of the disease?" The methods for answering these two questions, especially the first, include study of familial aggregation, comparison of concordance rates of monozygotic and like-sex dizygotic twins, comparison of different racial groups, study of the genetics of separate components in pathogenesis, search for blood group and disease association,* and genetic study of homologous disorders in experimental animals.

Discussion of the genetics of common connective tissue disorders, such as systemic lupus erythematosus, is beyond the scope of this book.

Eponyms

It is desirable to avoid eponyms whenever possible. It is preferable, at any rate, to use designations that indicate as precisely as possible the fundamental nature of the disease entity under consideration. In the present state of knowledge, however, there are good reasons to use eponyms for many syndromes. (1) Eponyms do not prejudice the search for the fundamental defect or conceal our ignorance of its nature. For the Hurler syndrome the name "lipochondrodystrophy" was used, with the erroneous notion that the basic defect is one of

*Blood group and disease association is often confused with genetic linkage. As stated earlier, genetic linkage produces no permanent association in the population. Although the locus for the gene determining the nail-patella syndrome is on the same pair of chromosomes as that for the ABO blood group genes, a large series of unrelated patients with the nail-patella syndrome would show the same distribution of ABO blood types as the population from which they came. The fact that as a group persons with duodenal peptic ulcer show a higher frequency of blood type O than does the general population of which they are a part is owing not to the location of an ulcer gene and a blood group O gene on the same chromosome but rather to a physiologic peculiarity of the type O person that renders him slightly but definitely more prone to duodenal ulcer.

cellular fat metabolism. (2) Since it does not use one feature of a complex syndrome as the designation, an eponym does not convey the impression that the presence of some one specific feature is a *sine qua non* for the diagnosis or that the feature mentioned occurs exclusively as a component of the particular syndrome. "Arachnodactyly" is a poor term for the Marfan syndrome, because the fingers of many of the patients are not more spidery than those of normal persons. "Cutis hyperelastica" is a poor term for the Ehlers-Danlos syndrome, since skin abnormalities may be relatively inconspicuous in patients who for one reason or another clearly have the disorder. The pity is not that eponyms are employed in these diseases but rather than no phonetically satisfactory or widely accepted eponyms are available for use in connection with syndromes such as osteogenesis imperfecta and pseudoxanthoma elasticum, in which the defect and its manifestations are much broader in their localization than bone or skin, respectively.

Eponyms are merely tags. They often have no justification from the standpoint of historical priorities, since frequently either someone else had described the condition earlier or the man whose name is used eponymously did not describe the full syndrome. Largely for the latter reason, it is preferable to say *the* Marfan syndrome or *the* Hurler syndrome rather than Marfan's syndrome or Hurler's syndrome.

REFERENCES

1. Beadle, G. W.: Genes and chemical reactions in neurospora, Science **129**:1715, 1959.
2. Bowen, P., Lee, C. S. N., Migeon, C. J., Kaplan, N. M., McKusick, V. A., and Reifenstein, E. C., Jr.: Hereditary male pseudohermaphroditism with hypogonadism, hypospadias and gynecomastia (Reifenstein's syndrome), Ann. Intern. Med. **62**:252, 1965.
3. Burnet, Sir Macfarlane: The riddle of influenza virus, Endeavour **14**:5, 1955.
4. Faber, K. H.: Nosography, ed. 2, New York, 1930, Paul B. Hoeber, Inc., Medical Book Department of Harper & Row, Publishers.
5. Gowers, W. R.: Abiotrophy, Lancet **1**:1003, 1902.
6. Grüneberg, H.: Animal genetics and medicine, New York, 1947, Paul B. Hoeber, Inc., Medical Book Department of Harper & Row, Publishers.
7. Jeghers, H., McKusick, V. A., and Katz, K. H.: Generalized intestinal polyposis and melanin spots of the oral mucosa, lips and digits, New Eng. J. Med. **241**:993 and 1031, 1949.
8. McKusick, V. A.: On the X-chromosome of man, Washington, D. C., 1964, American Institute of Biological Sciences.
9. Morton, N. E.: The detection and estimation of linkage between the genes for elliptocytosis and the Rh blood type, Amer. J. Hum. Genet. **8**:80, 1956.
10. Penrose, L. S.: Measurement of pleiotropic effects in phenylketonuria, Ann. Eugen. **16**:134, 1951.
11. Snyder, L. H.: Principles of gene distribution in human populations, Yale J. Biol. Med. **19**:817, 1947.
12. Stent, G. S.: The operon—on its third anniversary, Science **144**:816, 1964.
13. Vertue, H. St. H.: Medical mispronunciation, Guy's Hosp. Gaz. **68**:237, 1954.

2

The biology of normal connective tissue

If by some magic solution one could dissolve all the connective tissue of the body, all that would remain would be a mass of slimy epithelium, quivering muscle and frustrated nerve cells.
*—Arcadi**

Connective tissues, the supporting structures of the body, include cartilage, ligaments, tendons, fascia, joint capsules, the subepidermal portions (corium) of the skin, important elements of the heart valves and aorta and smaller blood vessels, and finally bone. In general, connective tissue consists of cellular and fibrous constituents embedded in the so-called ground substance. Reference is made to textbooks of histology (e.g. Fig. 45 of reference 67) for graphic presentation of the structural interrelationships of these elements.

In connection with his theory that organs are composed of a limited number of tissues, Bichat (1771-1802) distinguished fibrous tissue as one variety. About 1830 Johannes Müller (1801-1858) assigned the generally used designation "Bindegewebe." Schwann discovered the connective tissue cells.

The cellular elements

Virtually all the other endogenous elements of connective tissue are elaborated by the fibroblast, the main cellular constituent of connective tissue, or by its congeners, such as the osteoblast and the chondroblast. Sometimes the term "fibrocyte" is used and, in the older literature, "lamellar" or "fixed tissue cell." Other cellular elements include the mast cell and wandering cells such as macrophages. (The mast cell,[91] which has long been implicated in the formation of heparin, has been thought to be concerned also in the formation of hyaluronic acid.[1]) Some information has accumulated about the enzymatic processes involved in the formation of acid mucopolysaccharides.[19] Also information on the synthesis of collagen, a protein formed on the ribosomes of the fibroblast, is accumulating, as will be briefly reviewed later.

*Arcadi, J. A.: Bull. Hopkins Hosp. **90**:334, 1952.

The pedigree of the cells called fibroblasts is an uncertain matter in tissue culture, even though few other cells have been subjected to such extensive study by this technique. The spindle-shaped cells derived from various tissues and organs and referred to as fibroblasts have different functional properties in spite of identical morphology.[25,79]

Modulation and differentiation are important features of the biology of the fibroblast. Differentiation[23] indicates a maturation of the cell with specialization of function and usually increased structural complexity; with this specialization the potentiality to develop along certain lines is lost—a chrondroblast cannot, for example, develop into a fat cell even though both are descendants of a common mesenchymal cell. Modulation is the term used to indicate changes of such a type, as in a fat cell, let us say, that the fundamental nature of the cell is not lost although the functional capacity has been quantitatively altered and the structural features that permit identification of the precise species of the cell may be lost. Differentiation and modulation in the group of connective tissue cells are particularly complex matters.

The fibrous constituents

The fibrous constituents of connective tissue comprise two main groups: collagenous and elastic. The reticulin fiber would be classified by some as a separate category (p. 27), but most consider it a member of the collagen group although its precise relationship to the classic collagen fiber is moot.

*Collagen** must be defined in terms of its properties. It is a fibrous protein occurring in wide, straight, unbranching white bundles that possess high tensile strength and low elasticity.†

Collagen fibers at times have a tensile strength as high as 100 kg. per square centimeter, as high as some metals.[16] Collagen has characteristic 640 Å periodicity by small angle x-ray diffraction and by electron microscopy. It contains two unique amino acids, hydroxyproline and hydroxylysine.[42] The former is present in relatively large amounts and is used in quantitative determination of collagen.[64,75] It contains large amounts of glycine. Aromatic and sulfur amino acids are present only in low concentration.

The biologic importance of collagen in the individual organism and in the phylogenetic series is tremendous. Collagen represents approximately 30% of the total protein of the human body. In the vertebrate animal it is what cellulose is to plants. As the matrix of bone[7,87b] it was referred to as "ossein" in the older literature. Even the vitreous humor of the eye contains fibers with the properties of collagen, the so-called "vitrosin" of Gross.[35] That it is not limited to vertebrates is indicated (as merely one example) by the fact that collagen is the skeleton of the invertebrate sponge familiar in household and other usage.

The economic importance of collagen dates back to prehistory when the manufacture of leather[65] and glue was first undertaken. Isinglass, made from the swim bladder of fish such as the sturgeon, was also collagenous in nature. It was

---

*An annotated monthly bibliography of current literature on collagen research in chemistry, technology, and medicine was initiated in 1960 by the Research Division of Ethicon, Inc., Somerville, N. J.

†See p. 181 for a discussion of the several definitions of elasticity. As used here, the term refers principally to extensibility.

Table 2. Characteristics of collagen—a partial tabulation

Category based on method of study	*Characteristic features*
Histologic properties[86a]	Tinctorial characteristics: Acid fuchsin—bright red staining Periodic acid and Schiff's reagent—faint red staining Silver agents—staining poor or absent Dilute acids and alkalis—swelling
Electron microscopic features	640 Å periodicity
Chemical features	14% hydroxyproline by weight; hydroxylysine also a unique amino acid; low content of tyrosine, methionine, and histidine; absence of cystine and tryptophane; 1% hexosamine (associated carbohydrate)
Shrinkage characteristics	Temperature: 60°-65°C. (shrinkage to about one third original length) certain electrolyte solutions
Behavior toward enzymes	Attacked by pepsin Attacked by "collagenases" of *Clostridium histolyticum* and *Cl. welchii*[86b] Resistant to trypsin, chymotrypsin, papain, hyaluronidase
Isotope tracer studies of metabolic turnover rate	Relative metabolic inertia[74]
X-ray crystallography	Characteristic pattern(s)[3]
Immunology	Very low antigenicity of unaltered collagen,[97a,108] viz., use for suture material

in leather manufacture that one property of collagen, thermal shrinkage (at 60° to 65° C.), was discovered and used in judging adequacy of tannage. (Some of the best studies of collagen have been directly or indirectly supported by the leather industries. For example, Highberger[96] has been in the employ of the United Shoe Machinery Corporation of Beverly, Massachusetts, and Gustavson[36] works at the Swedish Leather Research Institute in Stockholm. Grassmann[28] works at the Max Planck Institute for Protein and Leather Investigation [Max Planck-Institut für Eiweiss- und Lederforschung] in Regensburg.) Gustavson[36] has demonstrated that thermal shrinkage is the result of breaking of cross-links in the collagen molecule that occur mainly through hydrogen bonding between hydroxyl groups of hydroxyproline and the keto-imide groups of adjacent helices. Gustavson[106q] has further suggested the intriguing possibility that *in vivo* "tanning" may be the basis of some changes seen with aging and in pathologic states.

The importance of collagen in pathology will be evident to a medical audience, since the concept of "collagen vascular diseases" has seemingly gained such wide acceptance. Further medical implications appear to be represented by certain of the hereditary disorders of connective tissue under discussion here.

These implications—biologic, economic, and medical—have been responsible for very extensive investigations of the nature of collagen[3,11,53,84,86] by scientists of diverse interests and perspectives. The result has been, in the past at least, a situation like the portrayal of the elephant that was examined by the six blind men. Recently several excellent symposia have effected a synthesis of the diverse bits of information.

The building blocks of collagen, the tropocollagen unit in the terminology of Gross and associates[34] are thought to have a length (and periodicity) of about 2,200 Å, and the 640 Å periodicity of the finished product is conceived by Schmitt and collaborators as the result of a staggering of the building blocks in their lining up side-to-side. The discovery that it is possible to solubilize collagen and then reconstitute it from solution was responsible for much of this concept. Physicochemical studies indicate that the tropocollagen unit is a thin, rigid rod with a molecular weight of 300,000 to 310,000, by osmolarity and by light scattering, and with dimensions of about 14 by 2,000 Å.[9] Although the larger collagen aggregates are only slightly extensible and in no way approach elastic fibers in this respect, electron optical observations of collagen fibrils[97] indicate that considable extensibility of the smaller units is possible. Abnormality in the fibrillar organization may be important in the genesis of the abnormal extensibility of tendons, joint capsules, and ligaments in certain of the hereditary disorders of connective tissue.

The work of Jackson and Smith[1d,52] has done much to help establish a view that has had some support hitherto: a collagen precursor is excreted by the fibroblast (or a congener) and transformed into the collagen fiber extracellularly. These workers used osteoblasts and grew them in a fibrin-free medium, thus disproving one theory of collagenesis. Appreciable amounts of protein-bound hydroxyproline appeared before typical collagen fibrils were demonstrable. Subsequently many fibrils appeared without a significant further rise in hydroxyproline. During the period of collagen fibrogenesis the osteoblasts displayed cytoplasmic granules that stained intensely with PAS. The osteoblast was found to be capable of converting L-proline to hydroxyproline.[102]

The collagen molecule is now known to have a three-stranded helical structure. The monomeric components, called alpha chains, are of two types, designated alpha-1 and alpha-2. They differ in amino acid composition but have identical molecular weights (about 90,000). Each molecule of collagen contains two alpha-1 chains and one alpha-2 chain.

Usage has dictated application of the designation beta component to dimers derived from denatured collagen and gamma component to trimers so derived. The beta components are of two types, beta-12 and beta-11, depending on whether the dimer is made up of two alpha-1 chains or of an alpha-1 and an alpha-2. Ordinarily the collagen molecule is gamma-112 according to this system of nomenclature.[58]

(The terminology is somewhat confusing to the student of the hemoglobins—in connection with which alpha, beta, and gamma designate separate polypeptide chains.)

Recent evidence[11a] indicates that all three polypeptide chains of collagen have a unique primary structure throughout their lengths. The alpha-1 chains, which were earlier thought to be of one type only, are shown by recent studies to be of two types.

By analogy to the biochemical genetics of hemoglobin, which has advanced much further, at least three structural genes are probably involved in determination of the collagen molecule, two for the two types of alpha-1 chains and one for the alpha-2 chain. The assembly of amino acids into the alpha subunits occurs in the cytoplasm of the fibroblast (or one of its congeners such as the osteoblast) on clusters of ribosomal particles, polyribosomes.[60] Some evidence suggests that hydroxyproline cannot be incorporated directly into collagen but must be derived from proline, which is hydroxylated after formation of sRNA-proline. Peterkofsky and Udenfriend[82] have demonstrated hydroxylation of proline in the ribosomal-RNA-bound peptide.

Best evidence seems to indicate that after the alpha-1 and alpha-2 chains are synthesized on polyribosomes in the cytoplasm of the fibroblasts, they are extruded as such into the extracellular area where the two types of two-stranded tropocollagen beta-12 and beta-11 are formed, followed by further condensation to form the three-stranded gamma-112 tropocollagen unit. The interactions of the alpha subunits can occur *in vitro* in a cell-free, experimentally controlled, aqueous system, suggesting that the same probably occurs extracellularly *in vivo.* The gamma-112 is soluble collagen. Insolubilization to produce mature collagen almost certainly occurs extracellularly.

Because of specific interchain ordering of the polypeptide chains by the formation of stable cross-linking bonds, such as ester and/or aldehyde linkages, the collagen molecule acquires characteristic clusters of polar amino acids in a precise stereochemical configuration at the "head" and "tail" ends of the tropocollagen molecule. (The basic and acidic amino side-chain residues in tropocollagen aggregates can be demonstrated by electron microscopy, using "electron stains" such as phosphotungstic acid and cationic uranium.) The specific cross-linkage, together with water molecule and secondary hydrogen bonds, which stabilize the helical configuration of three-stranded collagen, also account for its rodlike configuration (14 by 2,800 Å) and its molecular weight (360,000). (The dimensions cited above are, obviously, of the same order of magnitude, and the differences reflect differences in methods used for measurement. The incorporation of water and mucopolysaccharides accounts for the fact that the molecular weight of the three-stranded unit is greater than the sum of the weights of three alpha subunits.)

Hodge and Schmitt[48] have presented electron microscopic and chemical evidence to indicate the existence of end chains or telopeptides on each of the alpha chains. These seem to function particularly with reference to the aligning of the alpha components in the collagen molecule.

The carbohydrate content of collagen is low. What is present may be derived from ground substances playing the role of interfibrillary cement. In pure collagen, hydroxyproline is present is about 14 gm. per 100 gm. protein (8.6 gm. per 100 gm. amino nitrogen) and glycine in roughly twice as great a proportion. The polar side groups of collagen appear to be located at the areas of the bands displayed by x-ray diffraction and by electron microscopy. These are the reactive areas where stains and tanning agents operate.

The relative metabolic inertia of nonsoluble collagen is a very striking feature.[74] The turnover rate is slightly higher in bone than in tendon, and in younger animals, but is much lower than in proteins of cells and plasma. Soluble or extractable collagen,[76a] which according to the trinitarian categorization of connective tissue elements followed here must be considered part of the ground substance, has a considerably higher rate of turnover.[44] No collagenase comparable to that produced by clostridia has been demonstrated in man, with the exception of the extraction by Schmitt and Sizer[98] of material with the properties of collagenase from the cells around embedded collagenous sutures. Keech[55,56] has demonstrated interesting variability in the sensitivity of collagen from different human individuals to the action of collagenase. In a few cases a high degree of resistance to digestion was exhibited; others showed more digestion than the average. It would be very interesting to know whether or not sensitivity to collagenase is genetically determined and whether there are any correlations with disease. Is there any characteristic variation in collagenase sensitivity in the heritable disorders of connective tissue?

Reticulin fibers have most of the same properties as collagen fibers, most important being the 640 Å periodicity. The main difference is their small diameters, stainability by silver, and a relatively high concentration of associated polysaccharide. Reticulin fibers predominate in the embryo and in the adult animal are relatively abundant in parenchymatous organs, in lymph nodes and spleen, around muscle bundles and fat globules, and in association with amorphous material in epithelial basement membranes. The differences from collagen fibers may be a matter of fiber size or diameter of the individual fibrils in a bundle. Given a collagen bundle and a reticulin bundle of the same overall diameter, the reticulin bundle may stain with silver because it has a great many more component fibrils of small diameter and correspondingly greater total fibril surface area. Staining with silver is a surface phenomenon as demonstrated by Gross. Whether reticulin is precollagen or immature collagen (not to be confused with procollagen or soluble collagen) is perhaps not too important a consideration. The concept of Gross and others that it is not a progenitor of collagen is based on the fact that it is present in the adult organism, seemingly without ever being transformed into collagen, and that electron microscopic evidence for aggregation of reticulin fibers (of small diameter) into collagen fibers is lacking. Reticulin fibers are present in the adult organism, in the corium, for example, and are possibly present in as great absolute amounts as at any earlier stage in ontogeny. In the adult, however, the reticulin fibers are "swamped" by the preponderance of collagen fibers. Several observations[51] suggest that reticulin of granulation tissue is different from that of basement membranes.

Elastic fibers[46] are large branching refractile structures, light yellow or brown, depending on their age; with a high degree of extensibility; extreme insolubility; indestructibility in relation to heat, drastic pH changes, and enzymes; a low content of polar amino acids; and, finally, certain distinctive tinctorial characteristics. The nature of their staining by orcein and related dyes is not at all well understood; the staining bears no relationship to pH, and there is no other evidence that salt linkages are involved.[109]

Elastic fibers were first described in blood vessels by Hele in 1842. In 1902 Richards and Gies[89] discussed the chemical properties of elastin. It is sobering to note that there has been little improvement on their methods.

Whereas collagen is present in areas where a pliant but relatively nonextensible building material is necessary (ligaments, tendons, fascia, joint capsules), elastic fibers serve important functions in areas such as the media of the aorta (where they are responsible for the compression chamber, reservoir, or *Windkessel* hemodynamic function of that structure), in the elastic cartilage of the ear, and in ligaments with large elastic components such as those of the foot and the ligamenta flava of the spine. In the skin, elastic fibers are found mainly in the outermost layer of the corium. The leather industry has been a source of information on elastic fibers as well as on collagen. The outer part of the corium represents the grain layer of leather, so-called because it swells less with tanning and produces grain, which may or may not be desirable in the particular instance. Empirically, "bating"—treatment of the hides with pancreas—was practiced in order to remove the grain layer. Baló and Banga[5] subsequently found that the basis of the "bating" process is the presence of elastase in pancreas (see below).

Chemically, elastin is characterized by a dearth of acidic, basic, and hydroxy amino acids and an abundance of nonpolar amino acids. The peculiar staining characteristics of elastic fibers have their basis largely in these facts.

In degradation products from elastin, the group working with Partridge[105] demonstrated two new amino acids, desmosine and isodesmosine. These are apparently formed by the condensation of four lysine residues to form a pyrimidine ring structure.

Much less is known about the ultrastructure of the elastic fiber than of the collagen fiber. X-ray diffraction studies suggest that in the relaxed state the molecules of elastin are disorganized as in the case of unstretched rubber. Also as in rubber, positive areas of birefringence appear with stretching. Gross has found that the double helical structures earlier described by him[30] in electron photomicrographs of material derived from aorta were in fact not elastic fiber elements but trypsinogen[32] in the enzyme preparation used in removing nonelastic elements. One view[41] of the chemical constitution is that a pro-elastin core is embedded in a matrix of combined pro-elastin and elastomucin. There is produced, in the pancreatic islet tissue, an elastase[5,6] for which there is an inhibitor produced elsewhere in pancreas. Elastic fibers are moderately susceptible to digestion by trypsin, resistant to digestion by pepsin; this is the converse of the situation with collagen. From physicochemical studies of elastic fibers Lloyd and Garrod[62] concluded that lateral bonding between molecules must occur at infrequent intervals, resulting in a random configuration of the backbone of the fiber and consequent elasticity. The cross-links show high resistance to all the collagen solvents. Desmosine and isodesmosine may be important in the cross-linking. In experimental copper deficiency in pigs (p. 131) deficiency of desmosine in elastin is accompanied by failure of cross-links, with development of aneurysms or spontaneous rupture of the aorta.[110]

Because of the large size and inertness of the elastic fiber and by analogy to collagen it is likely that a monomeric unit or combination of subunits, a tropoelastin, is synthesized by fibroblasts. It is likely that the chemical methods for preparation of elastin destroy the postulated tropoelastin. Its isolation could be of great importance by permitting metabolic studies of elastin.

Studies with radioisotope tracer methods[99] indicate what is probably an even lower level of metabolic activity than in collagen. With aging there is a chemical alteration in elastin,[84IIb] including a change in the amino acid profile and an increased affinity for calcium and basophilic dyes.

Formation of elastic fibers in tissue culture is observed with more difficulty than in the case of collagen fibers.[8,77,78] Some workers[40] conclude that in several ways collagen participates in elastofibrogenesis and that there is an intimate interrelationship between the two. There appears to be evolving a general principle that the extracellular components of connective tissue are not the "free agents" they have generally been considered in the past. Increasingly, evidence accumulates for an intimate interrelationship between collagenous and elastic fibers. For example, Keech and Reed[56] demonstrate that by a variety of means—chemical, enzymatic, and physical—so-called "moth-eaten fibers" (MEF) can be produced from either type of fiber. The MEF are thought of as an intermediate form.

The ground substance

The term ground substance is a mistranslation of that used by the early German histologists, *Grundsubstanz,* meaning "fundamental substance." Although the ground substance has long been known (in 1861 there was enough information to justify a review of the subject by Köllicker), the most intensive investigations followed the discovery of the "spreading factor" by Duran-Reynals and Suner in 1929[22] and the studies of mucopolysaccharides of the ground substance and of hyaluronidase in the laboratory of Karl Meyer at Columbia University beginning in the early 1930's.[69]

The ground substance is the extracellular, extrafibrillar, amorphous matrix of connective tissue. It has components derived from the fibroblast, such as acid mucoprotein, acid mucopolysaccharide, and dispersed (soluble or pro-) collagen, and components not elaborated locally, such as water, ions, small organic molecules such as glucose, cell metabolites, plasma proteins, and others. It is important not to equate ground substance to acid mucoproteins and acid mucopolysaccharides, as has become a frequent practice, since on a quantitative basis, and possibly on a functional basis, some of the other constituents such as plasma proteins, soluble collagen, and neutral mucoproteins are as important. Another assumption that may be fallacious is that changes in serum mucoprotein (which is neutral) reflect changes in acid mucopolysaccharide of the ground substance; chemically the two are quite distinct.

There are several presumably distinct acid mucopolysaccharides in connective tissue (Table 3). All are polymers of high molecular weight and contain hexosamine and hexuronic acid moieties.[57] Hyaluronic acid, which has been identified in synovial fluid, vitreous humor, and umbilical cord, is composed, among other moieties, of glucosamine and glucuronic acid. It is digested by hyaluronidase. Chondroitin, which has been isolated only from cornea, differs from hyaluronic acid by the replacement of glucosamine by galactosamine; its properties are similar, however. Meyer distinguishes three chondroitin sulfates or ChS (A, B, and C) on the basis of solubility, optical rotation, and enzymatic properties. All contain galactosamine, not glucosamine. ChS A has been demonstrated in cartilage, bone, cornea, aorta, and ligamentum nuchae. ChS B, in which the hexuronic acid moiety is iduronic acid, not glucuronic acid, has been isolated from skin, tendon, heart valves, ligamentum nuchae, and aorta. ChS C has been found in cartilage, umbilical cord, tendons, and nucleus pulposus. Keratosulfate, the only sulfate mucopolysaccharide free of uronic acid, has been isolated from cornea, where it represents about 50% of total mucopolysaccharide. Heparitin sulfate, which as its name indicates has chemical, physical, and other properties resembling those of heparin, has normally been found only in aorta.

Metabolically mucopolysaccharides are rapidly turned over. The availability of S^{35} and description of its use in the study of acid mucopolysaccharides by Dziewiatkowski[18] in 1949 have permitted some insight into problems of the metabolism of these materials. Studies of mucopolysaccharide formation in microorganisms and in cell cultures have likewise been helpful. Production of components of the ground substance in tissue culture has been observed.[10,107]

Metachromatic staining of connective tissues, as by toluidine blue, is a function largely of mucopolysaccharides.[14,27] (Metachromasia is a term introduced by Ehrlich in 1877 to indicate the property of a tissue to stain one color when exposed to a dye of a different color.)

In the mammalian organism hyaluronidase has been identified with certainty only in testis.

The importance of the ground substance is evident when one considers that it must be traversed by all materials entering and leaving the cells.[93b] The concept[17,29,53] that mucopolysaccharides function like a reactive gel of the ion exchange resin group is an intriguing but as yet unproved concept. It is at least theoretically possible that changes in the concentration or state of polymerization might modify greatly the capacity of connective tissues to bind inorganic ions and water. Hyaluronic acid, highly hygroscopic in the purified state, may be concerned in water-binding by tissues. It may also serve as a lubricant and shock absorber. Chondroitin sulfate, because of its highly charged anionic groups, may function[76f] as a cation exchange resin.

Jackson[50] has presented data which he interprets as indicating an important role of mucopolysaccharide in the organization and certain properties of collagenous structures such as tendon. Trypsin will digest gelatin but not native collagen. The characteristic shrinkage temperature of native collagen is altered by treatment directed at the matrix.

The evidence[59,66,95] on the role, if any, of mucopolysaccharide in collagen

Table 3. Mucopolysaccharides of connective tissue

	Hexosamine	*Hexuronic acid*	*Source*
Nonsulfated			
Chondroitin	Galactosamine	Glucuronic	Cornea
Hyaluronic acid	Glucosamine	Glucuronic	Vitreous humor Synovial fluid Umbilical cord
Sulfated			
Keratosulfate	Glucosamine Galactose	None	Cornea Cartilage Nucleus pulposus
Heparitin sulfate	Glucosamine	Glucuronic	Aorta
Chrondroitin sulfate A	Galactosamine	Glucuronic	Cornea Cartilage
Chondroitin sulfate B	Galactosamine	Iduronic	Skin Heart Aorta
Chondroitin sulfate C	Galactosamine	Glucuronic	Cartilage Tendon
Heparin	Glucosamine	Glucuronic	

fibrogenesis is held by some[51] to be conflicting and inconclusive. However, some connection is thought to exist.[106a]

As outlined in Chapter 9, genetic disturbances of mucopolysaccharide metabolism have been related to three of the acid mucopolysaccharides listed in Table 3: chondroitin sulfate B, heparitin sulfate, and keratosulfate. The excessive urinary excretion of various ones of these substances is the biochemical characteristic of six genetic disorders that have been delineated by combined clinical, genetic, and biochemical study. The methods used by Kaplan in a collaborative study of the genetic mucopolysaccharidoses were as follows. (See reference 64a for technical references.)

Mucopolysaccharides were isolated from urine by a method which, in brief, consisted of (1) removing as much salt as possible by centrifugation in the cold, (2) diluting the urine with distilled water to reduce salt concentration further, (3) adjusting the pH to 5 to 6 with glacial acetic acid, and (4) precipitating the mucopolysaccharides with cetylpyridinium chloride. The precipitate, after washing with NaCl-saturated 95% ethanol, was dissolved in acetate buffer, pH 5.5, and stirred with a chloroform–amyl alcohol mixture to extract protein and peptides. The aqueous phase was precipitated with ethanol and then redissolved in acetate buffer and stirred with a mixture of Lloyd's reagent and kaolin to remove further traces of protein. The mucopolysaccharides were then reprecipitated with ethanol. The precipitate was dissolved in distilled water and treated again with Lloyd's reagent and kaolin. The clear solution was brought to 2.5% calcium acetate–0.5N acetic acid, and appropriate alcohol fractions were made, the precipitates from which were dried and weighed.

Analyses done on the isolated materials consisted of the following: carbazol and orcinol reactions for uronic acid, anthrone reaction for neutral sugar, determination of total hexosamine, column chromatography to determine relative amounts of glucosamine and galactosamine, paper chromatography to demonstrate the presence of galactose, measurements of optical rotation, elemental sulfur analyses, and incubation with testicular hyaluronidase to demonstrate resistance or susceptibility to this enzyme.

Chondroitin sulfate B was identified by its low alcohol solubility, a low carbazol and high orcinol value, no anthrone value, a high negative optical rotation, resistance to digestion by testicular hyaluronidase, and the presence of galactosamine. Heparitin sulfate was identified by a high carbazol and low orcinol value, no anthrone value, a high positive optical rotation, resistance to digestion by testicular hyaluronidase, and the presence of glucosamine. Keratosulfate was identified by its high alcohol solubility, no carbazol or orcinol value, a high anthrone value, the presence of glucosamine, the demonstration of galactose by paper chromatography, and resistance to testicular hyaluronidase. Chondrointin sulfate A and C, the major normal constituents of urine, were identified by a carbazol to orcinol ration of about 3 to 2, no anthrone value, susceptibility to digestion by testicular hyaluronidase, and the presence of galactosamine.

Further considerations

The indications of an intimate interrelationship between the several elements of connective tissue, e.g. between collagen and elastin, between mucopolysaccharide and collagen, etc., are numerous. The details of these interrelationships are not yet fully known.

In addition to these general features of connective tissue, which undoubtedly assist in the understanding of the heritable disorders to be discussed, there are some specific questions about the biology of connective tissue that come to mind with study of these diseases. A few examples follow. *In the Marfan syndrome:* What does the suspensory ligament of the ocular lens have in common with the media of the aorta? What controls longitudinal growth of bone? *In pseudoxanthoma elasticum:* What is the nature of Bruch's membrane of the eye and what does it have in common with the corium? *In the Ehlers-Danlos syndrome:* What is responsible for the tensile strength of the skin and for its elasticity? What is the organization of collagen bundles in ligaments, tendons, and joint capsules and what is the relationship between this organization and the stretchability of these structures? What determines the elastic properties of the collagen and elastin molecules, and of fibers of these proteins? *In osteogenesis imperfecta:* What is the normal organization of apatite on collagen, which accounts for the important structural properties of bone, and in this disease what change in collagen has occurred to disrupt the normal collagen-apatite relationship? In disorders such as osteogenesis imperfecta and the Ehlers-Danlos syndrome is there any abnormality of amino acid sequences[106z] comparable to the abnormalities demonstrated by Ingram[49] in the aberrant hemoglobins? In connection with the full discussion of each of the entities, what is known in answer to these questions and others will be presented. Unfortunately, much remains to be learned in all these areas.

REFERENCES

1. Asboe-Hansen, G.: The origin of synovial mucin. Ehrlich's mast cell—a secretory element of connective tissue, Ann. Rheum. Dis. **9**:149, 1950.
2. Asboe-Hansen, G., editor: Connective tissue in health and disease, Copenhagen, 1954, Ejnar Munksgaard Forlag.
   (a) Asboe-Hansen, G.: Introduction, p. 9. (b) Robb-Smith, A. H. T.: Normal morphology and morphogenesis of connective tissue, p. 15. (c) McManus, J. F. A.: Histochemistry of connective tissue, p. 31. (d) Meyer, K.: Chemistry of ground-substance, p. 54. (e) Kulonen, E.: Chemistry of collagen, p. 70. (f) Dorfman, A.: Metabolism of mucopolysaccharides, p. 81. (g) Boström, H.: Sulphate exchange of sulpho-mucopolysaccharides, p. 97. (h) Duran-Reynals, F.: The spreading reaction, p. 103. (i) Mathews, M. B., and Dorfman, A.: Inhibition of hyaluronidase, p. 112. (j) Iversen, K.: Hormonal influence on connective tissue, p. 130. (k) Banfield, W. G.: Aging of connective tissue, p. 159. (l) Howes, E. L.: Connective tissue in wound healing, p. 159 (m) Altschuler, C. H., and Angevine, D. M.: The pathology of connective tissue, p. 178. (n) Teihum, G.: Cortisone, ascorbic acid and changes in the reticulo-endothelial system, p. 196. (o) Sprunt, D. H.: Connective tissue and infection, p. 208. (p) Cavallero, C.: Influence of hormones on infection, p. 214. (q) Simpson, W. L.: Connective tissues and cancer, p. 225. (r) Rinehart, J. F.: Histogenesis and pathogenesis of arteriosclerosis, p. 239. (s) Klemperer, P.: Collagen diseases, p. 251. (t) Ragan, C.: Arthritis, p. 263. (u) Asboe-Hansen, G.: Systemic connective tissue disorders pertaining to dermatology, p. 274. (v) Godtfredsen, E.: Mesenchymal aspects in ophthalmology, p. 296. (w) Zacharias, L.: Fibroses due to injury, p. 308.
3. Bear, R. S.: The structure of collagen fibrils, Advances Protein Chem. **7**:69, 1952.
4. Baker, B. L., and Abrams, G. O.: The physiology of connective tissue, Ann. Rev. Physiol. **17**:61, 1955.
5. Baló, J., and Banga, I.: The elastolytic activity of pancreatic extracts, Biochem. J. **46**:384, 1950.
6. Banga, I., and Baló, J.: Elastin and elastase, Nature **171**:44, 1953.

7. Blackett, N. M.: On the organization of collagen fibrils in bone, Biochim. Biophys. Acta **16**:161, 1955.
8. Bloom, W.: Studies on fibers in tissue culture. II. The development of elastic fibers in cultures of embryonic heart and aorta, Arch. exp. Zellforsch. **9**:6, 1929.
9. Boedtker, H., and Doty, P.: On the nature of the structural element of collagen, J. Amer. Chem. Soc. **77**:248, 1955.
10. Bollet, A. J., Boas, N. F., and Bunim, J. J.: Synthesis of hexosamine by connective tissue (in vitro), Science **120**:348, 1954.
11. Borasky, R.: Guide to the literature on collagen, Philadelphia, 1950, Agricultural Research Administration, United States Department of Agriculture (Eastern Regional Research Laboratory).

11a. Bornstein, P., and Piez, K. A.: Collagen: structural studies based on the cleavage of methionyl bonds, Science **148**: 1353, 1965.

12. Bowen, T. J.: Physical studies on a soluble protein obtained by the degeneration of elastin with urea, Biochem. J. **55**:766, 1953.
13. Bowes, J. H., and Kenten, R. H.: Summary of published results (1900-1946) on amino acid composition of gelatin and collagen, 1947, Leather Manufacturers Research Association, pp. 1-22.
14. Braden, A. W. H.: The reactions of isolated mucopolysaccharides to several histochemical tests, Stain Techn. **30**:19, 1955.
15. Campani, M.: Function of mast cells, Lancet **1**:802, 1951.
16. Castor, C. W.: Approaches to the study of connective tissue, Bull. Rheum. Dis. **9**:177, 1959.
17. Day, T. D.: The mode of reaction of interstitial connective tissue with water, J. Physiol. **109**:380, 1949.
18. Dziewiatkowski, D. D.: Rate of excretion of radioactive sulfur and its concentration in some tissues of the rat after intraperitoneal administration of labeled sodium sulfate, J. Biol. Chem. **178**:197, 1949.
19. Dorfman, A.: Metabolism of the mucopolysaccharides of connective tissue, Pharmacol. Rev. **7**:1, 1955.
20. Dorfman, A.: The biochemistry of connective tissue, J. Chronic Dis. **10**:403, 1959.
21. Dorfman, A., and Mathews, M. B.: The physiology of connective tissue, Ann. Rev. Physiol. **18**:69, 1956.
22. Duran-Reynals, F., and Suner Pi, J.: Exaltation de l'activité du staphylocoque par les extracts testiculaires, Compt. Rend. Soc. Biol. **99**:1908, 1929.
23. Fawcitt, D. W.: Cell differentiation and modulation. In An introduction to cell and tissue culture, by the staff of the Tissue Culture Course, Cooperstown, N. Y., 1949-1953, Minneapolis, 1955, Burgess Publishing Co.
24. Fleischmajer, R., and Fishman, L.: Amino acid composition of human dermal collagen, Nature **205**:264, 1965.
25. Gerarde, H. W., and Jones, M.: The effect of cortisone on collagen synthesis in vitro, J. Biol. Chem. **201**:553, 1953.
26. Gersh, I., and Catchpole, H. R.: The nature of ground substance of connective tissue, Perspect. Biol. Med. **3**:282, 1960.
27. Gomori, G.: The histochemistry of mucopolysaccharides, Brit. J. Exp. Path. **35**:377, 1954.
28. Grassmann, W.: Unsere heutige Kenntnis des Kollagens, Das Leder **6**:241, 1955.
29. Gray, J.: The properties of inter-cellular matrix and its relations to electrolytes, Brit. J. Biol. **3**:167, 1926.
30. Gross, J.: The structure of elastic tissue as studied with the electron microscope, J. Exp. Med. **89**:699, 1949.
31. Gross, J.: Connective tissue fine structure and some methods for its analysis, J. Geront. **5**:343, 1950.
32. Gross, J.: Fiber formation in trypsinogen solutions: an electron optical study, Proc. Soc. Exp. Biol. Med. **78**:241, 1951.
33. Gross, J., Highberger, J. H., and Schmitt, F. O.: Some factors involved in the fibrogenesis of collagen in vitro, Proc. Soc. Exp. Biol. Med. **80**:462, 1952.
34. Gross, J., Highberger, J. H., and Schmitt, F. O.: Collagen structures considered as states of aggregation of a kinetic unit. The tropocollagen particle, Proc. Nat. Acad. Sci. **40**:679, 1954.

35. Gross, J., Matoltsy, A. G., and Cohen, C.: Vitrosin: a member of the collagen class, J. Biophys. Biochem. Cytol. **1**:215, 1955.
36. Gustavson, K. H.: The chemistry and reactivity of collagen, New York, 1956, Academic Press, Inc.
37. Hall, D. A.: The fibrous components of connective tissue with special reference to the elastic fiber, Int. Rev. Cytol. **8**:211, 1959.
38. Hall, D. A.: The chemistry of connective tissue, Springfield, Ill., 1961, Charles C Thomas, Publisher.
39. Hall, D. A.: Elastolysis and ageing, Springfield, Ill., 1964, Charles C Thomas, Publisher.
40. Hall, D. A., Keech, M. K., Reed, R., Saxl, H., Tunbridge, R. E., and Wood, M. J.: Collagen and elastin in connective tissue, J. Geront. **10**:388, 1955.
41. Hall, D. A., Reed, R., and Tunbridge, R. E.: Structure of elastic tissue, Nature **170**:264, 1952.
42. Hamilton, P. B., and Anderson, R. A.: Hydroxyproline in proteins, J. Amer. Chem. Soc. **77**:2892, 1955.
43. Harkness, R. D.: Biological functions of collagen, Biol. Rev. **36**:399, 1961.
44. Harkness, R. D., Marko, A. M., Muir, H. M., and Neuberger, A.: The metabolism of collagen and other proteins in the skin of rabbits, Biochem. J. **56**:558, 1954.
45. Harrington, W. F., and von Hippel, P. H.: The structure of collagen and gelatin, Advances Protein Chem. **16**:1, 1961.
46. Hass, G. M.: Elastic tissue, Arch. Path. **27**:334, 543, 1939.
47. Hlaváčková, V., and Hruoza, Z.: The role of mucopolysaccharides in the mechanism of contraction of collagen fibres in rats of various ages, Gerontologia **9**:84, 1964.
48. Hodge, A. J., and Schmitt, F. O.: Interaction properties of sonically fragmented macromolecules, Proc. Nat. Acad. Sci. **44**:418, 1958.
49. Ingram, V. M.: Gene mutations in human haemoglobin; the chemical difference between normal and sickle cell haemoglobin, Nature **180**:326, 1957.
50. Jackson, D. S.: The nature of collagen-chondroitin sulfate linkages in tendon, Biochem. J. **56**:699, 1954.
51. Jackson, D. S.: Some biochemical aspects of fibrogenesis and wound healing, New Eng. J. Med. **259**:814, 1958.
52. Jackson, S. F., and Smith, R. H.: Studies on the biosynthesis of collagen. I. The growth of fowl osteoblasts and the formation of collagen in tissue culture, J. Biophys. Biochem. Cytol. **3**:897, 1957.
53. Joseph, N. R., Engel, M. B., and Catchpole, H. R.: Interaction of ions and connective tissue, Biochim. Biophys. Acta **8**:575, 1952.
54. Keech, M. K.: The effect of collagenase on human skin collagen. Comparison of different age-groups and of cases with and without "collagen disease," Yale J. Biol. Med. **26**:295, 1954.
55. Keech, M. K.: Transformation of collagen to "elastin" in dermal collagens with varying sensitivity towards collagenase, Ann. Rheum. Dis. **17**:23, 1958.
56. Keech, M. K., and Reed, R.: Enzymatic elucidation of the relationship between collagen and elastin; an electron microscopic study, Ann. Rheum. Dis. **17**:23, 1958.
57. Kent, P. W., and Whitehouse, M. M.: Biochemistry of amino sugars, New York, 1955, Academic Press, Inc.
58. Kohn, R. R., Bensusan, H. B., and Klein, L.: Cross-linkages in collagen, Science **145**:186, 1964.
59. Kramer, H.: The nature and formation of normal and abnormal connective tissue (Ph.D. thesis, University of Oxford, 1952); cited by Robb-Smith.[2b]
60. Kretsinger, R. H., Manner, G., Gould, B. S., and Rich, A.: Snythesis of collagen on polyribosomes, Nature **202**:438, 1964.
61. Lillie, R. O.: Histopathologic technique and practical histochemistry, New York, 1954, Blakiston Co., chap. 16, p. 333.
62. Lloyd, D. J., and Garrod, M.: A contribution to the theory of the structure of protein fibres, with special reference to the so-called thermal shrinkage of the collagen fibre, Trans. Faraday Soc. **44**:441, 1948.
63. Lowry, O. H., Gilligan, D. R., and Katersky, E. M.: The determination of collagen and elastin in tissues with results obtained in various normal tissues from different species, J. Biol. Chem. **139**:795, 1941.

64. McKusick, V. A., Kaplan, D., Wise, D., Hanley, W. B., Suddarth, S. B., Serick, M. E., and Maumanee, A. E.: The genetic mucopolysaccharidoses, Medicine, November, 1965.
65. McLaughlin, G. D., and Theis, E. R.: The chemistry of the leather industry, New York, 1945, Reinhold Publishing Corp.
66. Mancini, R. E., and de Lustig, E. S.: Acción de la hialurinadasa sobre los fibroblastos in vitro, Rev. Soc. Argent. Biol. **26**:7, 1950.
67. Maximow, A. A., and Bloom, W.: A textbook of histology, Philadelphia, 1942, W. B. Saunders Co.
68. Meyer, K.: Nature and function of mucopolysaccharides in connective tissue. In Nachmanson, D., editor: Molecular biology, New York, 1960, Academic Press, Inc., p. 69.
69. Meyer, K., and Palmer, J. W.: The polysaccharide of the vitreous humor, J. Biol. Chem. **107**:629, 1934.
70. Meyer, K., and Rapport, M. M.: The mucopolysaccharides of the ground substance of connective tissue, Science **113**:596, 1951.
71. Meyer, K., and Rapport, M. M.: Hyaluronidases, Advances Enzym. **13**:199, 1952.
72. Milch, R. A., and McKusick, V. A.: Genes, molecules and deformities, Clin. Orthop. **33**:11, 1964.
73. Morrione, T. G.: The formation of collagen fibers by the action of heparin on soluble collagen, J. Exp. Med. **96**:107, 1952.
74. Neuberger, A., Perrone, J. C., and Slack, H. G. B.: Relative metabolic inertia of tendon collagen in the rat, Biochem. J. **49**:199, 1951.
75. Neuman, R. E., and Logan, M. A.: The determination of collagen and elastin in tissues, J. Biol. Chem. **186**:549, 1950.
76. New York Heart Association Symposium: Connective tissue: intercellular macromolecules, Biophys. J. (supp.) **4**:1964. Selected contributions: (a) Gross, J.: Organization and disorganization of collagen, p. 63. (b) Gallop, P. M.: Concerning some special structural features of the collagen molecule, p. 79. (c) Robertson, W. van B.: Metabolism of collagen in mammalian tissues, p. 93. (d) Schubert, M.: Intercellular macromolecules containing polysaccharides, p. 119. (e) Strominger, J. L.: Nucleotide intermediates in the biosynthesis of heteropolymeric polysaccharides, p. 139. (f) Dorfman, A.: Metabolism of acid mucopolysaccharides, p. 155 (g) Porter, K. A.: Cell fine structure and biosynthesis of intercellular macromolecules, p. 167. (h) Thomas, L.: The effects of papain, vitamin A, and cortisone on cartilage matrix *in vivo,* p. 207. (i) Dziewiatkowski, D. D.: Effect of hormones on the turnover of polysaccharides in connective tissue, p. 215. (j) Holtzer, H.: Control of chondrogenesis in the embryo, p. 239.
77. Odiette, D.: La fibre élastique dans les cultures de tissues in vitro. Étude histo-physio-pathologique, J. Physiol. Path Gén. **32**:715, 1934.
78. Odiette, D.: La fibre élastique dans les cultures de tissues in vitro (deuxième mémoire), J. Physiol. Path. Gén. **33**:475, 1935.
79. Parker, R. C.: The races that constitute the group of common fibroblasts, J. Exp. Med. **58**:401, 1933.
80. Partridge, S. M.: Elastin, Advances Protein Chem. **17**:227, 1962.
81. Perl, E., and Catchpole, H. R.: Changes induced in the connective tissues of the pubic symphysis of the guinea pig with estrogen and relaxin, Arch. Path. **50**:233, 1950.
82. Peterkofsky, B., and Udenfriend, S.: Conversion of proline to collagen hydroxyproline in a cell-free system from chick embryo, J. Biol. Chem. **238**:3966, 1963.
83. Piez, K. A., Eigner, E. A., and Lewis, M. S.: Chromatographic separation and amino acid composition of subunits of several collagens, Biochemistry **2**:58, 1963.
84. Ragan, C., editor: Josiah Macy Jr. Foundation Conferences on Connective Tissues.
I. (1950) (a) Angevine, D. M.: Structure and function of normal connective tissue, p. 13. (b) Bennett, G. A.: Pathology of connective tissue; fibrinoid degeneration, p. 44. (c) Meyer, K.: Chemistry of connective tissue; polysaccharides, p. 88 (d) Perlmann, G. E.: Enzymatically modified ovalbumins, p. 101. (e) Ragan, C.: Effect of ACTH and cortisone on connective tissues, p. 137.
II. (1951) (a) Gersh, I.: Some functional considerations of ground substance of connective tissues, p. 11. (b) Lansing, A. I.: Chemical morphology of elastic fibers, p. 45. (c) Travell, J.: Pain mechanisms in connective tissues, p. 86. (d) Porter, K. R.: Repair processes in connective tissues, p. 126. (e) Morrione, T. G.: Regression of scar tissue, p. 159.
III. (1952) (a) Lillie, R. D.: Connective tissue staining, p. 11. (b) Wyckoff, R. W. G.:

The fine structure of connective tissues, p. 38. (c) Robb-Smith, A. H. T.: The nature of reticulin, p. 92. (d) Fischel, E. E.: Hypersensitivity and the hyperadrenal state, p. 117.

IV. (1953) (a) Ashley, C. A., Schick, A. F., Arasimavicius, A., and Hass, G. M.: Isolation and characterization of mammalian striated myofibrils, p. 47. (b) Fell, H. B.: The effect of vitamin A on organ cultures of skeletal and other tissues, p. 142. (c) Meyer, K.: Outline of problems to be solved in the study of connective tissues, p. 185.

V. (1954) (a) Zweifach, B. W.: The exchange of materials between blood vessels and lymph. (b) Gaudino, M.: Interstitial water and connective tissues. (c) Asboe-Hansen, G.: Hormonal effects on connective tissue.

85. Ramanathan, N., editor: Collagen, New York, 1962, Interscience Publishers, Inc.
86. Randall, J. T., editor: Nature and structure of collagen (symposium), New York, 1953, Academic Press, Inc.
    (a) Jacobson, W.: Histological survey of the normal connective tissue and its derivatives, p. 6. (b) Robb-Smith, A. H. T.: Significance of collagenase, p. 14. (c) Cruickshank, B., and Hill, A. G. S.: Histochemical identification of a connective tissue antigen, p. 27. (d) Kramer, H., and Little, K.: Nature of reticulin, p. 33. (e) Slack, H. G. B.: Metabolism of collagen in the rat, p. 51. (f) Hoppey, F., McCrae, T. P., and Naylor, A.: X-ray crystallographic investigation of the changes with age in the structure of the human intervertebral disk, p. 65. (g) Armstrong, D. M. G.: Donnan membrane equilibrium in collagen-water systems, p. 91. (h) Robinson, C.: The hot and cold forms of gelatin, p. 96. (i) Jackson, S. F., Kelly, F. C., North, A. C. T., Randall, J. T., Seeds, W. E., Watson, M., and Wilkinson, G. R.: The byssus threads of Mytilus edulis and Pinna nobilis, p. 106. (j) Brown, G. L., Kelly, F. C., and Watson, M.: Quantitative paper chromatography of amino acids in collagen, p. 117. (k) Stack, M. V.: Properties of dentine collagen, p. 124. (l) Martin, A. V. W.: Fine structure of cartilage matrix, p. 129. (m) Jackson, S. F.: Fibrogenesis in vivo and in vitro, p. 140. (n) M'Ewen, M. B., and Pratt, M. I.: Scattering of light by collagen solutions, p. 158. (o) Brown, G. L., and Kelly, F. C.: Electrophoresis of collagen solutions, p. 169. (p) Jackson, D. S.: Chondroitin sulphate as a factor in the stability of tendon, p. 177. (q) Jackson, S. F., and Randall, J. T.: The reconstitution of collagen fibrils from solution, p. 181. (r) Consden, R.: Observations on the composition of human subcutaneous tissue, p. 196. (s) Bowes, J. H., Elliott, R. G., and Moss, J. A.: Some differences in the composition of collagen and extracted collagens and their relation to fibre formation and dispersion, p. 199. (t) Harkness, R. D., Marks, A. M., Muir, H. M., and Neuberger, A.: Precursors of skin collagen, p. 208. (u) Randall, J. T., Brown, G. L., Jackson, S. F., Kelly, F. C., North, A. C. T., Seeds, W. E., and Wilkinson, G. R.: Some physical and chemical properties of extracted skin collagen, p. 213. (v) Randall, J. T.: Physical and chemical problems of fibre formation and structure, p. 232. (w) Cowan, P. M., North, A. C. T., and Randall, J. T.: High-angle x-ray diffraction of collagen fibers, p. 241. (x) Seeds, W. E.: Infra-red absorption and collagen structure, p. 250.
87. (a) Reifenstein, E. C., Jr., editor: Metabolic inter-relations, with special reference to calcium. Transactions of the Fifth Conference, Josiah Macy Jr. Foundation, New York, 1953. (b) Robinson, R. A., and Watson, M. L.: Electron micrography of bone, p. 72.
88. Rich, A., and Crick, F. H. C.: The molecular structure of collagen, J. Molec. Biol. **3**:483, 1961.
89. Richards, A. N., and Gies, W. J.: Chemical studies of elastin, mucoid and other proteids in elastic tissue, with some notes on ligament extractives, Amer. J. Physiol. **7**:93, 1902.
90. Riley, J. F.: The riddle of the mast cells, Lancet **1**:841, 1954.
91. Riley, J. F.: Pharmacology and functions of the mast cells, Pharmacol. Rev. **7**:183, 1955.
92. Robb-Smith, A. H. T.: The relationship of reticulin to other "collagens." In Stainsby, G.: editor: Recent advances in gelatin and glue research, New York, 1958, Pergamon Press, p. 38.
93. Rothman, S.: Physiology and biochemistry of the skin, Chicago, 1954, University of Chicago Press. (a) Felsher, Z.: Collagen, reticulin and elastin, chap. 17, p. 391. (b) Wells, G. C.: Connective tissue ground substance, chap. 18, p. 418.
94. Schmitt, F. O.: Cell constitution. In Willier, B. H., Weiss, P. A., and Hamburger, V., editors: Analysis of development, Philadelphia, 1955, W. B. Saunders Co., p. 46.
95. Schmitt, F. O., Gross, J., and Highberger, J. H.: A new particle type in certain connective tissue extracts, Proc. Nat Acad. Sci. **39**:459, 1953.

96. Schmitt, F. O., Gross, J., and Highberger, J. H.: Tropocollagen and the properties of fibrosis collagen, Exp. Cell. Res. (supp.) **3**:326, 1955.
97. Schmitt, F. O., Hall, C. E., and Jakus, M. A.: Electron microscope investigations of the structure of collagen, J. Cell Comp. Physiol. **20**:11, 1942.
97a. Schmitt, F. O., Levine, L., Drake, M. P., Rubin, A. L., Pfahl, D., and Davison, P. F.: The antigenicity of tropocollagen, Proc. Nat. Acad. Sci. **51**:493, 1964.
98. Schmitt, F. O., and Sizer, I. W.: Personal communication.
99. Slack, H. G. B.: Metabolism of elastin in the adult rat, Nature **174**:512, 1955.
100. Slack, H. G. B.: Some notes on the composition and metabolism of connective tissue, Amer. J. Med. **26**:113, 1959.
101. Smith, J. G.: The dermal elastoses, Arch. Dermat. **88**:382, 1963.
102. Smith, R. H., and Jackson, S. F.: Studies on the biosynthesis of collagen. II. The conversion of ^{14}C-L-proline to ^{14}C-hydroxy-proline by fowl-osteoblasts in tissue culture, J. Biophys. Biochem. Cytol. **3**:913, 1957.
103. Stacy, M., and Barker, S. A.: Carbohydrates of living tissues, New York, 1962, D. Van Nostrand Co., Inc.
104. Starcher, B., Hill, C. H., and Matrone, G.: Importance of dietary copper in the formation of aortic elastin, J. Nutr. **82**:318, 1964.
105. Thomas, J., Elsden, D. F., and Partridge, S. M.: Degradation products from elastin, Nature **200**:651, 1963.
106. Tunbridge, R. E., and others, editors: Connective tissue, a symposium, Springfield, Ill., 1957, Charles C Thomas, Publisher.
(a) Astbury, W. T.: Introduction, p. 1. (b) Asboe-Hansen, G.: On the structure and function of the mast cells, p. 12. (c) Sylvén, B.: On the topographical cystochemistry of tissue mast cells, p. 27. (d) Neuberger, A.: Observations on the presence and metabolism of plasma proteins in skin and tendon, p. 35. (e) Gross, J.: Studies on the fibrogenesis of collagen. Some properties of neutral extracts of connective tissue, p. 45. (f) Jackson, D. S.: The formation and breakdown of connective tissue, p. 62. (g) Jackson, S. F.: Structural problems associated with the formation of collagen fibrils in vivo, p. 77. (h) Meyer, K., Hoffman, P., and Linker, A.: The acid mucopolysaccharides of connective tissue, p. 86. (i) Snellman, O.: Evaluation of extraction methods for acid tissue polysaccharides, p. 97. (j) Delaunay, A., and Bazin, S.: Combinaisons in vitro collagène-mucopolysaccharides et modifications apportés à ces combinaisons par des sels et des polyosides bactériens, p. 105. (k) Gillman, T., Hathorn, M., and Penn, J.: Micro-anatomy and reactions to injury of vascular elastic membranes and associated polysaccharides, p. 120. (l) Snellman, O., Ottoson, R., and Sylvén, B.: On the nature of the metachromatic ground substance polysaccharides of healing wounds, p. 136. (m) Schwarz, W.: Morphology and differentiation of the connective tissue fibers, p. 144. (n) Grassmann, W., Hofmann, U., Kühn, K., Hörmann, H., Endres, H., and Wolf, K.: Electron microscope and chemical studies of the carbohydrate groups of collagen, p. 157. (o) van den Hooff, A.: A few remarks on connective tissues rich in mucoid, p. 172. (p) Robb-Smith, A. H. T.: What is reticulin? p. 177. (q) Gustavson, K. H.: Some new aspects of the stability and reactivity of collagens, p. 185. (r) Verzár, F.: The ageing of collagen, p. 208. (s) Partridge, S. M., Davis, H. F., and Adair, G. S.: The composition of mammalian elastin, p. 222. (t) Hall, D. A.: Chemical and enzymatic studies on elastin, p. 238. (u) Banga, I., and Baló, J.: The structure and chemical composition of connective tissue, p. 254. (v) Bowes, J. H., Elliott, R. G., and Moss, J. A.: The composition of some protein fractions isolated from bovine skin, p. 264. (w) Orekhovitch, V. N., and Shpikiter, V. O.: Procollagens as biological precursors of collagen and the physio-chemical nature of these proteins, p. 281. (x) Muir, H. M.: The structure of a chondroitin sulphate complex from cartilage, p. 294. (y) Reed, R.: The architecture of the collagen fibril, p. 299. (z) Grassmann, W., Hannig, K., Endres, H., and Riedel, A.: amino-acid sequences of collagen, p. 308. (aa) Bear, R. S., and Morgan, R. S.: The composition of bands and interbands of collagen fibrils, p. 321.
107. Vaubel, E.: The form and function of synovial cells in tissue cultures, J. Exp. Med. **58**:85, 1933.
108. Waksman, B. H., and Mason, H. L.: The antigenicity of collagen, J. Immun. **63**:427, 1949.
109. Weiss, J.: The nature of the reaction between orcein and elastin, J. Histochem. **2**:21, 1954.
110. Weissman, N., Coulson, W. F., and Carnes, W. H.: The effect of copper deficiency on the amino acid content of swine aortic elastica, Abstracts, Sixth International Congress of Biochemistry, New York, 1964.

3

The Marfan syndrome

*In an era when slenderness and ectomorphy are being equated with long life, it may be wise to point out an exception**

Historical survey

In 1896[246] the gross skeletal manifestations of the syndrome that bears his name were described by Marfan,† who called the condition *dolichostenomelia* (long, thin extremities) (Fig. 3-2). The condition was renamed arachnodactyly by Achard in 1902.[3] (Marfan had used the simile "pattes d'araignée," spider legs.) Salle[317] in 1912 reported necropsy observations in the case of a 2½-month-old infant who died with cardiac symptoms and showed generalized dilatation of the heart and patent foramen ovale. Boerger[46] first clearly related ectopia lentis to the other manifestations. As is usually the case, vague references to cases of what was certainly this syndrome can be found in medical reports antedating the definitive descriptions. For instance, Williams,[414] an ophthalmologist in Cincinnati, in 1876 described ectopia lentis in a brother and sister who were exceptionally tall and had been loose-jointed from birth.

Weve of Utrecht,[407] publishing in 1931, first clearly demonstrated the heritable nature of the syndrome and its transmission as a dominant trait. Furthermore he conceived of this syndrome as a disorder of mesenchymal tissues and accordingly designated it *dystrophia mesodermalis congenita, typus Marfanis.*

The major cardiovascular complications, namely aortic dilatation and dissecting aneurysm, were first clearly described in 1943 by Baer and associates[17] and

---

*From Editorial: New Eng. J. Med. **256**:39, 1957.

†Antoine Bernard-Jean Marfan (1858-1942), Parisian professor of pediatrics, did much to establish pediatrics as a specialty in France and elsewhere. He was the author of several widely read textbooks and monographs on pediatric topics and editor of *Le Nourrisson* for a great many years. In addition to the syndrome under discussion here, his name is often attached to Marfan's law (that immunity to pulmonary phthisis is conferred by the healing of a local tuberculous lesion) and Marfan's subxiphoid method for aspirating fluid from the pericardial sac.[247] (For other biographic details, see references 9, 10, 11, 178; for portrait, see Fig. 3-1).

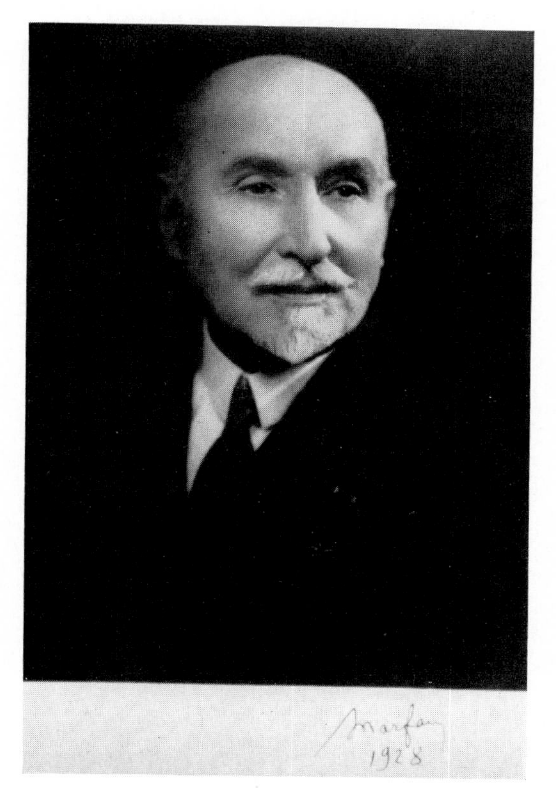

Fig. 3-1. Marfan. (Courtesy Académie de Médecine, Paris.)

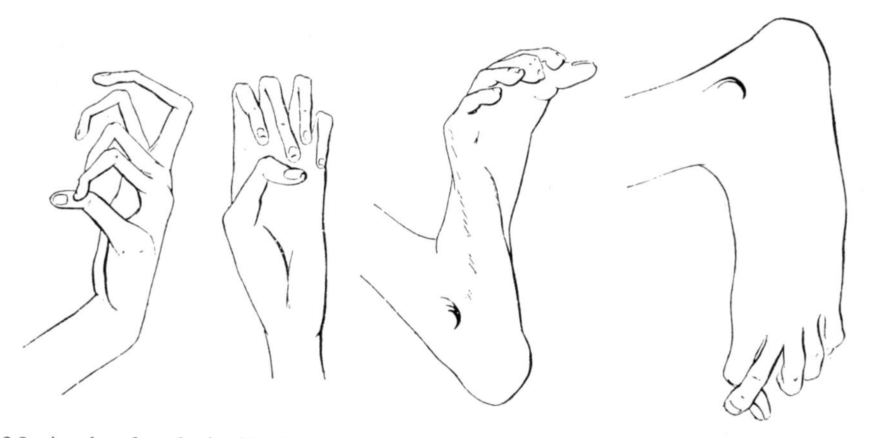

Fig. 3-2. Arachnodactyly in Marfan's case. (From Marfan, A. B.: Bull. Mém. Soc. Med. Hôp. Paris **13:**220, 1896.)

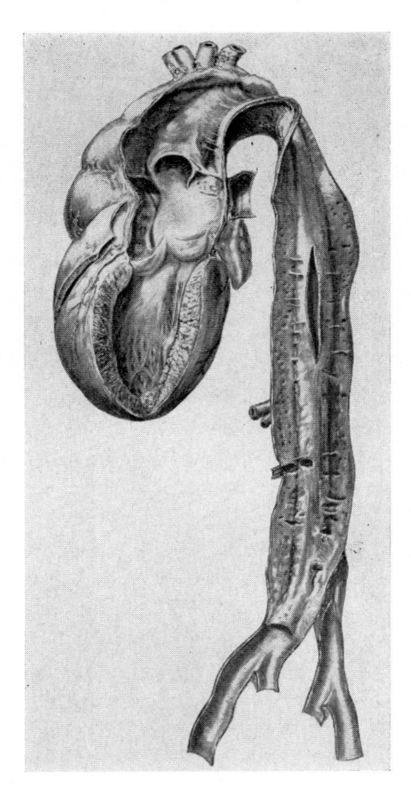

Fig. 3-3. An early reported case[227] of dissecting aneurysm in a patient who in retrospect appears to have had the Marfan syndrome. In 1909 MacCallum reported from the Johns Hopkins Hospital the case (Med. 15454; autopsy 2087) of "L. R., Negro, aged 30 . . . slender built." The man had been seen one year before death, at which time signs of aortic regurgitation were present. The patient was described in life as having a congenital umbilical hernia. A difference in the radial pulses was noted by Dr. Thomas McCrae. Dissecting aneurysm was not suspected, however, by Osler, Rufus Cole, and the other physicians who examined him. There was paralysis of the left recurrent laryngeal nerve. The mother and several brothers had died, as well as the patient's only child, who died at the age of 2 years. No definitely corroboratory features of the family history were recorded, however, and no note of ocular abnormality was made. The ascending aorta, as shown here, resembles that seen in Fig. 3-22*E*. Furthermore the pronounced dilatation in the region of the sinuses of Valsalva suggests the Marfan syndrome. (From MacCallum, W. G.: Bull. Hopkins Hosp. **20**:9, 1909.)

by Etter and Glover,[106] respectively. Again, although earlier reports of the aortic complications can be discovered (e.g. reference 62 and Fig. 3-3), these later authors first drew attention to them and opened the way for clearer recognition of the internal medical implications of this syndrome in adults.

It is difficult to imagine a better description of the Marfan syndrome than that given by Bronson and Sutherland[62] in 1918 in the case of a 6-year-old child with aneurysm of the ascending aorta which ruptured into the pericardium. "The unusual shape of his head and ears and the looseness of his joints attracted attention early in infancy." Inguinal hernia was repaired surgically at the age of 2 years, and a left diaphragmatic hernia was discovered by x-ray examination. He was always undernourished but was sensitive and mentally advanced for his age, with a quaint way of expressing himself and "a sense of humor of his own." The forehead was high and full, the palate highly arched. The ears were large without the normal folds of the pinnae. The joints were lax, the limbs flaillike, and the elbows showed definite subluxation. There were lordosis and pigeon breast with an increased prominence of the right side of the chest, which showed better expansion. A pulsating mass was discernible to the right of the sternum. Although no diastolic murmur was mentioned, the left ventricle was hypertrophied at autopsy. There was also partial coarctation proximal to the left subclavian artery. The authors presented a detailed review of reports made previous to that time; many of these cases also are reasonably clear instances of the Marfan syndrome.

"Marfan's syndrome," or better "the Marfan syndrome," is, in my opinion, the preferred designation until such time as the basic defect is known and an accurate name based thereon can be devised. (F. Parkes Weber[402] was of the same view.) Arachnodactyly is, on the one hand, not striking in some patients; on the other hand, it occurs with other developmental disorders, both acquired and genetic.

Probably at least 400 cases of the Marfan syndrome have been reported in the literature. By intensive searches of multiple sources, I was able in a six-year period to collect 74 kinships in which at least one bona fide affected person has occurred. Thirty-three of these definitely affected families are represented in Figs. 3-3 to 3-48. The total number of definitely affected persons in these pedigrees approaches 200. In this study, the Wilmer Ophthalmological Institute of the Johns Hopkins Hospital was the largest single source of propositi. However, other sources included pediatricians, orthopedists, endocrinologists, and cardiologists. The Medical Examiner's Office was another fruitful source; tracing the relatives of young individuals dying of dissecting aneurysm of the aorta revealed several affected kinships. Under continuing study are the following: survivorship, relative incidence of the several manifestations of the syndrome, intrafamilial and interfamilial variability, and other aspects, including incidence of sporadic versus familial cases, racial incidence, sex differences, etc.

Clinical manifestations

Fig. 3-56 (p. 129) presents a "pedigree of causes" in which the several manifestations of the Marfan syndrome are related to the hypothesized but, as yet, undefined fundamental defect of connective tissue.

The skeletal aspects. See Figs. 3-4*B* to 3-9 for the various body types encountered. Dolichomorphism characterizes the skeletal abnormality of the syndrome. The victim often suggests the subject of an El Greco painting.* The extremities are long, and characteristically the lower segment (pubis-to-sole) measurement is in excess of the upper segment (pubis-to-vertex) measurement and the arm span in excess of height. In general, the more distal bones of the extremities tend to demonstrate this excess length most strikingly. Arachnodactyly is the result (Fig. 3-14).

*Astigmatism is thought to have been the basis for El Greco's distorted representations, as in "St. Martin and the beggar" (National Gallery, Washington, D. C.). Actually the legs are not disproportionately long in El Greco figures. Furthermore, as Medawar[255] points out, if El Greco was astigmatic his paintings would look nonetheless normal to us, since they would have had to look normal to him.

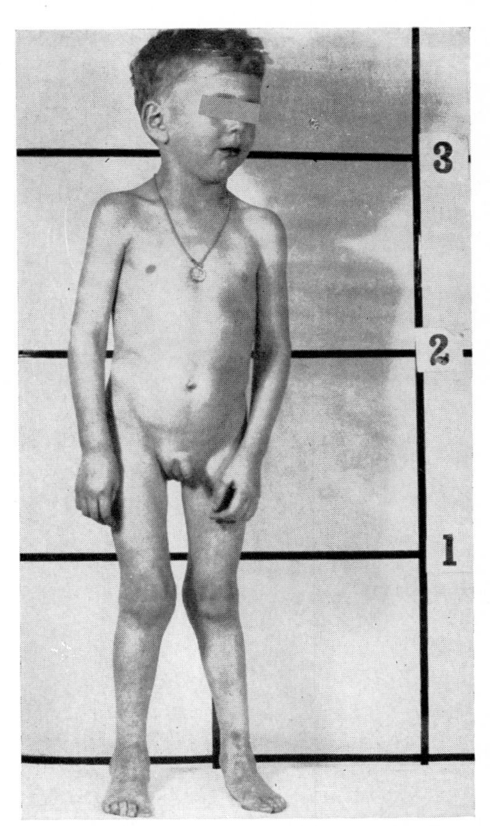

Fig. 3-4A. Photograph of M. D., affected male shown in **B** and **C,** taken in February, 1948 (3½ years of age). Dolichostenomelia is often less impressive at this age.

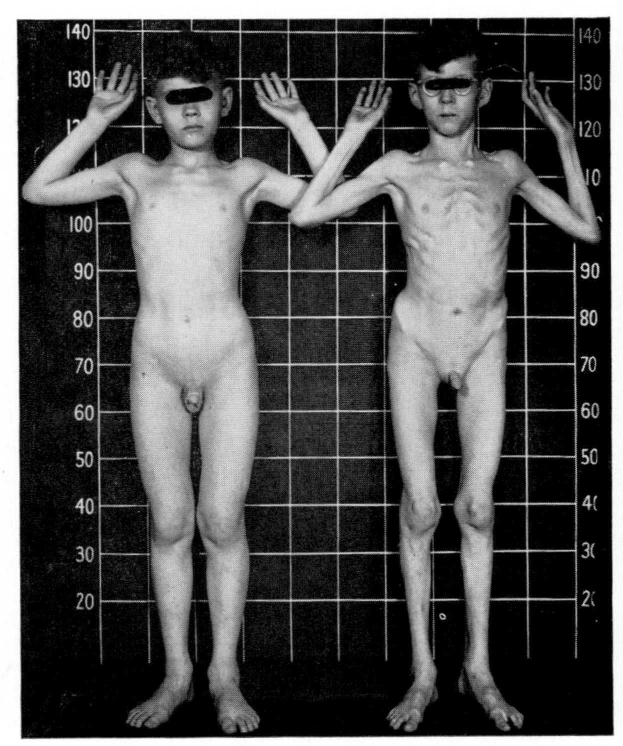

Fig. 3-4B. Brothers, one with Marfan's syndrome. The one on the left is normal, 10 years of age. M. D. (A59949), on the right, is only 8 years old. He shows ectopia lentis, contracture of the fifth fingers (Fig. 3-15*A*), heterochromia iridis (right iris, blue; left, light green), Horner's syndrome on left, lack of subcutaneous fat, high palate, scoliosis, thoracic deformity, and abnormal electroencephalogram. This is probably a sporadic case (original mutation). Contracture of the fifth fingers (clinodactyly or camptodactyly) occurred in other patients of this series (e.g. J. A. M., A65283). Photograph, May, 1953. Heterochromia iridis occasionally is found as an isolated hereditary abnormality, transmitted probably as a dominant.[68] It is sometimes due to birth injury to the cervical sympathetics.

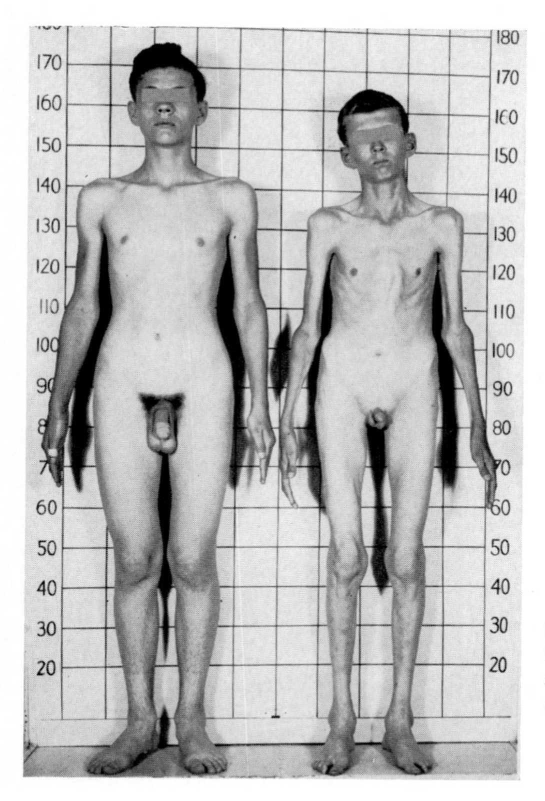

Fig. 3-4C. Same brothers as shown in **B.** Photograph, June, 1958. The older, unaffected brother has now outstripped the affected brother in height.

Skeletal proportions are more important than actual height. It is true that these patients are often very tall. One patient was 6 feet tall at the age of 12 years.[73] Another patient[410] was 7 feet tall. The tallest patient encountered in our investigation was 6 feet 7 inches. As indices of arachnodactyly it has been proposed[410] that the hand-height ratio should be greater than 11% and the foot-height ratio greater than 15%. Furthermore, it is stated that the finger, especially the middle finger, should be one and one half times greater than the length of the metacarpal. Excessive length of the inferior patellar ligament has been proposed as a useful diagnostic index. There is so much overlap with the normal that all measurements cannot be relied on as the sole diagnostic criterion in individual cases. More significance can be attached to them if they are particularly abnormal or if they represent marked deviations from the measurements in certain other members of the family.

Possibly the index of most usefulness, or at least one which is as reliable as any, is the ratio of upper segment (US) to lower segment (LS). The lower segment is measured from the top of the pubic symphysis to the floor. The upper segment is derived by subtracting this value from the height. As is indicated by the familiar illustration provided by Stratz in 1902 (Fig. 3-10), the legs grow relatively faster than the trunk during postnatal life. Resultingly, the midportion of the body moves progressively downward. The US-LS ratio is roughly 0.93 in the white adult, having higher in the prepubertal period. The individual born

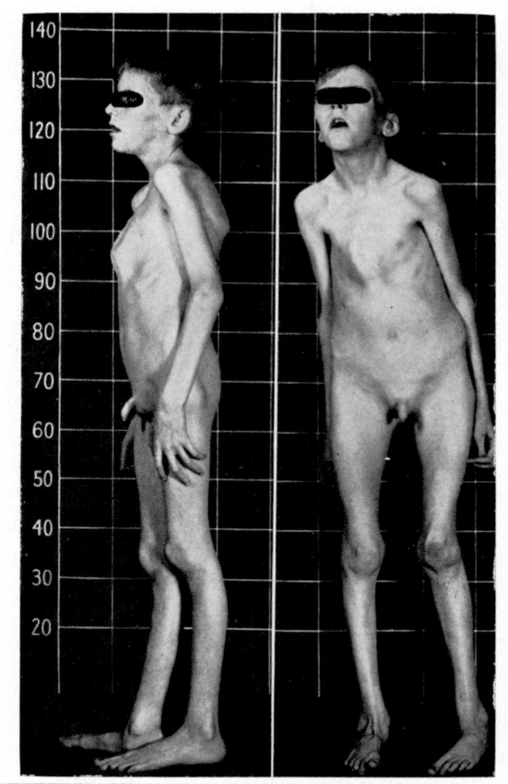

Fig. 3-5A. C. A. B. (B9912; 692938), 7 years old. Pronounced pectus carinatum. Normal mentality. Nystagmus. Bilateral ectopia lentis. "Rocker-bottom" feet. Sparse subcutaneous fat. Photograph, August, 1954.

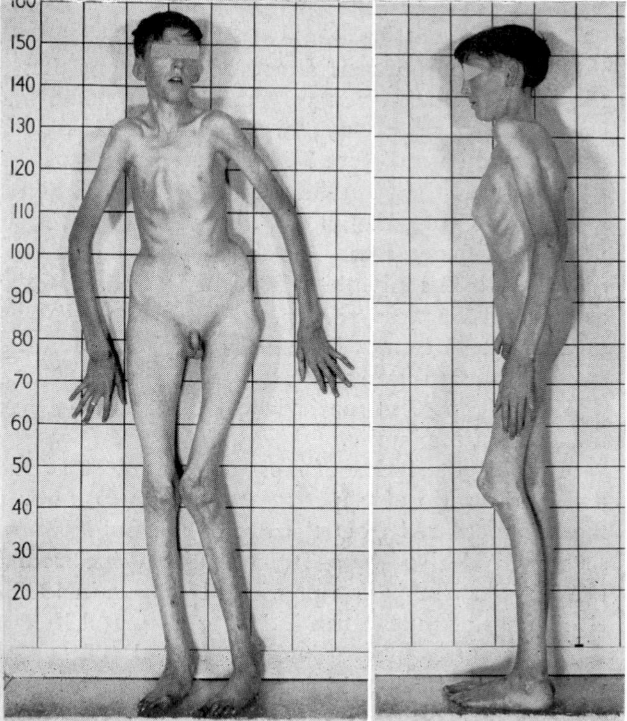

Fig. 3-5B. Same patient as shown in **A.** Photograph, August, 1958.

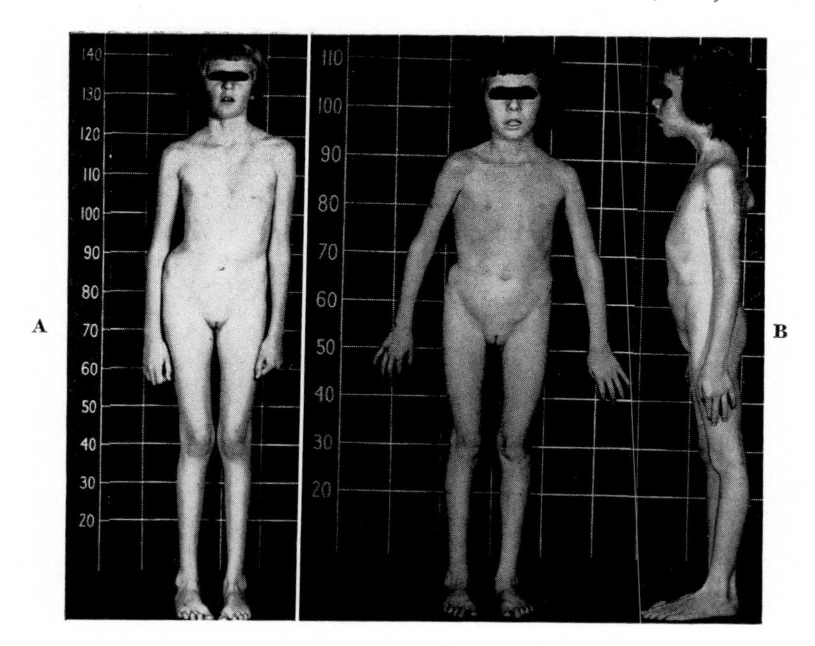

Fig. 3-6. A, M. McG. (A92675), 7 years of age. Bilateral ectopia lentis. Severe pectus excavatum. Highly intelligent. Frequent respiratory infections. Loud systolic murmur, of unclear origin. The mother has the full-blown syndrome and is sightless in one eye from spontaneous retinal detachment. This child died at the age of 10 years. The clinical picture was that of mitral regurgitation with progressive cardiac enlargement. Atrial fibrillation had its onset eight months before death. The mitral valve showed three cusps and abnormally short chordae tendineae. The left atrium was huge, with thickened endocardium. Both ventricles were grossly dilated. **B,** D. W. (B8430), 4 years 2 months of age, is thought to have minimal dilatation of the ascending aorta and mitral regurgitation. Also has kyphoscoliosis and ectopia lentis. Parents appear unaffected but paternal great grandfather was 6 feet 7 inches tall.

with the "Marfan gene" tends already to have an abnormally low segment ratio. Furthermore, he passes more rapidly through the sequence shown in Stratz' drawing, overshoots the mark, and ends with a segment ratio in the vicinity of 0.85.

Because there are no recent data on white persons and no published data whatever on Negroes, measurements of segments were made on 2,100 Baltimore school children of both races and sexes. The data are presented in Fig. 3-11. They should prove useful in the evaluation and follow-up of cases of the Marfan syndrome, as well as in the study of the hemoglobinopathies, endocrinopathies, and other disorders that influence body proportions. It is planned to increase the data at both ends of the age span shown in Fig. 3-11 and to extend them to about 30 years of age.

The photograph in the nude on the measured grid cannot be relied on for more than a rough estimate of body proportions. Errors in estimating the site of the pubic symphysis and parallax make for poor reproducibility and poor checks with direct measurements.

The dip in the US-LS ratio at the stage of puberty, with subsequent slight rise, is noteworthy.[362] If puberty is delayed, the dip may be even more striking. The possibility of the Marfan syndrome was raised in the patient (E. K., 766137) shown

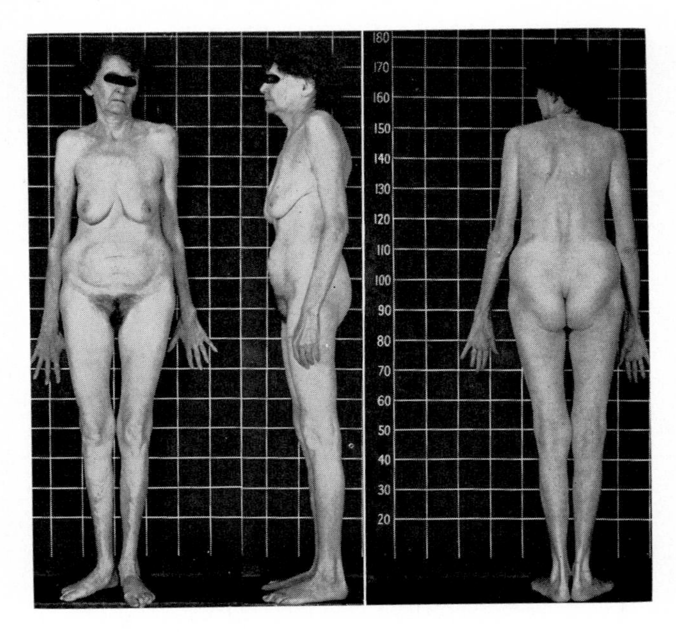

Fig. 3-7. M. P. (362804), 53 years old, one of the oldest patients with the Marfan syndrome I have had the opportunity to examine. I have in the past seen a 59-year-old man with the Marfan syndrome manifested by ectopia lentis, dolichostenomelia, and aortic aneurysm. One man with probable Marfan's syndrome was killed accidentally at the age of 82 years. He was still well preserved at that time. He was 75 inches tall and had fathered at least two offspring with full-blown Marfan's syndrome (see Fig. 3-46 for the x-ray film of one) and four probably affected individuals out of a sibship numbering twelve in all. Extensive pedigree of Marfan's syndrome. Systolic crunch (extracardiac sound) present for many years. The patient is now (1966) 65 years old.

in Fig. 3-50*B*. The presence of gynecomastia strengthens the impression of anomalous pubertal transition.

Sinclair and co-workers[335] suggested the metacarpal index as an objective indication of arachnodactyly. In the x-ray film of the right hand, the length (in millimeters) of the second, third, fourth, and fifth metacarpals is measured. At the exact midpoint of each shaft, the breadth is also measured and this value divided into the length. The figures for the four metacarpals are averaged. The metacarpal index is, then, the average ratio of length to breadth of metacarpals II to V. The data from twenty cases of the Marfan syndrome and a hundred normal subjects are plotted in Fig. 3-12. Since skeletal features alone were accepted in the diagnosis of Marfan's syndrome, some circular reasoning may have entered this study. The frequency distribution is distinctly peculiar; it suggests a continuous distribution with one class missing. Parish and associates[281] and Eldridge[99] reported metacarpal index data. It is doubtful that the metacarpal index is more specific than the US-LS ratio. It may be useful, however, to have another objective measure of skeletal peculiarity.

Sickle cell anemia is a recognized cause of growth disturbance that can result in body proportions resembling those of the Marfan syndrome. The patient (D. M., 659463) shown in Fig. 3-50*A* is an example. The osseous hyperemia that ac-

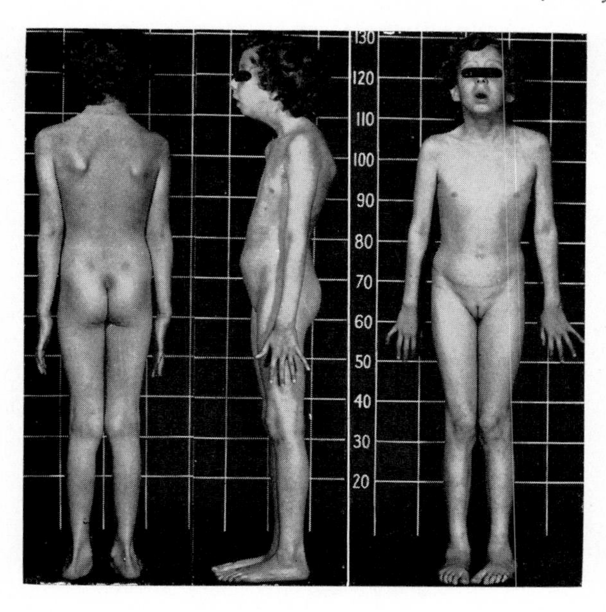

Fig. 3-8. D. L. F. (516670), 7 years of age. The ptosis was thought to be part of the general muscular hypotonia, which was so severe that amyotonia congenita was suspected when the patient was seen at the age of 4 years. Umbilical and bilateral inguinal hernias have been repaired surgically. The feet are very long, flat, and narrow. Kyphoscoliosis is evident. No ectopia lentis or ocular abnormality other than ptosis demonstrated. Intelligent. The ptosis has been corrected surgically since these photographs were taken. The patient may represent a new mutation. Possibly the bilateral ptosis is an independent mutation.

companies hyperactivity of the bone marrow in the long bones may be the mechanism.

In cases of the Marfan syndrome the occurrence of kyphoscoliosis with shortening of the trunk also reduces the segment ratio; two factors, trunk shortening and extremity lengthening, are collaborating in producing the low segment ratio. However, before the age of 10 or 12 years kyphoscoliosis is in most cases not of sufficient severity to be of major significance.

At times the great toes are elongated out of proportion to the others (Fig. 3-14*C*).[5,113,268,381] This may be related to the fact that the terminal center of ossification normally appears somewhat earlier in the metatarsus of the great toe than of the others. (The long bones of the hands and feet usually grow from one terminus only or predominantly. The first metatarsal has a proximal epiphyseal junction, whereas the epiphysis is distal in the other metatarsals—another point of difference in development of the first and other toes.) The ribs participate in the excessive longitudinal growth with formation of pectus excavatum (Fig. 3-6*A*), "pigeon breast" (Fig. 3-5), or less symmetric varieties (Fig. 3-16*A*) of thoracic cage deformity. The bones of the skull and face are likewise affected, with resulting dolichocephaly, highly arched palate, long, narrow face, and prognathism. There may be "spurring" of the heels as a result of excessive length of the os calcis.

Redundancy and "weakness" of joint capsules, ligaments, tendons, and fascia are responsible for a large group of manifestations, including pes planus, genu

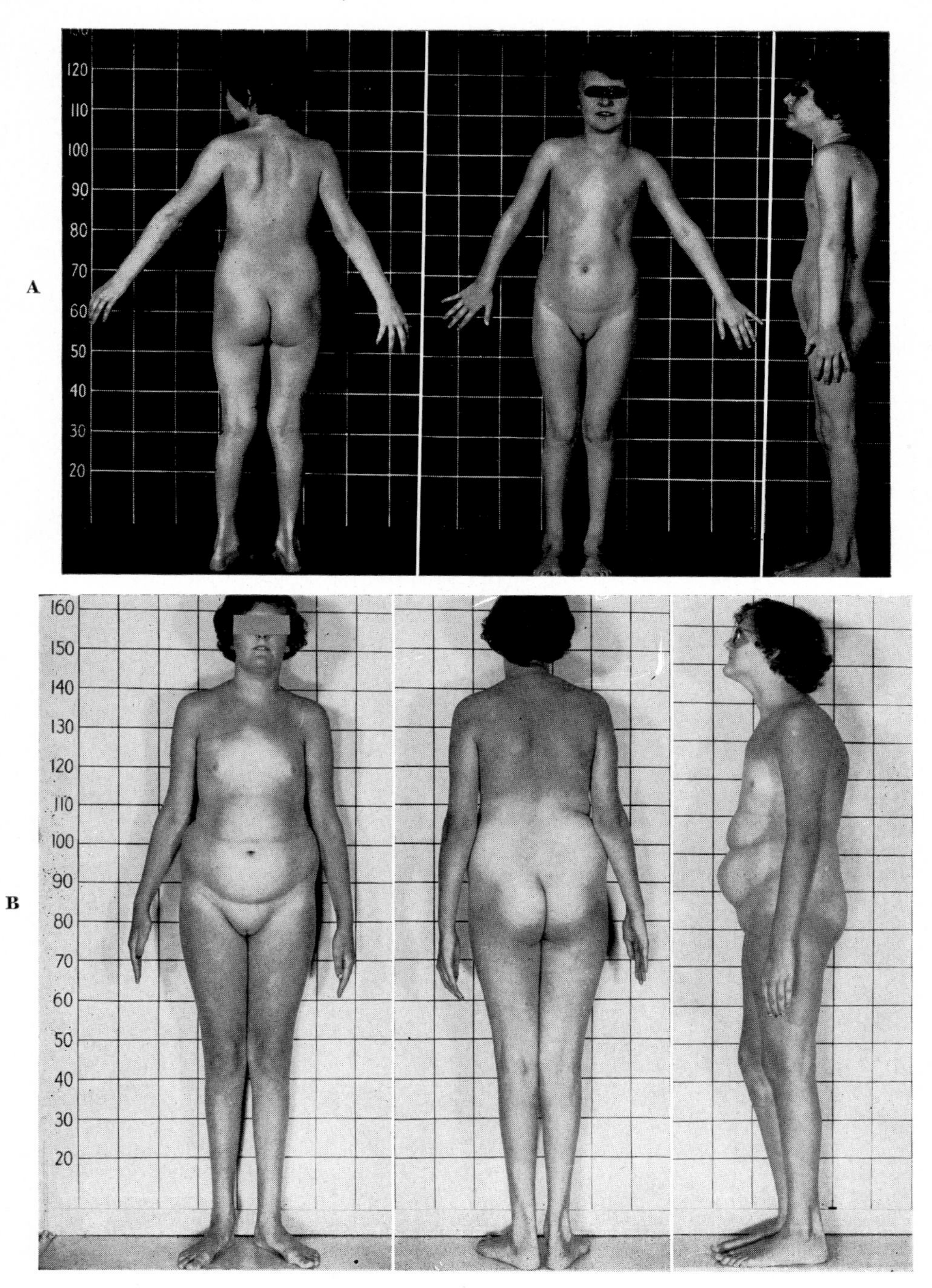

Fig. 3-9. A, J. A. L. (661948), 5 years 8 months of age. Ectopia lentis. Probably *de novo* mutation. Shown very well is the eversion of the feet with low position of the internal malleolus ("rocker bottoms"). Child bright, but highly nervous. Photograph, January, 1954. **B,** Same patient at age 10 years. Photograph, August, 1958. Sparsity of subcutaneous fat is not demonstrated in all cases of the Marfan syndrome.

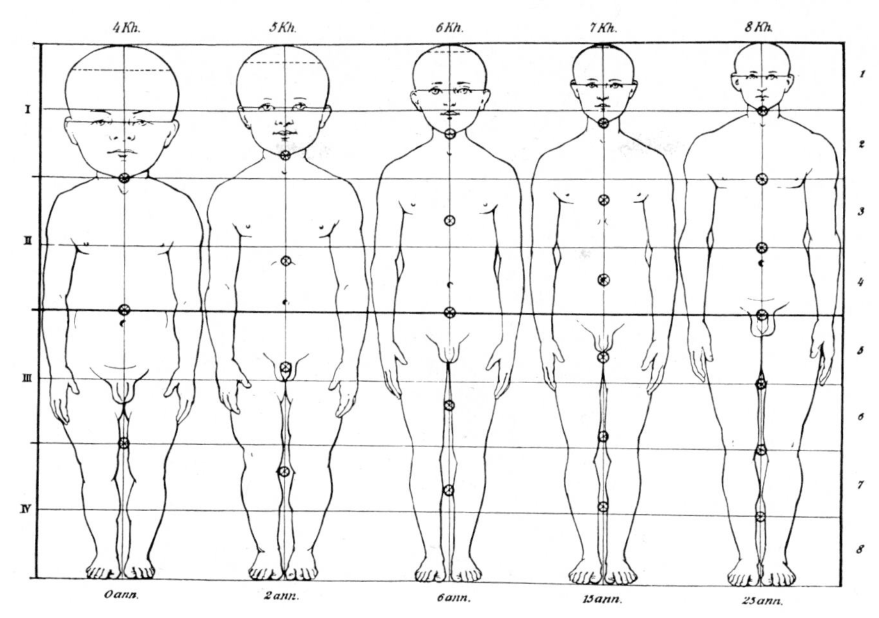

Fig. 3-10. Ordinarily the adult skeletal proportions are not attained until after puberty. There is evidence that the body proportions (as indicated by upper segment–lower segment ratio) are different now than at the turn of the century, when this diagram was made, and that the pattern differs in whites and Negroes. This diagram will require redrawing on the basis of the data presented in Fig. 3-11. (From Stratz, C. H.: Der Körper des Kindes, Stuttgart, 1902, Ferdinand Enke.)

recurvatum, hyperextensibility of joints, habitual dislocation of hips,[143] patella,[276] clavicles, mandible, and other joints, ganglia,* hernias, synovial diverticula,* and kyphoscoliosis. The "flat feet" are often so advanced that the internal malleolus almost literally rests on the floor (Fig. 3-15*B*). Much less commonly a pes cavus deformity is present.[416] Kyphoscoliosis can be very severe (Fig. 3-16*B*). In rare instances, hemivertebra is responsible in part for spinal deformity.[222] At times, the spinal deformity has been thought to be due to Scheuermann's epiphysitis.[242] Scoliosis is likely to increase rapidly during the years of maximal vertebral growth, from 11 to 15 years of age. Early recognition of scoliosis is assisted by examining the patient in a bending forward position. This maneuver renders asymmetry more obvious because of angulation of the ribs on one side.[308] While the deformity is still slight much can be accomplished by means of exercises and other measures. Nelson[268] emphasizes the presence of a large spinal canal, the enlargement being in depth or width or both.

Sinclair[334] found complaints of musculoskeletal nature of sufficient severity "to warrant medical attendance" in twenty of forty cases of the Marfan syndrome. Of the twenty patients, seven had low back pain. Two of these were at first considered to have ankylosing spondylitis. In five cases there were joint effusions; of these, three had been diagnosed as tubercular, one as rheumatic fever, and one

*In one case,[28] a peculiar pelvic cyst communicating with the lining of the sacral canal occasioned difficulties in delivery.

A

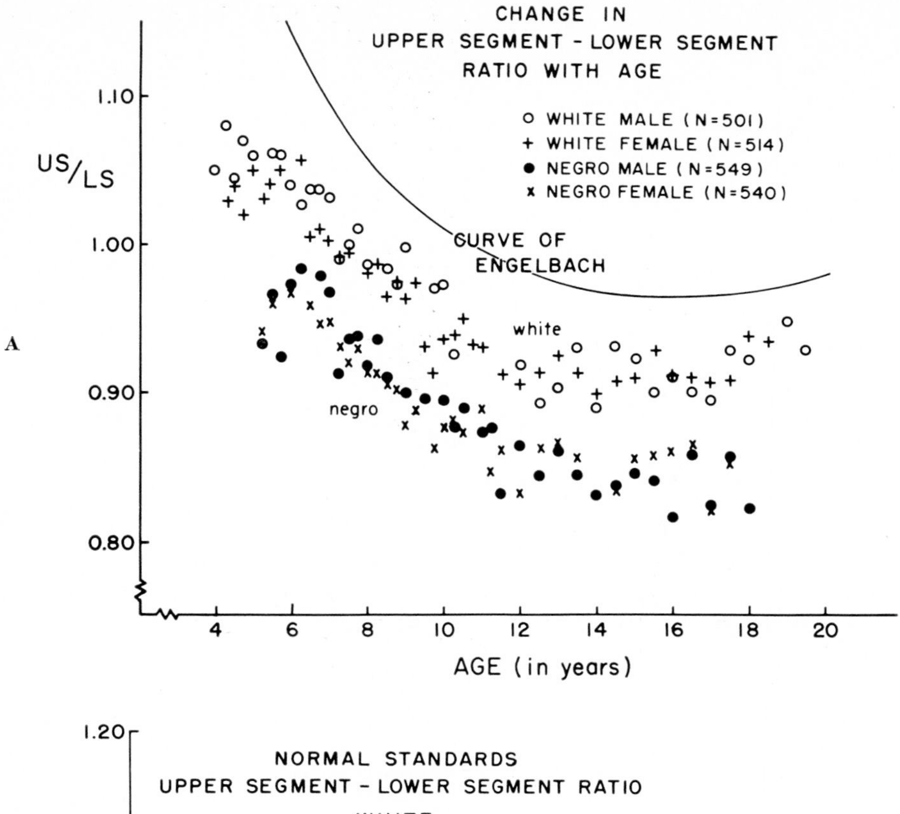

B

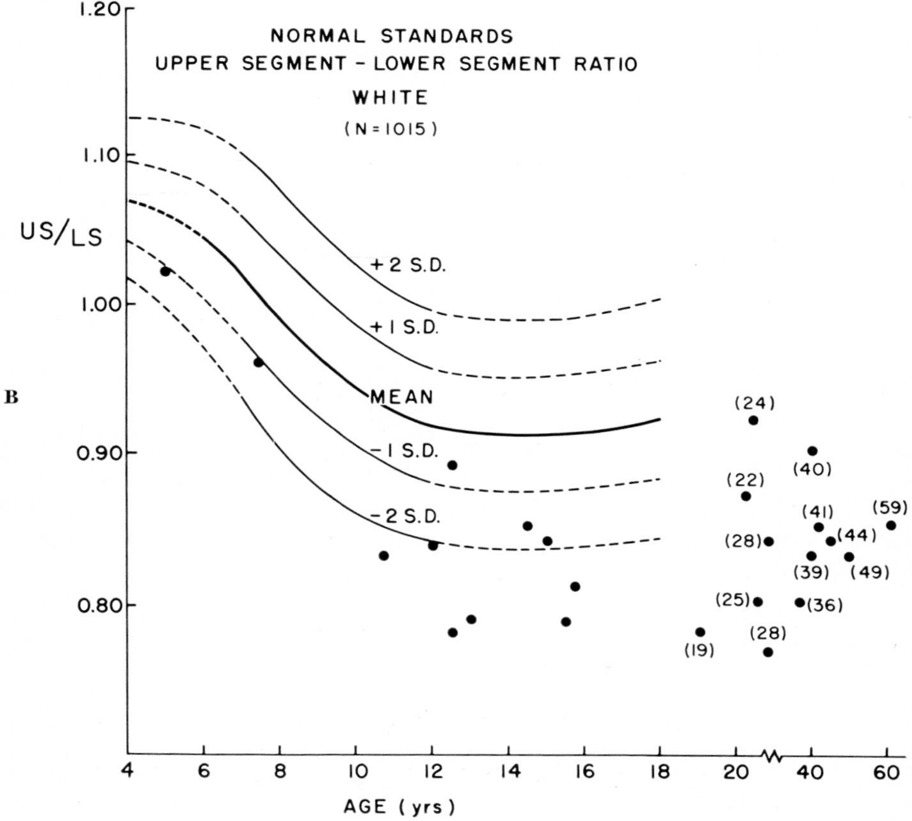

Fig. 3-11. For legend see opposite page.

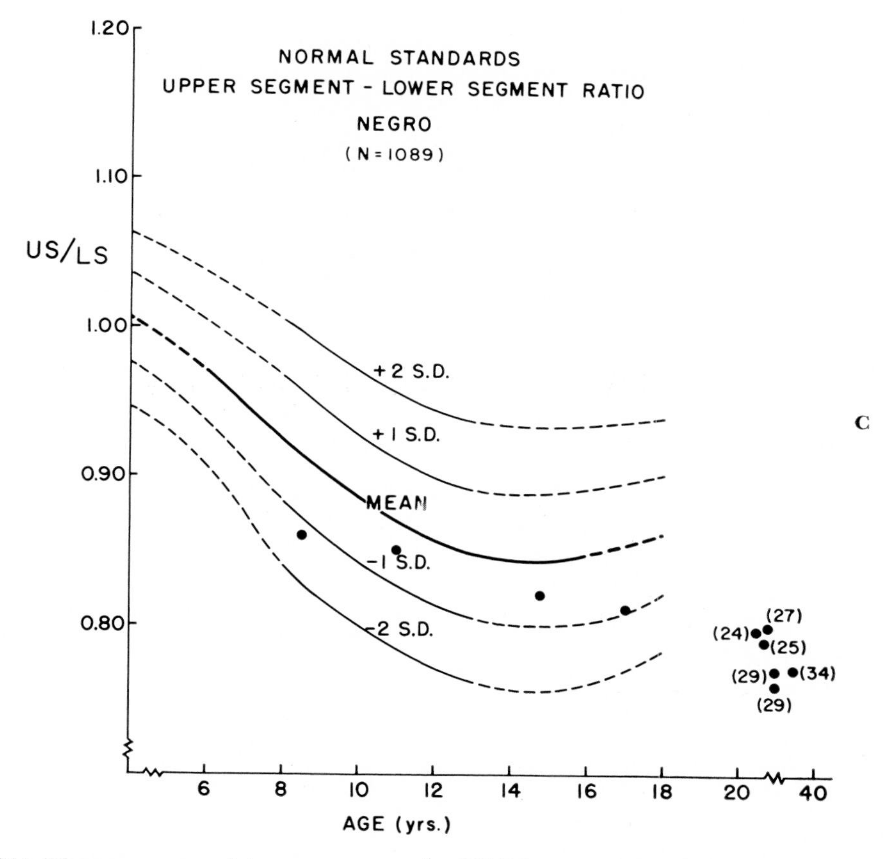

Fig. 3-11. The upper segment–lower segment ratio (US/LS) as a gauge of the skeletal changes in the Marfan syndrome. Because of the lack of recent data on US/LS in either whites or Negroes, measurements were made in 1959 on over 2,100 Baltimore school children. In brief, the findings were as follows: (1) Engelbach's data,[102] compiled from measurements made by various observers in whites only, between about 1860 and 1928, are not presently applicable for either race, **A.** (2) At all ages there is a significantly lower US/LS in Negroes than in whites, **A.** (3) Negroes have a slightly shorter upper segment and slightly longer lower segment than do whites. As a result the US/LS is strikingly different. (4) Within both racial groups no significant sex difference in the mean US/LS or the standard deviations of the means could be demonstrated, at least in the measurements up to the age of about 15 years. This is the rationale for considering the sexes together in **B** and **C.** It will almost certainly be necessary to consider the sexes separately in presenting data now being collected on persons 15 to 30 years of age. As shown in **B** and **C,** the US/LS of most patients with the Marfan syndrome fell in the abnormally low range. Measurements on thirty-four patients are shown. The number in the parentheses is the age in years. (From data of McKusick, V. A.: Ferguson-Smith, M. A., Leeming, J. T., and Merryman, C. F.)

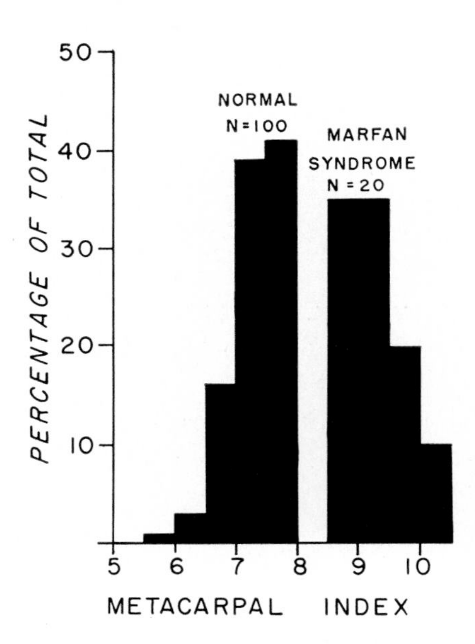

Fig. 3-12. Metacarpal index. (Data from Sinclair, R. J. G., Kitchin, A. H., and Turner, R. W. D.: Quart. J. Med. **29**:19, 1960.)

as rheumatoid arthritis. Hip joint pain was severe in two. Metatarsalgia was prominent in three patients.

Even femoral hernias occur rather commonly in men with Marfan's syndrome, and diaphragmatic hernia has been present in some of our patients and in some of those reported.[196] Hydrocele is occasionally present.

Muscular underdevelopment and hypotonia is a frequent[112,374] but by no means invariable feature. This feature has been so striking as to suggest a primary disorder of muscle in some instances. The converse error of diagnosis—primary muscular dystrophy called Marfan's syndrome—has occurred in isolated instances (Fig. 3-55*A* and *B*). It is probable that the muscular manifestations are secondary to the abnormality of bones and joints and to abnormality of the perimyal connective tissue and are not due to primary involvement of the muscle cell itself. This view is supported by the finding of a normal creatinine coefficient, an index of total muscle mass.[384]

Pronounced sparsity of subcutaneous fat is a striking feature of most cases (Figs. 3-4*B* and 3-5*A*) and is not easily reconciled with a fundamental defect of connective tissue. In children, it may be that the rapid growth accounts for the failure to store fat. One patient, who was thin as a child, has become exceedingly obese in recent years (she is now 35 years old), due in large part to inactivity associated with the blindness produced by bilateral retinal detachment (Fig. 3-17*A* and *B*). As demonstrated in Fig. 3-9*B*, others of these patients may have abundant subcutaneous fat.

Van Buchem[389] concluded that bone age is in advance of chronologic age and that the epiphyses tend to close earlier than normal. In our group of patients

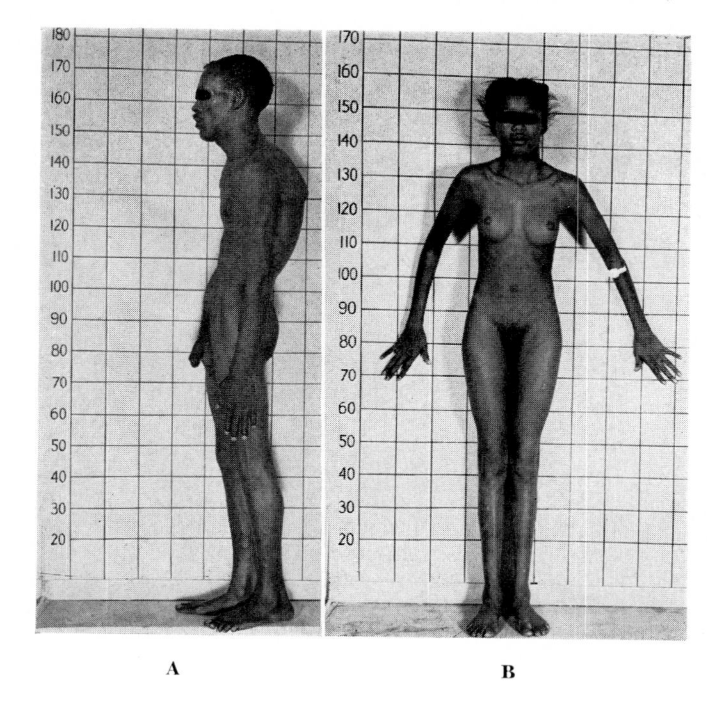

Fig. 3-13. Confusing and uncertain cases. **A,** L. M. (611512), 45-year-old Negro man, sustained an injury to his chest one year before this photograph. Shortly after the accident he began to have paroxysmal nocturnal dyspnea and was found to have profound aortic regurgitation. The left ventricle and first portion of the ascending aorta were enlarged. Spinal deformity became progressively more impressive in this patient. There was no ectopia lentis. For geographic reasons, the family investigation was not entirely satisfactory, but no suspicions of the Marfan syndrome were present. (The patient died two years after this photograph was taken. Unfortunately, autopsy was not performed.) **B,** W. F. (651498), 12 years old. Two years previously acute encephalitis occurred, followed by mental deterioration with positive neurologic signs. No ectopia lentis. The mother, who is normal, has the same skeletal proportions.

no marked deviation was observed, although no systematic controlled observations were undertaken. Certainly the excess length of the legs is not due to delayed closure of the epiphyses. The excess length is often demonstrable at birth (Fig. 3-18*I*) and throughout childhood and adolescence.

The eye. Ectopia lentis, almost always bilateral, is the hallmark of ocular involvement in this syndrome (Fig. 3-19). The suspensory ligaments, when visualized with the slit lamp, are redundant, attenuated, and often broken. The lower ligaments are more likely to be defective, with displacement of the lens upward as the usual finding. The lens is often abnormally small[120,216,217] and spherical. Iridodonesis, tremor of the iris, is often a tip-off to the presence of dislocation of the lens. Occasionally the edge of the dislocated lens is visible through the undilated pupil, or, of course, there may be complete dislocation of the lens into the anterior chamber. To exclude minor subluxation it is necessary to dilate the pupil fully and perform a slit-lamp examination. Bowers[56] describes an interest-

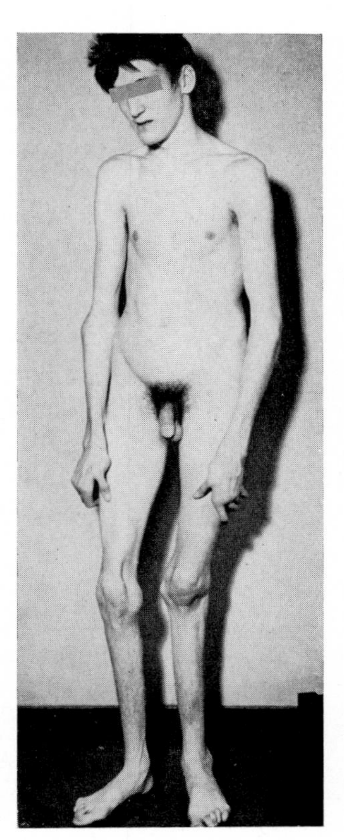

A

Fig. 3-14. H. W. (464314), 17 years old. Died suddenly at home eighteen months later. The patient was moderately crippled by the skeletal abnormality. Pain in the joints, especially those of the knees, seemed to be related to the loose-jointedness. A long follow-up in an orthopedic clinic. Ectopia lentis. Referred because of spontaneous retinal detachment. **A,** General view. **B,** Striking arachnodactyly with partial contractures of fingers. Children delight in doing contortions with their fingers but should not be permitted to do this, since serious damage may result. **C,** Extraordinary length of the great toes is well demonstrated. Even more pronounced excess of length of great toe shown in case illustrated by Whitfield and associates.[410]

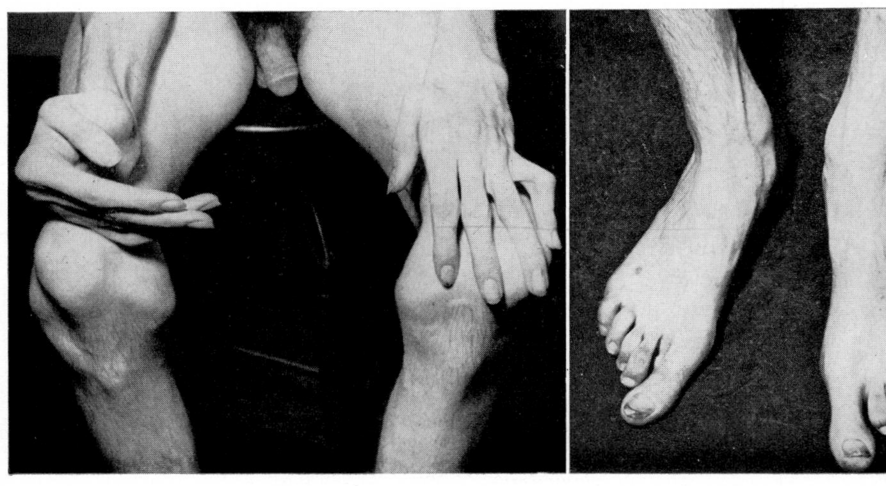

B C

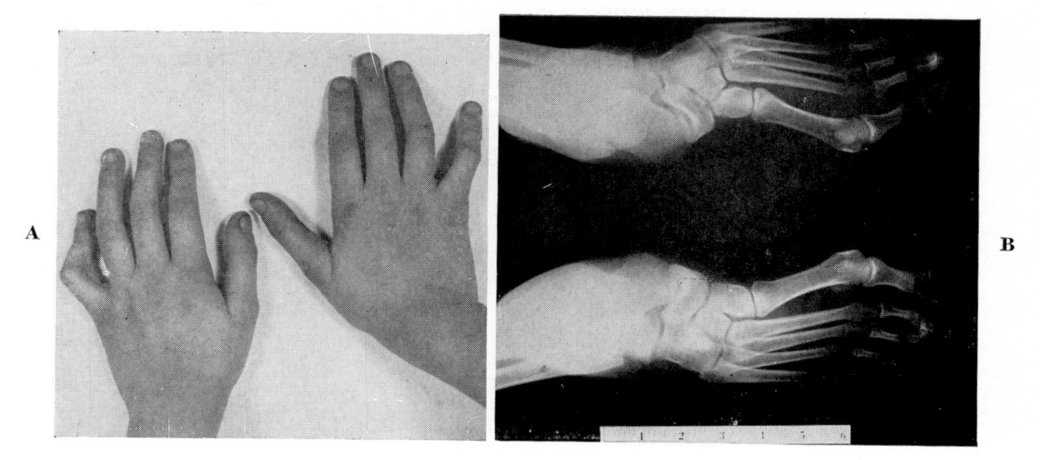

Fig. 3-15. A, Flexion deformity (clinodactyly) of fifth fingers, particularly on left. Taken at age of 38 months in M. D. (A59949), who is shown at a later age in Fig. 3-4*B*. Other patients in this series have shown this feature. **B,** X-ray films of feet in case with so-called "rocker bottoms," i.e. pronounced flat feet. Patient J. M. (544088); see also Fig. 3-27.

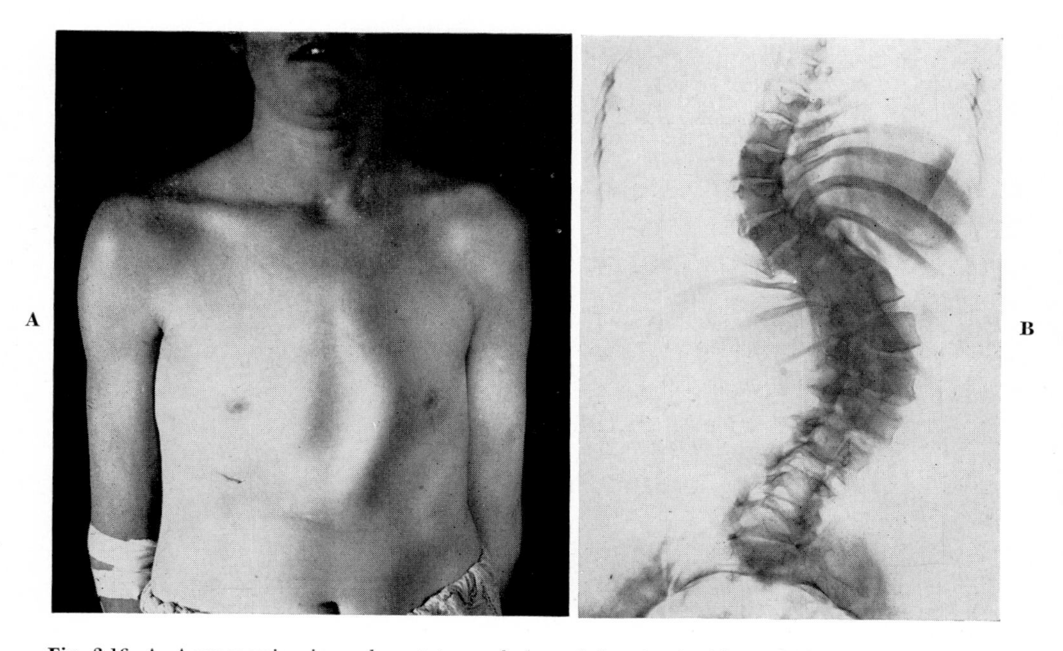

Fig. 3-16. A, Asymmetric pigeon-breast type of chest deformity in 14-year-old boy (J. S., 543026) with full Marfan's syndrome. This particular type of anterior chest deformity seems to be of frequent occurrence in Marfan's syndrome. At the age of 18 years, the patient was 73 inches tall. Incomplete right bundle branch block is present. The patient's father was 6 feet 7 inches tall, and at the age of 28 years died suddenly on a bus. He had been observed for two years for aortic regurgitation which had been considered rheumatic in origin. **B,** Marked spinal deformity in 14-year-old F. D., one of first cases of aortic aneurysm with arachnodactyly reported by Baer and co-workers.[17] (See reference 17 for photographs of the external appearance of this patient; also p. 356 of reference 412.)

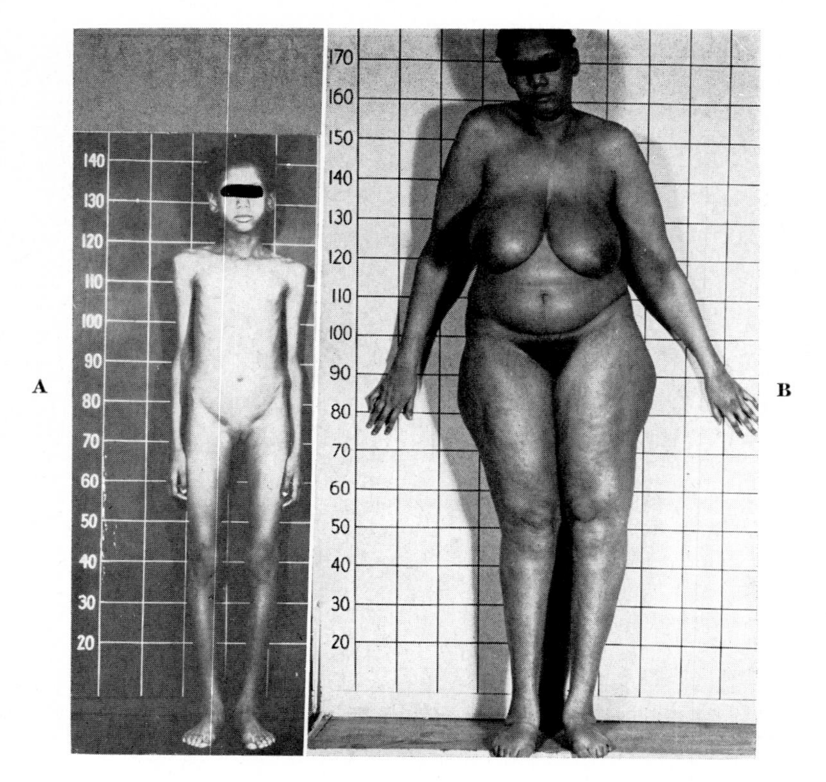

Fig. 3-17A and B. L. T. (221183), at the age of 8 years. **A,** and at age 23, **B.** At 8 years the patient is virtually the same height as M. D. (Fig. 3-4*B*), also 8 years old. The patient became almost completely blind from bilateral retinal detachment. With the inactivity associated therewith, she became very obese, as demonstrated in **B.** White atrophic striae appeared on the shoulders, upper arms, hips, and thighs, as has been described previously in obese patients with Marfan's syndrome.[402] The patient probably had rheumatic fever with carditis as a child, but no residua are detectable. She has demonstrated, in addition to ectopia lentis, accessory rudimentary sixth digit bilaterally, highly arched palate, and pupils that react poorly to mydriatics.

ing family in which members would seek the presence of dislocation by gently shaking the infant or small child while observing the eye in bright sunlight. The appearance of the dislocated lens was aptly compared to the bubble in a spirit level.

Heterochromia iridis was present in at least two patients in this series (Figs. 3-4*B* and 3-46).

Myopia is usually present in rather high degree. The excessive length of the eyeball, resulting in myopia, appears to indicate involvement of the sclera, fundamentally a ligamentous structure, in the basic connective tissue defect. The scleral defect is occasionally expressed in the cornea as keratoconus[14] or as megalocornea[356] (G. H., B50120).

The sclera may be impressively blue in the Marfan syndrome.[45] Clouding of the cornea occurs occasionally; this is probably not a primary element of the connective tissue disease but rather a result of the secondary iritis and glaucoma.

Spontaneous retinal detachment occurs with what is probably an unusually

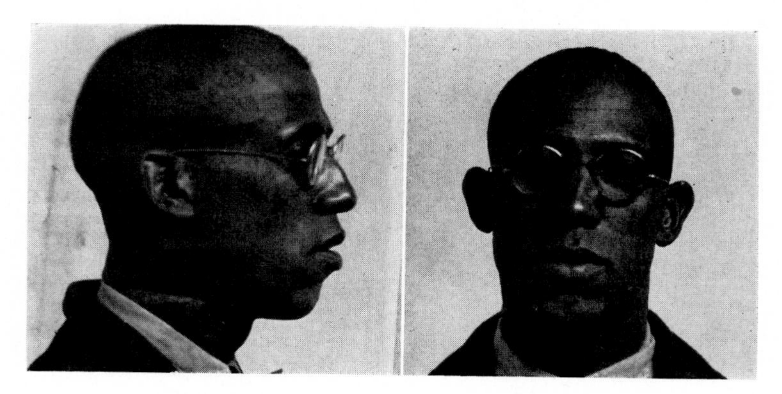

Fig. 3-17C. Prison photograph of the proposita's father (B. R.). The character of the spectacles suggests hyperopia, an unusual although occasional finding in the Marfan syndrome. He had several admissions to the Norfolk, Va., General Hospital (A46772) for hernia repair, for acute dissection of the aorta (age 38), for varicose veins, and for pain in the low back. The final hospital admission was to the St. Luke's Hospital, Newburgh, N. Y., because of severe pain up and down his back. Profound aortic regurgitation and a pulsating abdominal mass were discovered. Serologic tests for syphilis were negative. The patient died suddenly (age 39). Autopsy revealed old dissection of the aorta with recent rupture into the pericardial cavity, and tamponade. Both the father and the father's father of this man seem to have had the Marfan syndrome, making a total of four generations affected.

high incidence and is a frequent complication of lens extraction. Retinal detachment is probably related in part to the long myopic eyeball and therefore indirectly to the connective tissue defect; that there is a more direct relationship is strongly suspected[170] because of the high incidence in Marfan's syndrome even without more than a moderate degree of myopia. The pupil is often difficult to dilate in Marfan's syndrome, and the dilator muscle appears to be hypoplastic.[319]

Ectopia lentis per se would probably represent relatively little impairment of vision. Severe myopia (20 diopters in Boerger's[46] case), retinal detachment, and the iritis and/or glaucoma that may result from the ectopia lentis are often responsible for severe limitation of visual acuity or even for total blindness. The lens may become secondarily cataractous.

I was previously suspicious that estimations that only 50 to 70% of persons with clear-cut Marfan's syndrome have ectopia lentis were incorrectly low as a result of inadequate examination of the eyes and that virtually 100% of them would display at least minor redundancy of the suspensory ligament if subjected to maximal mydriasis and slit-lamp examination. It may be true that the first estimate above is indeed too low. However, we have now observed patients who showed advanced Marfan's disease with characteristic habitus, involvement of other members of the family, and dissection of the aorta, with autopsy demonstration of pathognomonic changes in the media, who did not have ocular abnormality on most careful examination. For example, in the two brothers shown in Fig. 3-27*A* and *B* there were characteristic changes discovered in the skeleton and aorta but no ectopia lentis. However, three of the five children of one of the men do show ectopia lentis, as well as skeletal changes. Furthermore, the older brother shown in Fig. 3-21 has no ectopia lentis although the diagnosis of Marfan syndrome is undoubted.

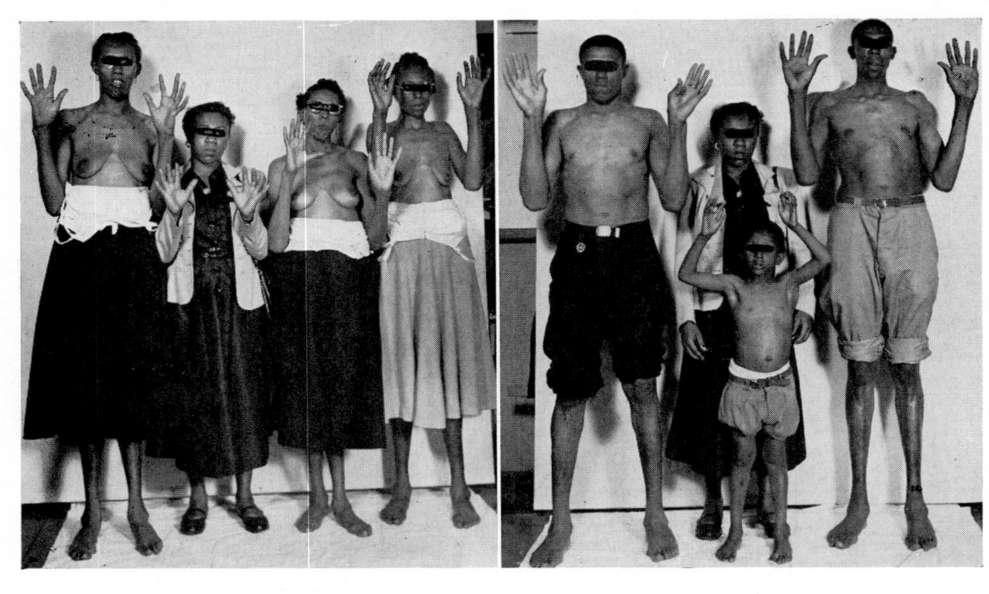

A B

Fig. 3-18A and B. A normal individual (III-12) and her five siblings affected by the Marfan syndrome (III-15, III-14, III-13, III-11, and III-8). In **B** is a 4-year-old affected member (IV-13) of the next generation, son of III-8. (The numbers correspond to those used in a pedigree shown in Fig. 3-35*A*.) Individual III-11 subsequently died of bacterial endocarditis engrafted on a mitral valve probably affected by connective tissue changes of the Marfan syndrome.[231] There was chromatropic degeneration of the ascending aorta and pulmonary artery, as well as advanced congenital cystic disease of the lungs. Individual III-14 is 78 inches tall. (History numbers: 176836, 176837, 176838, 103632, 637693, 637694, 392843.) The father of the sibship (W. R., 101043) died suddenly at home at the age of 43 years, presumably of aortic rupture. He was well known as a patient with Marfan's syndrome and had been under treatment for a cardiac ailment with aortic regurgitation for about two years. (Individual III-15 of the pedigree, the adult male on the far left in **B,** died in 1956 with aortic regurgitation.)

By gonioscopy, von Noorden and Schultz[396] detected changes in the angle of the anterior chamber of the eye, bridging pectinate strands, iris processes, irregularity and fraying of the iris root, etc. (Fig. 3-20). These findings are not specific for the Marfan syndrome, since they were found by Burian and associates[65] in a variety of conditions that may be construed as connective tissue disorders: severe idiopathic scoliosis, idiopathic genu varum, Legg-Perthes disease, slipped upper femoral epiphyses, and Osgood-Schlatter disease. When the angle changes are extreme in the Marfan syndrome, they may lead to glaucoma.[64]

The cardiovascular system.[140,231,239,333] Since most of the early autopsies in cases of this syndrome were in infants and children (who might have not yet developed the characteristic changes in the great vessels) and since interatrial septal defect was found (probably largely by coincidence) in several of the cases, this malformation and "congenital heart disease" in general came to be considered the usual form of cardiovascular involvement. As more adult cases were recognized, it became apparent (1) that an inborn weakness (with subsequent degeneration) of the media of the aorta and main pulmonary artery is of much greater

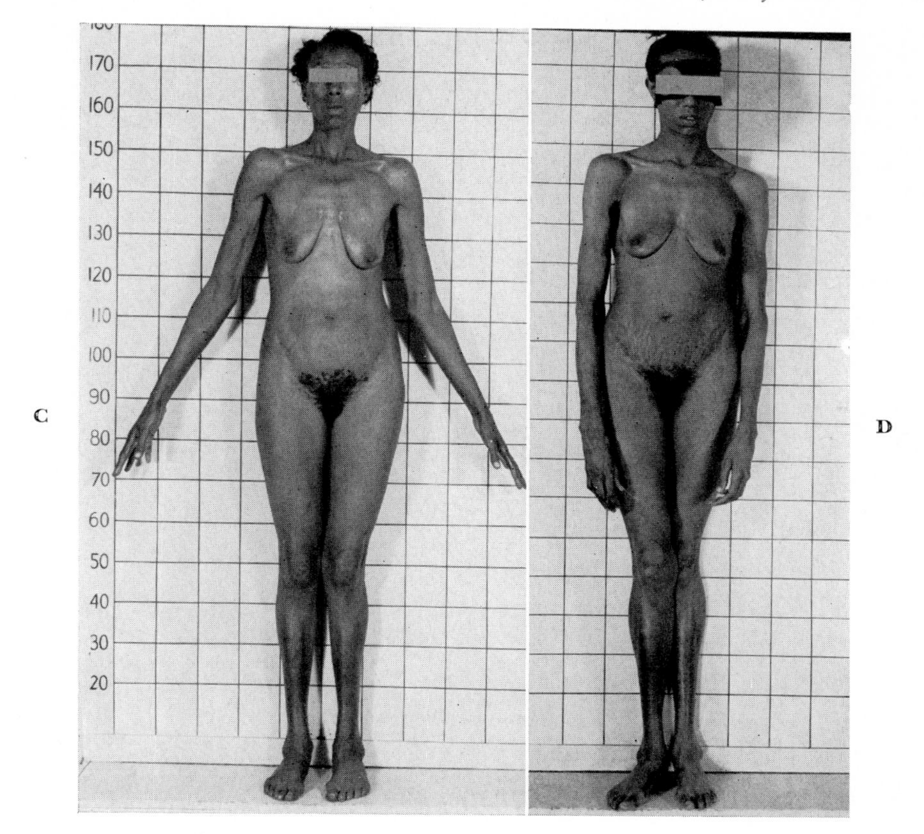

Fig. 3-18C and D. C, P. R. (103632), individual III-8 in Fig. 3-35*A*, 33 years of age. Bilateral ectopia lentis and dolichostenomelia. The patient died at the age of 34 years. Autopsy revealed pulmonary embolus. The base of the aorta was thin-walled. An anomalous flap of the mitral valve caused mitral regurgitation. **D,** H. R. (176837), individual III-13 in Fig. 3-35*A*, 29 years of age. Bilateral ectopia lentis and dolichostenomelia.

statistical importance and is of more functional importance in the individual patient and (2) that this abnormality is an abiotrophy, not a congenital malformation. The abnormality of the media may result in diffuse dilatation of the ascending aorta or pulmonary artery, in dissecting aneurysm, or in a combination of dilatation and dissection. Striking involvement of the pulmonary artery occurs[17,231,386] much less commonly than the corresponding involvement of the aorta. However, a clinical picture like that of so-called[190] "congenital idiopathic dilatation of the pulmonary artery" may occur,[74] as well as dissecting aneurysm of the pulmonary artery.[7,413] (See Figs. 3-36 and 3-44.)

In the aorta, dilatation usually begins in the aortic ring* and intrapericardial portion of the ascending aorta, as suspected clinically and as demonstrated in patients dying before further progression of their disease.[223,404] This, together with

*The term "aortic ring" is recognized to be inexact and difficult to define in precise anatomic terms. As used here it refers to the very base of the aorta, particularly the sinuses of Valsalva and the lines of attachment of the aortic cusps.

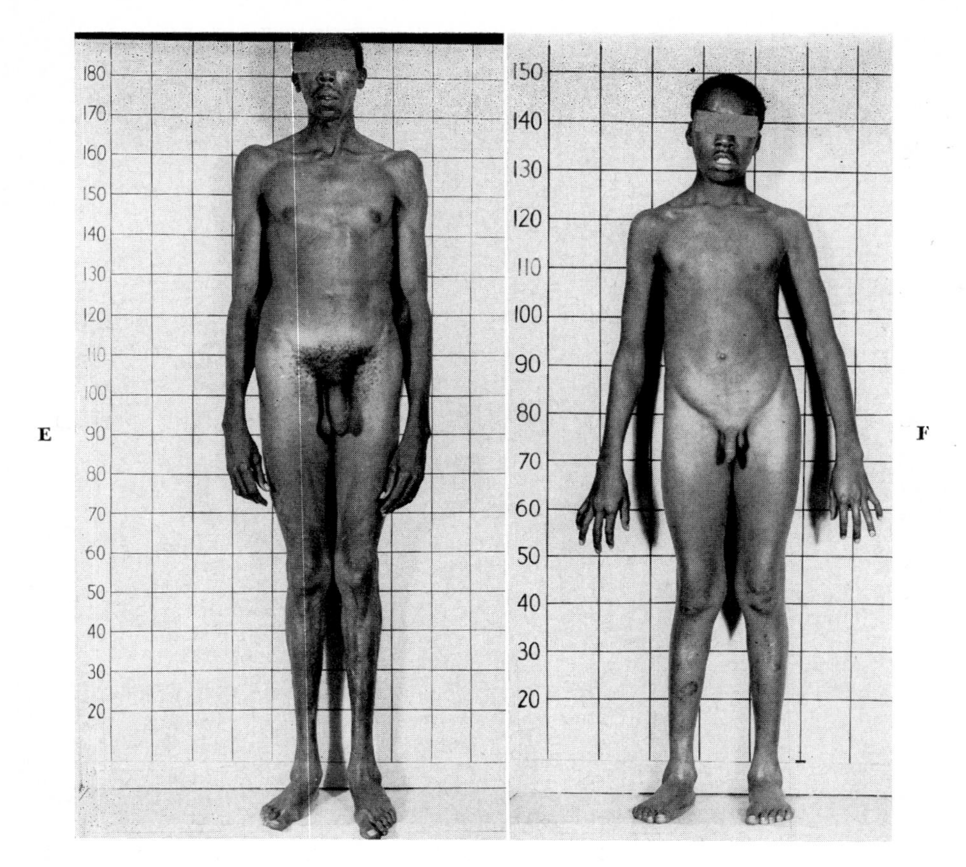

Fig. 3-18E and F. E, L. R. (176838), individual III-14 in Fig. 3-35*A*, 24 years of age. Bilateral ectopia lentis and dolichostenomelia. **F,** J. R. (637698), individual IV-8 in Fig. 3-35*A*, 11 years of age. Bilateral ectopia lentis and dolichostenomelia.

stretching of the aortic cusps, may produce profound aortic regurgitation before clear roentgenologic signs of aortic dilatation[385] are present (Figs. 3-22*B* and 3-27 to 3-29). If syphilis, rheumatism, and bacterial endocarditis can be excluded, traumatic rupture of an aortic cusp is often suspected.[29,231] (See Fig. 3-24.)

Furthermore, a deceptive prominence of the pulmonary conus and main pulmonary artery may be produced by the dilated aortic base and compound the confusion.[17,231,282] (Dilatation of the pulmonary artery itself contributes to the prominence). In a recent case (J. M., J.H.H. 544088) the aneurysm at the base of the aorta apparently caused partial obstruction of outflow from the right ventricle with the development of progressive right axis deviation by electrocardiogram. In these cases, the second heart sound in the pulmonary area may be unusually loud due to close proximity of the pulmonary artery to the anterior chest wall.

Aortic dilatation is usually progressive. The patient may be free of symptoms for five or more years after the development of aortic regurgitation, but once angina pectoris or symptoms of left ventricular failure have developed, he may live no more than two years. On the whole, the prognosis is quite similar to that of spyhilitic aortitis.[403] In fact, the similarities of the two diseases are in many re-

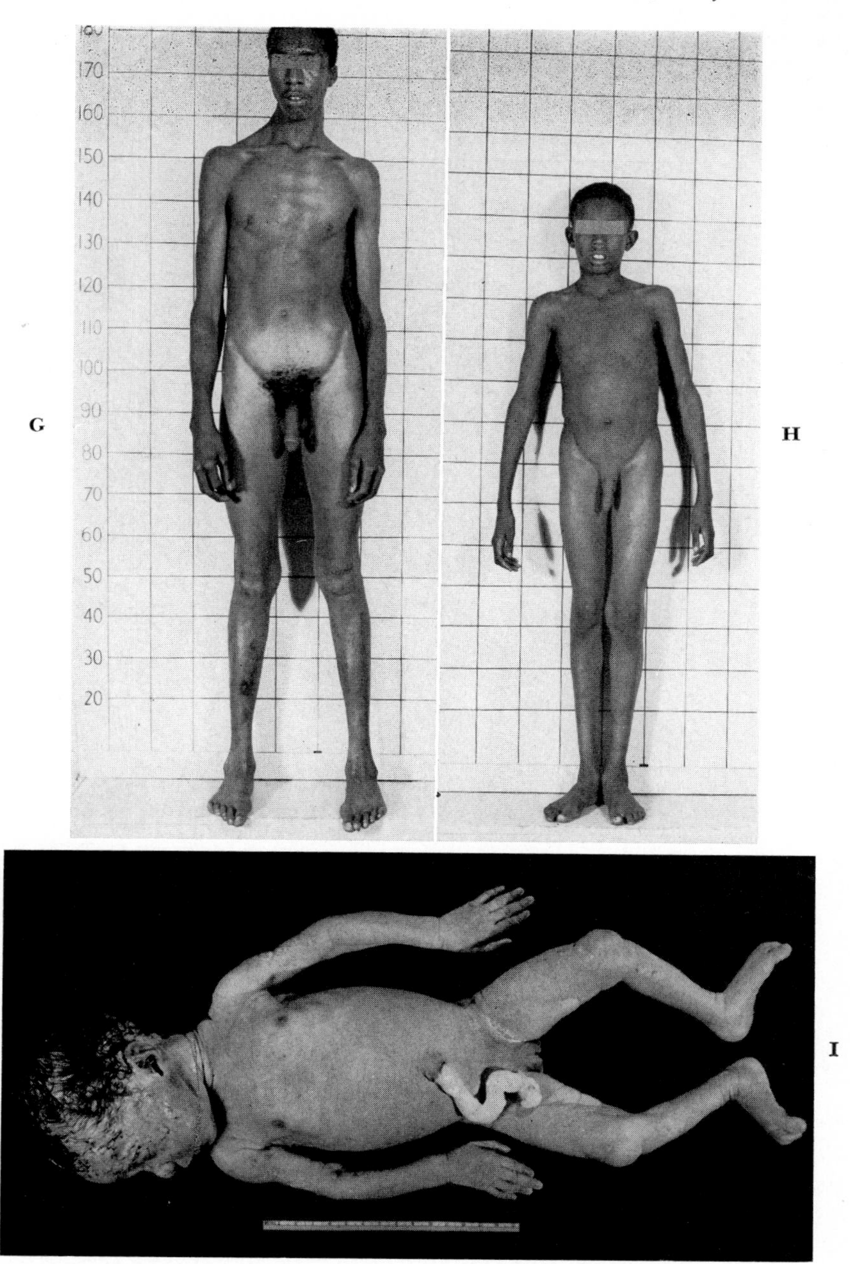

Fig. 3-18G to I. G, Same patient as shown in **F,** 15½ years of age. **H,** P. R. (637693), individual IV-13 in Fig. 3-35*A*, 9½ years of age. Bilateral ectopia lentis and dolichostenomelia. **I,** The stillborn infant (autopsy 29095) of patient shown in Fig. 3-35*B*. The infant is believed to be affected. For her age (8½ months) the foot was probably long (7.25 cm. as compared with 6.5). The crown-heel measurement was 46 cm. (usual, 43.5) and the crown-anus dimension 30.5 cm. (usual, 28 cm.). See reference 221 for normal standards used in these studies. The infant showed no other abnormality on gross and histologic study, except an abnormality of pulmonary lobation of the type described in cases of the Marfan syndrome. Specifically, the aorta was grossly and histologically normal!

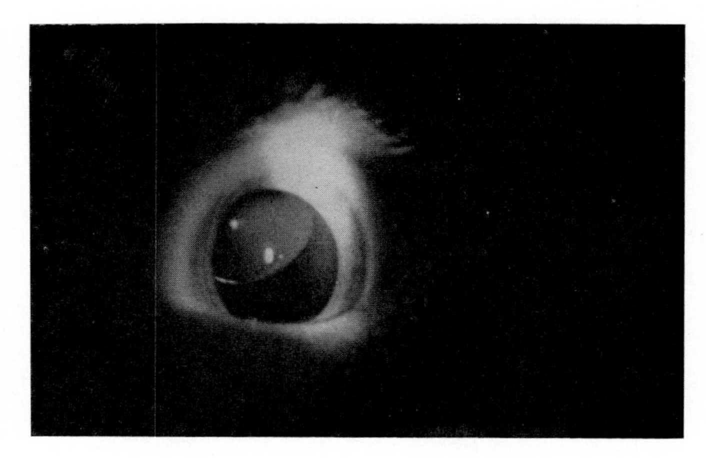

Fig. 3-19. Displacement upward and temporally of the lens in a case of the Marfan syndrome. (Courtesy Dr. Béla Varga, Eger, Hungary.)

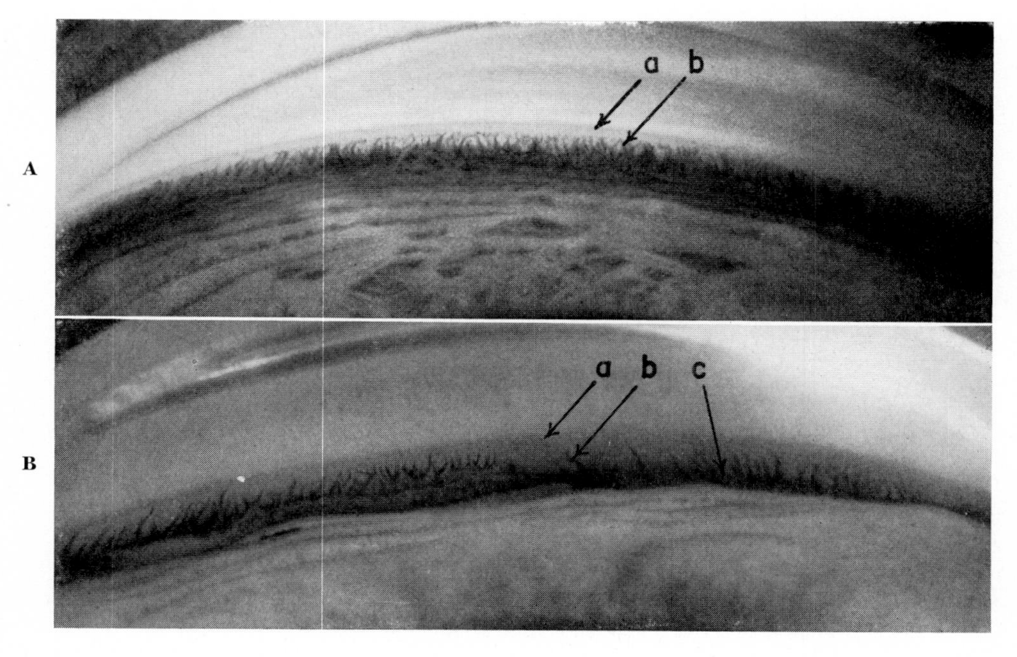

Fig. 3-20. The angle of the anterior chamber in two cases of the Marfan syndrome with ectopia lentis: **a,** Schwalbe's line; **b,** pectinate ligaments; **c,** ciliary body band. In both **A** and **B,** note the pectinate strands as described by von Noorden and Schultz.[396] In **B** note the irregular insertion of the peripheral iris. (Courtesy Dr. Gunter K. von Noorden.)

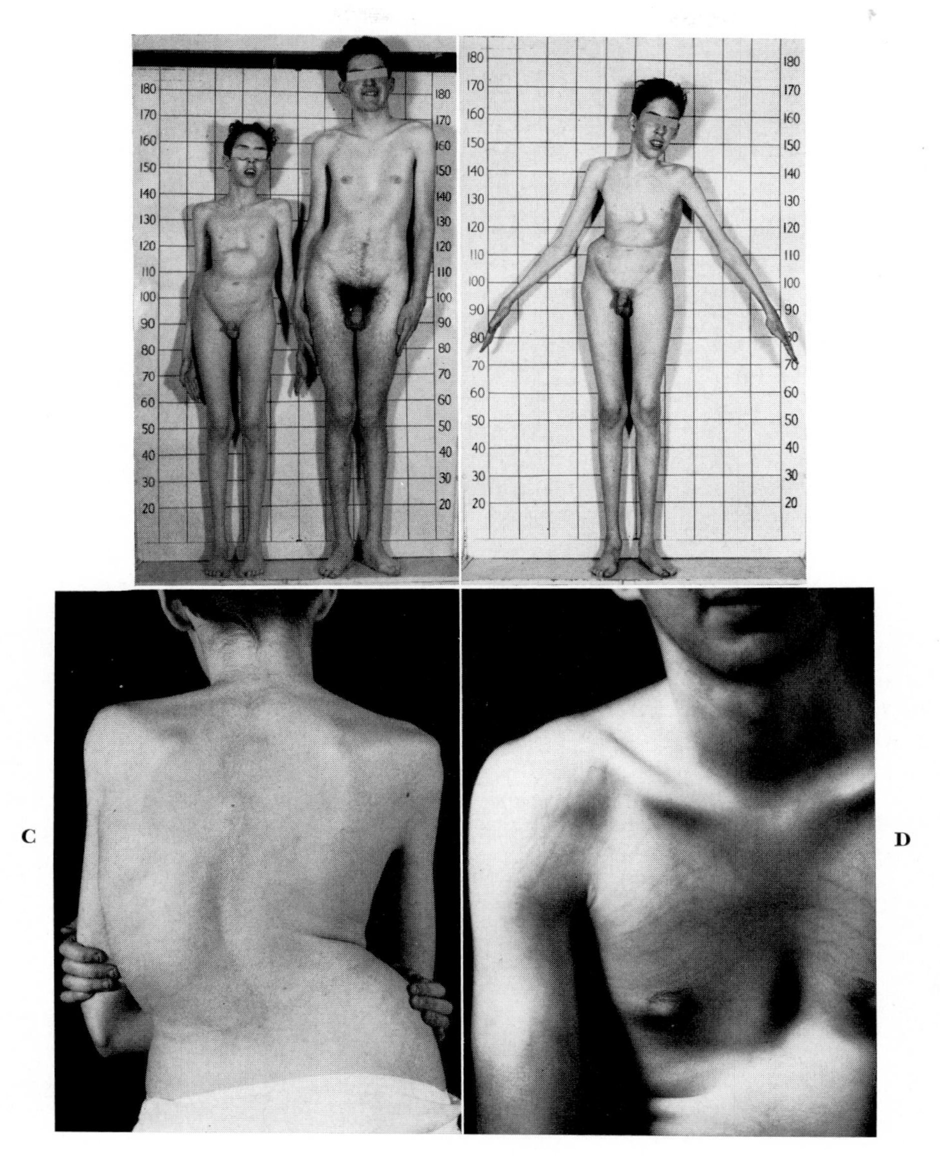

Fig. 3-21. Brothers with the Marfan syndrome (871800; 871801). **A,** The older brother (right), age 17, has no detectable ocular or intrinsic cardiovascular anomaly although the skeletal features, especially pectus excavatum, and scoliosis are pronounced. In him the diagnosis of the Marfan syndrome could not have been made with confidence but for the facts that his younger brother (left), age 13, has ectopia lentis and even more marked skeletal abnormalities and that the father, who had similar skeletal characteristics, died at 36 years, of aortic regurgitation. **B,** The younger brother at age 15. **C,** Severe scoliosis in the younger brother. **D,** Striae distensae in the older brother, in infrared photograph.

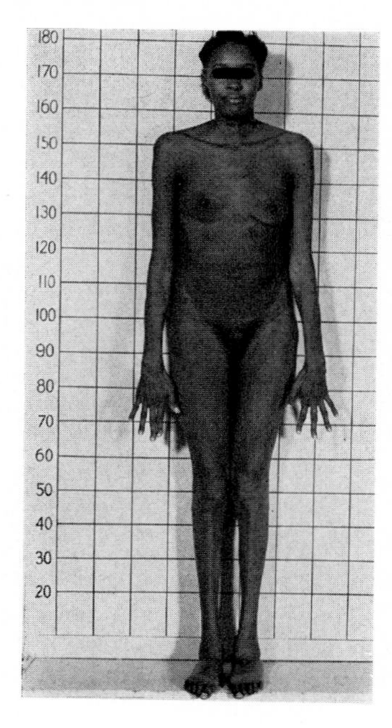

Fig. 3-22A. L. F. Y. (690823), 33 years old. Patient died of effects of severe aortic regurgitation. Autopsy revealed characteristic changes in the media of the aorta and pulmonary artery with old dissecting aneurysm of the ascending aorta. The dissection may have occurred during pregnancy.

spects striking. It seems to matter little whether the defect of the media is produced by the spirochete from without or the mutant gene from within.

As in syphilitic aortitis with aortic regurgitation, revision in the prognostic evaluation of aortic regurgitation in the Marfan syndrome is necessary on the basis of recent experience. From our own series it is now clear that the asymptomatic period may extend for appreciably more than five years. Furthermore, patients have survived five years or longer after the onset of major symptoms.

Chest pain that may have features usually associated with angina pectoris but more often is imperfectly relieved by nitroglycerin is a rather frequent finding in the Marfan syndrome. In some patients the pain may be due to relative coronary insufficiency and be of the same nature as the pain that occurs with aortic regurgitation, on a rheumatic basis, for example. In other cases, aneurysmal dilatation of the aorta, even before it is radiologically evident, may be the basis. Furthermore, chest pain may be striking before aortic regurgitation of hemodynamic significance develops. In one patient (A. S.) the pain was present for ten years before death occurred suddenly at the age of 35 years. In two other patients (R. C., 155970; A. D., 341643) chest pain was present for five and eight years, respectively, before death. Coronary ostial anomalies of apparently congenital type occur in some cases. Granting the importance of other factors in the angina pectoris of the Marfan syndrome, one cannot help but wonder if one factor may not be the pronounced dragging of the large blood-laden aortic cusps on the coronary ostia in diastole and the dilated aorta during systole.

The onset of aortic dilatation may be as early as the first year or at least as

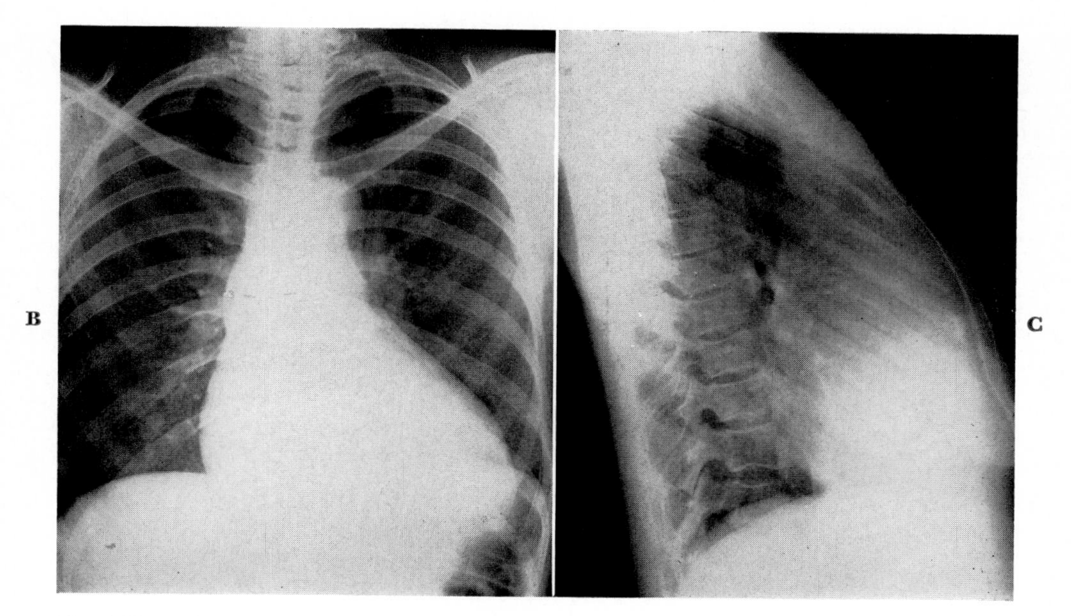

Fig. 3-22B and C. Posteroanterior and lateral views of chest in L. F. Y. It is remarkable that enlargement of the aorta is not more evident. In lateral view there is opacification behind the sternum.

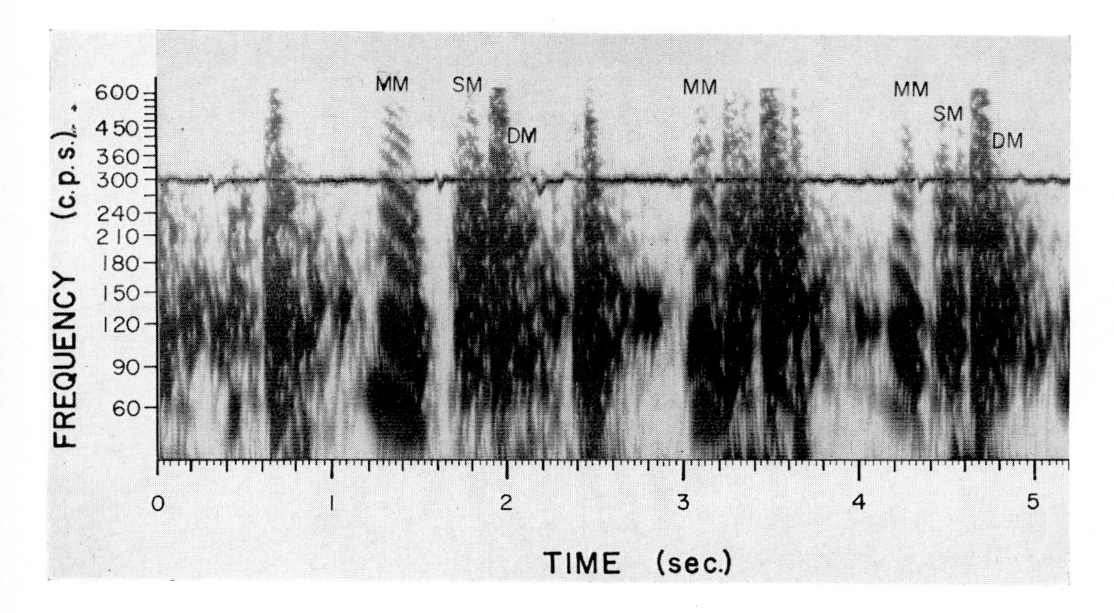

Fig. 3-22D. A spectral phonocardiogram of the sounds as recorded at the base of the heart in L. F. Y. Bigeminy was present as indicated by the electrocardiogram. There was a systolic murmur, **SM,** and a decrescendo diastolic murmur, **DM.** Near the end of the long diastolic periods that followed the extrasystoles there was a murmur, **MM,** that was strikingly musical as indicated by the conspicuous harmonics. When the bigeminy was absent and the rate higher, with short diastole, the murmur did not occur. (From McKusick, V. A., Murray, G. E., Peeler, R. G., and Webb, G. N.: Bull. Hopkins Hosp. **97:**136, 1955.)

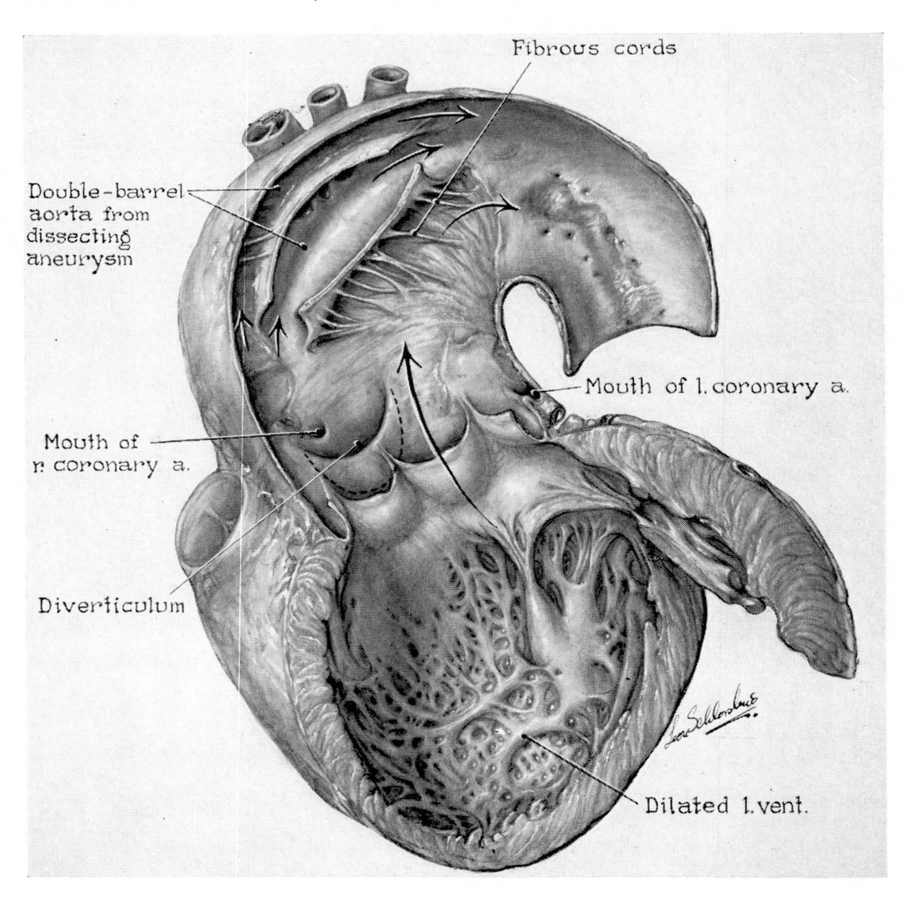

Fig. 3-22E. The autopsy specimen in patient L. F. Y. A chronic dissection of the ascending aorta is present. The patient died of heart failure. The drawing demonstrates three structures that might vibrate periodically, with production of a musical murmur as seen in **D:** (1) the fibrous cords that traverse the false channel, (2) the lip of the inner tube of the double-barrel aorta, and (3) the lip of the "diverticulum" above the sinuses of Valsalva. Why any one of these three structures should be incited in late diastole, with production of the musical murmur, is not clear. (From McKusick, V. A., Murray, G. E., Peeler, R. G., and Webb, G. M.: Bull. Hopkins Hosp. **97:**136, 1955.)

late as the sixth decade. The oldest reported patient with aortic insufficiency without evident aortic dilatation was 56 years of age.[188] In one reported case,[380] dilatation of the ascending aorta with aortic regurgitation and marked left ventricular hypertrophy resulted in the death of a 10-month-old infant; in another case,[341] death occurred at 55 years. Another report[279] described four children varying in age from 5 months to 26 months and demonstrating typical features of the Marfan syndrome, including aneurysms of the aortic sinuses of Valsalva and dilatation of the ascending aorta and main pulmonary artery. In my series the youngest patient with outspoken aortic regurgitation was 2 years old (Fig. 3-25*A*). The oldest patient with aortic regurgitation was 59 years old (H. B., 621760). He showed no radiologic evidence of dilatation of the ascending aorta.

The dilatation is almost always confined to the ascending aorta proximal to the innominate artery. However, in Case 3 of Thomas and co-workers[373] the descending aorta was also involved. Furthermore, several instances of fusiform aneurysm of the abdominal aorta have been described.[205]

One of our patients (H. B., 621760), 59 years of age, has what appears by ordinary radiography to be a well-circumscribed orange-sized aneurysm of the descending thoracic aorta. Aortograms show both the thoracic and abdominal aorta to be diffusely dilated, with buckling in the lower thoracic area as well as in the abdomen, creating a false impression of saccular aneurysm at these sites.

Fig. 3-26 describes another of our cases in which cylindric aneurysm was limited to the abdominal aorta. The ascending aorta was clinically unaffected. Van

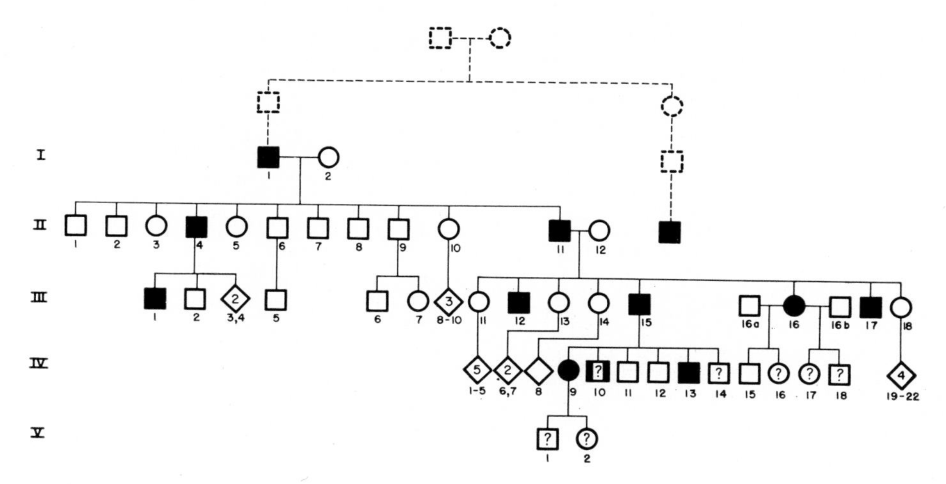

Fig. 3-23A. Pedigree of the F. kinship.

II. 1, Charles; died of acute indigestion at age 47 years. **4,** Grant; about 6 feet 4 inches tall; died at age 35 years; two of his children died at 8 and 12 months, respectively. **8,** Henry; examined; unaffected.

III. 1, James Aloysius; typical Marfan syndrome; 6 feet 4½ inches tall, size 13 shoe; ectopia lentis with secondary cataract formation; complete loss of vision from bilateral detachment of retina; early aortic diastolic murmur. **11,** Josephine; examined; unaffected. **12,** Clarence (352936); at age 32 years found to have complete detachment of right retina; left lens dislocated and cataractous; partial detachment of left retina; died at age 34 years, eighteen days after onset of congestive heart failure attributed to syphilitic heart disease, because of finding of aortic regurgitation. **13,** Blanche; examined; unaffected. **15,** Theodore (see **B**); typical Marfan syndrome, with cardiovascular death in 1952. **16,** Leona (see Fig. 3-22 *A* to *C*); typical Marfan syndrome, with autopsy confirmation of dissecting aneurysm of the aorta. **17,** James Leon (424834); ectopia lentis with severe secondary iridocyclitis and glaucoma; detachment of right retina; 75 inches tall, weight 172 pounds; kyphoscoliosis; varicocele; lax sternocleidomastoid joints, mobile patellae; flat feet; cardiomegaly with globular shape by x-ray examination; no murmurs. This individual and Theodore and Clarence "always looked just like twins." Positive serologic test for syphilis.

IV. 9, Mary Isabelle (844914), born 1939; definitely affected, with bilateral dislocation of lenses. **10,** James Leroy (844924), born 1940; possible slight lens dislocation. **11,** James Arthur (844925), born 1944; normal. **12,** John Edward (844922), born 1945; normal. **13,** David Theodore (844921), born 1950; definite Marfan syndrome; 38 inches tall at 30 months of age; long, peculiarly shaped head; dislocated lenses. **14,** Joseph Melvin (844923), born 1952; possibly affected.

V. 1, James Allen (844915), born 1945; uncertain status. **2,** Mary Anne, born 1947; uncertain status.

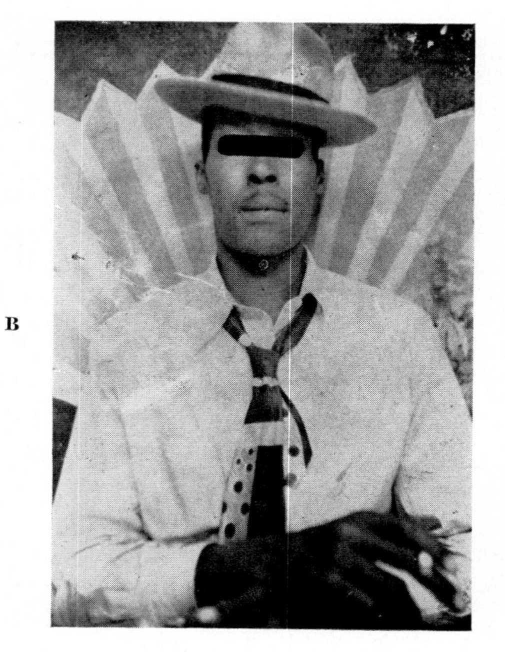

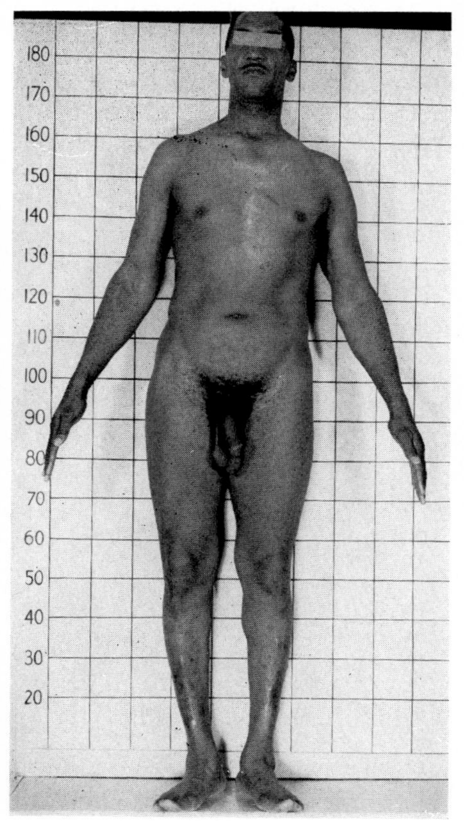

Fig. 3-23B and C. B, Carnival snapshot of III-15 (T. F.). Arachnodactyly is evident. In his left hand he holds his spectacles. He died suddenly at the age of 33 years, two weeks after consulting a physician for exertional dyspnea. Aortic regurgitation had been discovered. An optometrist reports that he had "a decided miosis and the ophthalmoscopy showed the media to be cloudy." He was myopic. Worked as farm laborer until a few days before death. **C,** J. A. F. (816419), individual III-1 in **A,** at 33 years of age. Bilateral ectopia lentis, dolichostenomelia, and mild aortic regurgitation.

Buchem[389] described rupture of the abdominal aorta with cystic medial necrosis in a 20-year-old man who, because of striking skeletal changes, probably had the true Marfan syndrome, although the rest of the family was unaffected and no subluxation of the lenses was discovered. Langeron and colleagues[205] described two cases of abdominal aneurysm in the Marfan syndrome. Hardin,[156] in a case of full-blown Marfan syndrome in a 21-year-old man, described a fusiform abdominal aneurysm extending from the level of the renal arteries to the bifurcation of the aorta. It had ruptured into the inferior vena cava. At autopsy, although the abdominal aorta showed the histologic changes characteristic of the Marfan syndrome, "the thoracic aorta, pulmonary artery, and remaining arteries showed intact elastic fibers." In another patient with the Marfan syndrome, a 43-year-old male, Hardin[157] successfully resected an abdominal aneurysm. See also the cases of ruptured abdominal aortic aneurysm reported by Irwin and associates[179] and by Heitzman and Bryant.[164] Davis and colleagues[87] performed a total replacement

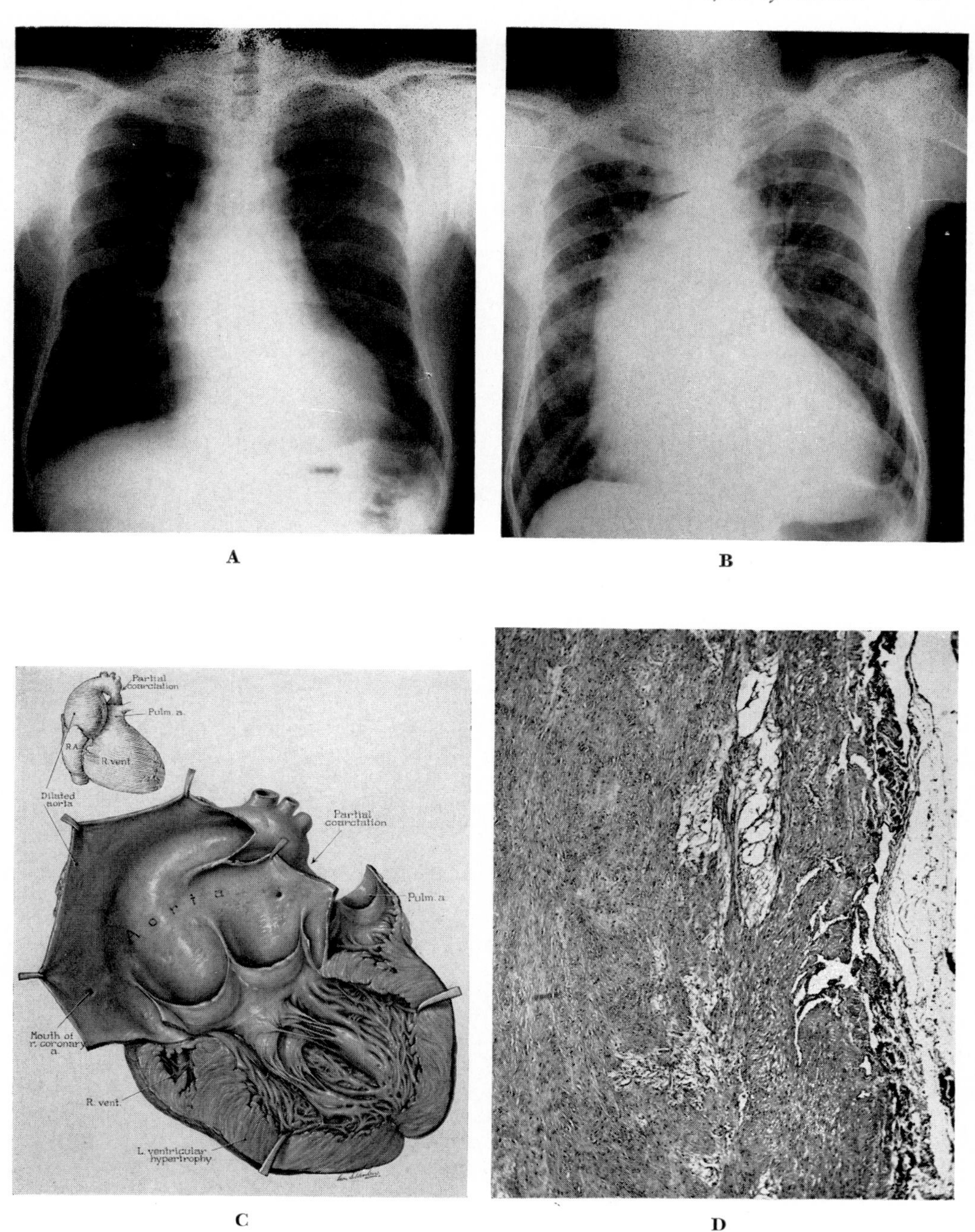

Fig. 3-24. A, Dilatation of the ascending aorta is present but is not impressive. Patient L. K. (film taken eighteen months before death). **B,** Film four months before death, same patient. **C,** Sketch of the heart and great vessels as visualized at autopsy in patient L. K. Mild coarctation was present. Dilatation limited to the ascending aorta and tremendous sacculation of the aortic cusps are conspicuous features. Note the relatively high position of the coronary ostia. **D,** Histologic section from the ascending aortic in same case.

Legend continued.

Legend to Fig. 3-24, cont'd

L. K. (J.H.H. 571745), a white man born in 1913, was first admitted to this hospital in May, 1951. On April 16, 1951, while riveting at an aircraft plant he noted the rather sudden onset of severe steady pain in his right chest, radiating down the right arm. This disappeared in a few hours, and he was essentially asymptomatic thereafter but was aware of profuse sweating, particularly of the hands and feet.

Examination revealed that the blood pressure was 195/40/0. He was a slightly built man of average height. There was alternating external strabismus, and the pupils were rather small but normally reactive. No other ocular abnormality was detected at that time. There were pronounced cardiac and peripheral signs of aortic regurgitation.

There was no history of rheumatic fever or syphilis and no laboratory or clinical evidence of syphilis or bacterial endocarditis. There was a story that in his work as a riveter the instrument which he held in front of his chest had, on several occasions, slipped, striking his chest forcefully. The possibility of traumatic rupture of an aortic cusp was considered most likely. In fact, this was considered so likely by his physicians that with their assistance the patient succeeded in making a $4,000 settlement with his employer! The history of his having been previously turned down for insurance was not elicited.

The patient was virtually asymptomatic until September, 1951, when he began to have attacks heralded by very profuse sweating and consisting of pain under the lower sternum, severe palpitation, and coughing. Rapid eating and excitement would precipitate the attacks. They occurred most often about midnight.

The patient's second admission was in May, 1952. At that time Dr. F. W. Dick first noted that the patient had iridodonesis bilaterally and that the edge of ectopic lenses could be seen with the ophthalmoscope. From the age of 10 years the patient had worn glasses for myopia, and bifocals from the age of 19 years. Examination revealed profuse sweating, even in a cool room. The lid slits were wide and there was lid lag; these were interpreted as probably being related to the effort to accommodate. (The excessive sweating was probably that frequently seen with left ventricular failure.) The head was round and the neck rather short. There was kyphosis without scoliosis. Muscular development was on the whole rather poor. The shoulders were rounded and scapulae moderately winged. His height was 5 feet 7 inches and fingertip-to-fingertip span 5 feet 11 inches. Pubic symphysis-to-heel dimension was 34 inches (over half his total height). There was syndactylism of the second and third toes bilaterally. There was a diastolic thrill at the right border of the sternum, and mediastinal dullness was increased to the right. It was then very apparent that the patient had Marfan's syndrome. Superannuated dissecting aneurysm of the aorta was considered likely.

The remainder of the patient's life was characterized by severe attacks of sweating, anginal pain, and orthopnea. At no time were there signs of right-sided failure. Comparison of early and late films are presented in **A** and **B.** The patient died Jan. 23, 1953.

At autopsy (24360) his height was determined to be 5 feet 6 inches. (There is a discrepancy among the various reported measurements.) The kyphosis was again described. The significant findings were limited to the heart, **C,** which weighed 980 grams. The increased weight was almost entirely the result of very marked left ventricular hypertrophy. The ascending aorta was the site of pronounced fusiform dilatation. The aortic valve ring was dilated to about four times the normal circumference. The sinuses of Valsalva were greatly dilated, and the aortic valve cusps themselves were relatively enormous baggy structures. The aortic dilatation stopped at the mouth of the innominate artery. Beyond the mouth of the left subclavian the aorta narrowed sharply in a typical, although only partial (about 40%), stenosis of the isthmus.

Microscopic sections of the aorta, **D,** revealed replacement of most of the media by scar tissue. There were some areas of cystic medial degeneration. Elastic tissue stains revealed marked disruption, fragmentation, and sparsity of elastic fibers.

After the death of the patient, an investigation revealed, in the records of an insurance company, information that the patient was turned down for insurance in 1944 because of aortic regurgitation. Therefore an aortic diastolic murmur had been present for at least nine years before death and for several years before symptoms of significance. It should also be noted that he had had varicose veins which required surgical treatment.

Comments. The aorta was not conspicuously dilated at the time the patient was first seen, in spite of the presence of striking aortic regurgitation. A possibly useful point may be a finding at fluoroscopy at the time of the first admission: "The lower right border of the heart in the region of the right atrium showed a marked increase in amplitude of pulsation. The pulmonary artery segment on the left side of the heart also pulsated vigorously, although the vascular markings of the lung were if anything decreased." In some of these cases the outflow tract of the right ventricle and base of the pulmonary artery are evidently displaced forward and to the left (by the dilatation of the base of the aorta), simulating enlargement of these structures.[282] On the other side the intrapericardial portion of the aorta may be responsible for displacement and active pulsations in the right atrium.

A feature of equal diagnostic significance and of considerable genetic interest is the relative submersion of the full-blown skeletal manifestations when the Marfan mutation occurred in this pyknic stock. When first seen the patient did not impress anyone as being beyond the normal range as to habitus. Discovery of ectopic lenses resulted in the observer being more impressed with the habitus. Comparison with his brothers and sisters would likewise have impressed the physician with the patient's abnormality. Other members of the family were about 5 feet 3 inches tall and were very heavily muscled, with short powerful extremities and stubby fingers. The moral to the diagnostician is obvious. Although extensive studies of the families were not undertaken, several cases in the literature probably illustrate this same phenomenon.[422]

This case bears many resemblances to Case 3 of Tung and Liebow.[386] The type of aortic involvement which they illustrate is almost identical to that in **C.** Their patient, who died of aortic insufficiency at the age of 42 years, had had two herniorrhaphies and had varicose veins. Although the authors state that "no suggestion of arachnodactyly nor of any other external sign of Marfan's syndrome [was] recorded by any of several senior physicians who were concerned with the care of this man," it must be noted that he died in 1932, which was before a single case of the Marfan syndrome had been reported in the internal medical literature of this country and over ten years before the association of aortic dilatation and arachnodactyly was first clearly described.[17]

(From McKusick, V. A.: Circulation **11**:321, 1955.)

---

of the abdominal aorta in a patient subsequently proved to have the Marfan syndrome. Dissection exclusively in the aorta beyond a mild coarctation at the usual site has been described.[388] In one reported case,[20] dissecting aneurysm was limited to the portion of the aorta between the mouth of the left subclavian artery and the level of the diaphragm; there seemed not to be other abnormality of the aorta.

Several cases (for example, see reference 264) have had cystic medial necrosis, dissection, and internal tears in the abdominal as well as the ascending aorta. Thrombosis of the abdominal aorta with production of the Leriche syndrome is described,[90] but such is more characteristic of homocystinuria (Chapter 4).

By examining a large number of patients with ectopia lentis and by studying the relatives in established cases of Marfan's syndrome, we discovered six patients who appeared to be in the early stages of aortic dilatation with aortic regurgitation.[231] In none was there then evident dilatation of the ascending aorta (Figs. 3-27*B*, 3-28*A* and *B*, and 3-29*B*). One of the six (Fig. 3-29*B*) died of aortic aneurysm about three years after first detection of aortic regurgitation. The others remained without particular cardiac symptoms, for periods as long as six years.

Recent years have witnessed a crescendo of interest in the subject of aneurysm of the sinuses of Valsalva.[30,118] Steinberg and Geller[353] have demonstrated such aneurysms, by means of angiocardiography, in patients with the Marfan syndrome, and we have had similar experiences (Fig. 3-30*A* to *C*). Actually the "aortic sinus aneurysms" that occur in the Marfan syndrome behave clinically in quite a different manner than do those to which this term is perhaps more legitimately

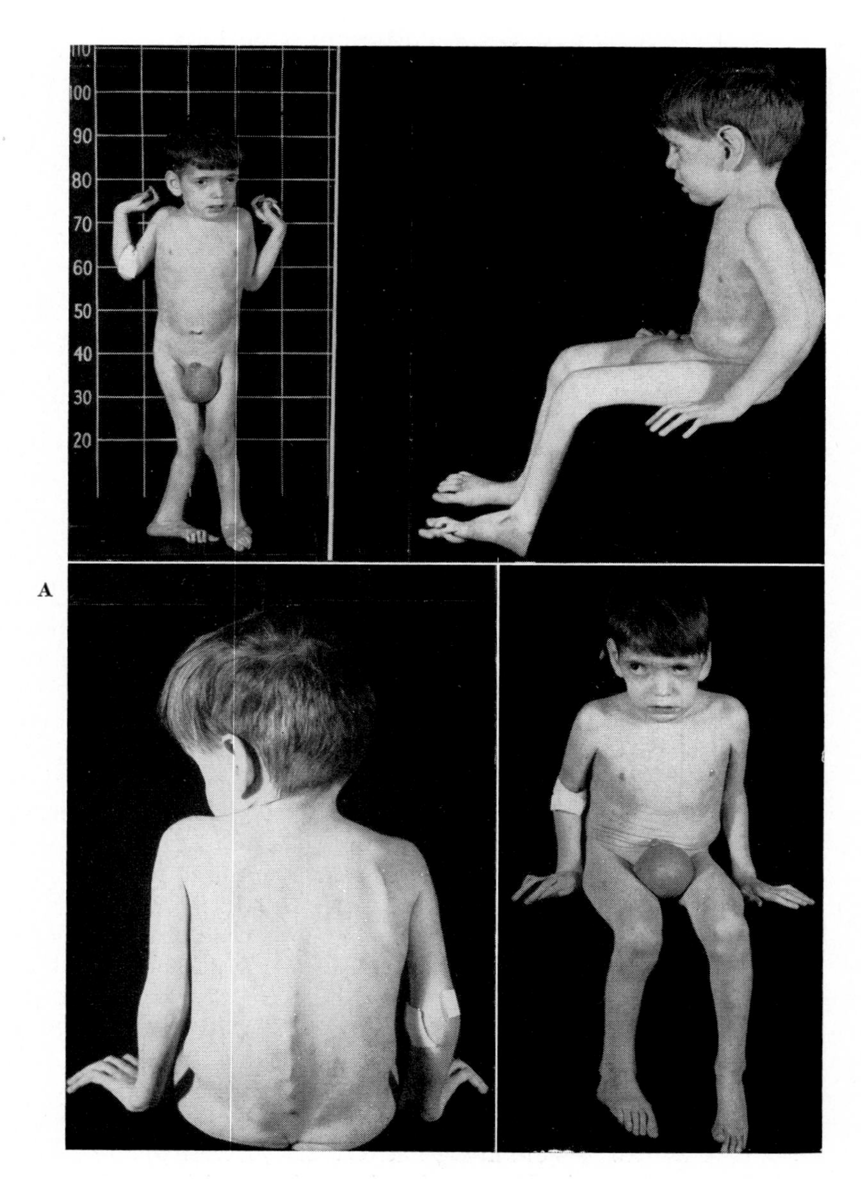

Fig. 3-25A. J. M. G. (795394), 26 months of age, has full-blown aortic regurgitation. The family history is negative. Dislocation of both lenses with striking iridodonesis, characteristically misshapen head and ears, kyphoscoliosis with "cat-back" in sitting, arachnodactyly, and a large left inguinal hernia are present. (From McKusick, V. A.: Ann. Intern. Med. **49**:556, 1958.)

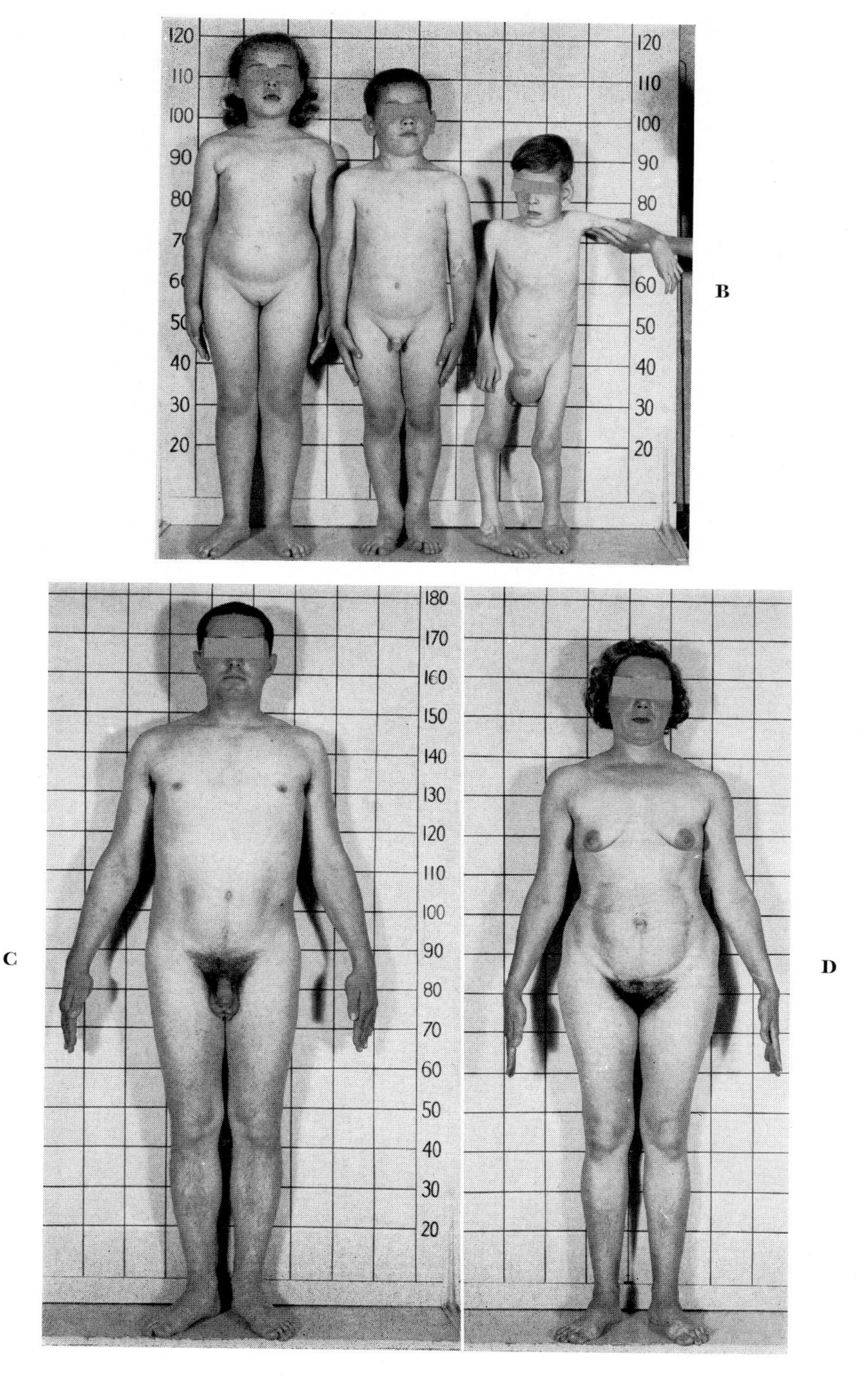

Fig. 3-25B to D. Two older children, **B,** and both parents, **C** and **D,** show no stigmata of the Marfan syndrome. The patient shown in **A** is probably the product of a new mutation. He died at the age of 3½ years. Autopsy revealed characteristic changes in the ascending aorta.

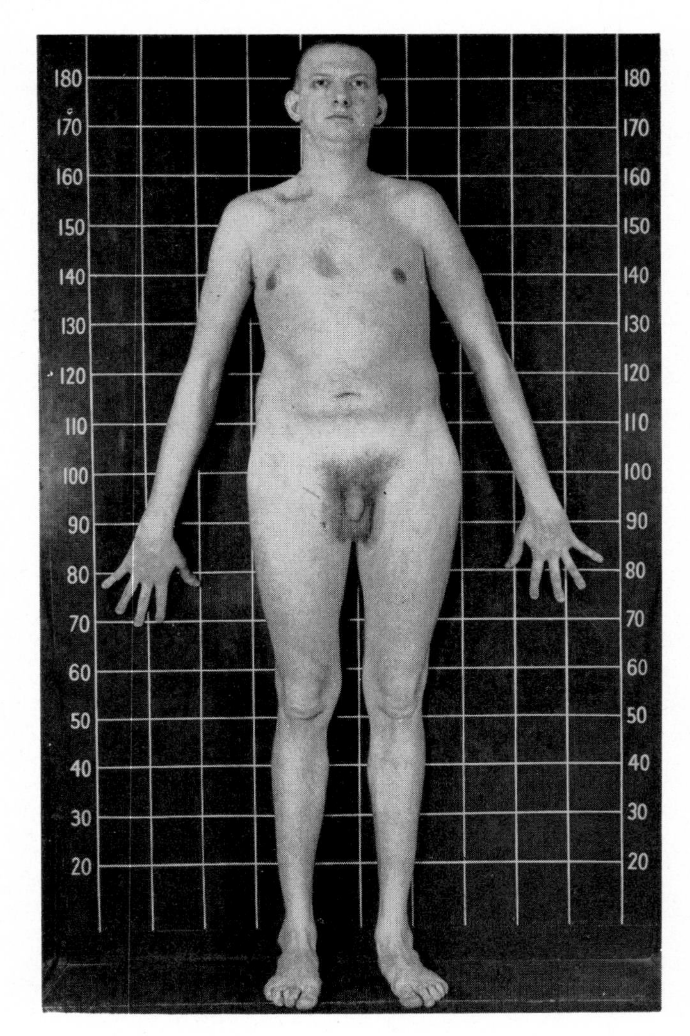

Fig. 3-26A. E. K. (760410), 26 years of age, was admitted for consideration of surgical correction of an abdominal aneurysm. The skeleton was considered to be typical of the Marfan syndrome. Both lenses were displaced upward and outward. The patient was partially deaf. but the hearing loss was of the conductive type, was largely limited to the left ear, and was readily accounted for on the basis of old otitis media. (From McKusick, V. A.: Ann. Intern. Med. **49**:556, 1958.)

applied. Rupture into the right side of the circulation has only rarely been observed; the aneurysm is not, with occasional exception, limited to one aortic sinus. The possibility of the Marfan syndrome should not be abandoned, however, in cases of rupture of an aortic sinus into the right side of the heart. In one reported case,[275] in a 36-year-old male, the following statement suggesting the Marfan syndrome was made: "Until his attack he was perfectly fit and served in the army during the Second World War in a low category on account of defective eyesight and flat feet." Rupture of dissecting aneurysm of the aorta into the right

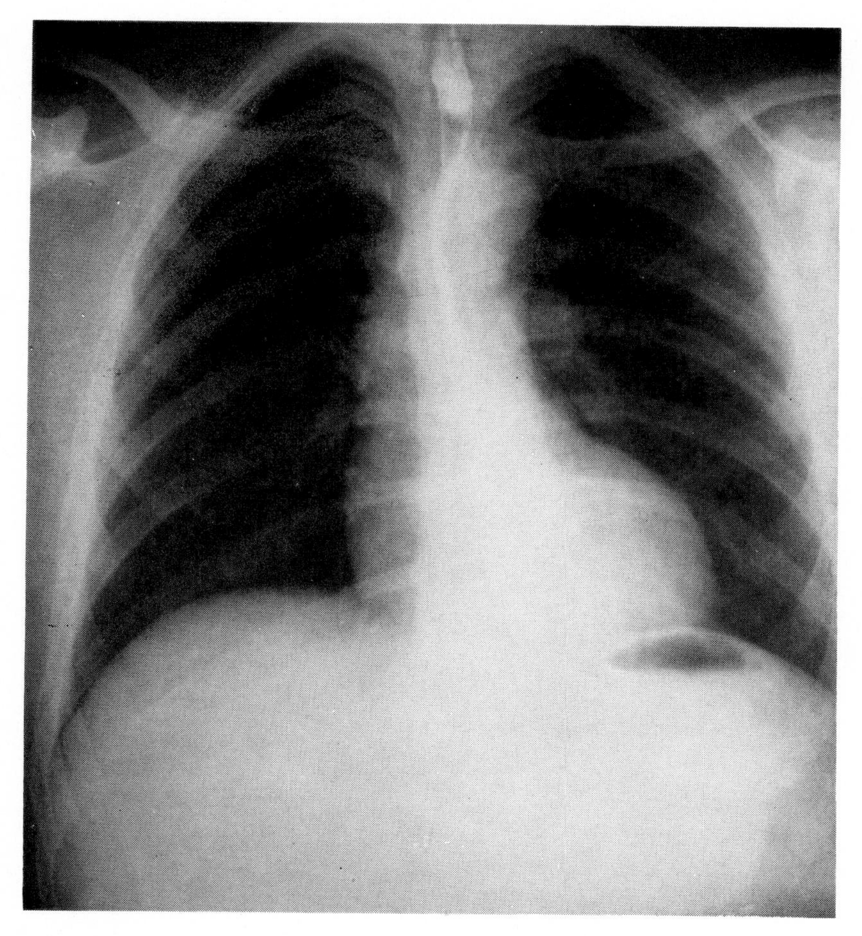

Fig. 3-26B. There was no aortic regurgitation. The thoracic aorta seems normal radiologically down to a point just above the diaphragm, where it became abruptly larger. (From McKusick, V. A.: Ann. Intern. Med. **49**:556, 1958.)

atrium[93] or the right ventricle[165] has been described in cases of the Marfan syndrome.

Dissecting aneurysm may occur as the first aortic complication or may be superimposed on diffuse dilatation of the ascending aorta.[241] There is evidence that dissection may occur in the first decade of life; Wong and associates[420] described fatal rupture of a dissecting aneurysm of the ascending aorta into the pericardial sac in a girl who was 4 years 9 months old. Possibly the oldest reported case of dissecting aneurysm in Marfan's syndrome was that of a 52-year-old woman.[114] The 59-year-old patient referred to earlier died of ruptured dissecting aneurysm.

The patient may survive for a number of years after first dissection of the aorta and even after a "leak" into the pericardium. Because of the aortic regurgitation, which results either from the dissection itself[153,304] or from the associated dilatation of the aortic ring, confusion with rheumatic[209] or syphilitic[139] heart

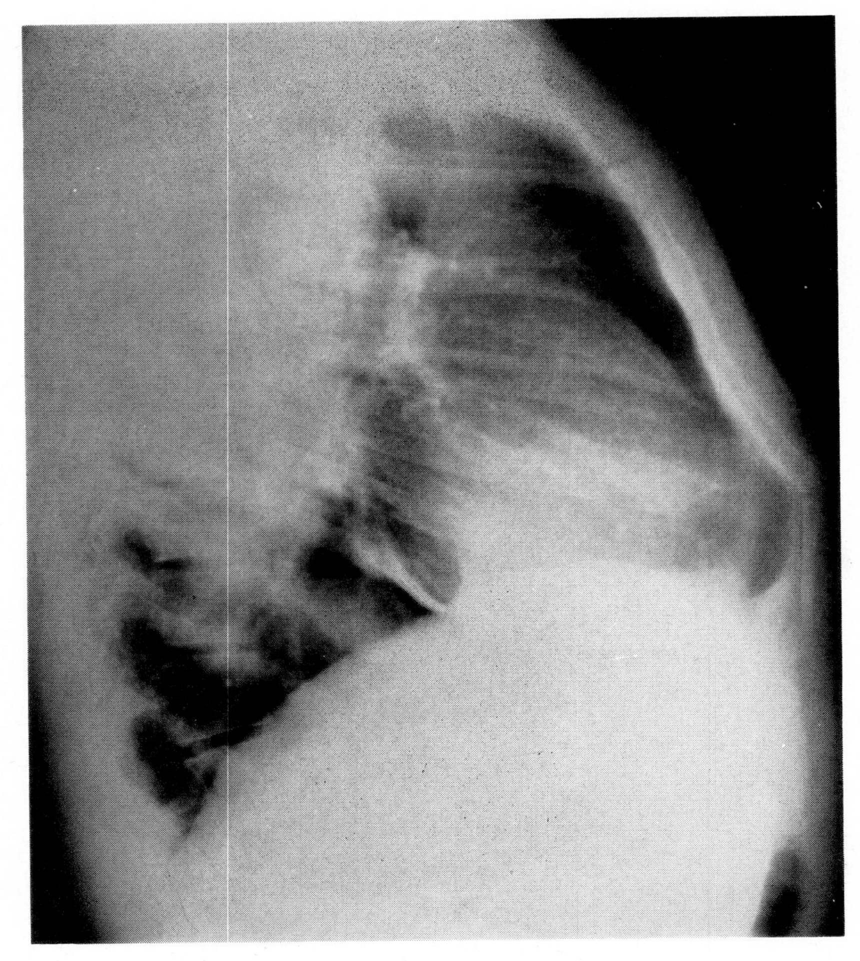

Fig. 3-26C. The deformity of the sternum is evident. (From McKusick, V. A.: Ann. Intern. Med. **49:**556, 1958.)

disease is frequent. In a recently autopsied case at this hospital, leaking of the original dissecting aneurysm into the pericardial sac led to the misdiagnosis of tuberculous pericarditis. The patient survived five years after the first pericardial episode. Dissection apparently occurs with increased frequency during pregnancy.[270,323,329] In chronic dissecting aneurysm of the aorta, there may be little enlargement of the aorta evident on x-ray examination (Figs. 3-22*B* and *C* and 3-27*C* to *E*). In our experience, when full family investigations are made, Marfan's syndrome is found to be a leading "cause" of dissecting aneurysm in persons under the age of 40 years. Gore[137] reported that three of twenty-two patients had arachnodactyly. This, however, was not a detailed clinicogenetic study. At least 17% of the reported cases of dissecting aneurysm in patients under the age of 40 years were recognized instances of the Marfan syndrome.[168] The true proportion is probably higher. For example, Spenser[347] described dissecting aneurysm during pregnancy in a "tall, thin" woman 32 years of age. Griffith and colleagues[146] reported on a dissecting aneurysm in a 34-year-old woman and in her

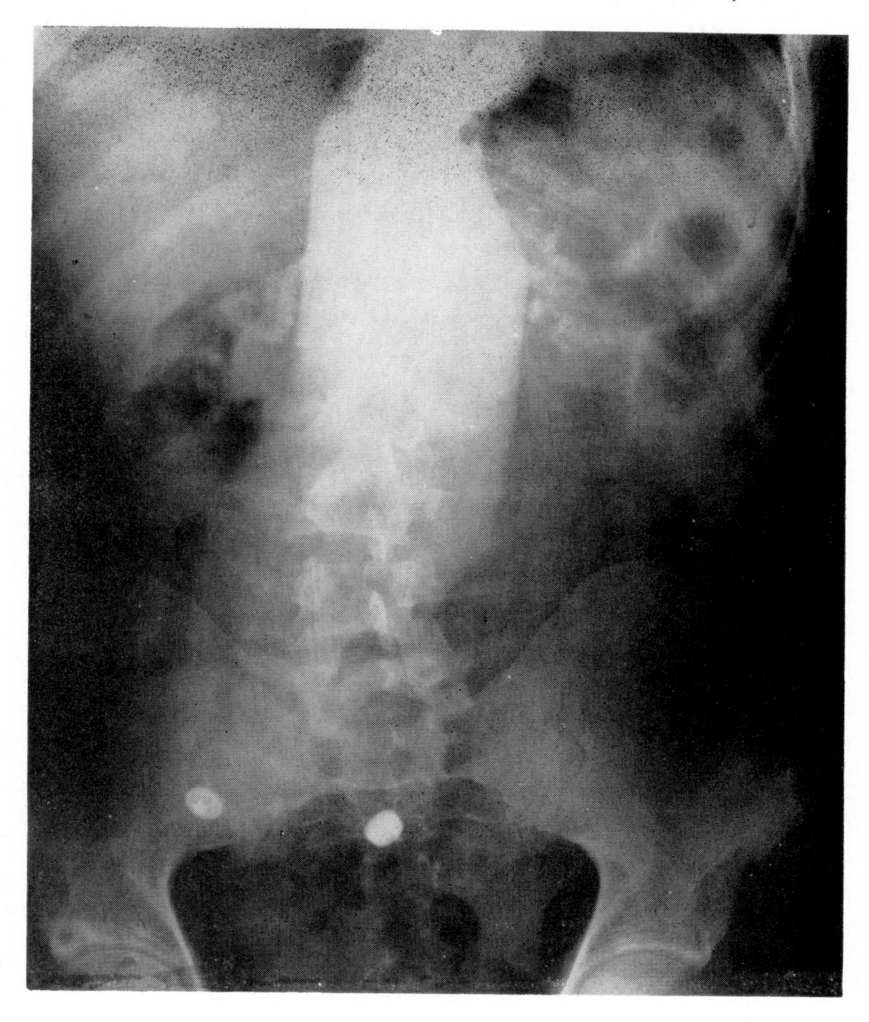

Fig. 3-26D. The enlargement of the aorta was shown by aortography to be cylindric and to extend the full length of the abdomen. The aneurysm was easily felt and seen on abdominal examination. (From McKusick, V. A.: Ann. Intern. Med. **49**:556, 1958.)

14-year-old daughter, both of whom were said to have been "delicate physically."

The occurrence of aortic regurgitation with dissecting aneurysm is well recognized in the English-speaking medical world since the publication of Resnik and Keefer[304] in 1925. Hamman and Apperly's[153] explanation that the aortic regurgitation results from deformation of the aortic ring by the intramural hematoma is the generally accepted one. Obviously another mechanism for the association is preexisting dilatation of the aortic ring, on the basis of the same defect of connective tissue that led to the dissecting aneurysm.

In patients with the Marfan syndrome the sudden development of a murmur, especially a musical buzzing murmur over the ascending aorta, may be a valuable clue to the presence of dissection. The murmur, which may be either systolic or, less commonly, diastolic (Fig. 3-22*D*), appears to be produced by vibrations excited in some of the anomalous structures—lips, fibrous cords, narrowed branches

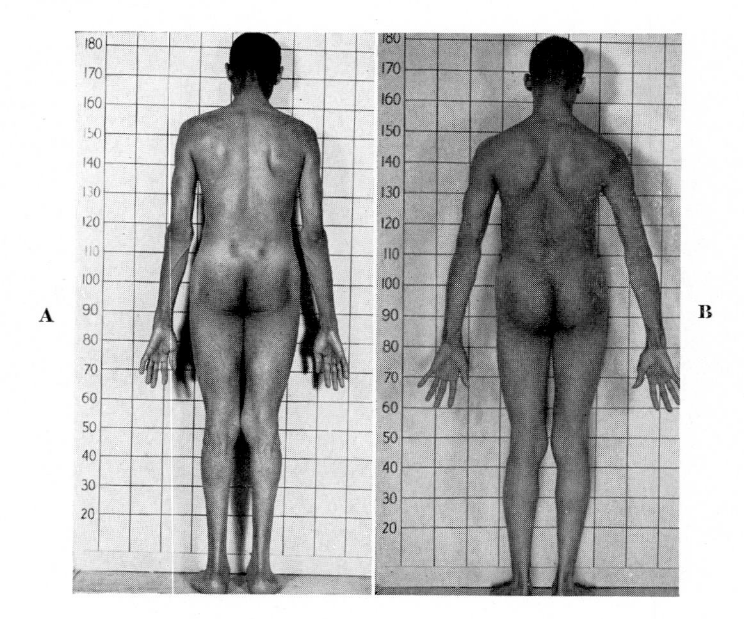

Fig. 3-27A and B. Brothers with the Marfan syndrome without ocular manifestations. **A,** J. M. (544088) had genu valgum, severe pes planus, and dolichostenomelia but no ectopia lentis. In 1950 an episode of chest pain accompanied by pericardial friction rub was interpreted as pericarditis and treated for presumed tuberculous etiology. Signs of aortic regurgitation developed thereafter. In 1953, there occurred at least one other episode of chest pain with pericardial friction rub. The effects of aortic regurgitation became progressively more severe and were the cause of death in April, 1955, at the age of 30 years. Autopsy revealed superannuated dissecting aneurysm of the ascending aorta and dilatation of the aorta above the aortic ring. The aorta had apparently "leaked" into the pericardial sac almost five years before death. (Known to us is a second case [S. T., 691351] in which the patient was still living following leakage about eighteen months before. The diagnosis of Erdheim's disease was established at operation for aneurysm of the ascending aorta. Sando and Helm[318] reported survival of a patient for four and one-half years after acute dissection accompanied by a pericardial friction rub.) **B,** W. M. (702409), 27 years of age, was discovered to have aortic regurgitation when examined in connection with his brother's illness. He had dolichostenomelia and spinal curvature. Although the left ventricle is large, no dilatation of the aorta is demonstrable. He is asymptomatic.

of the aortic arch—created by the dissection (Fig. 3-22*E*). The early diastolic murmur created at the aortic valve may be musical in quality[196] and, as in the case of many musical murmurs, may be very loud. Bean[27] had such a case in his series of precordial noises audible at a distance from the chest. Baer and associates[17] stated that one of their patients had a loud "systolic murmur" audible two inches from the chest. A diastolic murmur loudest at the *right* sternal border is more frequent in the Marfan syndrome than with aortic regurgitation of rheumatic causation.[162]

Another mechanism of aortic regurgitation in the Marfan syndrome is myxomatous transformation of the aortic valve itself.[299] This change may accompany aneurysm of the aorta with dilatation of the aortic ring and in occasional instances may be the sole factor in aortic regurgitation.

In general, the clinical picture of dissecting aneurysm in the Marfan syndrome is little different from that in persons without this syndrome, except that

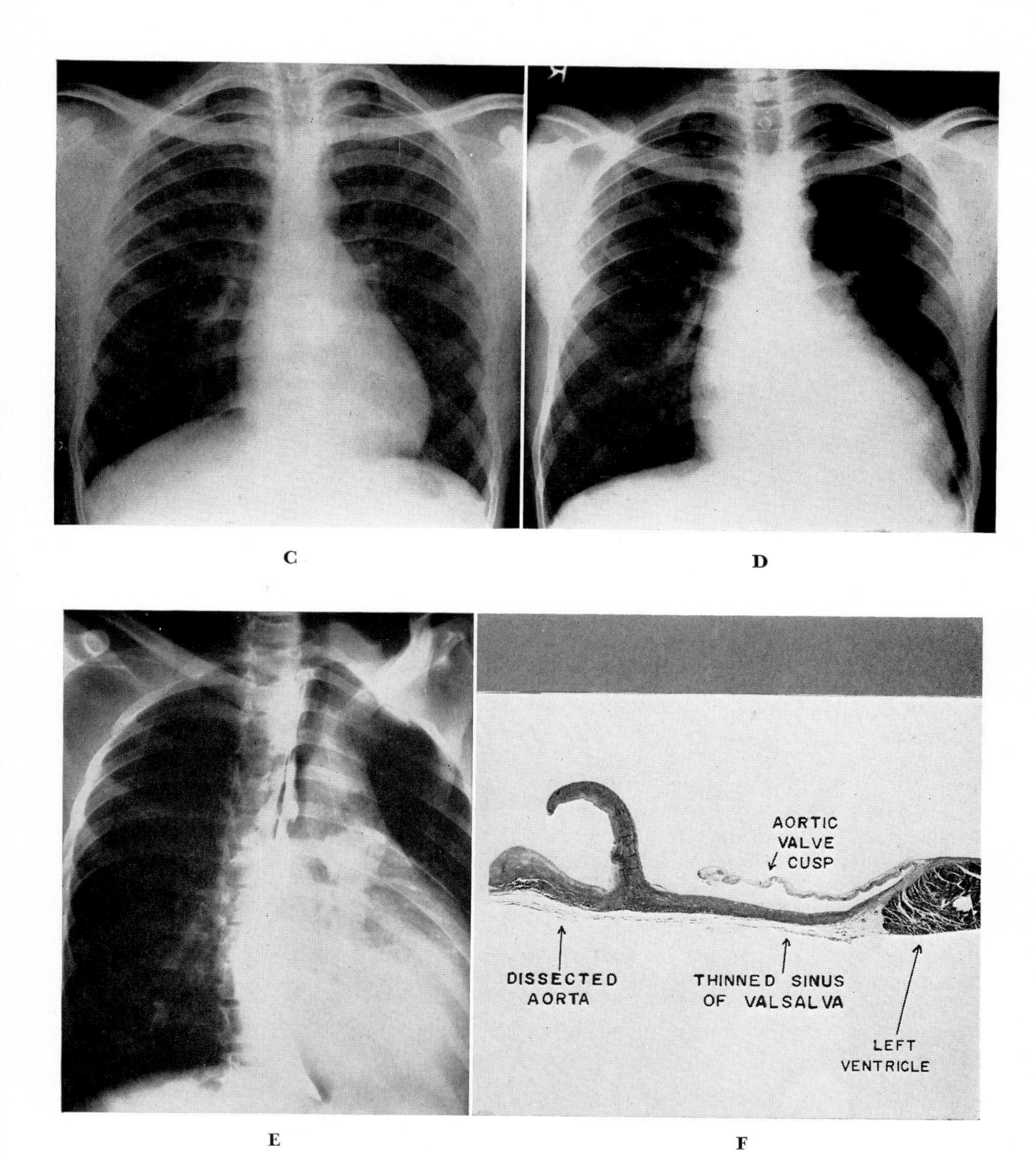

C D

E F

Fig. 3-27C to F. C to E, Series of x-ray films of J. M. **C,** Taken in 1950 about one month after the initial episode of leakage into the pericardial sac. **D** and **E,** The appearance in the last year of life. Enlargement of the aorta is not impressive in **D,** but the main pulmonary artery is prominent. In the right anterior oblique film, **E,** the barium-filled esophagus is displaced by a structure that necropsy demonstrated to be an aneurysm of the sinus of Valsalva. In the left anterior oblique (not shown here), again the aorta does not appear particularly dilated. **F,** Microscopic section (×4) of aortic valve area in J. M. (see **A**). The old dissection, the thinning of the sinus of Valsalva, and the minor fibrous thickening of the aortic valve are demonstrated.

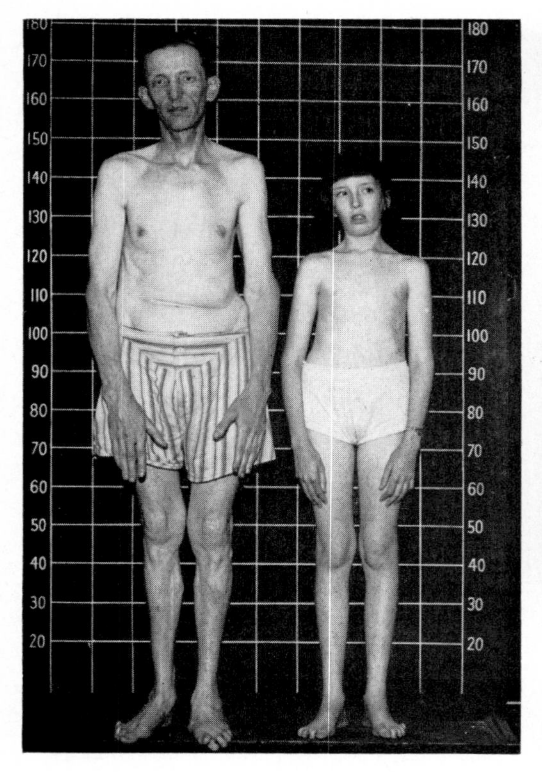

A

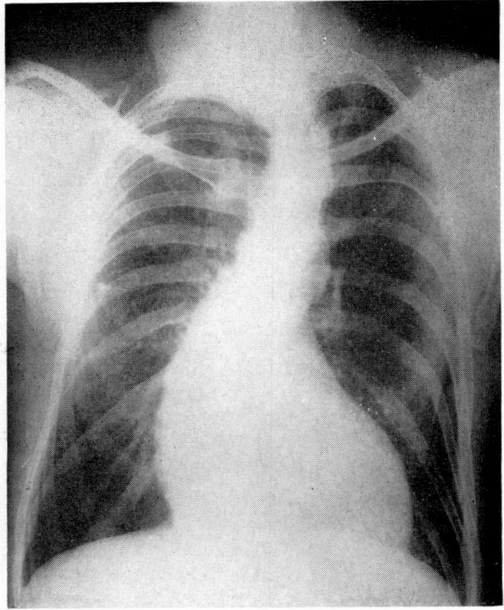

B

Fig. 3-28. A, Both the man (E. F., 194515) and his daughter (M. V. F., 565451) have bilateral subluxation of the lenses, spinal curvature, and dolichostenomelia (long, thin extremities). The man has had femoral and inguinal hernias repaired. The girl is only 9 years old. In 1950 the man had no cardiac murmurs. In 1953 he was found to have well-marked aortic regurgitation. Photograph, June, 1953. At this time the patient also had a crescendo holosystolic murmur of partially musical quality at the apex (see Fig. 317 in reference 232). **B,** The chest x-ray film of the man in **A** reveals no apparent dilatation of the ascending aorta. (The scoliosis obscures the picture.) Fluoroscopy likewise failed to establish dilatation of the aorta. **C,** Photograph of the daughter shown in **A,** August, 1958. (**A** and **B** from McKusick, V. A.: Circulation **11**:321, 1955.)

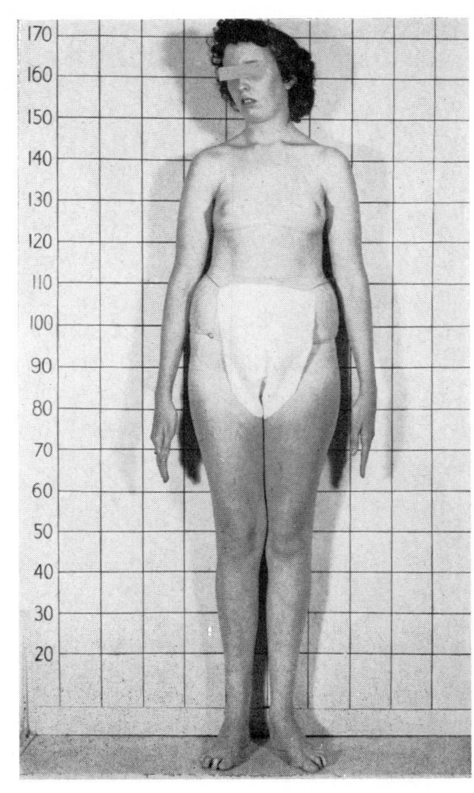

C

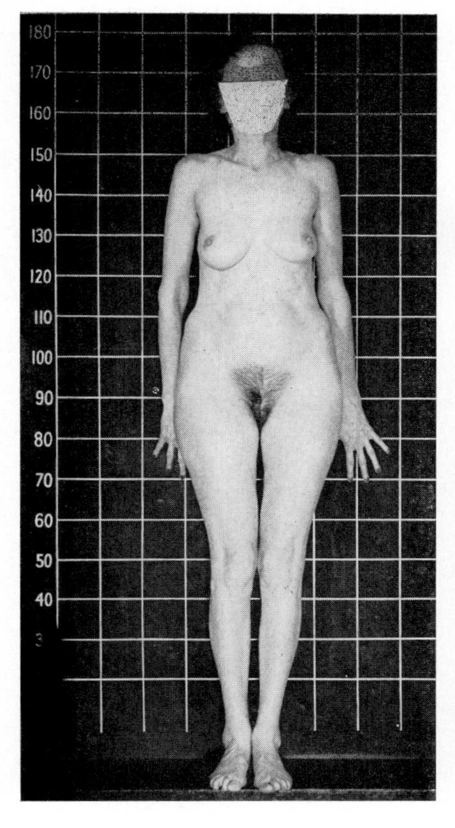

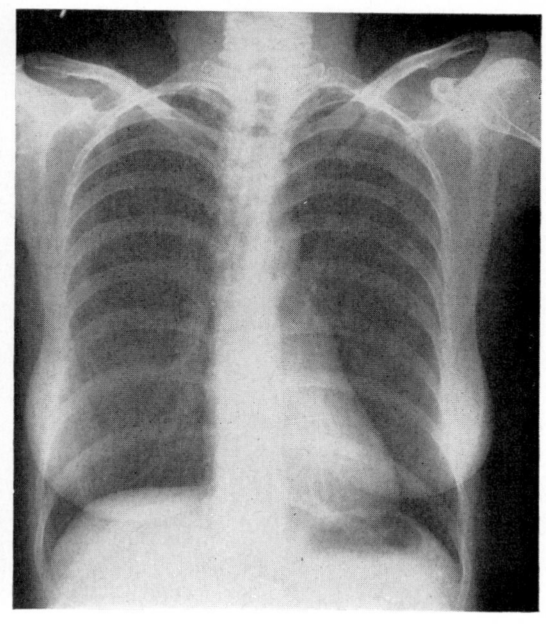

A B

Fig. 3-29. A, M. B. (697662), 46 years old. Ectopia lentis, moderate dolichostenomelia, and spinal curvature. **B,** Although at the time of these studies (February, 1955) the patient was asymptomatic and the cardiovascular silhouette normal, an aortic diastolic murmur was present. The patient died in December, 1957. Diagnosis: aortic aneurysm. (Systolic clicks were recorded at the apex in 1955. The multiple clicks were described by the stethoscopist as a systolic crunch. Because of the mild chest deformity and the general loose-jointedness, the clicks are thought to have been produced by movement of joints of the thoracic cage. See Fig. 146 in reference 232.)

in the Marfan syndrome aortic regurgitation is more likely to be present (as a result of preexisting dilatation in the first part of the aorta), the average age is about twenty years younger than that for other dissecting aneurysms, and hypertension is usually absent. As in any dissecting aneurysm, the patient may demonstrate inequality of the radial pulses.[280]

I have not observed calcification of the ascending aorta in the Marfan syndrome. This fact may be helpful in differentiating the aortic involvement of the Marfan syndrome from that of syphilis, in which calcification is frequent.[228]

McKeown[229] described a 21-year-old white man with arachnodactyly but "no other stigmata of Marfan's syndrome." The patient died from myocardial infarction resulting from dissecting limited to the right coronary artery.

Involvement of the aortic cusps has already been described. The aortic valve

A

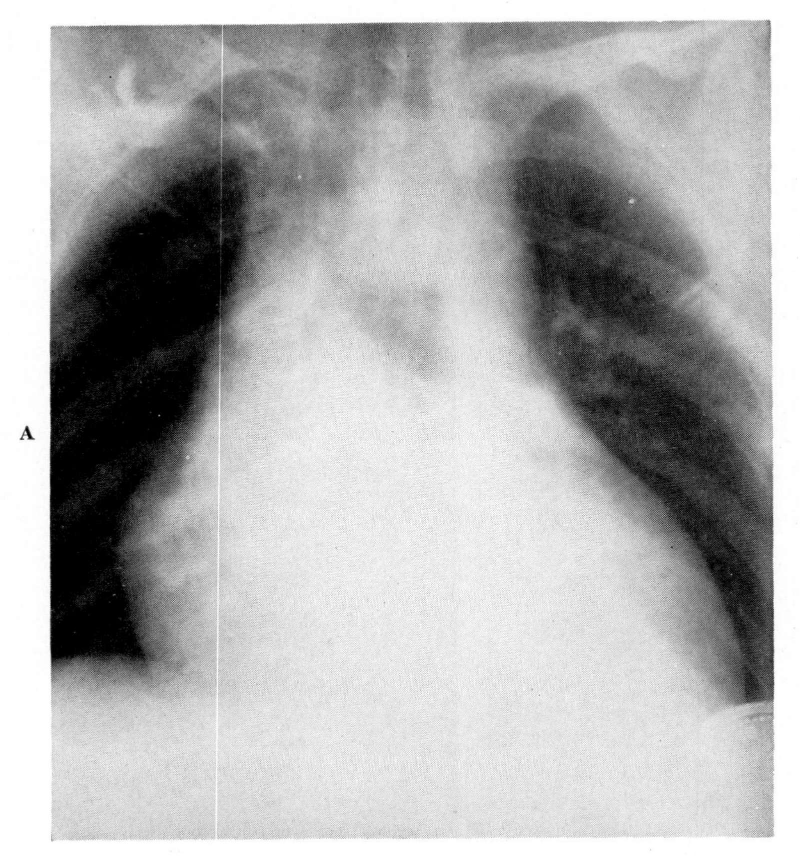

Fig. 3-30A and B. S. C. (575946), a veterinarian, had ectopia lentis and skeletal proportions of the Marfan syndrome. He died at the age of 37 years during an attempt at surgical repair of the ascending aorta. With the episode of dissection in October, 1955, a musical systolic murmur developed over the ascending aorta. This sign, a valuable diagnostic clue in such cases, probably owes its origin to vibration in intimal lip or fibrous bands in the ascending aorta. Angiocardiogram showed striking dilatation of the base of the aorta within the shadow of the heart, surprisingly little enlargement of the later portion of the ascending aorta, failure of opacification of the innominate artery, the lumen of which was tamponaded by a medial dissection, and finally, pseudocoarctation of the type so typical of the Marfan syndrome. (From McKusick, V. A.: Ann. Intern. Med. **49:**556, 1958.)

is sometimes bicuspid (Fig. 3-36); whether this is the case in the Marfan syndrome more often than one would expect with this relatively frequent abnormality is not certain. Frieden and co-workers[126] described ruptured aortic cusp in association with cystic medial necrosis of the aorta in a 42-year-old male patient with hyperextensible joints, chest deformity, severe flat feet, and bilateral retinal detachments—features strongly suggestive of the Marfan syndrome. Two of the man's children had blue sclerae and hyperextensible joints.

The mitral cusps and chordae tendineae may be redundant, with resulting mitral regurgitation. Subacute bacterial endocarditis may become engrafted on the valvular abnormality.[57,231,273,394,421] (See Fig. 3-26*A* and *B* for a case of bacterial endocarditis with the Marfan syndrome.) Murmurs of obscure origin are fre-

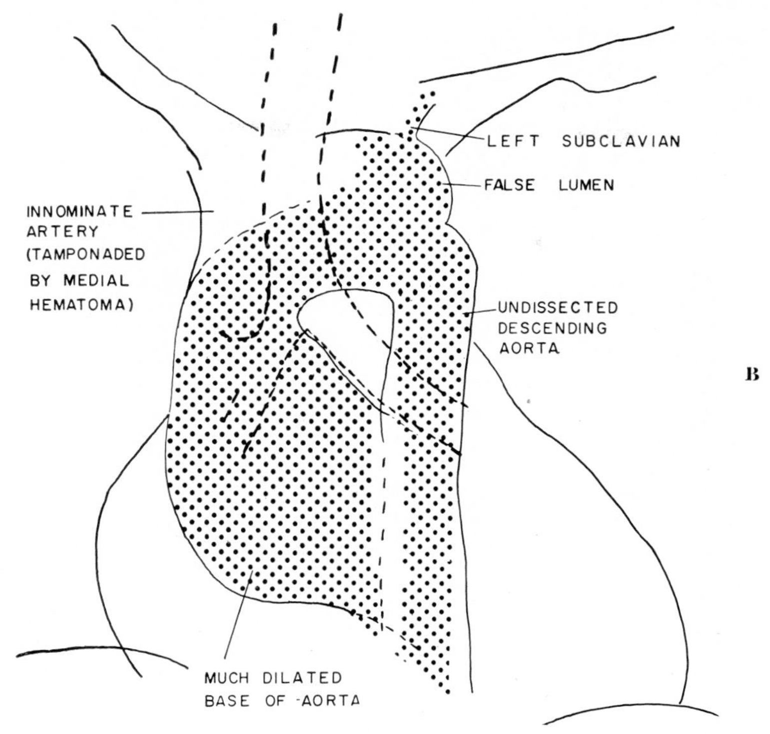

Fig. 3-30, cont'd. For legend see opposite page.

quently encountered. Some may be on the basis of redundant chordae tendineae with incompetence of atrioventricular valves. These murmurs may be partially musical. In one patient (S. C. 575946) with a musical mitral systolic murmur, autopsy revealed a tear at the insertion of the posterior mitral cusp, amounting to a partial avulsion of the cusp.

A striking early systolic click heard not only at the aortic area but also at the apex is a frequent sign of dilatation of the ascending aorta in the Marfan syndrome. It is thought to represent a snapping of the aortic wall early in systolic ejection.[232] Extracardiac clicks and other extraneous sounds are frequent and some may be attributable to a combination of thoracic deformity, the loose-jointedness of the bony thorax, and the cardiac enlargement. However, intracardiac origin of some systolic clicks, particularly those associated with a late systolic murmur, is supported by recent observations.

It is now clear that involvement of the mitral and possibly the tricuspid valve with regurgitation may be the predominant cardiovascular lesion in the Marfan syndrome and may lead to early death. Figs. 3-6*A* and 3-36 illustrate such cases. Redundancy of the chordae tendineae may be responsible, at least in part, for the valvular dysfunction. Tricuspid, or even quinquecuspid, mitral valves have been present in some cases. See Fig. 3-18*C* for reference to mitral anomaly.

It has been demonstrated in recent years[173] that a late systolic murmur is often produced by mitral regurgitation of a particular type. Retroversion of a redundant posterior mitral cusp, with leak from the left ventricle to the atrium in late

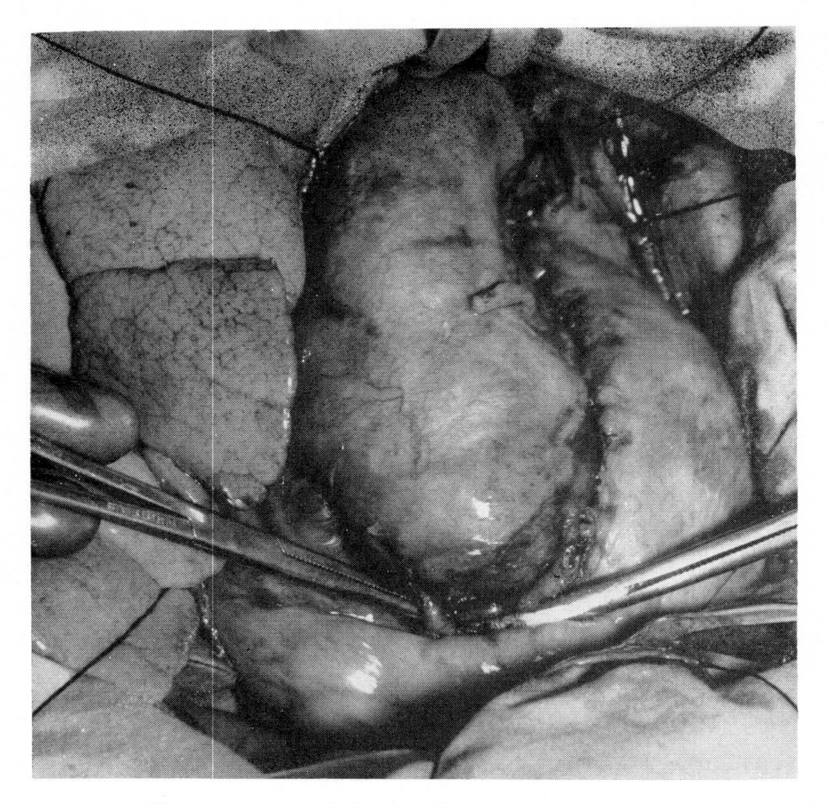

Fig. 3-30C. The gourdlike appearance of the ascending aorta as exposed through a surgical incision in the right interior thorax. A clamp lies under the right coronary artery. Unusually high displacement of this vessel made operation difficult, as did also the high extension of the aortic commissures. The patient died during surgery. The mother of this patient died of the cardiac complications of the Marfan syndrome at the age of 40 years. An older sister of the patient has the Marfan syndrome. (From McKusick, V. A.: Ann. Intern. Med. **49**:556, 1958.)

systole, has been demonstrated by cineangiocardiography (e.g. B. H. 941257). The murmur is of a type that was earlier interpreted as of extracardiac origin.[232] It often is of rather musical quality and in these instances may be quite loud, being audible over most of the back as well as the precordium centering around the apex. The musical quality may be present only intermittently and may be accentuated by exertion or excitement. Multiple systolic clicks in mid and late systole are frequent accompaniments of the late systolic murmur. These clicks may initiate the murmur. It is likely that they are also generated at the redundant posterior mitral leaflet.

Other organic causes of a late systolic murmur[327] include hypertrophic subaortic stenosis, coarctation of the aorta, and the postmyocardial infarction state. Bulging of the posterior or mural leaflet of the mitral valve toward the left atrium in late systole in a patient with the Marfan syndrome, accompanied by late systolic murmur, was demonstrated by Segal and associates.[326]

Major-grade mitral regurgitation as the predominant cardiovascular lesion in the Marfan syndrome has been recognized with increasing frequency in recent

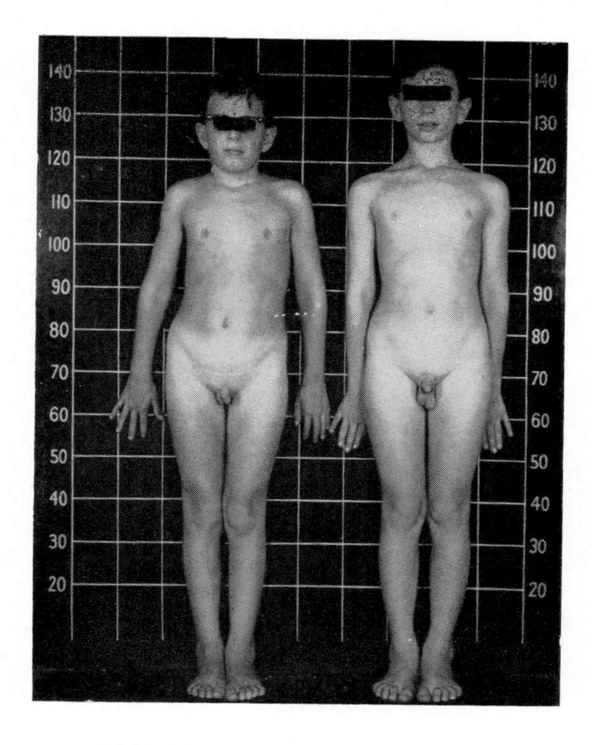

Fig. 3-30D. The proband's sons, one affected (left) and one unaffected, are seen here. R. C. (783343), the affected boy, $8\frac{3}{4}$ years old, has grossly visible dislocation of the lenses, myopia, and mild thoracic kyphosis. The normal brother is 12 years old; another brother, 4 years of age, is also normal. (From McKusick, V. A.: Ann. Intern. Med. **49:**556, 1958.)

years.[261,299,328] In Miller and Pearson's patient[261] the distribution of the systolic murmur simulated that of aortic stenosis, and at autopsy a jet lesion of the left atrial wall underlying the aortic ring was found. Read and co-workers[299] referred to the condition as the "floppy valve syndrome." Further study by Keech and colleagues[191a] tends to corroborate the diagnosis of the Marfan syndrome in these patients. Myxomatous transformation of the mitral valve was the anatomic basis for the mitral regurgitation. Most such patients are long considered to have rheumatic heart disease. It is undoubtedly relevant that the pathophysiologic effects of mitral valve involvement in the Marfan syndrome have been fully appreciated only in the era of left heart catheterization and contrast radiocardiography, as well as of prosthetic replacement of the mitral valve.

Calcification of the mitral annulus has been demonstrated in a number of instances.[43,261,373] We have observed one instance of calcified annulus fibrosus mitralis associated with "floppy" mitral valve and severe mitral regurgitation that was incorrectly interpreted as rheumatic (P. R., 559979). Although ocular stigmata of the Marfan syndrome were absent and the skeletal features only suggestive, the patient's son has the full-blown disorder.

I had previously thought that occasionally the pathophysiologic effects of interatrial septal defect can dominate the clinical picture. However, the only patient in my experience who might corroborate this impression (Fig. 3-36) proved on autopsy to have an intact atrial septum. Because of the gracile habitus that patients with atrial septal defect frequently display, the Marfan syndrome is frequently suspected. Such patients indeed have arachnodactyly; however, most do not have ectopia lentis or the characteristic family history to allow one to conclude that the true Marfan syndrome is present.

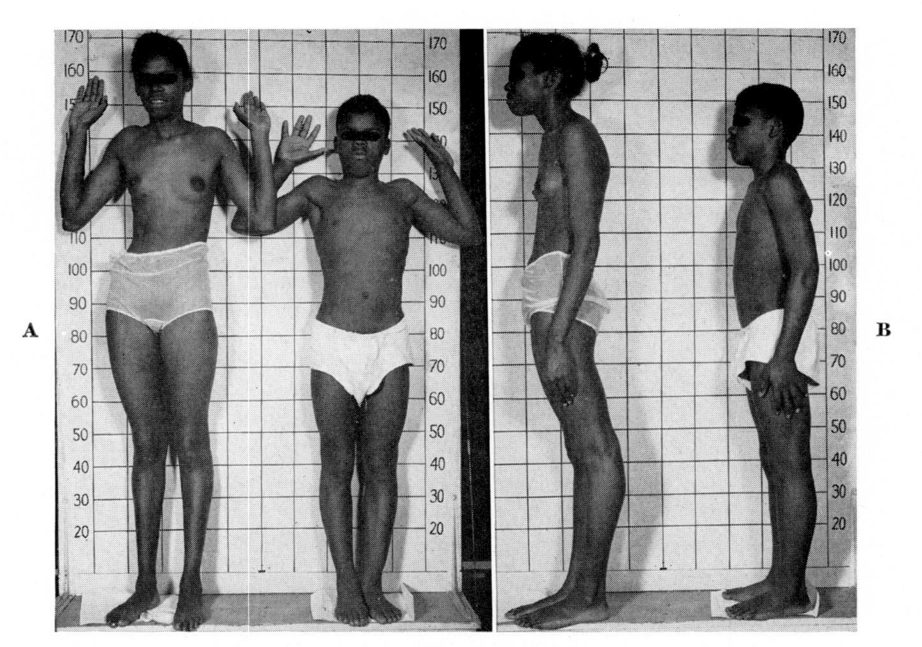

Fig. 3-31A and B. Fourteen-year-old S. S. (366788), II-6 of the pedigree (see **C**), and her normal 12-year-old brother, II-7. Note the kyphoscoliosis, genu recurvatum, excessively long legs, and strabismus. Ectopia lentis is present.

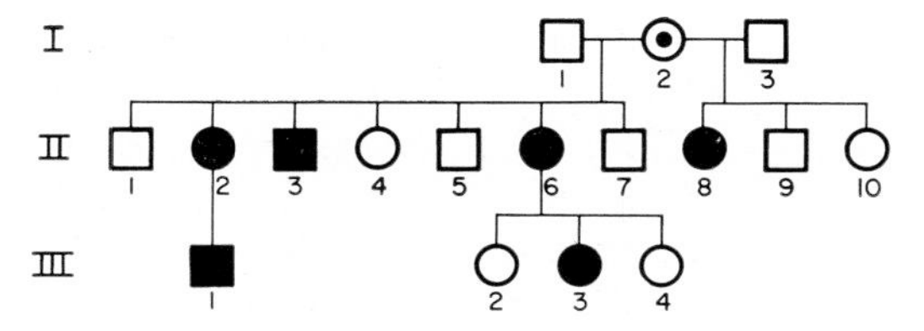

Fig. 3-31C. This pedigree illustrates how submerged the manifestations of Marfan's snydrome can be. Individual I-2 had had at least three affected offspring by one husband and one affected offspring by a second husband. Both husbands are unequivocally normal from the skeletal, ocular, and vascular points of view. The mother is 5 feet 8 inches tall, moderately long of limb, poorly muscled, and severely myopic (—6D), but has no ectopia lentis by careful ophthalmoscopic examination. (For the last I am indebted to Dr. J. E. Mishler of Atlantic City, N.J.) These manifestations are consistent with *forme fruste* of the Marfan syndrome but would not be recognizable as such without the knowledge of this pedigree. (Status of pedigree in 1959, six years after photographs in **A** and **B** were taken.)

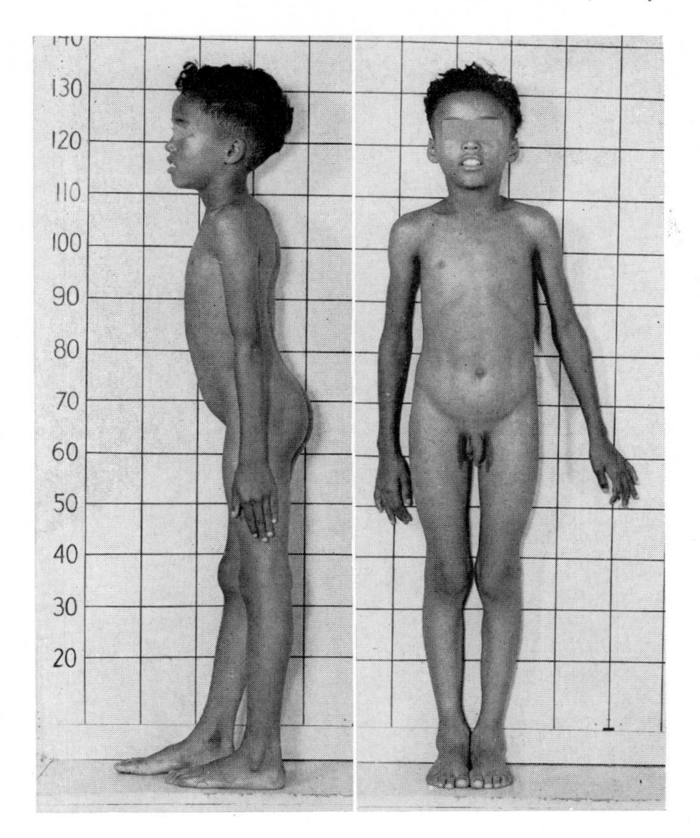

Fig. 3-31D. Two views of S. S. (719604), individual III-1 of the pedigree in **C.** Born March 1, 1948. Photograph, Aug. 6, 1956. When first examined at home in 1953, the patient was judged to be normal. It is now clear that slight bilateral lens dislocation is present. A faint aortic diastolic murmur was heard in 1958. The chest is asymmetrically deformed to a minor degree. Arachnodactyly and loose-jointedness are not impressive.

In 1955 I wrote as follows: "Notwithstanding careless statements of previous reviews, no autopsy-confirmed or even clinically convincing case of interventricular septal defect has been reported." Since that time, however, at least one case of autopsy-proved ventricular septal defect with the Marfan syndrome* has been reported,[378] and I have had an opportunity to study the patient in one such case, a 15-year-old girl with typical Marfan snydrome including ectopia lentis and clinically typical ventricular septal defect confirmed by cardiac catheterization (Fig. 3-39).† Ross and Gerbode[310] described a 15-year-old white girl with typical ocular and skeletal features of the Marfan syndrome. An unusual type of ventricular

*In this case[378] the diagnosis of the Marfan syndrome is in some question, since there was no ectopia lentis and no positive family history. The patient had both patent ductus arteriosus and ventricular septal defect. The habitus suggesting that of the true Marfan syndrome may have been merely that rather often seen with these lesions.

†I am indebted to Dr. Donald Nelson and Dr. Peter Luchsinger of the District of Columbia General Hospital, Washington, D. C., for calling this patient to my attention and providing catheterization data.

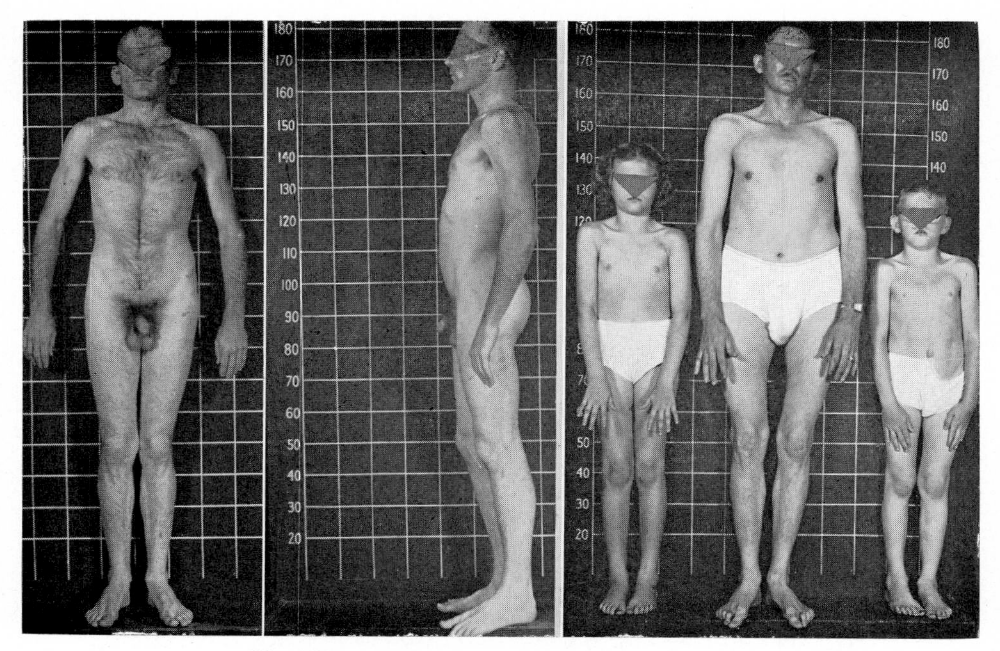

Fig. 3-32 **Fig. 3-33**

Fig. 3-32. C. H. (687485), 28 years old. Ectopia lentis. Lenses correcting for aphakia worn from age of 5 years. Brother, father, two paternal aunts, and two cousins are living and have the Marfan syndrome. Paternal grandmother and great grandmother likewise had it. Father blind in both eyes and aunt blind in one eye from secondary glaucoma. Patient in Army for forty-five months. Note deformity of knees. This and many of the other members of this group of photographs make it clear that on superficial inspection the habitus may not seem impressively or abnormally dolichostenomelic.

Fig. 3-33. Father, E. C., and two children, Anna (593933), 9 years of age, and Robert (441759), 7 years of age, all with ectopia lentis and skeletal proportions that, albeit not striking, are consistent with the Marfan syndrome. The father's brother had had a "leaky heart" for several years and died suddenly at the age of 35 years.

septal defect was repaired by open heart surgery. An aneurysm of the membranous septum bulged into the right ventricular outflow tract and displayed a fenestration (Fig. 3-38). It is attractive to suppose that the weakness of the membranous septum was part of the generalized disorder of connective tissue and that stress-fatigue was responsible for the fenestration. The murmur heard at an early age may have been produced by partial obstruction of right ventricular outflow, and the fenestration of the aneurysm may have occurred sometime after birth rather than being congenital. (Aneurysm of the membranous septum has been recognized in patients without stigmata of connective tissue disease.[21,70])

In Cockayne's case[78] the diagnosis of ventricular septal defect was only suspected clinically. There is a report[214] of possible tetralogy of Fallot with Marfan's syndrome. Two cases of tetralogy of Fallot with stigmata suggestive of the Marfan syndrome (see Fig. 3-40 for one of these) have come to my attention,[231] but the absence of involvement of other members of the family and the failure of ectopia lentis to be found in the patients make the diagnosis of the Marfan syn-

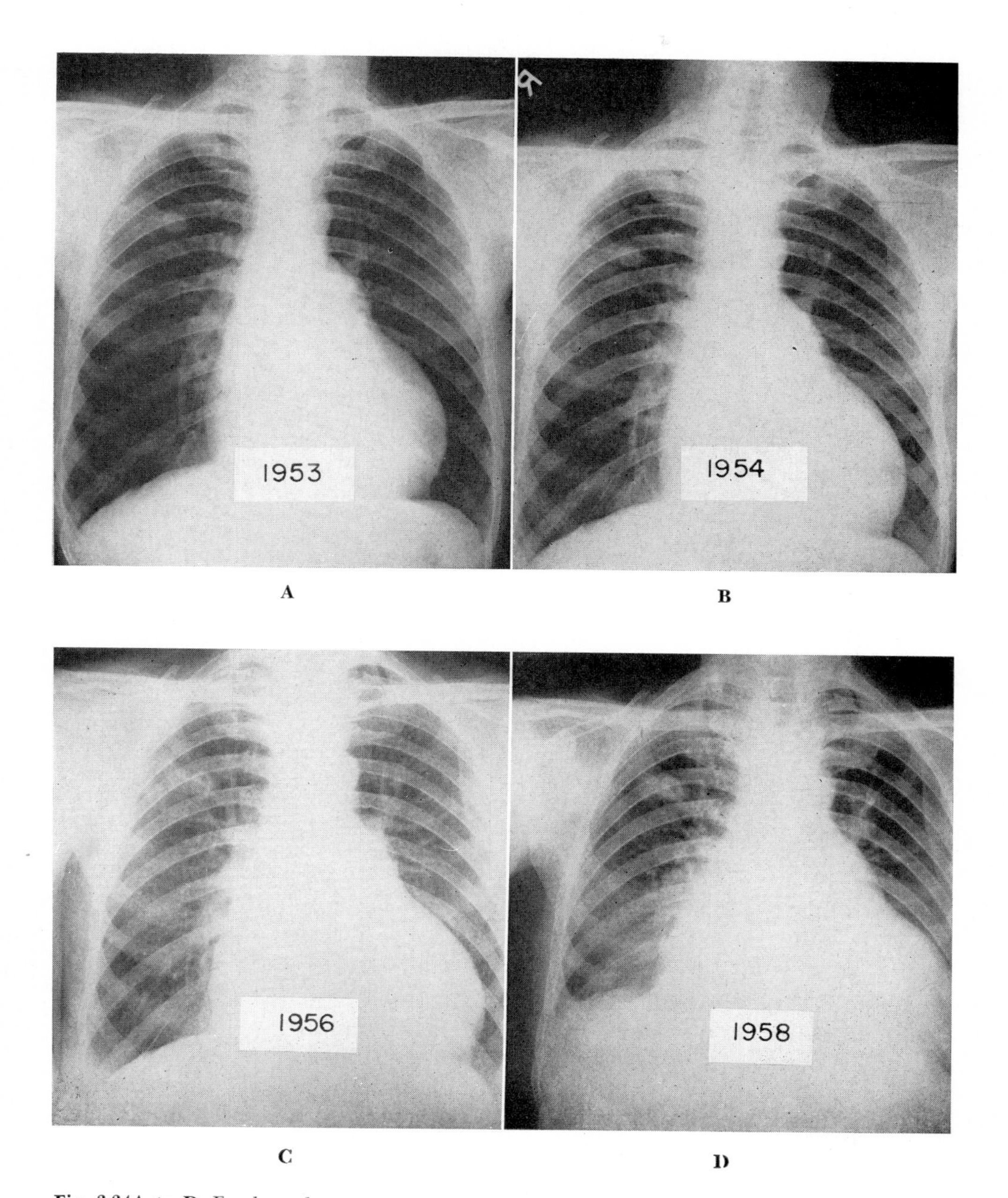

Fig. 3-34A to D. For legend see next page.

E

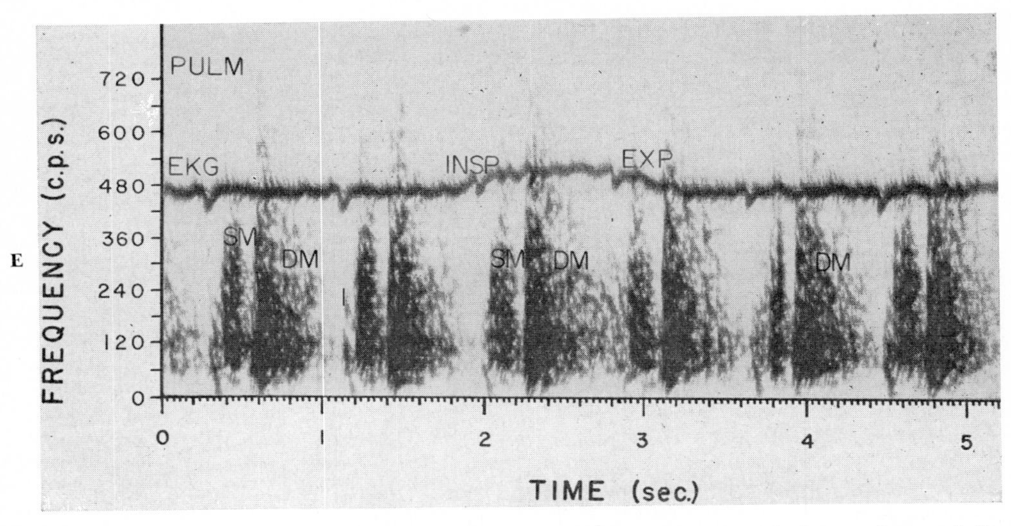

Fig. 3-34. Eight-year survival after onset of cardiac symptoms in the Marfan syndrome. A. D. (341643), a Negro male born in 1907, was well until 1950, when there was onset of chest pain and dyspnea. Late in 1951 chest pain and attacks of paroxysmal nocturnal dyspnea became especially frequent. The chest pain had the pattern typical of angina pectoris. At first it was relieved by nitroglycerin; later this drug seemed to have little effect. Throughout the eight years of observation the murmur and other signs of aortic regurgitation were present. Also, at the apex what was interpreted as an Austin Flint murmur was described. During the last three years of life a bizarre "crackling" systolic murmur was described at the apex. It was also described as "crunching" and compared to "footsteps in gravel." It disappeared on deep inspiration. Numerous serologic tests for syphilis and two treponemal immobilization tests were negative. Progressive widening of the QRS complexes, to a maximum of 0.13 second, occurred in the period of observation. Atrial fibrillation developed in the last two weeks of life. The patient died in 1958. The man was described as "tall," "thin," "asthenic," and "long-armed." His height was twice measured as 70½ inches. Visual acuity was essentially normal. Although no slit-lamp examination was performed, numerous standard ophthalmoscopic examinations showed no abnormality. There was no hernia or spinal deformity. The patient had had no children; his family was not available for study.

A to **D,** X-ray films: **A,** 1953; **B,** 1954; **C,** 1956; **D,** Three days before death in 1958. Dilatation of the aorta is conspicuous in its absence. The pulmonary artery segment is prominent throughout. **E,** Spectral phonocardiogram in pulmonary area, January, 1957. The findings are typical of severe aortic regurgitation, with no features pathognomonic for the Marfan syndrome.

Autopsy revealed findings similar to those shown in Fig. 3-24*C* except that the marked dilatation was limited more to the area of the sinuses of Valsalva. The histologic changes included loss of elastic fibers, spaces occupied by metachromatically staining material, whorls of disorganized smooth muscle fibers, and much dilated vasa vasorum.

drome uncertain. I am inclined to think that these are not cases of the Marfan syndrome. In yet another case (Fig. 3-41), dolichostenomelia (without, however, an abnormal segment ratio), congenital clouding of the cornea, and large interventricular septal defect are associated. Four siblings, two older and two younger, are unaffected as are all other members of the family, in so far as can be determined. Furthermore, no abnormality of the lens is detectable. This case seems most likely the result of infection or other abnormality of the intrauterine environment.

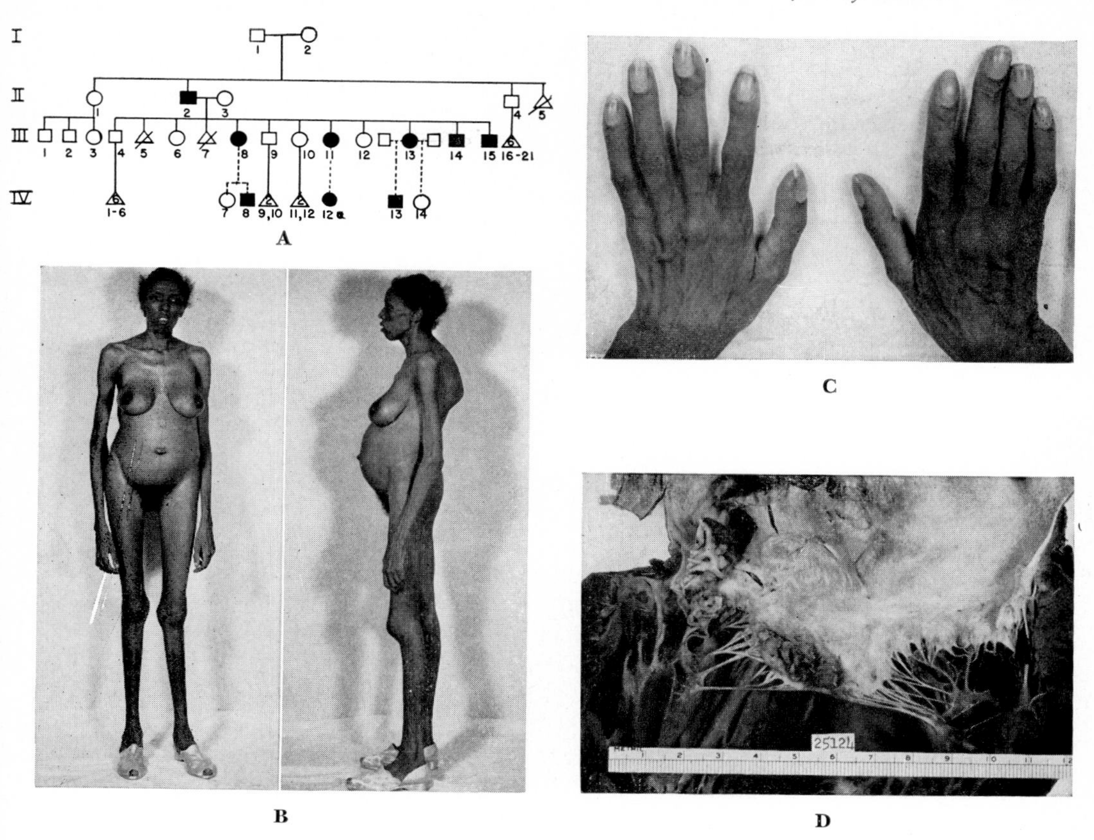

Fig. 3-35. A, Pedigree of the family of patient M. E. R. (III-11). Individual II-2 may have been the original mutant. However, illegitimacy is so much more frequent than mutation that one can never be certain. **B,** Patient M. E. R. **C,** The combination of arachnodactyly and clubbing of the fingers relates to Marfan's disease and subacute bacterial endocarditis from which the patient M. E. R. suffered. **D,** The mitral valve, showing bacterial vegetation.

M. E. R. (J.H.H. 176836), a Negro woman born in 1929, is a member of a family that has been known to Johns Hopkins Hospital for about twenty-five years and in which at least nine cases of Marfan's syndrome (including this patient) have occurred. (The patient is individual III-11 in the pedigree presented in **A.**) The father of the patient, a well-documented instance of this syndrome, died of dissecting aneurysm of the aorta at the age of 43 years. Of four siblings of the patient with this disease, three have signs consistent with interatrial septal defect.

The patient demonstrated bilateral ectopia lentis, severe myopia, pronounced dolichostenomelia, very poor muscular development, severe kyphoscoliosis, pes planus, and, by x-ray films, pulmonary emphysema with bleb formation. She recalled nothing suggestive of acute rheumatic fever. Most of her life she had been subject to exertional dyspnea.

The patient became pregnant early in November, 1953. After about four months there was increase in her lifelong exertional dyspnea and the appearance of ankle edema and orthopnea, which required two pillows. In early April, 1954, there was onset of evening fever, night sweats, and aching of joints, especially knees and ankles. Tender red spots appeared on the palms and soles.

Physical examination revealed as new findings, petechiae, embolic nodes of the palms, splinter hemorrhages of the nail beds, and clubbed fingers. A loud harsh systolic murmur was audible over the entire precordium, and the second pulmonic sound was accentuated.

Six blood cultures demonstrated a *Streptococcus viridans,* which was late in growing out and atypical in morphology due probably to streptomycin and penicillin that had been administered

Legend continued.

before admission to the Osler Medical Clinic. The patient's white blood cell count was 10,000 to 12,000 and hematocrit 26%. Treatment with penicillin in large doses was instituted with seemingly successful results.

On the patient's twentieth day in the hospital premature labor began as a result of septic infarction of the placenta, and an infant weighing 1,700 grams was born. The infant, which demonstrated pronounced dolichostenomelia, lived only a very few minutes. Autopsy in the case of the infant revealed no cardiovascular lesion, and the cause of death is not completely clear. There was an abnormality of pulmonary lobation such as is frequently seen in the Marfan syndrome. (See Fig. 3-18*I*.)

The patient died of uncontrollable heart failure about two weeks after delivery. **D** shows the mitral valve with its vegetations in this case. No evidence of rheumatism was discovered. The media of the aorta and the pulmonary artery showed extensive chromotropic degeneration.

Chest x-ray film in this patient (not illustrated) showed increased bronchovascular markings and evidences of bleb formation. At autopsy all lobes of the lungs, especially the upper ones, were cystic. Some of the cysts were as much as several centimeters in diameter. They were lined by columnar epithelium and contained strands of smooth muscle in the walls. (See Fig. 3-45.)

(From McKusick, V. A.: Circulation **11**:321, 1955.)

Van Buchem[389] concluded that mild pulmonary stenosis was present in one of his patients. However, the systolic gradient across the valve was only 35 mm. Hg. It is possible that there was only relative pulmonary stenosis from dilatation of the pulmonary artery (which was present).

Much has been written about cardiac disability in pectus excavatum[109,114,257,368] Furthermore, since originally proposed by Flesch[122] in 1873, excessive longitudinal growth of the ribs has been thought to be the mechanism in many cases. As stated above, this appears to be the pathogenesis of the pectus excavatum in the Marfan syndrome. The hereditary nature of pectus excavatum has been appreciated.[284,316,343,361] Many times the patients with pectus excavatum are described as being unusually tall and thin, with spinal curvatures. Despite all these considerations, it has not been properly appreciated that the pectus excavatum may be but one manifestation of a generalized disorder of connective tissue, in which primary involvement of the cardiovascular system may occur. In Fig. 3-43 we have presented the case of a 24-year-old man with severe pectus excavatum, who died of rupture of the aorta shortly after surgical repair of the chest deformity.[42] Autopsy revealed aortic changes typical of the Marfan syndrome. An aortic diastolic murmur had been present before operation. In the surgical literature, there are two cases that may have been instances of the Marfan syndrome. One patient[209] was 6 years old and was described as having "systolic and diastolic murmurs and cardiac incompetence." The other,[298] 23 years old and 74 inches tall, had congestive heart failure and atrial fibrillation and was specifically described by his physician as thin, gangling, loose-jointed, and round-shouldered. In another instance, a case reported by Sweet,[369] the patient has been discovered to have typical Marfan's syndrome.[409]

Wachtel and associates[397] suggest that cardiac disability in pectus excavatum can result from four factors: (1) Due to twisting and distortion of the great veins, venous return may be impeded. (2) Restriction of diastolic expansion may further limit delivery of more blood on demand. (3) Impingement on the atria leads to supraventricular arrhythmias. (4) Respiratory reserve is decreased from impairment of the intercostal component of respiration. The heart may appear

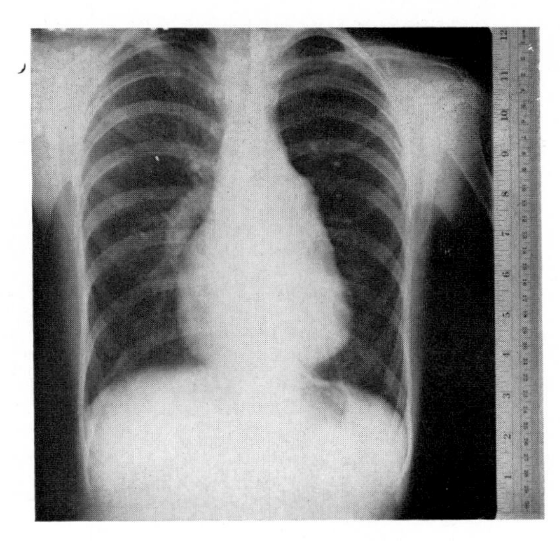

Fig. 3-36. X-ray film in case of Marfan syndrome in which atrial septal defect was incorrectly thought to be present.

M.E.C. (J.H.H. A98174), born in 1940, was first referred to Dr. Helen B. Taussig in November, 1952, for investigation of a congenital heart defect with paroxysmal tachycardia. The father was 76 inches tall and asthenic and had a spinal curvature and ectopia lentis but no evidence of cardiovascular abnormality. A single sibling, male, was unaffected.

In this case a heart murmur had been described before the age of 2 years. Except that she never gained weight well and could not keep up with the other children at play, the patient was relatively well until April, 1952, when she had a first attack of paroxysmal tachycardia lasting several hours. Two more attacks occurred, one in May and a second in September, 1952.

The patient was a tall, slender white girl of better than average intellect. She was 64 inches tall and weighed 79 pounds. She wore glasses for ectopia lentium, which had been discovered at the age of 5 years. The palate was high. The chest was long, with convex scoliosis of the thoracic spine toward the right. The heart was not enlarged. However, a loud systolic murmur accompanied by a thrill was heard in the second and third intercostal spaces to the left of the sternum. The patient stood with rather marked pronation of the feet at the heels and moderate abduction. There was minimal genu valgum.

On fluoroscopy the right atrium was seen to be enlarged and the main pulmonary artery was prominent and active. There was moderate hilar dance. The left atrium and the ventricles appeared to be normal in size. During the recording of the electrocardiogram short paroxysms of atrial tachycardia occurred. There was a higher degree of right axis deviation than would have been anticipated as normal for this age. Leads II and III showed changes in the ST-T complex, interpreted as "right ventricular strain pattern." The QRS complexes were notched in most leads. X-ray films revealed no structural abnormality of the vertebrae.

It was my previous impression that this patient had atrial septal defect (ASD). It was commented that surgical repair is probably worth while in such a patient, provided there is no evidence of involvement of other parts of the cardiovascular system or too severe skeletal involvement.

Subsequent events and the findings of autopsy proved the diagnosis of ASD to be incorrect. Late in 1955 a spinal operation for correction of deformity was performed. Thereafter, an infection with chronically draining sinuses necessitated readmission to the hospital. Following a debridement operation the patient died during a sudden bout of arrhythmia. The findings in the heart included bicuspid aortic valve and multicuspid mitral valve. The left coronary artery had two accessory ostia at the sinus of Valsalva. The mitral valve had five cusps, and the line of closure was thickened and nodular. Histologically this area showed "basophilic degeneration." The interatrial septum was perfectly intact. There was pulmonary emphysema. (I am indebted to Dr. John Franklin of Norfolk, Va., for information on this patient.)

(From McKusick, V. A.: Circulation **11**:321, 1955.)

A

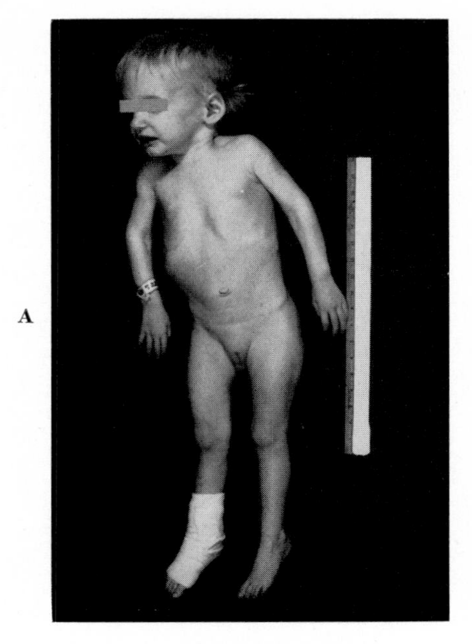

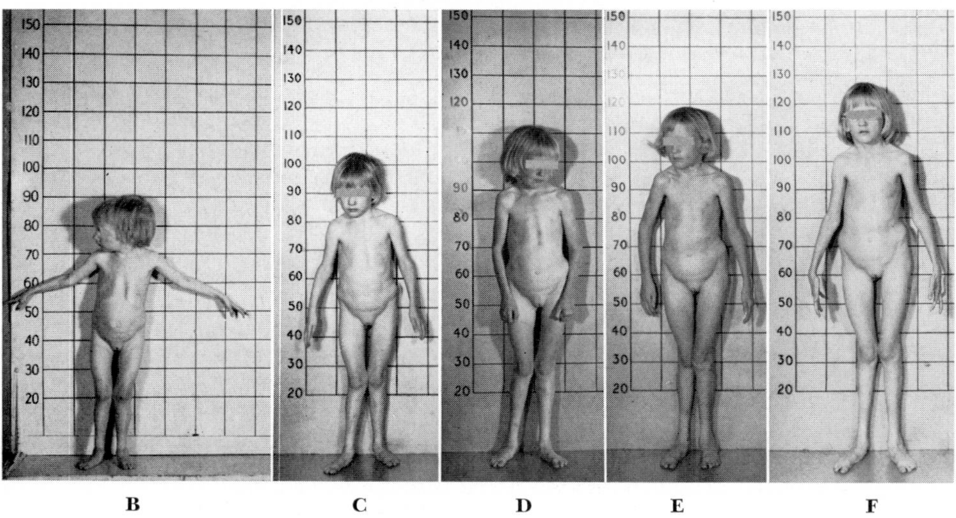

B C D E F

Fig. 3-37. Mitral regurgitation in Marfan syndrome (B.N., 941257). **A** to **F,** The appearance at ages, respectively, 14 months, 2 years, 3 years, 4 years, 5 years, and 6 years. Chest deformity—first pectus excavatum and later predominantly pectus carinatum—is shown. Dolichostenomelia and loose-jointedness are striking. Bilateral ectopia lentis is present. **G** to **I,** Auscultatory findings as demonstrated by spectral phonocardiograms. At the age of 14 months, the patient showed a loud musical late systolic murmur which was initiated by a click and which extended across the second heart sound, **G.** Later the findings were predominantly multiple clicks in the latter two thirds of systole, **H,** and in other areas a noisy late systolic murmur extending over the second sound, **I.** Selective left ventricular cineangiocardiography, **J,** at age 5 years demonstrated prolapsed posterior mitral leaflet and mitral regurgitation. The catheter was introduced in retrograde fashion via the femoral artery. In the right anterior oblique view, **J,** the sinuses of Valsalva are seen to be markedly dilated. (**LA,** Left atrium; **LV,** left ventricle; **NC** and **LC,** noncoronary and left coronary sinuses of Valsalva.) (No auscultatory evidence of aortic regurgitation has developed.) Toward the end of systole the posterior leaflet of the mitral valve bulged markedly into the left atrium (indicated by arrows), and there was mitral regurgitation. In **K** is shown a diagram of the normal heart as viewed in the right anterior oblique position. (Cineangiocardiographic view and diagram courtesy Dr. Michael J. Criley.)

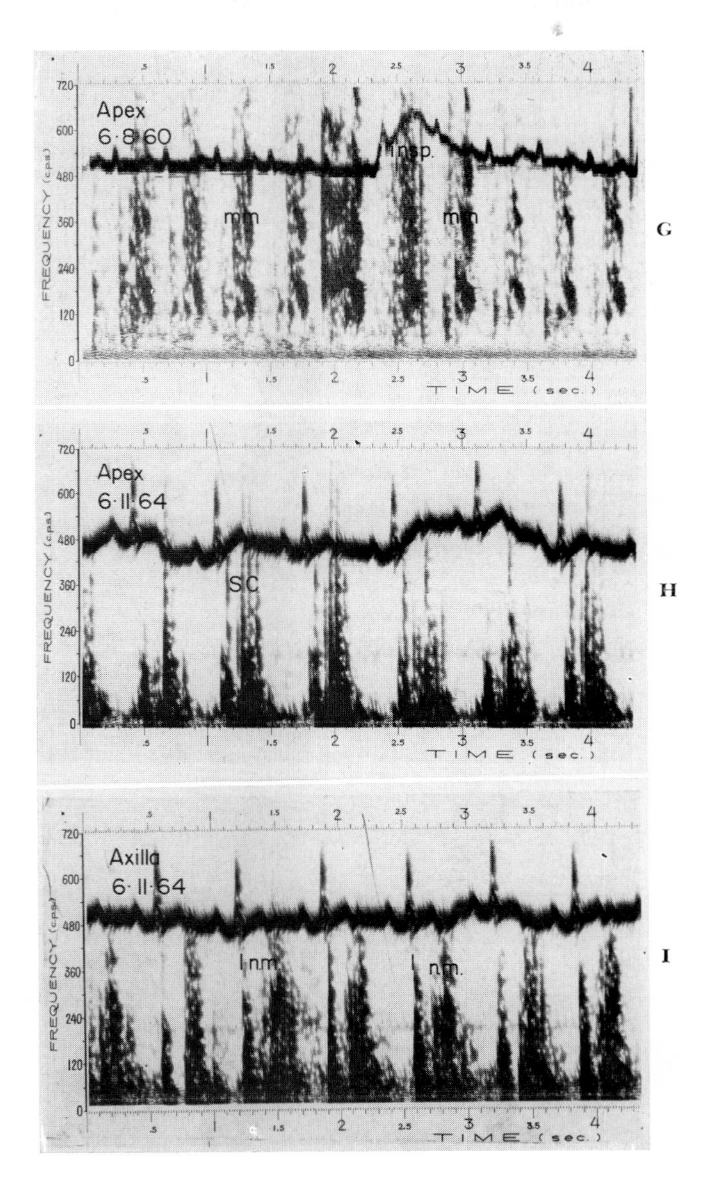

Fig. 3-37, cont'd. For legend see opposite page.

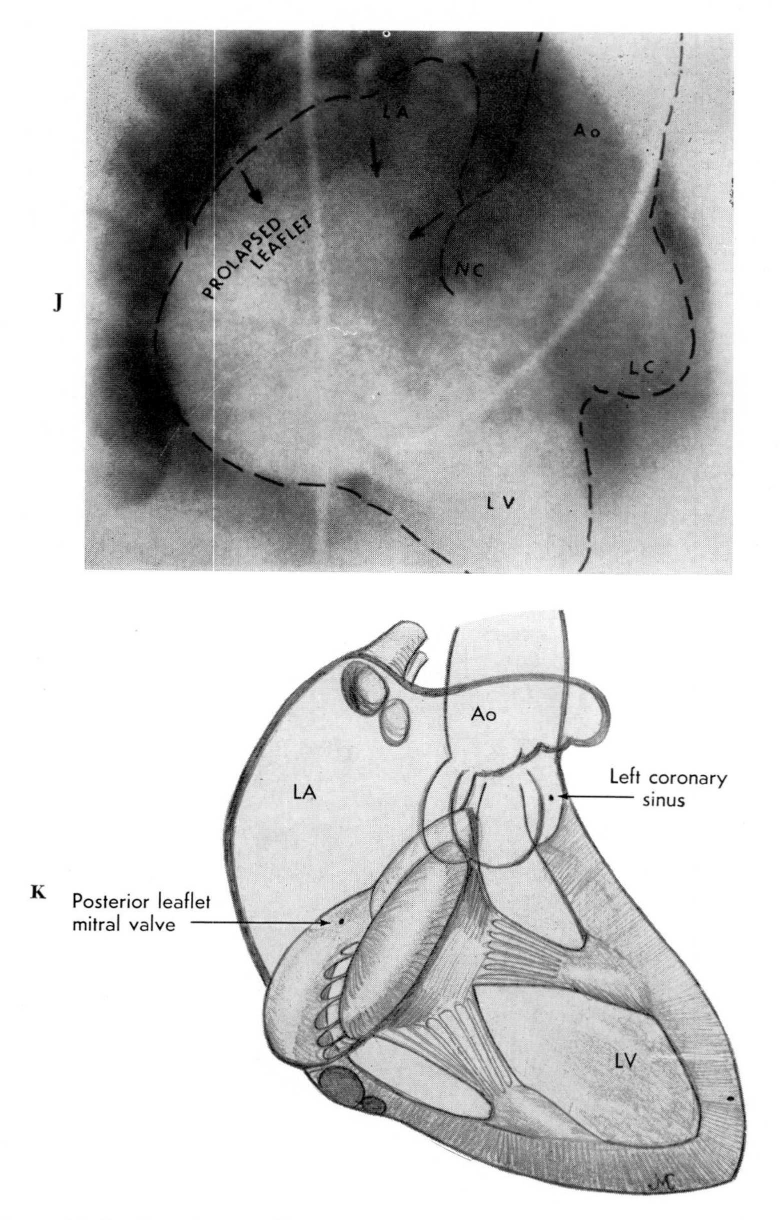

Fig. 3-37, cont'd. For legend see p. 94.

to be larger than it in fact is, because of (1) displacement of the heart into the left hemithorax with mild clockwise rotation and (2) pancaking of the heart with increase in the transverse dimension. Electrocardiographic variations, such as rSr′ or rSR′ pattern in V_1, are secondary to the influence of the chest deformity on cardiac position and rotation.

Prolongation of the P-R interval of the electrocardiogram occurs commonly in the Marfan syndrome[17,73,251] but is usually absent except in the presence of

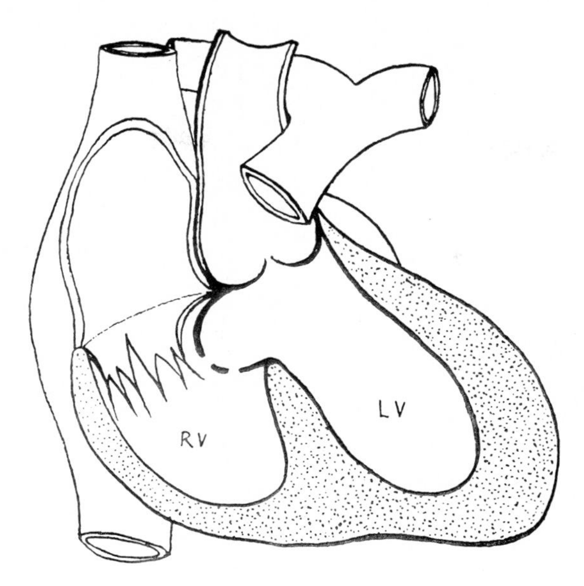

Fig. 3-38. Ruptured aneurysm of ventricular septum in the Marfan syndrome. Distortion of the septal leaflet of the tricuspid valve overlying the aneurysm is indicated. (From Ross, J. K., and Gerbode, F.: J. Thoracic Surg. **39:**746, 1960.)

aortic regurgitation. It is interesting to speculate that aneurysmal dilatation of the aortic ring may compromise atrioventricular conduction by pressure on the conducting tissue. Bundle branch block also occurs.[73,251,367] One patient (J. S., 543026), 18 years of age, with unequivocal ocular and skeletal signs of the Marfan syndrome has right bundle branch block as the only cardiovascular abnormality demonstrable by extensive studies, including cardiac catheterization. A brother of this patient, who probably suffers from a *forme fruste,* demonstrates inverted P waves bespeaking an ectopic pacemaker. The father, who was 78 inches tall, had aortic regurgitation and died suddenly at the age of 28 years; he had either ectopic pacemaker or polongation of the P-R interval with superimposition of P waves on T waves. Bowers[53,54] reviewed the electrocardiographic findings in a group of cases. Moretti and colleagues[263] observed complete heart block in the Marfan syndrome. The conduction abnormalities are of particular interest in connection with the pathologic changes in the vascular supply to the sinus and atrioventricular nodes, described by James and associates[181] (p. 126).

There is one report[214] of dilatation of the left external carotid artery. No histologic study was made. Dilatation of the ascending aorta was also present in that patient. Hardin[157] described a 73-year-old woman with the Marfan syndrome, from whom an aneurysm of the extracranial portion of the internal carotid artery was successfully resected. We have observed pronounced dilatation of the left common carotid in a 13-year-old boy (B. F., 724330), with skeletal changes characteristic of the Marfan syndrome and with ectopia lentis but no clinical evidence of change in the aorta. Except for these similar observations, no abnormalities of peripheral arteries have been described. Dissection may, of course, extend out branches of the aorta for an appreciable distance, but the media has usually appeared normal histologically.[213] In one case (S. C., 575946), the splenic artery

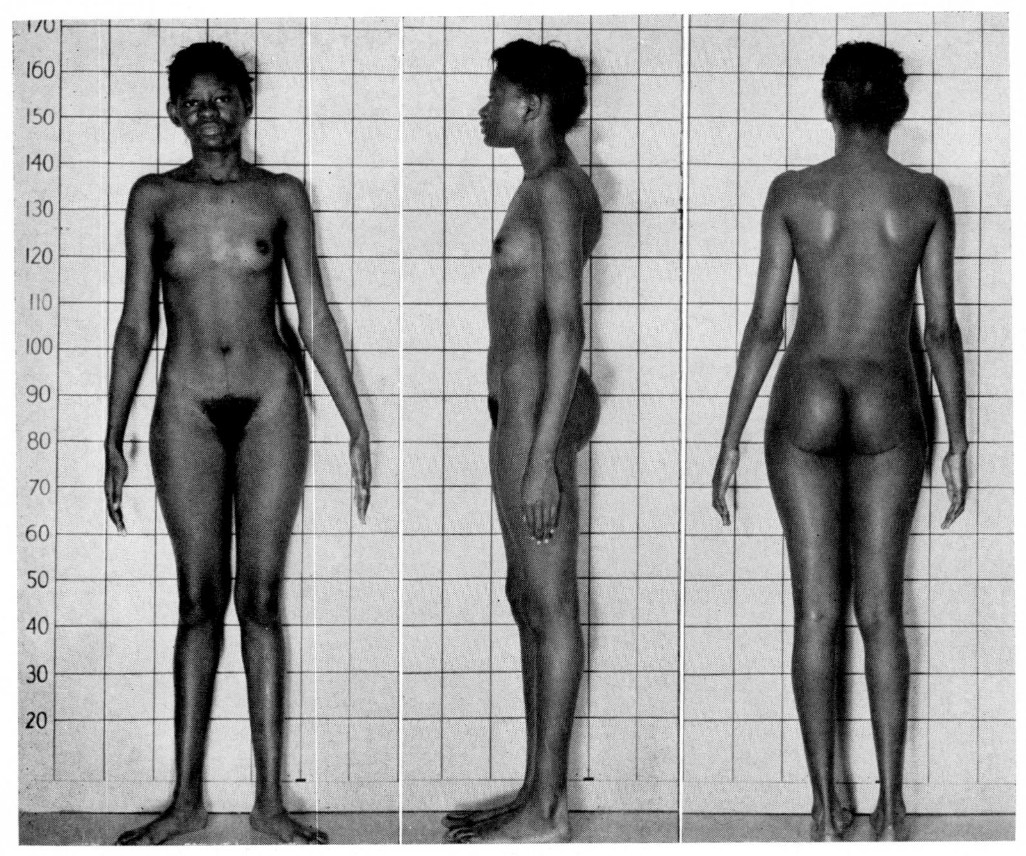

Fig. 3-39. G. H. (815634), 15 years of age, has bilateral subluxation of the lenses, spinal curvature, and the habitus typical of the Marfan syndrome. Clinical signs of ventricular septal defect are corroborated by the data of cardiac catheterization (courtesy Dr. Donald Nelson and Dr. Peter Luchsinger, District of Columbia General Hospital, Washington). In my personal experience this is the only case of ventricular septal defect in a patient with Marfan syndrome. (From McKusick, V. A.: Bull. N. Y. Acad. Med. **35:**143, 1959.)

was friable at autopsy and was found to be the site of cystic medial necrosis. Varicose veins probably occur more frequently and in more severe form in the Marfan syndrome than ordinarily would be expected.[416]

The coarctation[98] has rarely been of great functional significance. There is no reason, however, why it might not be in occasional instances. Seemingly the coarctation has not been resected in any case of the Marfan syndrome. Dissecting aneurysm occurs with increased frequency in coarctation,[159] and although the hypertension is doubtlessly a contributing factor, the possibility of a connective tissue abnormality being responsible for both the coarctation and the dissection must be considered. One patient in my series (L. Y., J.H.H., 392843) has hypertension and a small left radial pulse but no significant discrepancy in arm and leg pressures.

The changes at the aortic isthmus in the Marfan syndrome (Fig. 3-24*C*) have

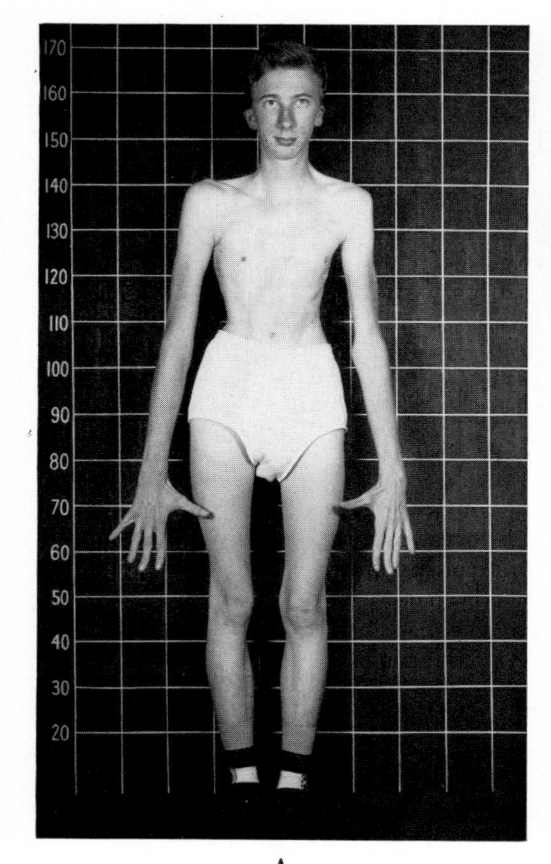

A

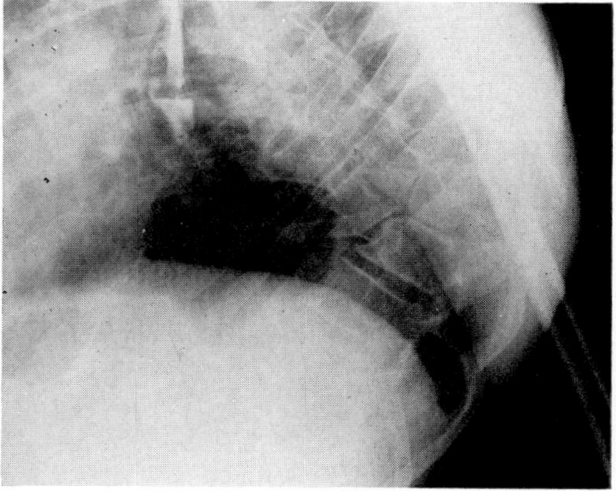

B

Fig. 3-40. A case (J.H.H. 525256) of tetralogy of Fallot with stigmata suggesting Marfan's syndrome. The absence of ectopia lentium and of other affected persons in the family makes the diagnosis of the Marfan syndrome dubious. There are malformed pinnae and long fingers, **A,** and hemivertebra, **B;** but these are nonspecific manifestations of the Marfan syndrome. Note also the facial asymmetry. (In yet another patient with tetralogy of Fallot [J.H.H. 482041] cleft palate, pes planus, talipes equinovarus, and long fingers are present, but in general the diagnosis of the Marfan syndrome is uncertain because of lack, as in the above patient, of ectopia lentis and positive family history.) (From McKusick, V. A.: Circulation **11:**321, 1955.)

many of the features of what the angiocardiographers, who are largely responsible for discovering the disorder, call "pseudocoarctation." Even the "figure-of-three" sign may be present on conventional radiography of the chest. One would be suspicious of the presence of the Marfan syndrome in a patient such as that described by Steinberg[350] in whom pseudocoarctation was associated with dilated sinuses of Valsalva.

The combination of aortic regurgitation with coarctation may confuse the diagnosis of coarctation. The pulses in the legs may seem normal unless the absence of the collapsing quality is noted.

Whitfield and associates[410] described a case of simple hypoplasia of the aorta with the Marfan syndrome. They suggested that the increased resistance resulting from the reduced aortic diameter might have been responsible, at least in part, for the cardiac hypertrophy observed in their case. Since hypoplasia of the aorta as a primary entity is a nebulous entity at the best, this interpretation is suspect.

Hypertension, presumably without coarctation, was present at the age of 12

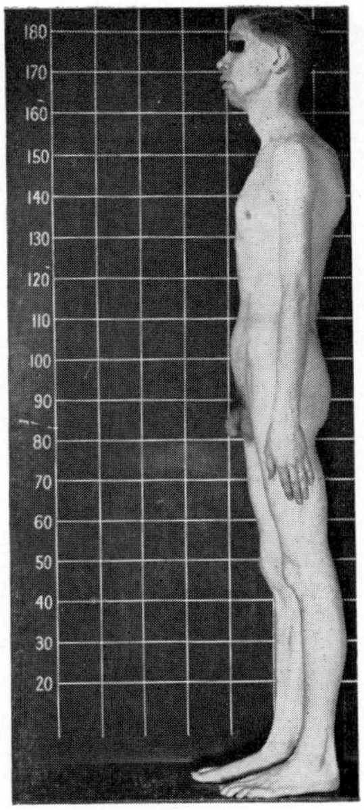

Fig. 3-41. The patient, R. R. (704121), 30 years of age, has clouding of the cornea, dolichostenomelia, and probable large interventricular defect. It is likely that this is due not to Marfan's syndrome but rather to intrauterine insult of unidentified variety. The upper segment–lower segment ratio does *not* suggest the Marfan syndrome.

years in one reported case.[149] In another patient,[48] hypertension had been present from at least the age of 24 years, and the Smithwick operation was performed at the age of 27 years. Hypertension has been present at least from the age of 26 years in two of our cases (L. Y., 392843; C. S., 596716). Presumably the presence of hypertension[250] places the patient in double jeopardy from rupture of the aorta.

In one reported case,[324] bacterial endaortitis was thought to be present.

Other cardiovascular abnormalities have been described, but in most the diagnosis of the Marfan syndrome is insecure. For example, Burry[66] described a 37-year-old mentally defective woman with negative family history and no ectopia lentis who did, however, have a moderate degree of myopia and had presumably characteristic skeletal proportion. Supravalvular aortic stenosis was present. Bingle[43] described a 32-year-old woman with patent ductus arteriosus, cystic medial necrosis of the aorta, dilatation of the aortic ring, and dissection of the ascending aorta with rupture into the pericardial sac. Grossly, there was an area of calcification and scarring in the wall of the left atrium and, histologically, fragmentation and sparsity of elastic fibers. Family history was not provided. Although the patient was 68½ inches tall, body proportions were not described. There were "no changes in eyes."

Other manifestations. Special attention is directed to certain manifestations which were indicated by dashed lines in the "pedigree of causes" presented in Fig. 3-56: in the cardiovascular system—coarctation* of the aorta,[99,108,111,120,231,388,389] patent ductus arteriosus,[†7,386] anomaly of valvular cuspation, interatrial

*Mild coarctation is common (Fig. 3-24). Occasionally severer, functionally significant coarctation is found.[389] Keech and colleagues[191a] observed complete coarctation in a 61-year-old Negro female with ectopia lentis and skeletal features of the Marfan syndrome.

†Patent ductus arteriosus must be very rare in the Marfan syndrome.[20] Apert[12] is frequently quoted as having described such a case; his patient in fact had "trou de Botal" (patent foramen ovale), not "ductus de Botal." Patent ductus arteriosus was present in one of the patients of Tune and Thal.[385]

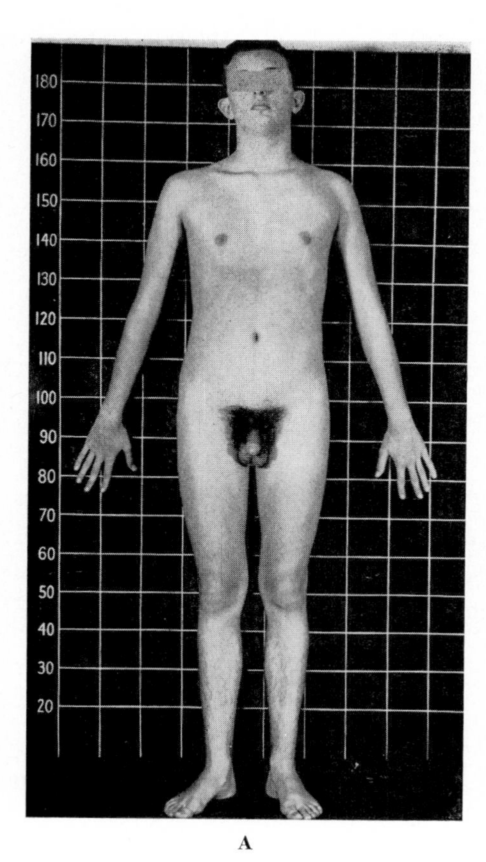

A

Fig. 3-42. D. D. (758872), 16½ years old, has skeletal proportions compatible with the diagnosis of the Marfan syndrome, **A,** slight bilateral ectopia lentis, very small posteroanterior dimension of the thorax, and asymmetric deformity of the anterior chest, **B.** Only mild pectus excavatum is present; however, its effects are greatly exaggerated by the small posteroanterior dimension, i.e. pronounced flat-chestedness. As in all cases of pectus excavatum, the thoracic spine is seen unusually clearly and little cardiac shadow is seen on the right of the midline, **C.** Both the spine and the sternum appear to impinge on the thoracic cavity, **D.** Multiple clicks in systole, **E,** were present in this, as in other cases of the Marfan syndrome.

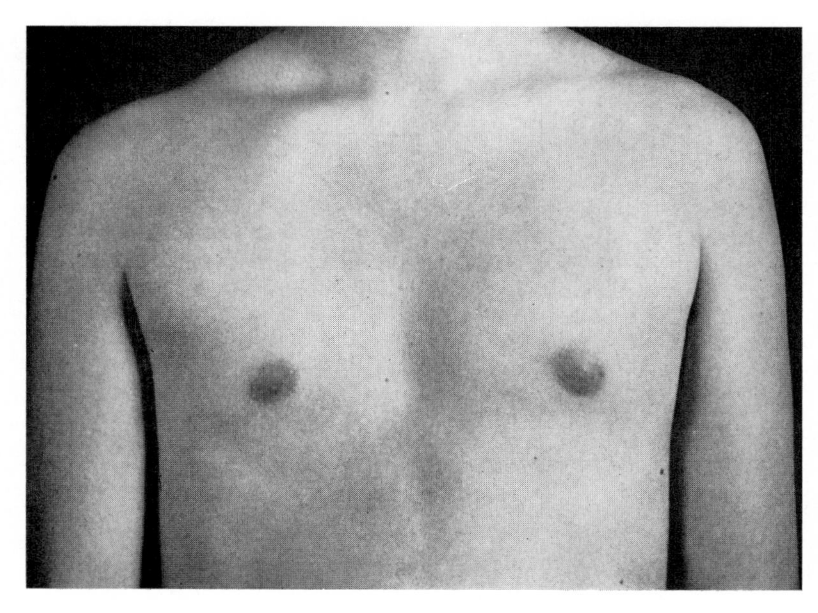

B

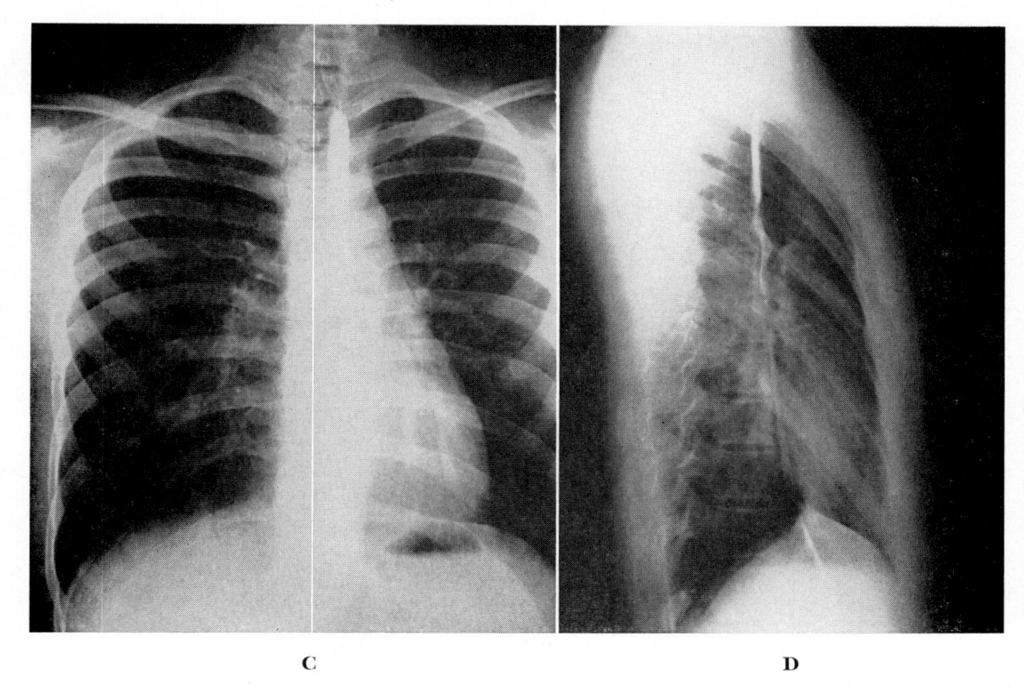

C D

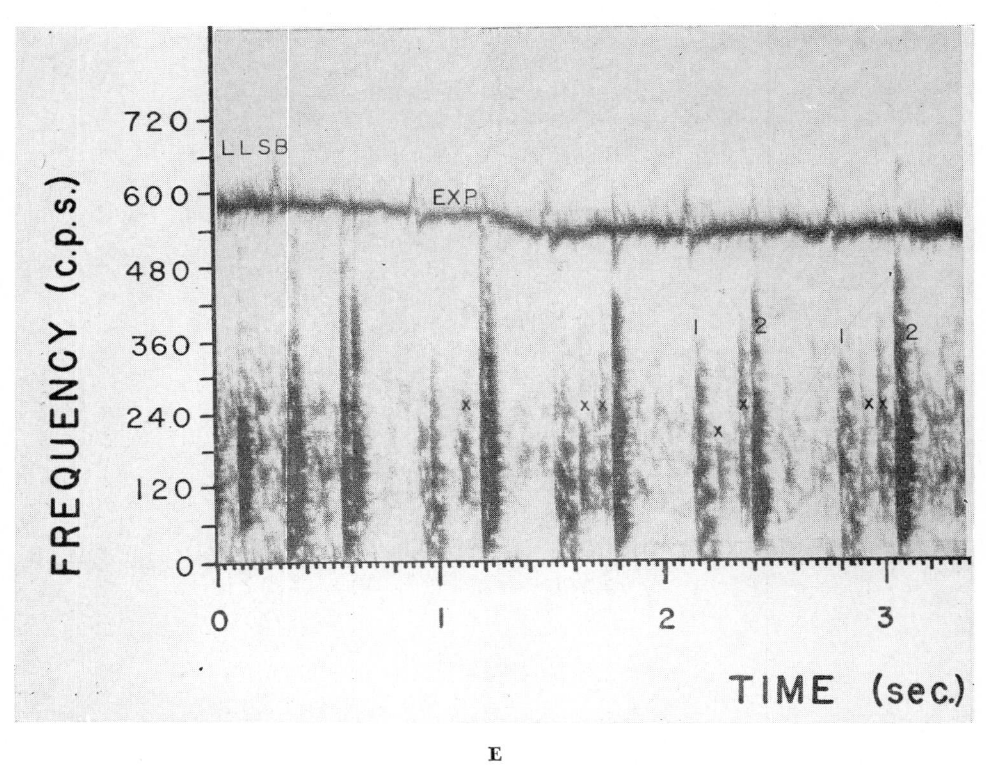

E

Fig. 3-42, cont'd. For legend see preceding page.

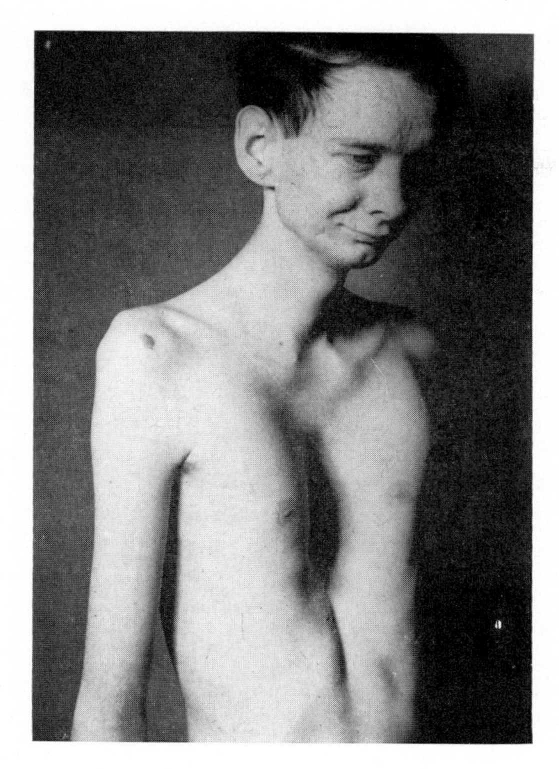

Fig. 3-43. Severe pectus excavatum in the Marfan syndrome. K. B., a 24-year-old white man, was admitted to the Medical College of Virginia Hospital after a year of increasing dyspnea. Twenty-four days before admission he had suddenly become markedly dyspneic and had severe palpitation and substernal pain. About two weeks before admission he had a second episode of pain and palpitation. Following the first attack his dyspnea progressed more rapidly than before and he also became orthopneic.

Physical examination revealed a slender, underdeveloped, undernourished man who was dyspneic even at rest. There was pronounced pectus excavatum. The heart was markedly displaced to the left with the point of maximum impulse in the midaxillary line and the seventh and eighth intercostal spaces. The left anterior chest wall heaved with each heartbeat. There was a loud continuous machinery-like murmur over the base of the heart, with a systolic thrill. Blood pressure was 90/40 in the right arm and 110/32 in the left.

On Nov. 5, 1949, surgical repair of the pectus excavatum was performed.[42] The patient withstood the operation well and remained in a satisfactory condition until forty-eight hours later, when he suddenly went into circulatory collapse and died in less than two hours after developing pronounced distention of the cervical veins.

At autopsy the body measured 72 inches in length. The arms and legs were very slender and long with poor muscular development. The left leg was shorter than the right and showed partial clubfoot. Bilaterally the first and second toes were unusually long but the fourth toes were shorter than normal. There were flexion deformities of the fingers, deformed teeth with malocclusion, bifid uvula, and lumbar kyphosis.

The heart weiged 550 grams. The increase in weight and size was the result of left ventricular hypertrophy and dilatation. The pericardial sac contained 880 ml. of blood. The ascending aorta and first portion of the arch were markedly dilated, and, in addition, there was a dissecting aneurysm of the wall extending from an intimal tear about 3 cm. above the aortic ring to the point where there was slight coarctation of the aorta between the left subclavian and left common carotid ostia. Just distal to the left subclavian a second dissection began and extended throughout the rest of the aorta to involve the first portion of both iliac arteries. A small rent

Legend continued.

on the anterolateral surface of the ascending aorta represented the spot where perforation into the pericardial sac had occurred.

Histologically both dissections were endothelialized and showed some atheroma formation. In addition, the media showed pronounced changes of the type described in other cases of aortic abnormality in this series.

Siegenthaler[333] reports an equally severe instance of pectus excavatum in the Marfan syndrome.

(From McKusick, V. A.: Circulation **11**:321, 1955.)

---

defect,[12,205,288] and possibly pulmonary stenosis[389]; in the skeletal system—spina bifida occulta,* hemivertebra, and cleft palate[311,416]; in the eye—microphakia, hypoplasia, or aplasia of the dilator pupillae muscle, coloboma lentis, and coloboma iridis.[196] These are not among the more common manifestations, yet they occur sufficiently often in the Marfan syndrome to be considered more than coincidental associations. Their occurrence is difficult to reconcile with a unitary theory of a connective tissue defect unless one assumes that the presence of said defect during embryogenensis provides an abnormal environment in which these anomalies, congenital malformations in the usual sense, occur with increased incidence. In accordance with this last and not improbable proposition, these particular manifestations can be considered *secondary* ones.

Whether deafness is a specific manifestation of the Marfan's syndrome and, if so, what its mechanism is,[216] cannot be stated at present. It is said to occur in 6% of cases.[296] Everberg[110] concluded that deafness is an integral feature and that it is of nerve (perceptive) type.

Pulmonary malformations are described in autopsy reports and various pulmonary complications in clinical reports.[143,191,231,277,288,297,317,376] (Fig. 3-44). Repeated spontaneous pneumothorax has been described.[4,183,191,149] Spontaneous pneumothorax sometimes occurs as a familial disorder in the absence of evident Marfan syndrome[40,58] and also occurs in association with the Ehlers-Danlos syndrome (p. 199). Brock[61] favored the presence of hereditary lung cysts as the anatomic substrate.

Occasionally, congenital cystic disease of the lung occurs, probably as an integral part of the Marfan syndrome. In patient M. R. (J.H.H. 176836; see Fig. 3-45), very extensive disease of this type was discovered at autopsy. The stillborn child of this patient showed abnormal lobation of the lungs but no congenital cystic disease. Without an exhaustive review of the literature, it was possible to find three cases of cystic disease of the lung in which stigmata suggestive of the Marfan syndrome were described.

Case 1. A 26-year-old male medical student (Case 9 in reference 277) had had three attacks of spontaneous pneumothorax. He died following an attack of severe chest pain. Dissecting aneurysm of the aorta with rupture into the pericardium was discovered. Histologically there was cystic medial necrosis. Both lungs showed diffuse cystic changes regarded as congenital.

Case 2. A 26-year-old housewife (Case 13 in reference 277) with striking dolichostenomelia had had increasing dyspnea and, at the end of her second pregnancy, frank congestive failure. X-ray examination showed dilatation of the outflow tract of the right ventricle; electrocardio-

---

*Encephalocele in the forehead area occurred in one patient (J. D., 184805). Internal hydrocephalus is also reported.[283,297]

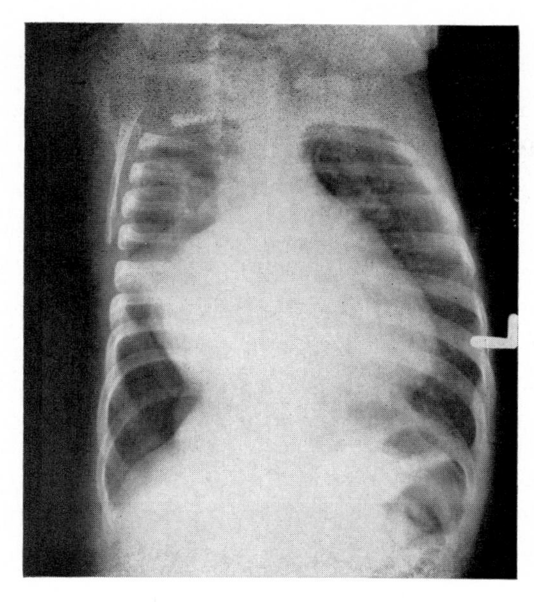

Fig. 3-44. X-ray film of the chest in infant B. J. P. A pulmonary anomaly is evident, as well as pronounced cardiomegaly.

B. J. P. (H.L.H. A93754) was born Nov. 9, 1951. She weighed 6 pounds 11 ounces and was thought to be healthy. The mother had had no pregnancies in the nineteen years between this one and that which occurred in 1933. The mother first learned of the child's heart murmur when the child was 4 months old. The child was never able to sit up or roll over by herself. When first seen at the age of 6 months, the following findings were recorded. The left side of the face was smaller than the right. Respirations were rapid (about 50 per minute). There was a pigeon-breast deformity of the thorax. The pulse was regular at a rate of 150 per minute. Femoral pulses were full. The heart was enlarged beyond the left midclavicular line. A systolic thrill was palpable over the entire precordium but was maximum in the left midprecordium. A harsh systolic murmur had the same location. The liver edge was 1.5 cm. below the right costal margin. There was no clubbing or cyanosis.

Fluoroscopy revealed great cardiac enlargement to both left and right, with globular shape. The right ventricle was definitely enlarged in the oblique views. The right lower lung field had a distinctly abnormal appearance. It lacked the usual lung markings and was unusually radiolucent. There was a question of atelectatic lung (? right middle lobe) at the right heart border. By electrocardiogram the P waves were broad and notched. The P-R interval was 0.16 second, which is long, considering the patient's age and heart rate of 150 per minute. Very large R waves in the leads from the left of the precordium suggested left ventricular hypertrophy. The hematocrit was 29.5%, with hypochromic, microcytic cell indices.

Late in May, 1952, the patient developed physical and x-ray signs of consolidation in the right upper lobe and became febrile. These signs were altered little by the administration of several different antibacterial agents. The heart was extremely overactive and shook the whole bed. Occasionally the murmur assumed a to-and-fro quality, especially at the lower left sternal border. The liver enlarged in size. Subsequently, signs of consolidation of the entire right lung appeared. On July 31, 1952, it was noted that both lenses were displaced mediad and that dilatation of the pupil with phenylephrine was only partially successful. Ophthalmologic consultants observed that the patient was extremely myopic with small lenses. In the last weeks of life there was an episode of hematuria related, perhaps, to sulfadiazine therapy. Death occurred on July 10, 1952, when the patient was only 8 months old.

Autopsy (23761) revealed that the right lung was partially atelectatic. The left lung was normal. The pulmonary artery was larger in circumference than the aorta. The foramen ovale was imperfectly closed. All chambers of the heart showed hypertrophy of their walls, and dilatation. The hypertrophy of the right atrium was particularly marked. Microscopically there were

Legend continued.

no lesions of the myocardium. However, the wall of the pulmonary artery and, to a lesser extent, that of the aorta showed typical changes of Marfan's syndrome. The media contained vacuoles filled with the metachromatically staining material, and there were derangement and relative sparsity of elastic fibers. The wall of the pulmonary artery was thicker than that of the aorta. At the time of the gross examinations the bronchial tree was injected with radiopaque material and radiograms were made. To the surprise of the prosector, no abnormality was identified.

Comments. Obviously the most informative feature of this case is the advanced change in the pulmonary artery, which undoubtedly resulted in pulmonary regurgitation and was a leading factor in the infant's death at the age of only 8 months. Ectopia lentium, myopia, microphakia, arachnodactyly, and retardation of ability to sit or roll over complete the picture of Marfan's syndrome.

This kinship illustrates one of the difficulties of genetic research in man. The illegitimacy of this infant and the presence of a legitimate wife of the father of the proposita made the utmost tact and resourcefulness necessary for collecting even these few data. The father of the infant is about 74 inches tall, has long hands and feet, and wears spectacles. Examination was not possible and no further pedigree information was obtained.

(From McKusick, V. A.: Circulation **11**:321, 1955.)

---

grams showed right axis deviation and the so-called P-pulmonale. Postmortem examination disclosed diffuse cystic changes in both lungs and widely patent foramen ovale.

Case 3. A 12-year-old child[313] was found at autopsy to have multiple simple cysts throughout both lungs, patent ductus arteriosus, aneurysm of the pulmonary artery, and anomalous coronary artery.

The case of Lillian[212] showed lung cysts, but the diagnosis of the Marfan syndrome is not completely certain.

Congenital cystic lung disease is probably a secondary component of this syndrome; that is, the presence of the connective tissue defect during embryogenesis conditions its development but is not as directly responsible for it as for some of the other manifestations. The Marfan syndrome can join Hand-Schüller-Christian disease[344,382] and tuberous sclerosis[37,38] in the group of systemic abnormalities associated with a type of cystic disease of the lung.

Bolande and Tucker[48] discussed the pathogenesis of emphysema in patients with the Marfan syndrome. Six patients in one group of seven cases had evidence of pulmonary dysaeration: two showed compression of the left main bronchus by a giant left atrium, with atelectasis of the lung and compensatory emphysema of the right lung, two showed chronic pulmonary emphysema, three had apical bullae bilaterally, and one developed pneumothorax. Bolande and Tucker suggested that emphysema, sometimes cystic, in young patients with the Marfan syndrome and without evidence of pulmonary infection, fibrosis, bronchitis, or bronchiolitis, is a result of the generalized disorder of connective tissue. No histologic changes leading to emphysema were found. Increased deposition of elastic fibers in the alveolar septa was interpreted as a response to mechanical stress and is seen in other comparable situations in non-Marfan patients. Flaccidity of the walls of the respiratory and terminal bronchioles may, they suggested, predispose to collapse during expiration and result in air trapping and emphysema. Pulmonary function was studied by Fuliehan and colleagues.[127]

The voice in patients with the Marfan syndrome sometimes is rather high pitched, with a timbre sufficiently characteristic that one author[56] thought he could recognize affected persons over the telephone.

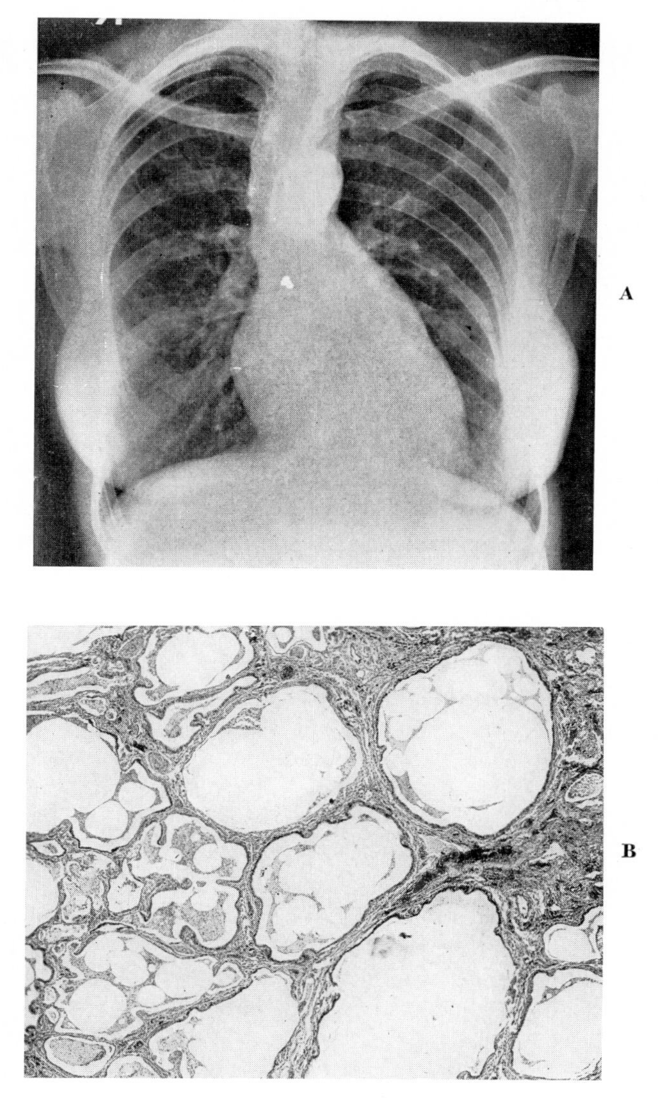

Fig. 3-45. A, X-ray film of the chest in M. R. (176836), from whom other illustrative materials are demonstrated in Figs. 3-18 and 3-35. Scoliosis, cardiac enlargement, increased pulmonary markings, and questionable bleb formation in the lungs are demonstrated. **B,** Same patient. At autopsy the lungs weighed 1,350 grams. There was exudation of copious edema from the cut surfaces. Bilaterally the upper lobes were involved by large, bleblike cavities filled with large amounts of greenish fluid. To a lesser extent, the middle lobe and both lower lobes were cystic. Histologically the cysts were large and conglomerate and lined with columnar epithelium. Some of the cysts were several centimeters in diameter. In the walls of many, thin strands of smooth muscle were identified. This photomicrograph was made at a magnification of ×25, reduced ⅓. The pulmonary cysts are clearly demonstrated.

Congenital cystic kidneys were described[49] in one case of arachnodactyly, but the evidence presented is inadequate for the reviewer to be certain that the genuine Marfan syndrome was present.

There are other manifestations that occur less frequently, often in no more than single reported cases, than those termed "secondary" above. In the case of these, it is more likely that the anomaly occurs only coincidentally with the bona fide features of Marfan's syndrome. When the case in question is a sporadic one, it may be valid to assume that the mutagenic factor might have caused more than one mutation simultaneously. Furthermore, in a given family, if the anomaly in question occurs in only one of the persons affected by Marfan's syndrome, or, better yet, if the anomaly also occurs in one or more members of the family unaffected by the Marfan syndrome, the manifestation in question should not be considered part of the Marfan syndrome.

Contrary to previous emphasis,[88,216,283,322] mental retardation is not, in my opinion, a component of this syndrome. Usually the patients are at least as bright as their siblings. Sometimes their innate intelligence is not fully realized because of the limitation of opportunities imposed by severe visual impairment and other physical handicaps. One patient in our series (F. D.), who died at the age of 14 years, wrote a book of verse, which was published, and composed short dramas for enacting by her playmates. In severe sporadic cases in infants and children, there may be mental retardation, but this has, in my opinion, a separate basis, possibly an independent mutation. Another basis for confusion is the fact that a picture including arachnodactyly and suggesting the Marfan syndrome occurs with acquired developmental abnormalities such as those due to rubella and other maternal illness, maternal exposure to x-ray, and Rh incompatibility. These patients are likely to show mental retardation. The occurrence of mental retardation as a conspicuous feature of homocystinuria (p. 150), which in several other respects simulates the Marfan syndrome, may be another reason that mental retardation has been thought to be a feature of the Marfan syndrome.

Haber[150] points out that a rare but characteristic *skin lesion* may be associated with the Marfan syndrome. It is called Miescher's elastoma, or elastoma intrapapillare perforans verruciforme. The lesions occur particularly on the neck and grossly appear as small nodules or papules. Histologically these are cysts occupied by whorls of material, which have the tinctorial characteristics of elastic fibers and which seem to have erupted into the epidermis from the upper corium. In 1952 Storck[364] of Zurich described a patient with typical Marfan syndrome and skin lesions he classified as Kyrle's hyperkeratosis follicularis et perifollicularis in cutem penetrans. However, Miescher reported to Haber[150] that the skin lesions were histologically more characteristic of Miescher's elastoma. In 1958 Anning[8] of Leeds, England, described a young man in whom the diagnosis of Miescher's elastoma was made at the age of 18 years and who died at the age of 20 years of dissecting aneurysm of the aorta. (From the report of Meara[254] one can conclude that Miescher's elastoma may occur also with the Ehlers-Danlos syndrome.)

Striae of the skin in the pectoral and anterior deltoid areas[187,220,262,321] are frequently found in Marfan patients. They are observable in the teens and cannot be attributed to weight loss. (See Figs. 3-17 and 3-21*D*.)

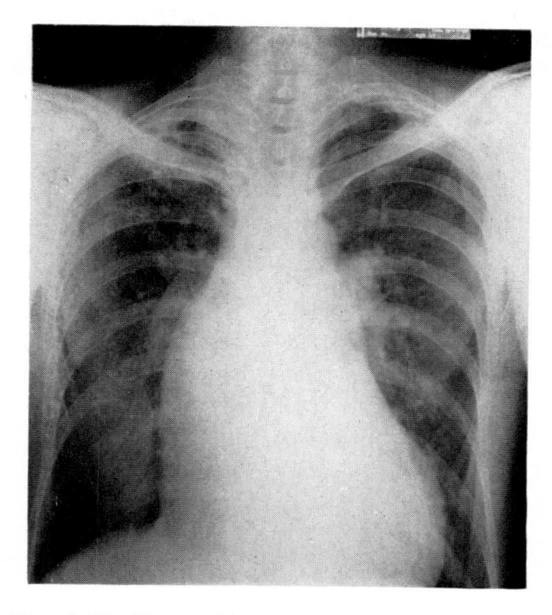

Fig. 3-46. The x-ray film of this 49-year-old man (B. L., 195805) shows prominence of the pulmonary artery and inconspicuous dilatation of the ascending aorta. These features, together with the murmur of aortic regurgitation and the associated Austin Flint murmur, led to the diagnosis of rheumtaic heart disease with combined aortic and mitral lesions. This was the case in spite of the fact that the patient was 75½ inches tall, had spinal and thoracic deformities (a suggestion of which is indicated by the figure), and had had ectopic lenses removed ten and thirteen years previously. The patient had pneumonia twice in youth and had an operation for varicose veins at the age of 25 years. Scholastic performance was outstanding, with graduation from college at the age of 18 years. A bout of iritis prompted removal of the right lens in 1937. In 1940 the left lens was removed because of dislocation into the anterior chamber. Detachment of the retina on the left was discovered at that time. There was heterochromia iritis with normal brown pigmentation on the right and greenish coloration on the left. The patient was accepted for service in the Army and, while there (1947), had his first bout of severe chest pain with extension to the arms, neck, and epigastrium. A second episode of probable aortic dissection occurred later in 1947 and a third in 1948. The episode in 1948 was characterized by severe low back pain radiating into the lower abdomen and genitalia. The diagnosis of rheumatic heart disease was based on the prominence of the pulmonary artery segment (due actually to displacement by the dilated aorta), a diastolic murmur at the apex (which was probably either radiation of the murmur of aortic regurgitation or an Austin Flint murmur or both), and displacement of the esophagus by what was interpreted as left atrium (possibly indeed left atrium enlarged from chronic left ventricular failure or possibly the aortic aneurysm, Fig. 3-27*E*). The patient died at home in 1950. The father, 6 feet 3 inches tall, was killed by a bus at the age of 82 years. He probably had the Marfan syndrome in mild form; he sired several affected children; his wife appears to have been unaffected. Of eleven siblings of the proband, two, always puny, died at 8 and 10 years, of unknown causes; two had the same habitus as the proband; a fifth has definite Marfan syndrome. This man, now 49 years old, is 70½ inches tall, weighs 178 pounds, and wears an 11½C shoe. He was discharged from the Army when he lost the sight in one eye. Detachment of the retina was discovered at the age of 40 years. He has severe myopia and flat feet, is stoop-shouldered, is said to have a heart murmur, and has had left inguinal herniorrhaphy. (From McKusick, V. A.: Circulation **11**:321, 1955.)

Prognosis

One man almost certainly affected with the Marfan syndrome (Fig. 3-46) was killed accidentally at the age of 82 years. One of our oldest patients was 59 years old (H. B., 621760). He had severe aortic regurgitation. Bowers[56] described two patients with the Marfan syndrome still living at 61 and 66 years of age. Among sixteen dead affected members of a large family, Bowers[56] found the average age at death to be 43 years in the males and 46 years in the females. One individual survived to 73 years; another died at 9 years. We have a patient who is 65 years old.

Prevalence and inheritance

The sexes are equally affected.[223,296] The aortic complications do seem to occur more frequently in men.[231] Manual labor may be responsible for this. There is no racial or subracial concentration of cases. The syndrome has been reported in Negroes,[128,231] Chinese,[75,158] Japanese,[269,338] Hindus,[41] and Jews.[223] It has, furthermore, been reported in natives of virtually every European country. Its incidence in the American Negro is probably essentially the same as in the white population. It has occurred in American Indians.[132]

The Marfan syndrome is an uncommon, but by no means rare, disorder. Its incidence is certainly far greater than indicated in the general conception of the medical public. The connective tissue defect of the Marfan syndrome is a leading cause of dissecting aneurysm of the aorta in the younger decades. There is reason to believe that there is an appreciable number of very mild cases *(forme fruste)*, in which the connective tissue defect has little or no effect on health or longevity.

Preposterously high estimates of the number of sporadic cases (those derived presumably from *de novo* mutation), as opposed to inherited cases, have been made. My own experience would indicate that no more than 15% of all cases are new ones. Higher estimates, up to 70% by some writers, are the result of incomplete family studies. How often this mutation occurs in a total population is hard to determine. Attempts at estimation of gene frequency or of mutation rate are beset by difficulties, such as diagnostic doubts in mild cases, the impossibility of ascertaining mild cases unless severe cases are present in the family, variability in the age of onset of the aortic manifestations, and the mimicry of phenocopies. These difficulties attend the study of other incomplete dominant traits, such as dystrophia myotonica. On the basis of as complete ascertainment as possible and using Haldane's method,[152,225] which assumes that mutation replaces those genes lost because of reduced effective fertility of affected persons, Lynas[224] estimated the mutation rate to be 5 per million genes per generation in the population of northern Ireland:

$$\mu = \tfrac{1}{2}(1 - f)\,x = \tfrac{1}{2}(1 - \tfrac{1}{2})\,\frac{36}{1{,}370{,}921}$$

x = proportion of persons with the Marfan syndrome in the population
f = the effective fertility of affected persons, when unity is the average fertility

When the mutation rate was estimated from the incidence of sporadic cases a similar estimate was obtained. A minimal figure for prevalence of the Marfan syndrome was 1.459 per 100,000 of the population and for gene frequency, one-half this value, 0.729 per 100,000 genes.

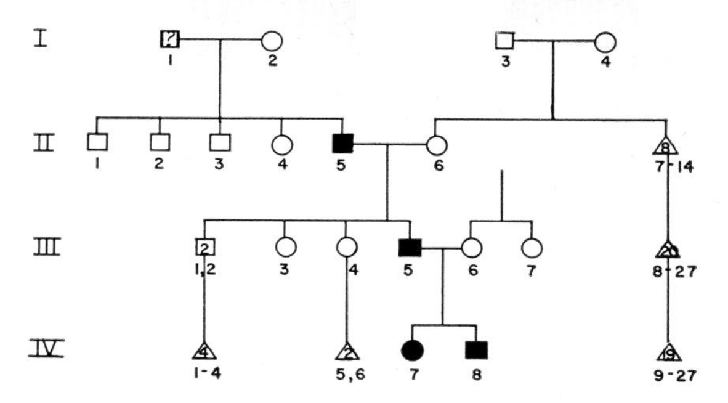

Fig. 3-47. By way of summary of the aortic complications of the Marfan syndrome, I present the story and pedigree of a family that was unusually heavily affected. Individual I-1 died suddenly in 1897 at the age of 47 years, presumably of apoplexy. This may have been dissecting aneurysm. A son of this man (II-5) died at the age of 27 years after a very brief illness of undiagnosed nature. He was 6 feet tall, was always very thin, and had been sent to Texas at one time, for suspected tuberculosis. He became ill at noon one day and was dead at 5 A.M. the following day. He was said to have had no pain but developed hematuria in the last afternoon of the day he became ill.

Most of the remainder of the story of this family is told in the words of individual III-6, an intelligent observer and cooperative informant. Her husband (III-5) died in 1945 at the age of 32 years. "His heart condition was diagnosed as endocarditis by a heart specialist. He was apparently in good health up to two months prior to his death. He was 6 feet 2½ inches tall and in the last two years of his life he weighed more than ever before—175 pounds—and appeared to be in excellent health, except for his failing eyesight. He was working exceptionally hard due to the wartime manpower shortage. He was appointed to a job that necessitated a great deal of coast-to-coast flying at high altitudes. It was on one of these trips that he was taken ill. He returned home, was put to bed and given medicine, to which he responded beautifully. He insisted on going on another trip and lived one month after his return. He was hospitalized, but his case was pronounced hopeless. He had a hernia operation two years before his death. A routine checkup before the anesthesia showed no heart condition then."

The daughter of this man (IV-7) "was born May 17, 1937. She was always frail. She and her brother had whooping cough when they were 6 and 5 years old. Her heart started enlarging at that time. She was extremely nearsighted and wore glasses from the age of 3 years. She had a bad spinal curvature that we first noticed when she was 10 years of age. The family doctor did not advise a brace or cast, as she was so frail and her heart was getting increasingly worse. During her last illness, which lasted six weeks, the doctor said that her heart was just as it would have been in a person in his forties who had had rheumatic fever in his youth, that her heart was just worn out. She died at the age of 12½ years and was 5 feet 2 inches tall in spite of a very bad curvature. She had a brilliant mind and was at the top of classes in spite of her many handicaps. Both of the children were thin to the point of looking emaciated."

The brother of this girl (IV-8) "was born Nov. 27, 1938. He and Catherine looked like twins and were as nearly like their father as was possible. He was well as a baby and up to the time that he had whooping cough at the age of 5 years. After that long siege of coughing the doctor discovered that he had a heart murmur. His heart enlarged so that his chest protruded. He complained of chest pain occasionally. He died suddenly in August, 1946. His sister said after he died that he had complained of severe chest pains a couple of days before but he didn't tell anyone else. He developed hernia when he was about 2 years old, but it never seemed to bother him. He had a bad case of influenza the winter before he died and had a bad cough that lingered all winter and we felt hastened his death."

At age 7 years, this last patient was 53 inches tall and weighed 51 pounds. He showed arachnodactyly, hypotonia, hammertoes, thin and translucent skin, ectopia lentium, cardiomegaly, dilatation of the aorta, aortic systolic and diastolic murmurs, left axis deviation (by electrocardiogram), deformity (not described in detail) of the hip joints and skull (by x-ray examination). The lenses in this case were displaced downward and outward.

(From McKusick, V. A.: Circulation **11**:321, 1955.)

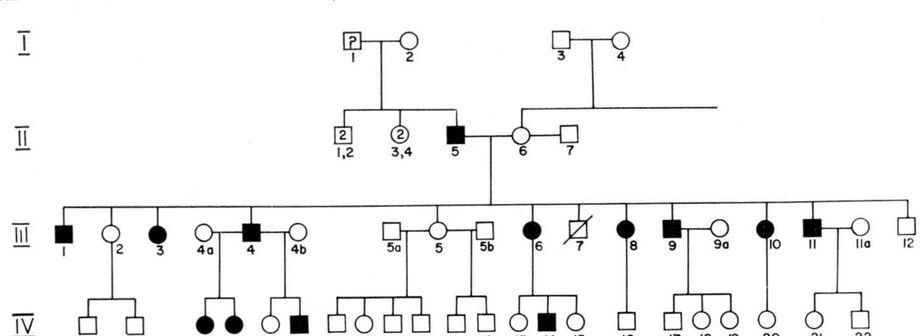

Fig. 3-48A. The Marfan syndrome in three and probably four and more generations. **I-1,** Died at 39 years of age after brief illness. **II-5,** John Peter S., died at age 50 years, of dissecting aneurysm of aorta; had bad eyes. **III-1,** John A. S., born Sept, 29, 1913; has ectopia lentis and severe myopia; strabismus. **III-2,** Elizabeth S. M., born 1915; unaffected; requires hearing aid. **III-3,** Hilda S. S., born 1918; ectopia lentis, severe myopia, chest deformity, and dolichostenomelia. **III-4,** Joseph William S., born 1921; ectopia lentis, left myopia, and dolichostenomelia (see **B**). **III-5,** Frances S. Z. O., born May 9, 1922; small left posterior pole cataract; one of her six children deaf; probably unaffected. **III-6,** Naomi S. M., born Jan. 27, 1924; ectopia lentis, severe myopia, and "tongue-tied," with indistinct speech, **III-7,** Died at one year of "summer complaint." **III-8,** Mildred S. D., born July 10, 1928; ectopia lentis and severe myopia. **III-9,** Frank Martin S., born April 9, 1931; ectopia lentis, severe myopia, dolichostenomelia, severe pneumonia twice as child, slight sternal depression and left chest deformity, and hernia. **III-10,** Nancy Patricia S. M., born 1932; ectopia lentis and myopia. **III-11,** Walter Raymond S., born Feb. 5, 1934; ectopia lentis, myopia, dolichostenomelia, history of severe pneumonia, and chest deformity. **III-12,** Jerome S., born 1935; unaffected apparently, but had operation for severe strabismus in 1949. **IV-3,** Katherine S.; affected. **IV-4,** Mary Dorothy Diane S., born Dec. 19, 1943; bilateral immature cataract and ectopia lentis; affected. **IV-6,** Probably affected. **IV-14,** Harry Douglas M., Jr., born 1945; trouble, like mother, in talking, chicken breast and myopia. **IV-15,** Sophronia M., born 1947; apparently unaffected; trouble talking distinctly. (In a family of twelve children—see generation III—the chance of eight or more children being affected is almost one in four.) (From McKusick, V. A.: Ann. Intern. Med. **49:**556, 1958.)

The pattern of inheritance is that of a simple Mendelian autosomal dominant (Figs. 3-22, 3-23, 3-28, 3-35, 3-47, and 3-48). Parental consanguinity has not been an impressive feature, but exceptions are described.[51] In a few instances, a recessive mode of inheritance seemed to be indicated by the presence of multiple affected members of one sibship with ostensibly normal parents. In only one of the pedigrees of this type that have come to my attention has it been practicable to do thorough investigations of parents and patients (Fig. 3-31). In the one kinship in which this was possible, I was forced to conclude that the mother was probably affected by a *forme fruste.* This woman had had at least three affected children by one man and one affected child by a second. The occurrence in one male and three females excluded the possibility of a sex-linked recessive trait. There was, therefore, no question but that each of the victims inherited the disease rather than developed it through *de novo* mutation and that the mother carries the gene. On examination, she was found to be 5 feet 8 inches tall, to be moderately long of limb without typical arachnodactyly, and to be myopic but free of ectopia lentis on careful ocular examination. This pedigree demonstrates how it is possible for the student of the full clinical and genetic picture to recognize cases which would be missed otherwise. (There are risks, of course, of

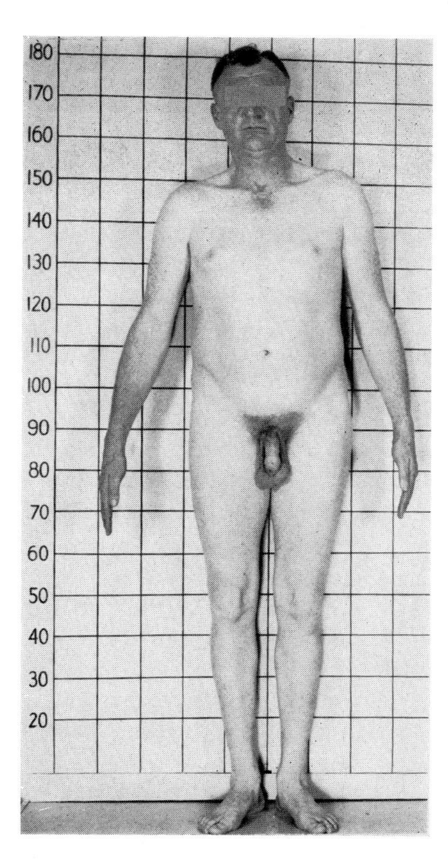

Fig. 3-48B. Individual III-4 (810977) in **A,** 38 years of age. The skeletal proportions are certainly not strikingly dolichostenomelic. The patient has substernal pain, suggesting angina, but no cardiac abnormality by x-ray or electrocardiographic examination. He has suffered also from back pain following a fall at work. Bilateral ectopia lentis is present.

counting cases as affected that are in fact not.) Recessive inheritance of a disorder characterized by ectopia lentis, vascular abnormalities, and skeletal features somewhat similar to those of the Marfan syndrome should suggest homocystinuria (Chapter 4). In Hungary, for example, Varga[391] found six families in which both parents were normal and nine out of twenty-seven sibs were affected with what was interpreted as the Marfan syndrome. The families lived in villages with a highly inbred population. Tests for homocystinuria and more details on the clinical picture would be of interest.

Lynas[224] observed one pedigree (A2) of three affected children from apparently normal parents. Two of the three were, however, not definite cases. In another pedigree (A9) each of two unaffected brothers produced one affected child. Again, however, only "slight signs" were present in one of these.

Capotorti and co-workers[71] described an Italian kindred in which sixteen members of three generations showed the Marfan syndrome. The family contained the first known instance of marriage of two affected persons, who were first cousins. Of their nine children, four were affected, one was normal, three died in infancy, and one was stillborn. Two of the four living affected children showed more severe manifestations than any of the other patients in the pedigree. Some members of this sibship may have been homozyzous for the Marfan gene.

Skipping of generations has never been observed in any thoroughly studied pedigree.[160]

Steinberg and colleagues[354] have reported on 2-year-old identical twins with the Marfan syndrome and "unperforated aortic sinus aneurysm." Becker[31] described identical twins, both affected, in a family with multiple cases of the Marfan syndrome. Papaioannou and associates[279] reported triplets, of whom two may have the Marfan syndrome.

Bowers[56] has traced the disease through six generations of a single family with a total of about thirty-three affected persons.

Lynas and Merrett[226] could find no evidence of genetic linkage between the Marfan trait and the following traits: sex, color vision, phenylthiocarbamide tasting, and ABO, Rhesus, Lewis a and b, Luther, Kell, P. and MNS blood groups.

Partial submersion of the manifestations of this syndrome, depending apparently on the rest of the genetic milieu in which the mutant gene is operating, has been observed.[231] For instance, when the mutation occurs in unusually pyknic stock, the victim's habitus may be much less impressively unusual (Fig. 3-24).* No protection against ocular or aortic abnormality seems to be afforded thereby, however. Lynas[224] seems also to have observed the modifying effects of other genes. In one pedigree a woman with the Marfan syndrome married twice. By the first husband, a "non-Marfan" but tall man with tuberculosis, there were two children: one died in infancy and one had a severe complete form of the Marfan syndrome. By the second husband, "a small square-built man," one child was normal and a second had only mild skeletal and cardiac manifestations.

The fact that in some families pronounced aortic and skeletal abnormalities occur without demonstrable abnormality of the lens seems to be further evidence of the operation of the genetic milieu on expression of the syndrome. Differences in the severity of the several components of the syndrome, including absence of some cardinal ones, is not inconsistent with the view that a single mutant gene is primarily responsible for the abnormality.

Differential diagnosis

Given stigmata suggestive of the Marfan syndrome, one can be most confident of the diagnosis if ectopia lentis is present in the patient or if other members of the family are unequivocally affected (Fig. 3-13).[248]

For example, how can one be certain of the diagnosis of the Marfan syndrome in the case reported as such by Sinha and Goldberg,[336] when the patient "did not have tall features or long fingers," there was no ectopia lentis, "the family history

*By assigning, to affected and unaffected individuals, a score for upper segment–lower segment ratio based on the number of standard deviations by which each individual deviates from the mean for his race, age, and sex (Fig. 3-11), it will probably be possible to test this clinical impression. From initial observations it appears that when the scores for patients with the Marfan syndrome are lower (that is, deviate more on the negative side of the mean), then the average score for his normal first degree relatives is in the low normal range. When the normal relatives have high normal scores, the Marfan patients do not have as markedly low US/LS values.

was noncontributory," and the histologic changes possibly typical of the aorta in the Marfan syndrome p. 124 were not described? Rather numerous uncertain cases are being reported.[43,49,66,133,224,302] Note that the Marfan syndrome can undoubtedly exist in sporadic, nonfamilial cases and that ectopia lentis can occasionally be absent in patients who, because of family data, are known to be affected. It is merely pointed out that usually one cannot be certain of the diagnosis when neither ocular nor familial features are present.

The possibility of the Marfan syndrome is encountered in many situations such as that of aortic regurgitation, otherwise unexplained, in an individual of asthenic and possibly dolichostenomelic habitus. Measurements alone are indicative but not completely conclusive. Measurements must be evaluated in the light of a rough evaluation of the average habitus of the family of which the possibly

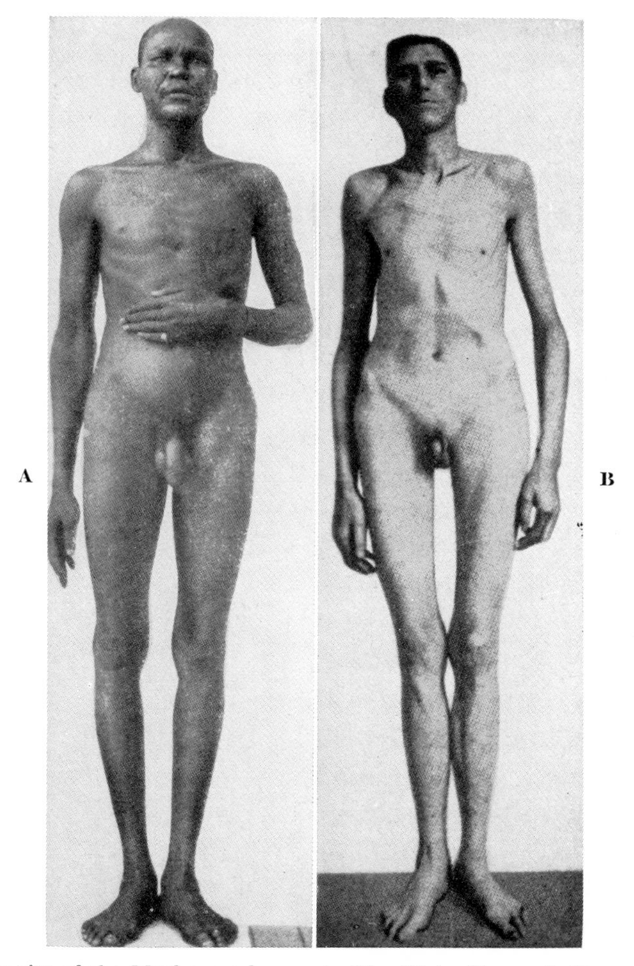

Fig. 3-49. Phenocopies of the Marfan syndrome. **A,** The Dinka Negro. **B,** Eunuch. Brief clinical description given by Bauer and the skeletal proportions suggest the Klinefelter syndrome. (**A** from Martin, R.: Lehrbuch der Anthropologie, ed. 2, Jena, 1928, Gustav Fisher, p. 343; **B** from Bauer, J.: Innere Sekretion, ihre Physiologie, Pathologie und Klinik, Berlin, 1927, Julius Springer.)

affected individual is a member. In the first decade of life, comparison of upper and lower segment measurements and of arm span with height is of greater significance because of the relatively short extremities during this period.[365] (For normal values for these measurements during this period see references 102 and 412 or, better, Fig. 3-11.) The lack of complete specificity of such measurements is indicated by the occurrence of excessively long extremities on an anthropologic basis in the Dinka Negro[249] and on a pathologic basis in the eunuch,[25,134,260] in the Klinefelter syndrome (Fig. 3-49), and in patients with sickle cell anemia. In Wilkins' textbook[412] he pictures in the nude a Negro female patient who had had prepubertal castration for strangulated dermoid cysts. The skeletal proportions are strikingly suggestive of the Marfan syndrome. The rule of thumb for identification of arachnodactyly—longest digit at least 50% longer than the longest metacarpal—has proved to have both positive and negative error. In the Negro in particular, the Marfan syndrome is often suggested by skeletal proportions (Fig. 3-11). Sheldon[331] refers to this habitus as Nilotic dysplasia, since, according to him, inhabitants of the upper Nile area and their descendants display it most often. Members of the Watusi tribe of Uganda are very tall.

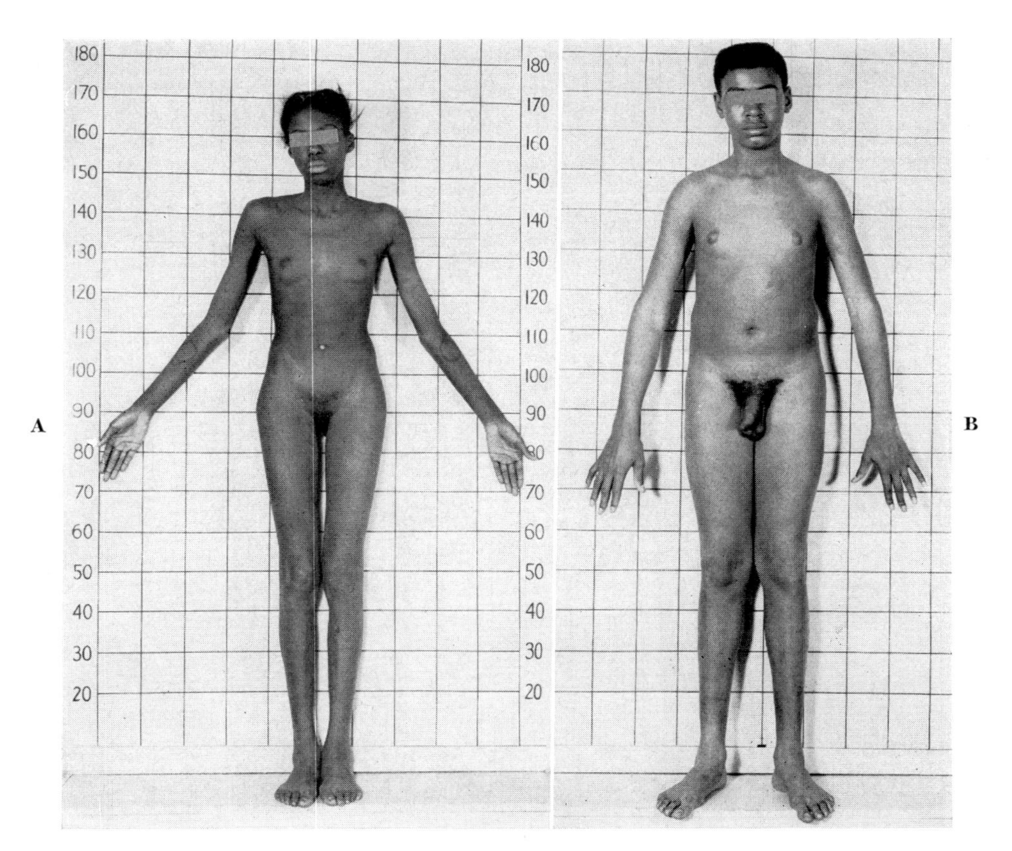

Fig. 3-50A and B. A, Sickle cell anemia. D. M. (659463), 14½ years old, has no ectopia lentis or family history suggesting the Marfan syndrome but does have well-documented sickle cell anemia. **B,** Adolescence. E. K. (766137) was referred because of gynecomastia. There is no ectopia lentis or family history suggesting the Marfan syndrome.

The habitus of successful basketball players suggests that of the Marfan syndrome. Although I have made no systematic study of athletes in this group, one Negro all-state basketball star, previously a member of a champion university team, is 79½ inches tall and has myopia, high narrow palate, deformed chest, genu recurvatum, and the typically flat feet; at 24 years of age he shows profound heart failure and aortic regurgitation with characteristically dilated base of the aorta by aortography. Mitral regurgitation is also present.

Delayed puberty may be accompanied by Marfan-like body proportions. In one individual (E. K., Fig. 3-50*B*) adolescent gynecomastia was also present. As noted earlier, the gracile habitus of many patients with atrial septal defect often leads to a mistaken diagnosis of the Marfan syndrome (Fig. 3-50*D*). The high incidence of chest deformity in patients with congenital malformations of the heart[253] may further increase the confusion with the Marfan syndrome.

A picture mimicking in some respects that of the Marfan syndrome can result from Rh incompatibility and from intrauterine rubella infection. Ectopia lentis does not occur in these cases. However, deafness, ocular and cardiac defects, hypo-

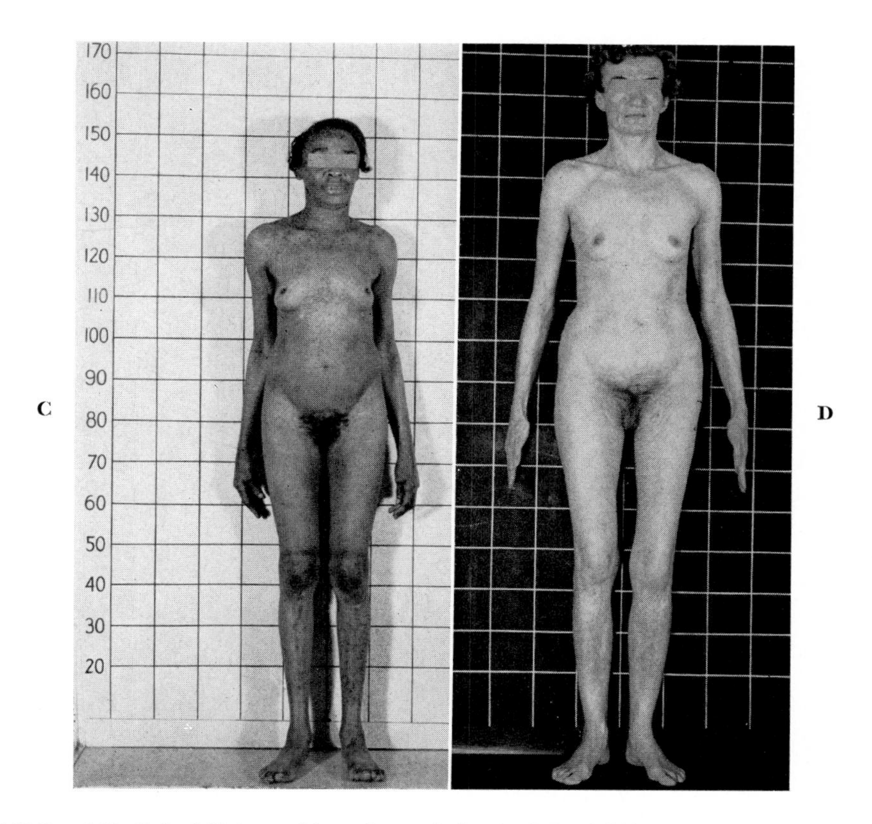

Fig. 3-50C and D. C, Syphilitic aortitis and ectopia lentis. S. J. (802999), 58 years old, has atrophy of the irides, bilateral ectopia lentis, optic atrophy, choroiditis, and secondary glaucoma. Aortic regurgitation is accompanied by blood pressure of 170/60 mm. Hg and enlargement of the left ventricle and left atrium. The family history is not indicative of the Marfan syndrome. **D,** Dolichostenomelia in atrial septal defect. M. L. (713241), 50 years of age, had a secundum type of ASD repaired surgically. There is no ectopia lentis or family history to suggest Marfan syndrome.

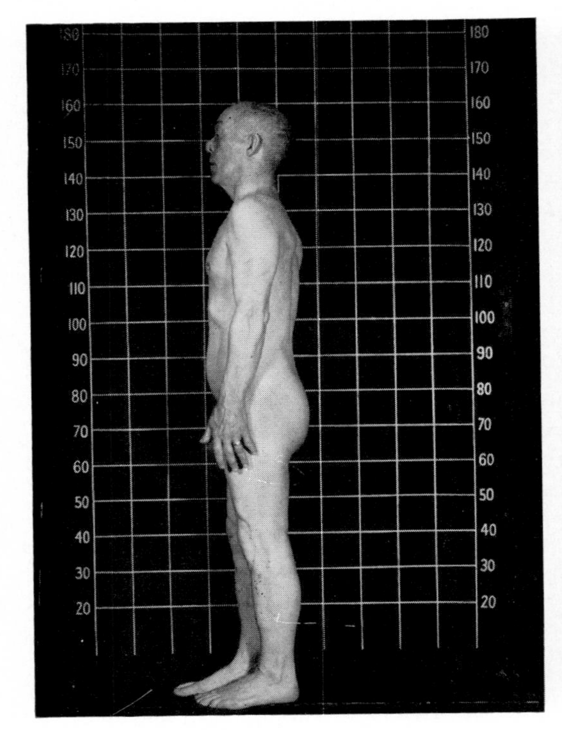

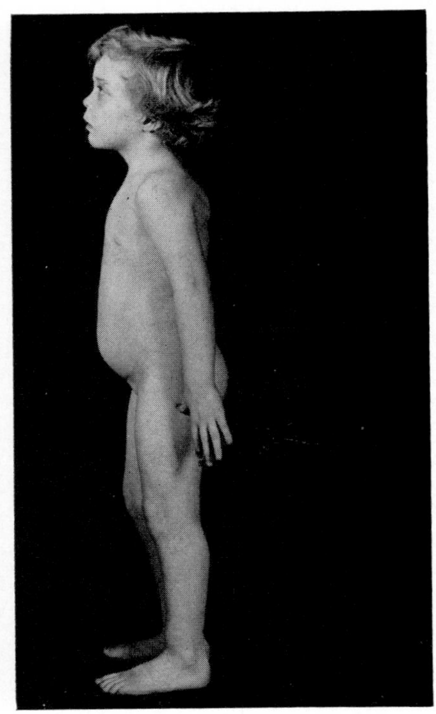

Fig. 3-51. Shown here are father and daughter, both probably examples of the Weill-Marchesani syndrome (ectopia lentis and brachymorphism). The skeletal manifestations are the antithesis of those of Marfan's syndrome. The daughter has a cleft palate and is mentally defective. No definite cardiovascular abnormality has been identified in cases of this syndrome. Compare these father-daughter pictures with that in Fig. 3-28*A*. (From McKusick, V. A.: Circulation **11**:321, 1955.)

tonia, and even arachnodactyly may occur. The presence of some manifestations, such as anophthalmos, which is never encountered in the Marfan syndrome, is a point in favor of one of these other possibilities. Cases simulating Marfan's syndrome have occurred apparently as a result of the occurrence during early pregnancy of febrile illness of unspecified type[129] and of x-ray therapy.[357] (See Fig. 3-41.)

Institutions for mental defectives often list an unbelievably high percentage of patients with arachnodactyly. This should not be taken to indicate Marfan's syndrome, in the majority of instances at any rate, since other evidence indicates that mental retardation is not an integral component of this syndrome and since it is clear that arachnodactyly is a nonspecific manifestation with many possible causes. The patient described by Benda,[35] for example, does not appear to have had the true Marfan syndrome. I would question the correctness of the diagnosis of the Marfan syndrome in the proband of family A5 of Lynas.[224] The patient, a female, was the only one of five children affected. She was a mental defective and "inclined just to sit and drool." The hands and fingers were very long and slender and showed marked clubbing due to bronchiectasis. The feet were abnormally small, however. Very severe kyphoscoliosis was present. The palate was broad

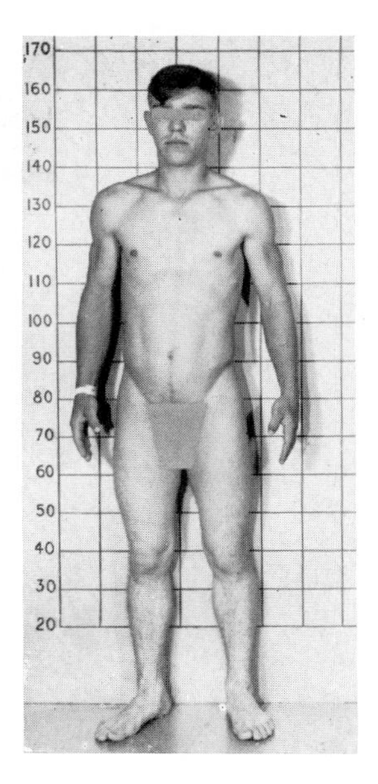

Fig. 3-52. Weill-Marchesani syndrome. R. L. U. (1122410) and two of his four sibs have high-grade myopia and ectopia lentis. No other ocular abnormality is known in the family. All three affected sibs are short of stature as compared with unaffected members of the family. The right eye in the proband showed central serous retinopathy resulting in a rather abrupt drop in vision.

and domed, not high and arched, and there were no eye and cardiac signs. "However, the clinicians are satisfied that she should be included as a case of arachnodactyly." Although by definition arachnodactyly was present, it is very doubtful that this is a case of the true Marfan disease.* (Fig. 3-53 demonstrates another patient with familial mental retardation and arachnodactyly. This is also not the true Marfan syndrome, although the nature of the disorder is unknown.)

Several of the individual components of the Marfan syndrome occur alone or as part of other heritable syndromes and on a genetic basis distinct from the Marfan syndrome. Pectus excavatum,[284,316,343] scoliosis,[130,314] myopia,[92,169] and hernia[108,406] are cases in point. Scoliosis is an important feature of von Recklinghausen's neurofibromatosis, which is inherited as a dominant.[82] Erdheim's cystic medial necrosis is almost certainly not a homogeneous entity from the etiologic standpoint (p. 125). Marfan's disease is but one cause, there being other genetic (e.g. Ehlers-Danlos syndrome) and possibly acquired causes.

Several genetic varieties of ectopia lentis have been described.[33] One variety of isolated ectopia lentis is inherited as a simple Mendelian recessive.[124,387] I have observed[230] eight children of a first-cousin marriage, of whom four had ectopia lentis and four had ateleiotic dwarfism (a condition usually inherited as a recessive). Coincidence of the two anomalies occurred in two of the individuals. An-

*This statement, written in 1959, has been proved true by the demonstration that this patient has homocystinuria.[131]

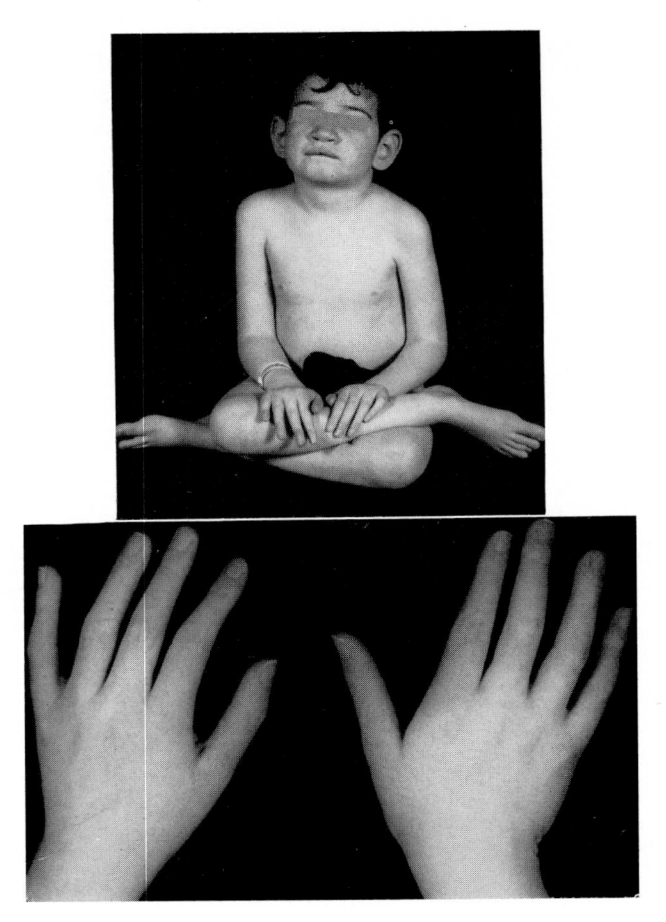

Fig. 3-53. Arachnodactyly with mental retardation. T. C. (1060982) was 6½ years old at the time of this study. Three sibs were unaffected; a brother, age 17 months, was apparently affected in an identical manner. The proband showed marked generalized hypotonia with hyperactive deep tendon reflexes and extensor plantar responses. Pneumoencephalogram suggested cerebellar atrophy. Precise classification of the disorder was impossible.

other variety of ectopia lentis is part of the Weill-Marchesani syndrome.[231,244,245,259,404] The habitus of the victim of the Weill-Marchesani syndrome is diametrically opposite to that of the Marfan syndrome, since he is brachymorphic and short of stature, with round head, pug nose, depressed nasal bridge, and short, pudgy hands and fingers. This syndrome is inherited as a dominant with low penetrance or as a recessive with partial expression in the heterozygote.[195] Feinberg,[117] who suggested the cumbersome designation "congenital mesodermal dysmorpho-dystrophy, brachymorphic type," described two affected sisters who also had patent ductus arteriosus. The occurrence of affected father and daughter, as suggested in the cases shown in Fig. 3-51, is unusual. Ectopia lentis sometimes occurs with aniridia,[69] which is usually inherited as a dominant.

In approximately 70% of instances of congenital ectopia lentis, the anomaly occurs as a component of the Marfan syndrome. The skeletal manifestations of

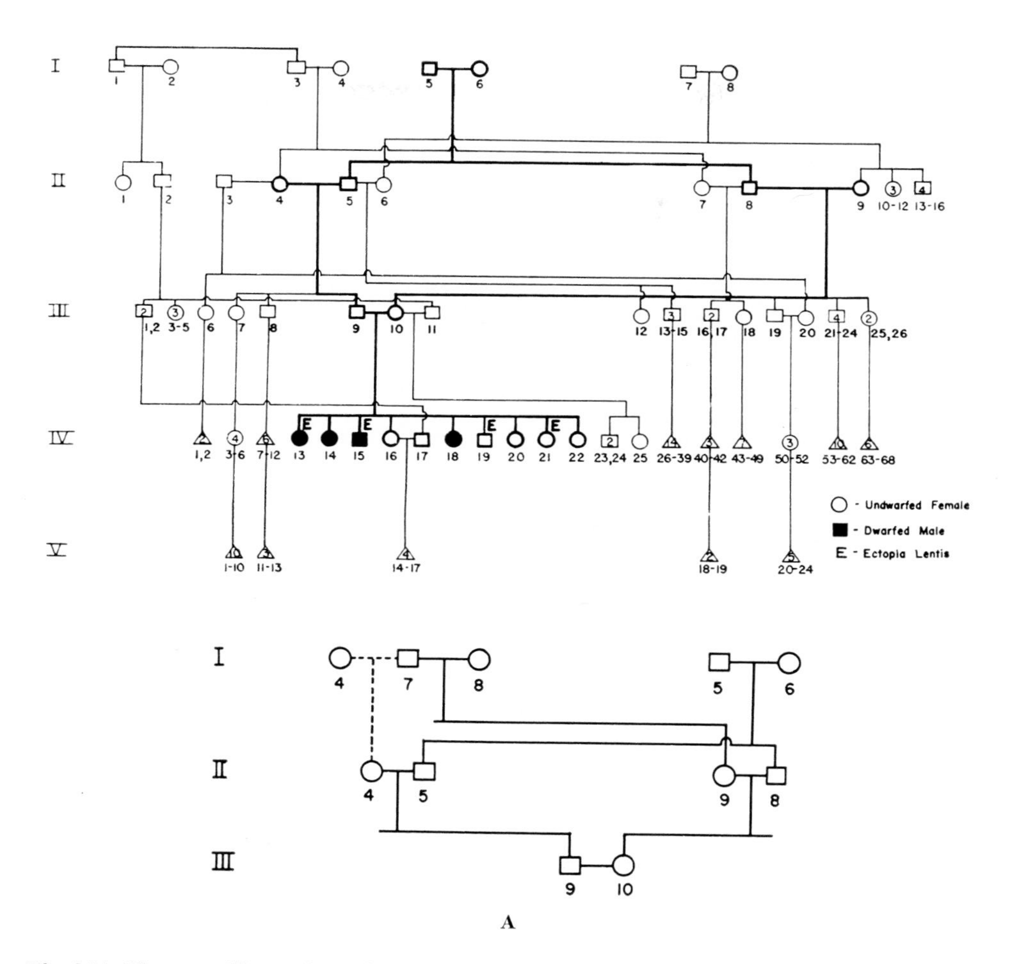

Fig. 3-54. These are illustrations of a sibship,[230] children of a consanguineous marriage, in which four of eight members had ectopia lentis and four had primordial, or ateleiotic, dwarfism. In two individuals there was coincidence of the two pathologic traits. The pedigree is consistent with the view that the two traits were independently inherited as autosomal recessives. In the past, observations on the inheritance of primordial dwarfism have been consonant with this theory of inheritance and it has been thought that ectopia lentis, as an isolated trait, is at times inherited as an autosomal recessive. This material is included to illustrate, along with the example of the Weill-Marchesani syndrome (Fig. 3-51), that the ectopia lentis of the Marfan syndrome is not the only genetic variety of this ocular anomaly. "The phenotype is not necessarily an indication of the genotype." **A,** The pedigree. The parents of the affected sibship were either first cousins or intermediate double first cousins. **B,** Left to right, individuals IV-15, IV-13, and IV-18 of the pedigree. The first two also have ectopia lentis with complicating glaucoma. Not photographed is individual IV-14 who, next to IV-15, is the shortest member of the family. The ages of these individuals are 31, 35, and 24 years, respectively, and their heights 39, 40, and 43¾ inches. **C,** These subjects, of approximately the same age, are 72 and 39 inches tall, respectively. Other than the proportionate dwarfism, the only abnormality revealed by radiographic study of the entire skeleton in individuals IV-15, IV-13, and IV-18 was delayed fusion of the epiphyses at the iliac crests in IV-15, who is 31 years old. (From McKusick, V. A.: Amer. J. Hum. Genet. 7:187, 1955.)

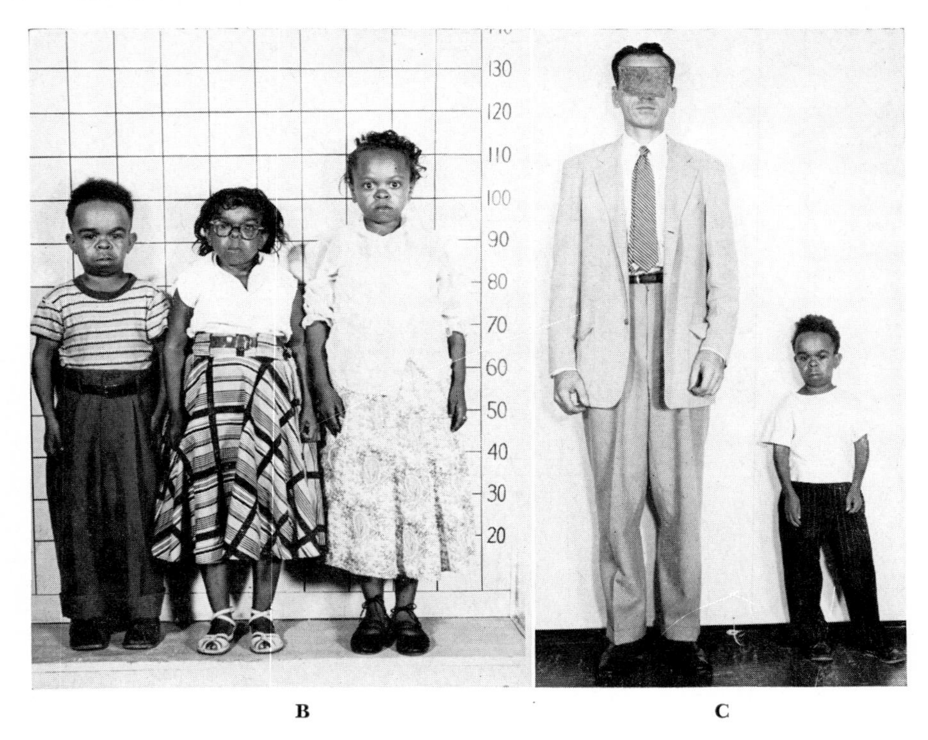

Fig. 3-54, cont'd. For legend see preceding page.

the Marfan syndrome may be so unconvincing in many cases that the presence of ectopia lentis in a patient with cardiovascular signs consistent with the Marfan syndrome should lead one to suspect the diagnosis even though the skeletal changes per se cannot be considered pathognomonic.

Muscular dystrophy was confused for Marfan's syndrome in the patient shown in Fig. 3-55*A* and *B*. Unusually pronounced spinal deformity and long fingers were apparent. The patient presented with bacterial endocarditis and aortic regurgitation—additional features suggesting the Marfan syndrome. Autopsy revealed no histologic evidence for this diagnosis but did show changes consistent with a rheumatic basis for the bacterial endocarditis. A brother, subsequently studied (Fig. 3-55*C* and *D*), shows unequivocal evidence of muscular dystrophy. In children, the pronounced muscular hypotonia may result in a picture suggesting Oppenheim amyotonia congenita or Werding-Hoffmann muscular atrophy.[144] Arachnodactyly has been described[194] with amyoplasia congenita. In brief, then, it is possible to make errors of diagnosis, in either direction, between the primary muscular disorders and the Marfan syndrome.

The relationship, if any, of the Marfan syndrome to "status dysraphicus" is obscure.[287] The latter condition is too ill-defined to make an analysis of relationship possible. We (Fig. 3-15*A*) and others have observed bent fifth fingers, so-called camptodactyly or clinodactyly,[166] and heterochromia iridis,[88] both manifestations that are said to be characteristic of status dysraphicus. Apparently identical clinodactyly is sometimes inherited as an isolated anomaly.[166]

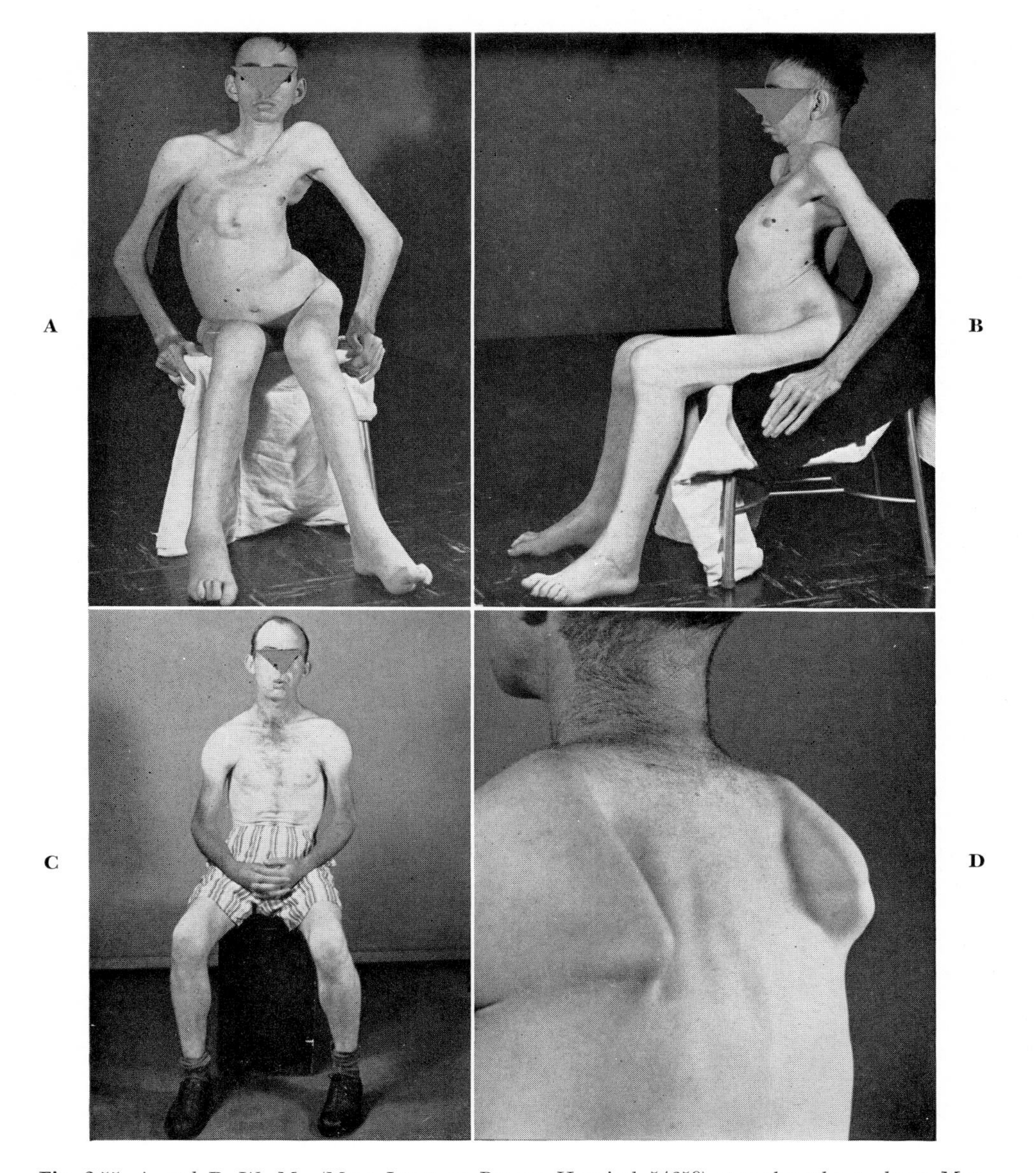

Fig. 3-55. A and **B,** W. M. (Mary Imogene Bassett Hospital 54659) was thought to have Marfan's syndrome because of aortic regurgitation, severe spinal deformity, and arachnodactyly. Clinical evidence for bacterial endocarditis was present. At autopsy the heart lesions appeared to be rheumatic with superimposed valvular infection. (I am indebted to Dr. James Bordley, III, for knowledge of this patient and permission to include him here.) Numerous pigmented nevi were present in this patient. **C** and **D,** D. M., brother of W. M. The finding of muscular dystrophy in this brother makes it likely that W. M. (in **A** and **B**) likewise had muscular dystrophy. The disease trait appears to be recessive in this family. In D. M. note the wasting of the upper arms, especially the left, the asymmetry of the face in whistling, and the winging of the scapulae. There is no arachnodactyly. Spinal deformity as severe as that in W. M. is sometimes seen with muscular dystrophy.[355] The proper classification of the muscular dystrophy in these brothers is uncertain. The parents are living and well. No other cases are known in the family. The brother in **C** and **D** has four children who show no sign of disease. This is probably an autosomal recessive form of muscular dystrophy, which is thought by Becker[32] and others[359] to occur at times. (I am indebted to Dr. Charles Ellicott for studying this patient.)

Parish and associates[281] suggested that arachnodactyly with mandibulofacial dysostosis, particularly receding lower jaw, is a syndrome separate from Marfan's and properly called Achard's syndrome. In the patient described, a 40-year-old woman, joint laxity was confined to the hands and feet.

We have observed two patients (L. E., 677290; S. J., 802999) with ectopia lentis and syphilis. Is it possible that syphilis can cause or predispose to ectopia lentis? The association of syphilitic aortitis with ectopia lentis might occasion diagnostic confusion. Aside from the diagnostic implications the theoretic ones are great, since, as previously indicated, the clinical behavior of the aortic involvement in syphilis has certain parallels to that in the Marfan syndrome. (The rarity of dissecting aneurysm in syphilitic aortitis is a conspicuous difference, however.)

It has been emphasized above that profound aortic regurgitation may be present in patients with the Marfan syndrome for many years before dilatation of the ascending aorta becomes evident by x-ray examination. Some patients with severe aortic regurgitation (Figs. 3-22, 3-23*A* and *B*, and 3-34) never show dilatation of the aorta. The differential diagnosis of the aortic lesion can, therefore, be confusing. Syphilis, rheumatism, or bacterial endocarditis is often suspected first. When these appear unlikely from collateral evidence and when, as is so often possible in all sorts of disorders, a history of trauma is elicited, traumatic rupture of a normal aortic cusp is postulated (Fig. 3-24 and reference 29). Furthermore, a deceptive prominence of the pulmonic conus and main pulmonary artery may result from displacement of these structures by the dilated intrapericardial portion of the ascending aorta. Or the pulmonary artery may be dilated because of intrinsic involvement of its media. As in any severe, prolonged aortic regurgitation with chronic left ventricular failure, the left atrium is likely to become dilated. The prominence of the pulmonary artery and left atrium, the prolongation of the P-R interval (p. 96), and the Austin Flint murmur of aortic regurgitation conspire to lead to the incorrect diagnosis of rheumatic heart disease with combined aortic and mitral lesions.

Pathology

Roark,[309] in 1959, estimated that at least seventy-one autopsies had been reported in the literature. Autopsy was performed in eighteen of the seventy-four probands in my first series; necropsy information was available in at least ten other affected members of these families. The gross changes in the aorta, as demonstrated in Fig. 3-24*C* and Fig. 3-25*E*, are the most dramatic. There are numerous reports of dissecting aneurysm in cases of the Marfan syndrome.[6,67,73,106,140,167,213,214,248,295,300,348,373,376,411]

With the exception of the changes in the media of the great vessels and in the heart valves, no specific histologic abnormalities have been detected in this syndrome. In the media of the aorta, the most advanced changes are seen in cases of diffuse dilatation of the ascending aorta in which the process has gone on over several years' time and the patient succumbed to the effects of aortic regurgitation. In such cases, there are frequently early changes in the pulmonary artery. The early changes in the aorta are best demonstrated in those patients dying of dissecting aneurysm.

The advanced changes consist of fragmentation and sparsity of elastic fibers, irregular whorls of seemingly hypertrophied and perhaps hyperplastic smooth muscle, increase in collagenous tissue, pronounced increase in the vascularity of the media with wide dilatation of the vasa vasorum in both the adventitia and the media and cystic spaces occupied by metachromatically staining material. The net result is an aorta which is thicker (but weaker) than normal.

The early changes are those described by Erdheim[103] as cystic medial necrosis. There is mild to moderate degeneration of elastic fiber elements, with more or less striking cystic areas filled with metachromatically staining material.

The predominant involvement of the ascending aorta is not inconsistent with a generalized defect of some element of connective tissue, since it is the ascending portion of the aorta that bears the main brunt of hemodynamic stress. Reynolds and associates[306] concluded that, with physiologic pulse pressures, it is only the ascending aorta that shows dilatation (i.e. increase in diameter) with each ventricular ejection. Other observers, while disagreeing with Reynolds' claim that virtually no expansile pulsation occurs beyond the arch, corroborate the finding that much greater expansion occurs in the ascending aorta (15 to 20% increase over diastolic diameter in the ascending aorta and 5% in the distal aorta). Engineers, textile scientists, and others concerned with testing the "strength of materials" are familiar with the fact that cyclical application of a stressing force results in structural disintegration much sooner than does steady application of the same force.

Another factor in the predominant localization in the ascending aorta may be implicit in Laplace's law (wall tension = pressure × radius). Since both pressure and radius find their largest values in the ascending aorta, the tension on the wall of that portion is greater than anywhere else in the vascular tree. In the case of aneurysm there is, by the same token, a vicious cycle or self-perpetuating action—the greater the radius, the greater the wall tension, the greater the radius, and so on.

Changes similar to the early ones in the aorta are not uncommon in the main pulmonary artery. Occasionally the changes there are as advanced as are ever seen in the aorta.[386]

The predominant localization of the pathologic changes of Marfan's syndrome, of other varieties of Erdheim's cystic medial necrosis (p. 134), and of syphilis, in the ascending aorta, probably has its basis in the physical and hemodynamic considerations outlined above. The pulmonary artery has the same defect of its media but rarely gives trouble of clinical significance, probably because both blood pressure and pulse pressure are lower in the pulmonary artery than in the aorta. (In syphilis, other theories for preferential thoracic localization of the spirochete have been invoked, such as difference in the distribution of the vasa vasorum and a slightly cooler environment of the thoracic aorta. Proponents of the latter theory point to the difficulties in inducing syphilis in rabbits during hot weather and the preferential localization of spirochetes in parts of rabbit skin that have been shaved.)

Minor changes in the heart valves, in the form of marginal thickening or fibromyxomatous excrescenses, have been described grossly in many of the autopsied cases,[317,341,380,404] including Salle's[317] case, the first autopsied. Histologically, one case[386] was found to show "numerous lacunas in the collagenous substance of the mitral valve that were filled with a homogeneous basophilic material." This lesion resembles closely that which occurs in the media of the aorta. Fig. 3-27*F* represents the changes in the aortic valve in one of our cases. The pronounced sacculation and stretching of the aortic cusps is probably per se evidence of weakness of the connective tissue stroma of the valve. In the process of the stretching, breaks with fenestration of the cusp may occur.[388] Corresponding to the redundant and subluxating posterior leaflet of the mitral valve demonstrated by cineangiocardiographic studies and correlated with a late systolic murmur (p. 83), this cusp was described at autopsy as "ballooned out like a billowing sail," by Tung and Liebow.[386] In a 34-year-old Marfan patient with aneurysm of the ascending aorta, Edynak and Rawson[97] found ruptured aneurysm of the mitral valve. "Diaphanous" appropriately describes the gross appearance of the valves at operation or autopsy in many cases.[299] Olcott,[273] Tobin and co-workers,[376] and Read and associates,[299] among others,[14,36] also described myxomatous transformation of the heart valves, especially the mitral. There are now numerous experiences (p. 82) indicating that the myxomatous valve transformation of the Marfan syndrome can be the basis for bacterial endocarditis.

Calcification and even ossification of the mitral annulus were detected radiologically and/or pathologically by several workers,[43,261,373] and we have observed one such case (P.R., 559979).

James and co-workers[181] studied the cardiac conduction system in two patients with the Marfan syndrome dying at ages 20 and 19. Significant narrowing of the nutrient arteries to the sinus node and atrioventricular node was demonstrated, as well as evidence of old and recent injury to these structures. The vessels showed medial degeneration and hyperplasia and intimal proliferation. In both patients the terminal illness was characterized by arrhythmias and conduction disturbances. Similar pathologic changes were present in the small arteries of the ventricular myocardium and lungs.

In one case (S. C., 575946) the splenic artery was grossly friable and showed advanced cystic medial necrosis on histologic examination. The splenic, iliac, innominate, both subclavian, both common carotid, both renal, and mesenteric arteries showed characteristic cystic medial necrosis in one well-studied case.[309] The intracranial arteries, inferior vena cava, and common iliac veins were normal. Austin and Schaefer[14] described a case in which both common carotids were extensively involved by cystic necrosis with subsequent dissection. Biopsy of the femoral artery during surgical repair of the heart or aorta under cardiopulmonary bypass has shown cystic medial necrosis in cases of the Marfan syndrome.[299]

The pathologic studies of the eyes[201] have not been very helpful from the fundamental standpoint. Hypoplasia of the dilator muscle of the iris provides explanation for the miosis and poor response to mydriatics.[319]

In the histopathologic study of an eye removed at autopsy from a 27-month-old infant Theobald[372] found incomplete separation between the iris and trabeculum. The dilator pupillae and the circular muscle of the ciliary body were not developed. Reeh and Lehman[300] reported similar findings in an older patient. The chamber angle contained numerous iris processes and strands extending from the anterior portion of the trabeculum to the iris, similar to pectinate ligaments seen in lower animals. Prominent blood vessels were seen to cross through some of the larger processes. The dilator pupillae muscle was thinner than in the normal eye.

Joint capsules, ligaments, tendons, and periosteum have shown no abnormality, but studies in these areas are distressingly few. Roark[309] could find no definite abnormality in the anterior spinous ligament or intervertebral discs.

The basic defect

Bacchus[15] reported low levels of serum seromucoid in patients with the Marfan syndrome. However, comparing forty persons having undoubtedly affected with this disorder with an equal number of normal subjects matched for age, sex, and race, Leeming and McKusick[207] could demonstrate no abnormality of serum seromucoid. Lehmann[208] could demonstrate no abnormality of serum mucoproteins or urinary amino acids in the numerous affected members of a family.

Prockop and Sjoerdsma[294] found that whereas normal subjects excrete in the urine 16 to 34 mg. of peptide-bound hydroxyproline per day, three patients with the Marfan syndrome excreted 38 to 90 mg. Low hydroxyproline diet, isocaloric low protein diet, and state of hydration had no effect on hydroxyproline excretion, and no diurnal variations were found. Since hydroxyproline is an amino acid unique to collagen, the findings in the Marfan syndrome were greeted as of fundamental importance, suggesting that the primary defect involves collagen. Although such may indeed be the case, the work with hydroxyproline perhaps cannot be taken as proof, since (1) many conditions of increased growth are accompanied by elevated urinary hydroxyproline[182,185] and (2) adult Marfan patients may have normal urinary excretion of this amino acid.[337] (Jones and colleagues[186] did find elevation of urinary hydroxyproline in five adult patients, 23 to 38 years of age.) In the present view, the increased urinary excretion of hydroxyproline in patients with the Marfan syndrome under 20 years of age is merely a reflection of their increased growth.[256,342]

In what element of connective tissue is the defect of the Marfan syndrome located? The histologic appearance of the aorta suggests that the primary defect may be in the elastic fiber. The pathogenic chain of events might be this[136]: The elastic fibers, constitutionally inadequate, undergo degeneration, particularly at the site of maximum hemodynamic stress, the ascending aorta. The smooth muscle elements, which normally have origin and insertion on the elastic lamellae, collapse together into disorganized whorls and undergo hyperplasia and hypertrophy. Reparative processes leave the media scarred. Secondary to the frantic hypertrophy of smooth muscle fibers and the scarring process, dilatation of the vasa vasorum occurs. (In 1933 Wolff[419] suggested that Erdheim's cystic medial necrosis might be a generalized weakness of elastic fibers. He demonstrated abnormalities in larger peripheral arteries and in the main pulmonary artery.)

What the suspensory ligament of the lens has in common with the media of the aorta is obscure. If that were known, the basic defect of the Marfan syndrome might be understood. Most information suggests that the suspensory ligament is collagenous in nature.[258] However, it cannot be like most collagen (Table 2, p. 24), because it is digested by chymotrypsin, as demonstrated by the surgical technique developed by Dr. Joaquin Barraquer of Spain and introduced into the United States by Dr. Derrick T. Vail. Furthermore, the zonular fibers are not digested by collagenase.[289]

The histologic changes in the aorta in the Marfan syndrome are not inconsistent with the possibility that the primary defect involves collagen. There is more collagen in the aorta than elastic tissue,[258] and by interconnecting the elastic lamellae the collagen fibers may be important to the structural integrity of the skeleton of the aortic media.

It is possible to reconcile with a generalized connective tissue defect many of the other manifestations: the lax joint capsules, the weak ligaments, especially those with large elastic fiber representation such as the ligamenta flava of the spine, the malformed elastic cartilages of the pinnae, and the deformity of the foot where elastic fibers are abundant in the ligaments.[366] But how is one to explain the most striking feature of this syndrome, dolichostenomelia, and the other dolichomorphic features? One gets the impression that the factor that is missing during morphogenesis and growth of bone in victims of this syndrome is a binding force that places a rein on longitudinal growth. Whether it is elastic fiber as such or some element with the properties of the elastic fiber matters not at the moment. Is some such element missing from the ground material of the cartilaginous precursors of bone? Or is the location of the defect in the periosteum? Longitudinal growth of the large bones of the extremities occurs at the epiphyseal-diaphyseal junctions. The periosteum, attached as it is to the epiphyseal cartilage, may exercise control over longitudinal growth.[400] Experiments of Ollier in 1867[274] and of others[203] more recently, although not without flaw, suggest such to be the case: If a cuff of periosteum is removed from the circumference of a growing long bone, that bone will grow longer than its untampered counterpart. An inborn weakness of the periosteum might have a similar effect. The bony abnormality does not appear to be one of simple overgrowth, since the excess is limited to longitudinal growth. The bones are abnormally small in cross section. Osteogenesis may be proceeding at a normal rate in the periosteum, which slides along the diaphysis, adding bone to the circumference; the diaphysis may not attain normal transverse dimensions because the periosteal bone is spread over a greater total area.*

The failure to find abnormality of elastic tissue in the trachea, skin, spinal ligaments, and intervertebral disc[309] is disturbing to the theory implicating elastic tissue.

The report[15] that the affected members of one family showed abnormally low levels of serum mucoproteins was received with great interest. If confirmed, not only would the observation have diagnostic usefulness but also it might assist in pin-pointing the basic defect. Note that as stated on p. 28 the elastic fiber is, in one view, composed in part of "elastomucin." Unfortunately, Dr. James T. Leeming and I have been unable to demonstrate any abnormality of serum mucoprotein in forty-six Marfan patients as compared with controls matched for age, sex, and race.[207]

---

*Lacroix[203] writes (p. 59) as follows: "A fibro-elastic membrane, the periosteum grows, while yielding to a traction imposed upon it, by stretching over its entire extent. Where only one zone of growth exists, as in the case of the long bones of the hand and foot, the periosteal sheath is attracted in only one direction; it is pulled in two opposite directions on the two sides of a 'neutral' zone in bones with two zones of growth. Since the diaphysis elongates only at the level of the growth cartilage, the periosteum during development slides along the bone surface at a rate and in a direction specific to each level." Later (p. 67), he writes: "Since the periosteum slides along the diaphysis which it encloses, the youngest trabeculae, those in formation at the moment of examination are not deposited at exactly the same level as those which the same zone of periosteum elaborated in the preceding days." The obliquity of the canals of the nutrient arteries has its origin in this phenomenon.

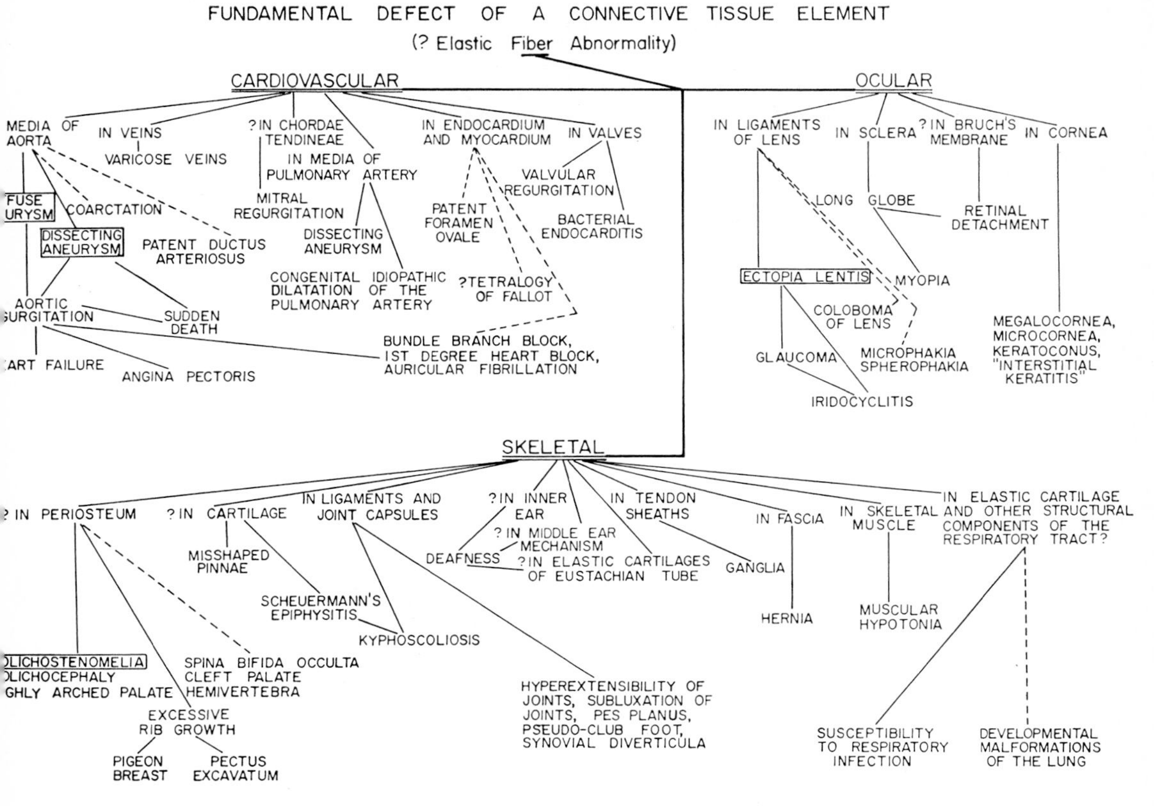

Fig. 3-56. Marfan's syndrome, a pedigree of causes. The chart reviews the components of this syndrome. Special attention is directed to those manifestations indicated by interrupted lines: in the skeletal system, spina bifida occulta and hemivertebra; in the heart, interatrial septal defect and coarctation of the aorta; in the eye, coloboma of the lens and microphakia. In the present state of our knowledge these congenital anomalies of the more conventional type are difficult to explain on the basis of a unitary defect of connective tissue unless one assumes that the presence of this defect during embryogenesis produces an abnormal setting in which these particular anomalies occur with increased incidence. If this is true, these less frequent manifestations indicated by the interrupted lines may be considered secondary ones. (From McKusick, V. A.: Circulation 11:321, 1955.)

The precise element of connective tissue that is defective in the Marfan syndrome awaits identification. Nonetheless, it is possible to describe the behavior of the defect in considerable detail. (See the "pedigree of causes" in Fig. 3-56.)

The production in rats of a somewhat analgous, but *acquired,* syndrome has been of great interest, for obvious reasons. Kyphoscoliosis, hernia, and aneurysm of the aorta (dissecting, diffuse, or saccular) can be produced in rats (Fig. 3-57) fed a toxic agent contained in the seed of *Lathyrus odoratus.*[60,291,293] The toxic material has been crystallized[94] and identified[320] as β (γL-glutamyl) aminopropionitrile $(HOOC{-}CH(NH_2){-}CH_2{-}CH_2{-}C({=}O){-}NH{-}CH_2{-}CH_2{-}C{\equiv}N)$.

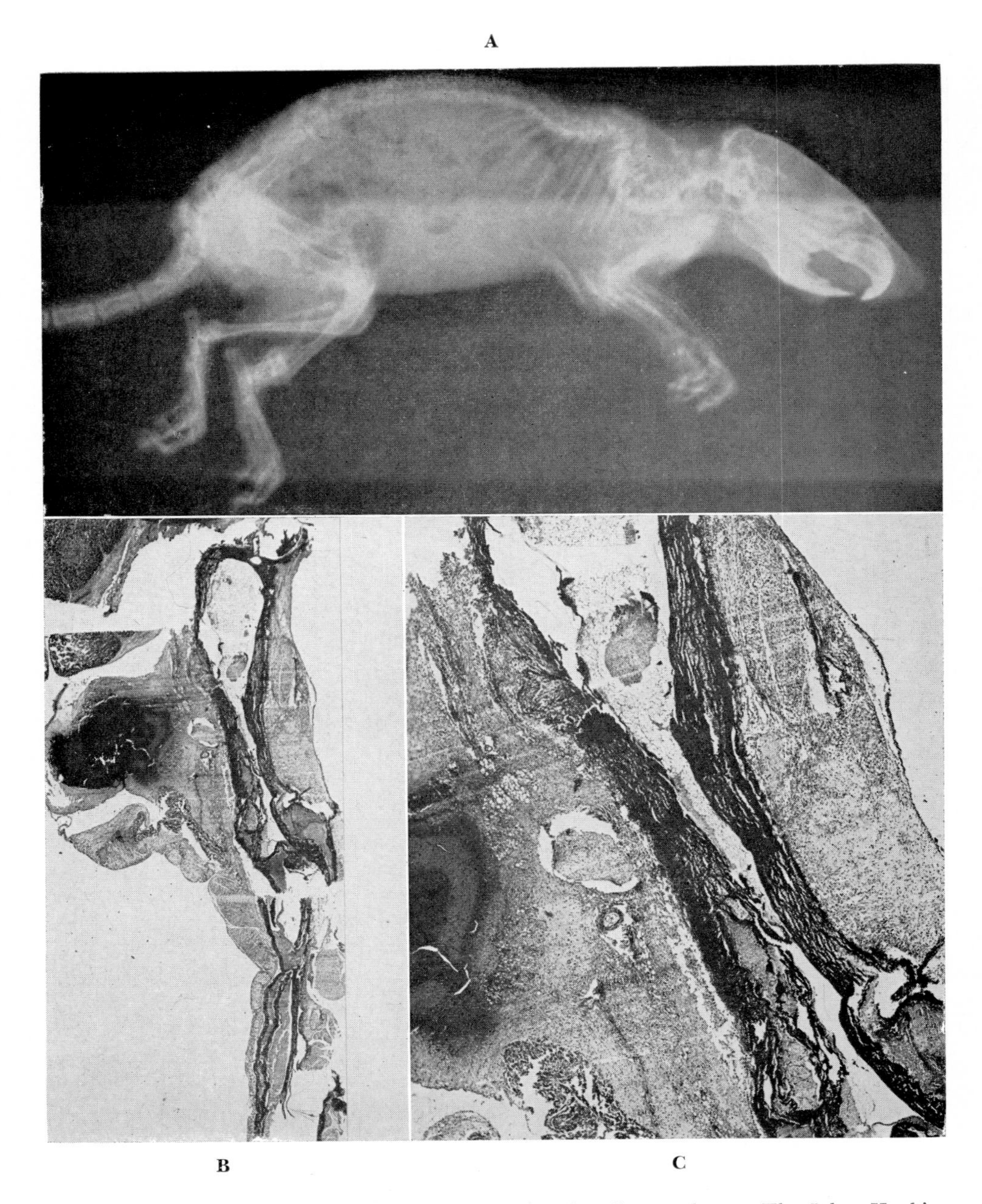

Fig. 3-57. Experiments conducted by Dr. James R. Brayshaw,[60] as student at The Johns Hopkins University School of Medicine. **A,** Deformity and pathologic fracture of spine and other bones in rat fed seeds of *Lathyrus odoratus.* **B,** Dissecting aneurysm of the aorta with rupture in rat fed seeds of *L. odoratus.* Shown is the dissection of the media and the large mediastinal hematoma. Elastic tissue stain. The elastic lamellae are black. (×10; reduced 1/5.) **C,** Same at higher magnification. On the left below, the wall of the aorta is grossly scarred through almost its entire thickness. (×30; reduced 1/5.)

The aminopropionitrile will also cause skeletal changes and dissecting aneurysm of the aorta.[401] Gelatin and casein appear to afford partial protection against the effects of these toxins.[85] Whether the primary difficulty is in the elastic fibers or in the intermediate material is not clear.[16,77] Possibly significant with reference to the predominant male sex incidence of dissecting aneurysm in man is the finding[397] that aortic rupture occurs much more frequently in male rats fed sweet pea seeds than in female rats. Furthermore, the simultaneous administration of androgen considerably enhanced the incidence and severity of aortic medionecrosis[399] in sweat pea–fed rats. The demonstration of increased mucopolysaccharide[77] is of interest in light of the metachromatically staining material seen in human cases of Erdheim's cystic necrosis, including that caused by Marfan syndrome (p. 125). Although the basic defect in this acquired syndrome is probably not the same as that in Marfan's syndrome, studies of this sort should be helpful in elucidating some of the many mysteries that surround dissecting aneurysm in particular[199] and disorders of connective tissue in general. Clinically, Bean and Ponseti[130] have been impressed with a relatively high incidence of kyphoscoliosis in the group of cases of dissecting auerysm of the aorta.

If the defective connective tissue element in the Marfan syndrome is indeed collagen, the elucidation of the molecular defect in lathyrism, which simulates the Marfan syndrome rather closely, is of obvious pertinence. The amino-nitriles, the toxic component of *Lathyrus odoratus* seeds, interfere with collagen cross-linking mechanisms.[147]

Another possible model or phenocopy for the aortic lesion in the Marfan syndrome may be copper deficiency in swine.[81,215,332,405] Rupture of the aorta occurs at the age of 3 or 4 months in these animals. A defect in the elastica of the media has been demonstrated mechanically, histologically, and biochemically. Linker and associates[215] demonstrated a threefold increase in the mucopolysaccharide content of the aorta.

Tjio and co-workers[375] described the presence of a chromosome with giant satellites in each of two patients designated as having familial Marfan's disease. They stated that "while the present data do not prove the given abnormalities to be the underlying cause of Marfan's syndrome, a relationship is definitely suggested." Because of doubts about the diagnosis of Marfan's syndrome in the two patients, the failure to find giant satellites in a third undoubted case of Marfan's syndrome, and the observation of giant satellites in persons either without phenotypic abnormality or with features other than those of the Marfan syndrome, it seemed unlikely that a causal relationship existed.[235] Furthermore, Ford,[123] Böök (cited by Ford), and Handmaker[155] could find no abnormality of the chromosomes in a considerable number of Marfan patients. In four such patients Källén and Levan[189] found that chromosomes 21 and 22 were relatively shorter than those of normal persons. Of the three male patients one had an abnormally long Y chromosome and one an abnormally short Y chromosome. The findings in chromosomes 21 and 22, which apparently have not been sought by other workers, were interpreted by Källén and Levan[189] as a phenotypic expression at the level of the chromosomes, rather than a casual feature. The XYY sex chromosome constitution found by Hustinx and van Olphen[176] was apparently only coincidental.

Other considerations

There is, of course, no definitive treatment for this disorder. It should be noted that healing after surgical operations is normal. Herniorrhaphy, orthopedic procedures, and correction of pectus excavatum can be performed with success. (One patient went through a lienorenal shunt procedure for unrelated hepatic cirrhosis.[386]) Correction of pectus excavatum should probably be postponed until after puberty, since an imperfect result may follow if there is still opportunity for excessive longitudinal growth of the ribs. The current philosophy in regard to ectopia lentis seems to favor performing lens extraction only if iritis or glaucoma develops. Hufnagel's plastic valve operation[172] was performed in a case of aortic regurgitation on this basis; because of the nature of this disease and the physiologic effects of the operation, its practicability is very questionable. Evidence is presented elsewhere[237] that the Hufnagel operation produces widening of the pulse pressure (due both to increase in the systolic level and to decrease in the diastolic level) proximal to the valve. This might well increase the strain on the already weakened ascending aorta and accelerate the process of dilatation or predispose further to dissection. One might fear that the valve would tear out of the aorta. This has indeed been observed.[192] In this instance the tear occurred at the junction of the aorta with the prosthesis, some months after operation. The gross appearance suggested the wear with cracking which occurs in stethoscope tubing at the junction with the metallic parts of the stethoscope. Support for the view that "wear-and-tear" is a factor in the pathogenesis of the changes observed in the aorta in the Marfan syndrome may be provided by this observation. Thrombosis with occlusion of the valve has been described in two cases of the Marfan sydrome,[67,91] but this is a complication not unique to this hereditary disorder.

During the last decade several surgical groups[89,148,266,346,363] have acquired experience with treatment of the aortic complications of the Marfan syndrome. It is thought that the most frequent lesion—aneurysm of the ascending aorta, with or without dissection, in association with severe aortic valve dilatation—is best treated by replacing the ascending aorta up to the first branch at the arch by a fabric prosthesis and reconstituting the aortic valve by some type of valvuloplasty such as bicuspidization or replacement with a Starr-Edwards prosthetic ball valve. In those instances in which dissection extends beyond the arch, cross-sewing in the most distal areas may suffice, especially if the intimal rent is identified in the resected portion of the ascending aorta.

Baker and co-workers[20] reported the successful use of an aortic homograft in a patient having the Marfan syndrome with dissection limited to the descending thoracic aorta. Replacement of the abdominal aorta has been performed in cases of the Marfan syndrome, with varying success, by Davis and colleagues,[87] Van der Hyde and Zwaveling,[390] Heitzman and Bryant,[164] and by others.

In cases of idiopathic cystic medial necrosis without extravascular stigmata of the Marfan syndrome, graft replacement of the ascending aorta,[19,89,171,346] as well as the earlier procedure of plication and periaortic binding,[18,116] is attended with more success because the involvement of the aortic valve mechanism is not so extreme as in cases of the Marfan syndrome.

A point of medicolegal importance is the relationship of trauma to the development of various manifestations of the Marfan syndrome. The development of hernia, detachment of the retina,[56,236,322] dissecting aneurysm,[50,67,91,286,384] and total dislocation of the lenses may be intimately related to trauma as a precipitating factor. In Choyce's case[76] dislocation of the lenses into the anterior chamber occurred when the patient leaned forward to pick something up from the floor. Wilson[416] suggested that the strain of sexual intercourse may contribute to deterioration of the aorta. In one of his patients, death occurred five days after marriage; in another, symptoms of left ventricular failure began after intercourse. On the other hand, a murmur of aortic regurgitation is known to have been present for sixteen years in an unmarried affected sister. It has been said that in the Marfan syndrome a sedentary spinster may outlive an athletic husband.[416]

In connection with the relation of the Marfan syndrome to other diseases or special physiologic states, rheumatic fever, syphilis, hypertension, and pregnancy might be mentioned. The suggestion of Futcher and Southworth[128] that rheumatic fever may occur with increased incidence in these patients has not been confirmed by further observations. Syphilis and hypertension, if combined with the Marfan disease, might have particularly dire effects on the aorta.

There is now convincing evidence of a strikingly increased incidence of dissecting aneurysm of the aorta in pregnancy.[168,243,270,323,329] Conceivably, this is related to the hormone "relaxin" and to the general relaxation of ligaments and other joint structures during pregnancy.[1,2,161,285,290,303,423] Against this hypothesis is the fact that my colleagues and I[174,236] have been unable to induce aortic dissection in animals treated with large doses of "relaxin," with or without challenge with vasopressor agents. Rupture of the splenic artery, another rather frequently reported[330,377] accident of pregnancy, may be on a similar basis. The reduction of tensile strength of the skin during pregnancy (reference 242, p. 175) is further evidence of a generalized change in connective tissue.

We have observed three patients in whom pathologic changes occurred in the aorta in association with pregnancy. There is no evidence of the Marfan syndrome in any of these. (In addition, dissection may have occurred during pregnancy in the patient illustrated in Fig. 3-22*A*.)

Case 1. A. P. (621953), Negro female, at the age of 36 years had a difficult labor with her sixth child. During a period of hard straining in labor she suddenly "felt something snap" inside her body at the level of the lower back, and an excruciating pain spread over most of the trunk. The baby was delivered by Cesarean section. A laparotomy five months later showed abdominal aneurysm, for which no treatment was attempted. She was aware of a pulsating mass in the abdomen. Palpitation, dyspnea, and profuse sweats developed. She was examined at the Johns Hopkins Hospital six years later. There was a pulsating abdominal mass, auscultatory signs of aortic regurgitation, and marked cardiomegaly. Serologic test for syphilis was negative. The patient died elsewhere; no autopsy was performed.

Case 2. C. T., a 41-year-old mother of seven, was found six weeks before her death to have a blood pressure of 180/100 mm. Hg. She was 6 months or more pregnant. She refused hospitalization at that time. On the morning of the day of death the patient had the onset of substernal pain and profuse perspiration. The blood pressure was 225/120 mm. Hg. On the way to the University Hospital the patient was suddenly seized with severe chest pain, collapsed in the car and became very "blue." She was dead on arrival at the hospital. A postmortem Cesarean section delivered a full-term live male child which weighed 5,089 grams. Autopsy of the mother revealed dissecting aneurysm of the aorta with rupture. (The case reported by Spenser[347] is rather similar, in that postmortem Cesarean delivery was done in a woman dead of dissecting aneurysm.)

Case 3. D. W. (706005), a 33-year-old woman, sustained rupture of a coronary sinus into the right side of the heart, in the early puerperium.

Lindeboom and Bouwer,[213] Husebye and colleagues,[175] Novell and associates,[272] and Baker and colleagues[20] reported on dissecting aneurysm in pregnant or recently pregnant women with the Marfan syndrome, and Spenser's case[347] may be another example. Avoidance of pregnancy seems indicated, especially by more severely affected women.

Relation to Erdheim's cystic medial necrosis[315]

Erdheim's disease is probably not a single entity from the etiologic standpoint. There are probably a number of possible "causes"—some genetic (like the Marfan syndrome) and some acquired in nature. With the control of syphilis and rheumatic fever, cystic medial necrosis will assume increasing importance as a cause of aortic regurgitation. It must be kept in mind particularly when there is no history of syphilis, rheumatism, and bacterial endocarditis and must *not* be excluded from consideration on the grounds that there is no radiologic evidence of aortic dilatation. Unfortunately, the diagnosis of idiopathic Erdheim's disease (Erdheim's disease without the Marfan syndrome) will for the present need to be a diagnosis of exclusion.

Some pathologists such as Dr. A. R. Rich and Dr. Ella Oppenheimer[307] feel that the aorta in the Marfan syndrome has histologic features—specifically, large whorled bundles of disorganized smooth muscle and greatly dilated vasa vasorum —that are not seen in ordinary Erdheim's disease. The changes that are considered specific for the Marfan syndrome are most likely to occur in the first part of the aorta, the part that first undergoes dilatation. Further on in the aorta the changes are indistinguishable from those of idiopathic medial necrosis. It is uncertain whether this histologic picture indicates a fundamental difference. It seems to me possible that merely the prolonged evolution or some other feature of the Marfan syndrome permits or dictates the occurrence of this particular change.

The experience with Marfan's syndrome should prove very useful in the cases of idiopathic Erdheim's disease. In both, dissecting aneurysm or fusiform dilatation* or a combination can occur. In both, the ascending aorta is most severely affected. In both, the process seems to pursue an unrelenting progression to death from rupture of the aorta or from the effects of aortic regurgitation.

There is now convincing evidence[340] that the metabolic turnover rate in the elastic skeleton of the aorta is so low† as to raise serious suspicions of complete metabolic inertia. The elastic structures of the aorta can be looked on as intended to outlive the rest of the organism. In certain unfortunate individuals, however, the elastica "gives out" prematurely. The result is Erdheim's cystic medial necrosis. Genetic inferiority is probably most frequently the basis. It has been described in brothers,[141,395] in father and son,[121] and in mother and daughter,[146] but the clinical information provided is too scant to permit exclusion of the Marfan syndrome. Erdheim's medial necrosis may be the cause of death in the first months of life or not until the ninth decade. Rupture of the aorta, possibly on a

*Erdheim's disease is very familar as a cause of dissecting aneurysm. That it can also cause diffuse or fusiform dilatation of the aorta is indicated by the surgically proved cases referred to above and by reports in the literature.[86,159,312,418,422,423,427] In some of these, insufficient clinical information is provided to permit exclusion of the Marfan syndrome.

†Labella[202] suggests there may be a component of elastic fiber that is metabolically fairly active.

comparable basis, is said to occur in horses and occurs in epidemic fashion in turkeys,[240] where dietary factors may be responsible.

The treponemal immobilization test for syphilis has created a clinical problem in connection with patients with dilatation of the ascending aorta and aortic regurgitation, who often in the past would have been considered to be syphilitic in spite of negative serologic tests for syphilis of the conventional type. In coming years, cystic medial necrosis of the aorta, previously the exclusive property of the pathologists, will be discussed much more frequently in the clinical literature.

Gordon[135] and Schwartz[325] have suggested that Abraham Lincoln had the Marfan syndrome. Both based the impression in part on Lincoln's long extremities and statements of his contemporaries that he was unusually loose-jointed. Nathaniel Hawthorne described him as a "tall, loose-jointed figure." The Washington correspondent of the London *Times* described Lincoln as a "tall, lank, lean man, considerably over six feet in height, with stooping shoulders, long pendulous arms terminating in hands of extraordinary dimensions, which, however, were far exceeded in proportion by his feet." Lincoln's mother, Nancy Hanks, who in the opinion of Gordon had the Marfan syndrome, was of unknown paternity. (Her death is more usually attributed to "milk sickness," hypoglycemia from milk from cows that have fed on white snake root.) On the other hand, Schwartz[325] believes he has evidence that Lincoln inherited the Marfan gene from his father; he has a patient named Lincoln, with seemingly typical Marfan syndrome, who is a descendant of Lincoln's grandfather.

Gordon suggested that Thomas Lincoln, who resembled his father closely and died at 18 years of age of "dropsy of the chest," had the Marfan syndrome with cardiovascular complications.

Because of the obvious general interest, the conclusions of Gordon and Schwartz found their way into the lay press. The public reaction has had interesting features. For example, in a letter-to-the-editor (*Newsweek,* June 11, 1962), one reader insisted that Lincoln could not have suffered from such a "loathsome disease." The statement reflects an unfortunate and uninformed attitude toward hereditary disease, which is no more (or less) loathsome than poliomyelitis, sarcoma, myocardial infarction, alcoholism, and cerebral arteriosclerosis, with which other Presidents have been afflicted.

SUMMARY

The cardinal manifestations of the Marfan syndrome are skeletal, ocular, and aortic. Dolichostenomelia (long, thin extremities) and redundant ligaments and joint capsules characterize the skeletal changes. Ectopia lentis is the hallmark of the disorder in the eye. In the aorta, predominantly the ascending aorta, diffuse dilatation and/or dissection occur.

The only histopathologic changes described to date are those in the aorta, where degeneration of the elastic lamellae appears to be primary in the pathogenetic chain. Whether the basic defect resides in the elastic fiber or, as seems somewhat more likely, in collagen is unknown.

The pedigrees are consistent with inheritance of this trait as a simple Mendelian dominant with a relatively high grade of penetrance.

Although certainly there are some persons having true cases of the Marfan syndrome without ectopia lentis and without other less equivocally affected members in the family, the lack of both of these features leaves the diagnosis in question in many instances.

REFERENCES

1. Abramson, D., Hurwitt, E., and Lesnick, G.: Relaxin in human serum as test of pregnancy, Surg. Gynec. Obstet. **65**:335, 1937.
2. Abramson, D., Roberts, S. M., and Wilson, P. D.: Relaxation of pelvic joints in pregnancy, Surg. Gynec. Obstet. **58**:595, 1934.
3. Achard, C.: Arachnodactylie, Bull. Mém. Soc. Méd. Hôp. Paris **19**:834, 1902.
4. Adams, R. A., and Porter, W. B.: Marfan's syndrome. Report of a case, Southern Med. J. **42**:844, 1949.
5. Albanese, A.: Sulla dolichostenomelia, Arch. Ortop. **47**:539, 1931.
6. Anderson, A., Spencer, H., and Staffurth, J. S.: Dissecting aneursym and medial degeneration of the aorta in Marfan's snydrome, St. Thomas's Rep. **7**:146, 1951.
7. Anderson, M., and Pratt-Thomas, H. R.: Marfan's syndrome, Amer. Heart J. **46**:911, 1953.
8. Anning, S. T.: Elastoma intrapapillare perforans verruciforme (Miescher), Proc. Roy. Soc. Med. (Sect. Dermat.) **51**:932, 1958.
9. Anon.: Marfan's biography, Brit. J. Med. **2**:175, 1942.
10. Anon.: A. B. Marfan, Presse Méd. **50**:301, 1942.
11. Anon.: A. B. Marfan, Union Méd. Canada **73**:1706, 1944.
12. Apert, E.: Les formes frustes du syndrome dolichosténomélique de Marfan, Nourrisson **26**:1, 1938.
13. Atta, A. G., and Hoch, J.: Marfan's syndrome and dissecting aneurysm of the aorta, Arch Intern. Med. **108**:781, 1961.
14. Austin, M. G., and Schaefer, R. F.: Marfan's syndrome, with unusual blood vessel manifestations. Primary medionecrosis dissection of right innominate, right carotid, and left carotid arteries, Arch. Path. **64**:205, 1957.
15. Bacchus, H.: A quantitative abnormality in serum mucoproteins in the Marfan syndrome, Amer. J. Med. **25**:744, 1958.
16. Bachhuber, T. E., and Lalich, J. J.: Effect of sweat pea meal on the rat aorta, Arch. Path. **59**:247, 1955.
17. Baer, R. W., Taussig, H. B., and Oppenheimer, E. H.: Congenital aneurysmal dilatation of the aorta associated with arachnodactyly, Bull. Hopkins Hosp. **72**:309, 1943.
18. Bahnson, H. T., and Nelson, A. R.: Cystic medial necrosis as a cause of localized aortic aneurysms amenable to surgical treatment, Ann. Surg. **144**:519, 1956.
19. Bahnson, H. T., and Spencer, F. C.: Excision of aneurysm of ascending aorta with prosthetic replacement during cardiopulmonary bypass, Ann. Surg. **151**:879, 1960.
20. Baker, C. B., Wilson, T. K., and Woods, J. M.: Marfan's syndrome; a successful aortic homograft for a dissecting aneurysm of the thoracic aorta, Canad. J. Surg. **1**:371, 1958.
21. Baron, M. G., Wolf, B. S., Grishman, A., and van Mierrop, L. H. S.: Aneurysm of the membranous septum, Amer. J. Roentgen. **91**:1303, 1964.
22. Barraquer, J., and Rutllán, J.: Alpha-chymotrypsin in cataract surgery, Postgrad. Med. **35**:57, 1964.
23. Barrett, J. S., Helwig, J., Jr., Kay, C. F., and Johnson, J.: Cineangiographic evaluation of aortic insufficiency: unsuspected idiopathic aneurysmal dilatation of the aortic root as a possible indication of the Marfan syndrome, Ann. Intern. Med. **61**:1071, 1964.
24. Barron, A. A.: Arachnodactyly (Marfan's syndrome), N. Carolina Med. J. **3**:353, 1942.
25. Bauer, J.: Innere Sekretion, ihre Physiologie, Pathologie und Klinik, Berlin and Vienna, 1927, Julius Springer, p. 361.
26. Bawa, Y. S., Gupta, P. D., and Goel, B. G.: Complete heart block in Marfan's syndrome, Brit. Heart J. **26**:148, 1964.
27. Bean, W. B.: Precordial noises heard at a distance from the chest. In Monographs in medicine, Baltimore, 1952, Williams & Wilkins Co., p. 22.
28. Bean, W. B., and Fleming, J. G.: Arachnodactyly; report of a case complicating pregnancy at term, Ohio Med. J. **36**:155, 1940.
29. Bean, W. B., and Mohaupt, F. X.: Rupture of the aortic valve, J.A.M.A. **150**:92, 1952.

30. Bean, W. B., and Ponseti, I. V.: Dissecting aneurysm produced by diet, Circulation **12:**185, 1955.
31. Becker (Naumberg): Linsenektopie in der I., (II.), und III. Generation, Klin. Mbl. Augenheilk. **94:**547, 1935.
32. Becker, P. E.: Dystrophia musculorum progressiva; eine genetische und klinische Untersuchung der Muskeldystrophien, Stuttgart, 1953, Georg Thieme Verlag.
33. Bell, J.: Anomalies and diseases of the eye, the treasury of human inheritance, Cambridge, 1932, Cambridge University Press, vol. 2, part V, p. 477.
34. Benavides, P.: Sindrome de Marfan, Principia Cardiologica **3:**193, 1956.
35. Benda, C. E.: Developmental disorders of mentation and cerebral palsies, New York, 1952, Grune & Stratton, Inc., p. 159.
36. Berenson, G. S., and Greer, J. C.: Heart disease in the Hurler and Marfan syndromes, Arch. Intern. Med. **111:**58, 1963.
37. Berg, G., and Vejlens, G.: Cystic disease of the lung in tuberous sclerosis, Acta Paediat. **36:**16, 1939.
38. Berg, G., and Zachrisson, C. G.: Cystic lungs of rare origin—tuberous sclerosis, Acta Radiol. **22:**425, 1941.
39. Bergstrand, C. G.: Arachnodactylia: pathological anatomy in connection with a case, Acta Paediat. **30:**345, 1943.
40. Berlin, R.: Familial occurrence of pneumothorax simplex, Acta Med. Scand. **137:**268, 1950.
41. Bhat, P. K.: Bilateral ectopia lentis with arachnodactyly. Marfan's syndrome with report of case and review of literature, Antiseptic **43:**651, 1946.
42. Bigger, I. A.: The treatment of pectus excavatum or funnel chest, Amer. Surg. **18:**1071, 1952.
43. Bingle, J.: Marfan's syndrome, Brit. Med. J. **1:**629, 1957.
44. Binion, J. T.: Marfan's syndrome, Amer. Pract. & Digest Treat. **5:**135, 1954.
45. Black, H. H., and Landay, L. H.: Marfan's syndrome; report of five cases in one family, Amer. J. Dis. Child. **89:**414, 1955.
46. Boerger, F.: Ueber zwei Fälle von Arachnodaktylie, Zschr. Kinderheilk. **12:**161, 1914; Mschr. Kinderheilk. **13:**335, 1914.
47. Bolande, R. P.: The nature of the connective tissue abiotrophy in the Marfan syndrome, Lab. Invest. **12:**1087, 1963.
48. Bolande, R. P., and Tucker, A. S.: Pulmonary emphysema and other cardio-respiratory lesions as part of the Marfan abiotrophy, Pediatrics **33:**356, 1964.
49. Booth, C. C., Louchbridge, L. W., and Turner, M. D.: Arachnodactyly with congenital lesions of the urinary tract, Brit. Med. J. **2:**80, 1957.
50. Bornstein, F. P.: Dissecting aneurysm of the thoracic aorta due to trauma, Texas J. Med. **50:**720, 1954.
51. Bortree, L. W.: Discussion of Strayhorn and Wells.[367]
52. Bowden, D. H., Favara, B. E., and Donahoe, J. L.: Marfan's syndrome. Accelerated course in childhood associated with lesions of mitral valve and pulmonary artery, Amer. Heart J. **69:**96, 1965.
53. Bowers, D.: The electrocardiogram in Marfan's syndrome, Amer. J. Cardiol. **7:**661, 1961.
54. Bowers, D.: An electrocardiographic pattern associated with mitral valve deformity in Marfan's syndrome, Circulation **23:**30, 1961.
55. Bowers, D.: Marfan's syndrome: the S family re-visited, Canad. Med. Ass. J. **89:**337, 1963.
56. Bowers, D. (Kelowna, British Columbia) Unpublished observations.
57. Bowers, D., and Lim, D. W.: Subacute bacterial endocarditis and Marfan's syndrome, Canad. Med. Ass. J. **86:**455, 1962.
58. Boyd, D. H. A.: Familial spontaneous pneumothorax, Scot. Med. J. **2:**220, 1957.
59. Bramwell, C., and King, J. T.: The principles and practice of cardiology, London, 1942, Oxford University Press, p. 29.
60. Brayshaw, J. R., and McKusick, V. A.: Unpublished observations.
61. Brock, R. C.: Recurrent and chronic spontaneous pneumothorax, Thorax **3:**88, 1948.
62. Bronson, E., and Sutherland, G. A.: Ruptured aortic aneurysms in childhood, Brit. J. Child. Dis. **15:**241, 1918.
63. Burian, H. M.: Chamber angle studies in developmental glaucoma. Marfan syndrome and high myopia, J. Missouri Med. Ass. **55:**1088, 1958.
64. Burian, H. M.: A case of Marfan's syndrome with bilateral glaucoma: with description of

a new type of operation for developmental glaucoma (trabeculotomy ab externo), Amer. J. Ophthal. **50**:1187, 1960.

65. Burian, H. M., von Noorden, G. K., and Ponseti, I. V.: Chamber angle anomalies in systemic connective tissue disorders, Arch. Ophthal. **64**:671, 1960.
66. Burry, A. F.: Supra-aortic stenosis associated with Marfan's syndrome, Brit. Heart J. **20**:143, 1958.
67. Cabot Case No. 43011: Marfan's syndrome with old and recent dissecting aneurysm, fibrinous pericarditis with effusion, Hufnagel operation two months before death, thrombosis of valve, New Eng. J. Med. **256**:30, 1957.
68. Calhoun, F. P.: Causes of heterochromia iridis with special reference to paralysis of the cervical sympathetics, Amer. J. Ophthal. **2**:255, 1919.
69. Callahan, A.: Aniridia with ectopia lentis and secondary glaucoma, Amer. J. Ophthal. **32**:28, 1949.
70. Campbell, R. W., Steinmetz, E. F., and Helmen, C. H.: Congenital aneurysm of the membranous portion of the ventricular septum. A cause for holosystolic murmurs, Circulation **30**:223, 1964.
71. Capotorti, L., Gaddini de Benedetti, R., and Rizzo, P.: Contribution to the study of the heredity of Marfan's syndrome. Description of a family tree of 4 generations with marriage between consanguineous patients, Acta Genet. Med. (Roma) **8**:455, 1959.
72. Cartellieri, L., and Kleinsorge, H.: Neurologische Störungen beim Marfan-Syndrom, Nervenartz **24**:376, 1953.
73. Case Records of the Massachusetts General Hospital, New. Eng. J. Med. **243**:346, 1950.
74. Castellanos, A., Jr., Ugarriza, R., de Cardenas, A., and Cano, L. A.: Sindrome de Marfan. Reporte de seis casos en una misma familia, Arch. Hosp. Univ. (Habana) **9**:353, 1957.
75. Chang, C. E.: Marfan's syndrome. Review of literature and report of one case, Chin. Med. J. **68**:433, 1951.
76. Choyce, D. P.: Anterior dislocation of the lens in Marfan's syndrome, Brit. J. Ophthal. **41**:446, 1957.
77. Churchill, D. W., Gelfant, S., Lalach, J. J., and Angevine, D. M.: Alterations in the polysaccharides and elastic fibers in the aortas of rats fed toxic lathyrus factor, Lab. Invest. **4**:1, 1955.
78. Cockayne, E. A.: Arachnodactyly with congenital heart disease (patent interventricular septum), Proc. Roy. Soc. Med. **29**:120, 1935.
79. Coffey, J. H., Barker, D. E., and Friedlander, J. H.: Dissecting aneurysm with Marfan's syndrome, Texas J. Med. **51**:79, 1955.
80. Consul, B. N., Kutshrestha, O. R., and Kasliwal, R. M.: Marfan's syndrome, J. Indian Med. Ass. **35**:218, 1960.
81. Coulson, W. F., and Carnes, W. H.: Cardiovascular studies on copper-deficient swine. II. Mechanical properties of the aorta, Lab. Invest. **11**:1316, 1962.
82. Crowe, F. W., Schull, W. J., and Neel, J. V.: A clinical, pathological and genetic study of multiple neurofibromatosis, Springfield, Ill., 1956, Charles C Thomas, Publisher.
83. Crump, J., Mikelberg, R. M., and Recknagel, E. M. S.: Arachnodactyly (Marfan's syndrome), J. Amer. Med. Wom. Ass. **13**:62, 1958.
84. Das Gupta, B. K., and Basu, R. K.: Bilateral dislocation of the lens under voluntary control in Marfan syndrome with cardiovascular anomaly, Brit. J. Ophthal. **39**:566, 1955.
85. Dasler, W.: Partial protection against odoratism (sweet pea lathyrism) by diets high in gelatin or casein, Proc. Soc. Exp. Biol. Med. **85**:485, 1954.
86. Davies, D. H.: Idiopathic cystic medial necrosis of aorta, Brit. Heart J. **3**:166, 1941.
87. Davis, J. H., Benson, J. W., and Miller, R. C.: Thoracoabdominal aneurysm involving celiac, superior mesenteric and renal arteries. Report of a case successfully treated by resection and nylon-graft replacement, Arch. Surg. **75**:871, 1957.
88. Dax, E. C.: Arachnodactyly, J. Ment. Sci. **87**:434, 1941.
89. DeBakey, M. E., Henly, W. S., Cooley, D. A., Morris, G. C., Jr., Crawford, E. S., and Beall, A. C., Jr.: Surgical management of dissecting aneurysm involving the ascending aorta, J. Cardiov. Surg. **5**:200, 1964.
90. Dexter, M. W., Lawton, A. H., and Warren, L. O.: Marfan's syndrome with aortic thrombosis, Arch. Intern. Med. **99**:485, 1957.
91. Dimond, E. G., Larsen, W. E., Johnson, W. B., and Kittle, C. F.: Post-traumatic aortic insuf-

ficiency occurring in Marfan's syndrome, with attempted repair with a plastic valve, New Eng. J. Med. **256**:8, 1957.

92. Duke-Elder, W. S.: Textbook of ophthalmology, St. Louis, 1949, The C. V. Mosby Co., vol. 4, p. 4265.
93. Dulake, M., and Ashfield, R.: Dissecting aneurysm of the aorta with rupture into the right atrium, Brit. Heart J. **26**:862, 1964.
94. Dupuy, H. P., and Lee, J. G.: The isolation of a material capable of producing experimental lathyrism, J. Amer. Pharm. Ass. (Scient. Ed.) **43**:61, 1954.
95. Düx, A., Hilger, H. H., Schaede, A., and Thurn, P.: Zum Marfan-Syndrom, Z. Kreislaufforsch. **50**:492, 1961.
96. Editorial: Marfan's syndrome, New Eng. J. Med. **256**:39, 1957.
97. Edynak, G. M., and Rawson, A. J.: Ruptured aneurysm of the mitral valve in a Marfan-like syndrome, Amer. J. Cardiol. **11**:674, 1963.
98. Eldridge, R.: Coarctation in the Marfan syndrome, Arch. Intern. Med. **113**:342, 1964.
99. Eldridge, R.: The metacarpal index, a useful aid in the diagnosis of the Marfan syndrome, Arch. Intern. Med. **113**:248, 1964.
100. Ellis, F. W. B.: Four cases of fragilitas ossium and blue sclerotics, Proc. Roy. Soc. Med. **24** (part 2):1054, 1931.
101. Ellis, R. W. B.: Arachnodactyly and ectopia lentis in father and daughter, Arch. Dis. Child. **15**:267, 1940.
102. Engelbach, E.: Endocrine medicine, Springfield, Ill., 1932, Charles C Thomas, Publisher.
103. Erdheim, J.: Medionecrosis aortae idiopathica cystica, Virchows Arch. Path. Anat. **276**:187, 1930.
104. Erdohazi, M., Cowie, V., and Lo, S. S.: Case of haemophilia with Marfan's syndrome, Brit. Med. J. **1**:102, 1964.
105. Esteve, R.: Idiopathic scoliosis in identical twins, J. Bone Joint Surg. **40-B**:97, 1958.
106. Etter, L. E., and Glover, L. P.: Arachnodactyly complicated by dislocated lens and death from rupture of dissecting aneurysm of the aorta, J.A.M.A. **123**:88, 1943.
107. Euzière, J., Pagès, P., Lafon, R., Mirouze, J., and Salvaing, J.: Myopathie scapulo-humérale d'Erb et dolichosténomélie; cas., Arch. Franç. Pédiat. **6**:651, 1949.
108. Evans, P. A.: A hereditary tendency to hernia, Lancet **2**:293, 1942.
109. Evans, W.: The heart in sternal depression, Brit. Heart J. **8**:162, 1946.
110. Everberg, G.: Marfan's syndrome associated with hearing defect. Report of a case in one of a pair of twins, Acta Paediat. **48**:70, 1959.
111. Fabre, J., Veyrat, R., and Jeanneret, O.: Syndrome de Marfan avec anevrysme et coarctation de l'aorte; étude anatomo-clinique, Schweiz. Med. Wschr. **87**:49, 1957.
112. Fahey, J. J.: Muscular and skeletal changes in arachnodactyly, Arch. Surg. **39**:741, 1939.
113. Fairbank, T.: Atlas of general affections of the skeleton, Baltimore, 1951, The Williams & Wilkins Co., p. 175.
114. Faivre, G., Frenkiel, Pernot, C., and Hueber: Le coeur des dépressions sternales congénitales, Arch. Mal. Coeur **47**:322, 1954.
115. Falls, H. F.: A gene producing various defects of the anterior segment of the eye, with a pedigree of a family, Amer. J. Ophthal. **32**:41, 1949.
116. Fay, J. E., Horlick, L., Merrimban, J. E., and Nanson, E. M.: A case of Marfan's syndrome with an aneurysm at the ascending aorta, with physiologic, operative and postmortem studies, Canad. Med. Ass. J. **78**:862, 1958.
117. Feinberg, S.: Congenital mesodermal dysmorpho-dystrophy, Radiology **74**:218, 1960.
118. Feldman, L., Friedlander, J., Dillon, R., and Wallyn, R.: Aneurysm of right sinus of Valsalva with rupture into right atrium and into the right ventricle, Amer. Heart J. **51**:314, 1956.
119. Ferguson, M. J., and Clemente, A. R.: Rupture and dissection of the aorta in Marfan's syndrome, Amer. J. Cardiol. **4**:543, 1959.
120. Fischl, A. A., and Ruthberg, J.: Clinical implications of Marfan's syndrome, J.A.M.A. **146**:704, 1951.
121. Fleming, J., and Helwig, F. C.: Medionecrosis aortae idiopathica cystica with spontaneous rupture, J. Missouri Med. Ass. **38**:86, 1941.
122. Flesch, M.: Ueber eine seltene Missbildung des Thorax, Virchow Arch. Path. Anat. **57**:289, 1873.

123. Ford, C. E.: Human cytogenetics: its present place and future possibilities, Amer. J. Hum. Genet. **12**:104, 1960.
124. Franceschetti, A.: Ectopia lentis et pupillae congenita als rezessives Erbleiden und ihre Manifestierung durch Konsanguinität, Klin. Mbl. Augenheilk. **78**:351, 1927.
125. Frei, C.: Ueber das Aneurysma dissecans aortae, Inaugural Dissertation, Zürich, 1962, J. J. Meier.
126. Frieden, J., Hurwitt, E. S., and Leader, E.: Ruptured aortic cusp associated with an heritable disorder of connective tissue, Amer. J. Med. **33**:615, 1962.
127. Fuleihan, F. J. D., Suh, S. K., and Shepard, R. H.: Some aspects of pulmonary function in the Marfan syndrome, Bull. Hopkins Hosp. **113**:320, 1963.
128. Futcher, P. H., and Southworth, H.: Arachnodactyly and its medical complications, Arch. Intern. Med. **61**:693, 1938.
129. Ganther, R.: Ein Beitrag zur Arachnodaktylie, Z. Kinderheilk. **43**:724, 1927.
130. Garland, H. G.: Hereditary scoliosis, Brit. Med. J. **1**:328, 1934.
131. Gibson, J. B., Carson, N. A. J., and Neill, D. W.: Pathologic findings in homocystinuria, J. Clin. Path. **17**:427, 1964.
132. Gilston, R. J.: Marfan's syndrome, Med. Ann. D.C. **24**:127, 1955.
133. Golden, R. L., and Lakin, H.: The *forme fruste* in Marfan's syndrome, New Eng. J. Med. **260**:797, 1959.
134. Gordan, G. S., and Lisser, H., editors: Endocrinology in clinical practice, Chicago, 1953, Year Book Medical Publishers, Inc.
135. Gordon, A. M.: Abraham Lincoln—a medical appraisal, J. Kentucky Med. Ass. **60**:249, 1962.
136. Gore, I.: The pathogenesis of dissecting aneurysm of the aorta, Arch. Path. **53**:142, 1952.
137. Gore, I.: Dissecting aneurysm of the aorta in persons under forty years of age, Arch. Path. **55**:1, 1953.
138. Gore, I., and Seiwert, V. J.: Dissecting aneurysm of the aorta: pathologic aspects, an analysis of eighty-five fatal cases, Arch. Path. **53**:121, 1952.
139. Gouley, B. A., and Anderson, E.: Chronic dissecting aneurysm of aorta simulating syphilitic cardiovascular disease; notes on associated aortic murmurs, Ann. Intern. Med. **14**:978, 1940.
140. Goyette, E. M., and Palmer, P. W.: Cardiovascular lesions in arachnodactyly, Circulation **7**:373, 1953.
141. Graham, J. G., and Milne, J. A.: Dissecting aneurysm of the aorta: review of 29 cases, Glasgow Med. J. **33**:320, 1952.
142. Gray, H.: Arachnodactyly (spider fingers), Arch. Intern. Med. **75**:215, 1945.
143. Green, H., and Emerson, P. W.: Arachnodactylia, Arch. Pediat. **60**:299, 1943.
144. Greenfield, J. G., Cornman, T., and Shy, G. M.: The prognostic value of the muscle biopsy in the "floppy infant," Brain **81**:461, 1958.
145. Griffin, J. F., and Koman, G. M.: Severe aortic insufficiency in Marfan's syndrome, Ann. Intern. Med. **48**:174, 1958.
146. Griffith, G. J., Hayhurst, A. P., and Whitehead, R.: Dissecting aneurysm of aorta in mother and child, Brit. Heart J. **13**:364, 1951.
147. Gross, J.: An intermolecular defect of collagen in experimental lathyrism, Biochim. Biophys. Acta **71**:250, 1963.
148. Groves, L. K., Effler, D. B., Hawk, W. A., and Gulati, K.: Aortic insufficiency secondary to aneurysmal changes in the ascending aorta: surgical management, J. Thorac. Cardiov. Surg. **48**:362, 1964.
149. Gupta, S. K., and Sharma, V. N.: Chronic pneumothorax in Marfan's syndrome, Brit. J. Tuberc. **51**:346, 1957.
150. Haber, H.: Miescher's elastoma (elastoma intrapapillare perforans verruciforme), Brit. J. Derm. **71**:85, 1959.
151. Haik, G. M., Kalil, H. H., Ferry, J. F., and Childers, M. D.: Subluxations and luxations of the lens: with a special note on the Barraquer operation and on Marfan's and Marchesani's syndromes, Southern Med. J. **54**:642, 1961.
152. Haldane, J. B. S.: The rate of spontaneous mutation of a human gene, J. Genet. **31**:317, 1935.
153. Hamman, L., and Apperly, F. S.: Spontaneous rupture of the aorta with aortic insufficiency, Int. Clin. Series 43, **4**:251, 1933.
154. Hamwi, G. J.: Marfan's syndrome (arachnodactyly), Amer. J. Med. **11**:261, 1951.

155. Handmaker, S. D.: The satellited chromosomes of man with reference to the Marfan syndrome, Amer. J. Hum. Genet. **15:**11, 1963.
156. Hardin, C. A.: Ruptured abdominal aneurysm occurring in Marfan's syndrome. Attempted repair with the use of a nylon prosthesis, New Eng. J. Med. **260:**821, 1959.
157. Hardin, C. A.: Successful resection of carotid and abdominal aneurysm in two retarded patients with Marfan's syndrome, New Eng. J. Med. **267:**141, 1962.
158. Haridas, G.: Arachnodactylia in a Chinese infant, Arch. Dis. Child. **16:**257, 1941.
159. Harrison, F. F.: Coarctation of the aorta of the adult type, associated with cystic degeneration of the media of the first portion of the arch, Arch. Path. **27:**742, 1939.
160. Harrison, J., and Klainer, M. J.: Arachnodactyly; its occurrence in several members of one family, New Eng. J. Med. **220:**621, 1939.
161. Hartman, C. G., and Straus, W. L.: Relation of pelvic ligaments in pregnant monkeys, Amer. J. Obstet. Gynec. **37:**498, 1939.
162. Harvey, W. P., Corrado, M. A., and Perloff, J. K.: "Right-sided" murmurs of aortic insufficiency, Amer. J. Med. Sci. **245:**533, 1963.
163. Headley, R. N., Carpenter, H. M., and Sawyer, C. G.: Unusual features of Marfan's syndrome, Amer. J. Cardiol. **11:**259, 1963.
164. Heitzman, E. J., and Bryant, R. B.: The Marfan syndrome, gigantism and ruptured abdominal aneurysm, New York J. Med. **64:**436, 1964.
165. Henderson, J. W.: Marfan's syndrome: report of a case with congenital aneurysm of the coronary sinus and perforation into the right ventricle, J. Indiana Med. Ass. **54:**325, 1961.
166. Hersh, A. H., DeMarinis, F., and Stecher, R. M.: On the inheritance and development of clinodactyly, Amer. J. Hum. Genet. **5:**257, 1953.
167. Hirst, A. E., Jr., and Bailey, H. L.: Arachnodactyly with associated healing dissecting aneurysm, Calif. Med. **84:**355, 1956.
168. Hirst, A. E., Jr., Johns, V. J., Jr., and Kime, S. W., Jr.: Dissecting aneurysm of the aorta; a review of 505 cases, Medicine **37:**217, 1958.
169. Hofmann, W. P., and Carey, E. T.: Congenital myopic astigmatism in identical twins, Amer. J. Ophthal. **25:**1495, 1942.
170. Hudson, J. R.: Marfan's syndrome with retinal detachment, Brit. J. Ophthal. **35:**244, 1951.
171. Hufnagel, C. A., and Conrad, P. W.: Dissecting aneurysms of ascending aorta: direct approach repair, Surgery **51:**84, 1962.
172. Hufnagel, C. A., Harvey, W. P., Rabil, P. J., and McDermott, T. F.: Surgical correction of aortic insufficiency, Surgery **35:**673, 1954.
173. Humphries, J. O., and McKusick, V. A.: The differentiation of organic and "innocent" systolic murmurs, Prog. Cardiov. Dis. **5:**152, 1962.
174. Humphries, J. O'N., and Pusch, A. L.: Effect of the hormone relaxin on the aorta of the guinea pig and rat, Clin. Res. **6:**233, 1958.
175. Husebye, K. O., Wolff, H. J., and Friedman, L. L.: Aortic dissection in pregnancy; a case of Marfan's syndrome, Amer. Heart J. **55:**662, 1958.
176. Hustinx, T. W. J., and van Olphen, A. H. F.: An XYY chromosome pattern in a boy with Marfan's syndrome, Genetica **34:**262, 1963.
177. Huston, W. H.: The Marfan syndrome. A report of an atypical case, Henry Ford Hosp. Med. Bull. **5:**90, 1957.
178. I.A.A.: Bernard Jean Antoine Marfan, M.D., Amer. J. Dis. Child. **64:**354, 1942.
179. Irwin, J. W., Hancock, D. M., and Sharp, J. R.: Ruptured abdominal aortic aneurysm in Marfan's syndrome, Brit. Med. J. **1:**1293, 1964.
180. Jain, S. R., and Sepaha, G. C.: Marfan's syndrome. Report of 4 cases with brief review of literature, Indian J. Med. Sci. **14:**418, 1960.
181. James, T. N., Frame, B., and Schatz, I. J.: Pathology of cardiac conduction system in Marfan's syndrome, Arch. Intern. Med. **114:**339, 1964.
182. Jasin, H. E., and colleagues: Relationship between urinary hydroxyproline and growth, J. Clin. Invest. **41:**1928, 1962.
183. Jequier, M.: Observations sur le syndrome de Marfan, Helv. Med. Acta **10:**233, 1943.
184. Jervey, J. W., Jr.: Lens dislocation in Marfan's syndrome. A case report, Amer. J. Ophthal. **57:**484, 1964.
185. Jones, C. R., Bergman, M. W., Kittner, P. J., and Pigman, W. W.: Urinary hydroxyproline excretion in normal children and adolescents, Proc. Soc. Exp. Biol. Med. **115:**85, 1964.

186. Jones, C. R., Bergman, M. W., Kittner, P. J., and Pigman, W. W.: Urinary hydroxyproline excretion in Marfan's syndrome as compared with age matched controls, Proc. Soc. Exp. Biol. Med. **116**:931, 1964.
187. Kachele, G. E.: The embryogenesis of ectopia lentis, Arch. Ophthal. **64**:135, 1960.
188. Kahrs, T.: Three cases of arachnodactylia, Acta Med. Scand. **121**:240, 1945.
189. Källén, B., and Levan, A.: Abnormal length of chromosomes 21 and 22 in four patients with Marfan's syndrome, Cytogenetics **1**:5, 1962.
190. Kaplan, B. M., Schlichter, J. G., Graham, G., and Miller, G.: Idiopathic congenital dilatation of the pulmonary artery, J. Lab. Clin. Med. **41**:697, 1953.
191. Katz, H. L.: Thoracic manifestations in Marfan's syndrome, Quart. Bull. Sea View Hosp. **13**:95, 1952.
191a. Keech, M. K., Wendt, V. E., Read, R. C., Bistue, A. R., and Bianchs, F. A.: Family studies of the Marfan syndrome, J. Chronic Dis., 1966. In press.
192. Killip, T., III (New York City): Personal communication.
193. Killip, T., III, and Holmquist, N. D.: Aortic surgery in Marfan's syndrome. Hemodynamic and histologic response, Ann. Intern. Med. **54**:431, 1961.
194. Kingsley-Pillers, E. M.: Arachnodactyly with amyoplasia congenita, Proc. Roy. Soc. Med. **39**:696, 1946.
195. Kloepfer, H. W., and Rosenthal, J. W.: Possible genetic carriers in the spherophakia-brachymorphia syndrome, Amer. J. Hum. Genet. **7**:398, 1955.
196. Knight, A. M., Jr.: The Marfan syndrome, J. Med. Ass. Georgia **46**:413, 1957.
197. Knight, A. M., Clark, S. W., and Terry, D. B.: Case presentation: Marfan syndrome, dissecting aneurysm, intermittent occlusion of both coronary arteries, J. Med. Ass. Georgia **49**:222, 1960.
198. Kohn, J. L., and Strauss, L.: Marfan's syndrome (arachnodactyly). Observation of a patient from birth until death at 18 years, Pediatrics **25**:872, 1960.
199. Kountz, W. B., and Hempelmann, L. H.: Chromatrophic degeneration and rupture of the aorta following thyroidectomy in cases of hypertension, Amer. Heart J. **20**:599, 1940.
200. Kravitz, D.: Marfan's syndrome, Amer. J. Ophthal. **39**:576, 1955.
201. Kvorak-Theobald, G.: Histologic study of an eye from a child with arachnodactyly, Arch. Ophthal. **24**:1046, 1940.
202. Labella, F. S.: Elastin, a metabolically active lipoprotein, Nature **180**:1360, 1958.
203. Lacroix, P.: The organization of bone; translated by Stewart Gilder, Philadelphia, 1951, The Blakiston Co.
204. Lampen, H.: Das Marfan-Syndrom als kardiologisches Problem, Deutsch. Med. Wschr. **87**:2250, 1962.
205. Langeron, T., Girard, P., Liefooghe, J., and Masson, C.: Maladie de Marfan et anéurysme abdominal, Bull. Soc. Méd. Hôp. Paris **70**:374, 1954.
206. Lavoie, R. G., and Boulanger, J.: Le syndrome de Marfan, Laval Méd. **25**:453, 1958.
207. Leeming, J. T., and McKusick, V. A.: Serum seromucoid levels in the Marfan syndrome, Bull. Hopkins Hosp. **110**:38, 1962.
208. Lehmann, O.: A family with Marfan's syndrome traced through an affected newborn, including analysis of the mucoproteins in serum and urinary excretion of amino acids, Acta Paediat. **49**:540, 1960.
209. Lester, C. W.: The surgical treatment of funnel chest, Ann. Surg. **123**:1003, 1946.
210. Levine, E., Stein, M., Gordon, G., and Mitchell, N.: Chronic dissecting aneurysm of the aorta resembling chronic rheumatic heart disease, New Eng. J. Med. **244**:902, 1951.
211. Liboro, A., Torralba, T. P., Perez, A. P., Basa, G., and St. Ana, D.: The Marfan syndrome, J. Philipp. Med. Ass. **36**:513, 1960.
212. Lillian, M.: Multiple pulmonary artery aneurysms; endocarditis of ductus arteriosus and congenital pulmonary cysts, Amer. J. Med. **7**:280, 1949.
213. Lindeboom, G. A., and Bouwer, W. F.: Dissecting aneurysm (and renal cortical necrosis) associated with arachnodactyly (Marfan's disease), Cardiologia **15**:12, 1949.
214. Lindeboom, G. A., and Westerveld-Brandon, E. R.: Dilatation of the aorta in arachnodactyly, Cardiologia **17**:217, 1950.
215. Linker, A., Coulson, W. F., and Carnes, W. H.: Cardiovascular studies on copper-deficient swine. VI. The mucopolysaccharide composition of aorta and cartilage, J. Biol. Chem. **239**:1690, 1964.

216. Lloyd, R. I.: Arachnodactyly, Arch. Ophthal. **13**:744, 1935.
217. Lloyd, R. I.: A second group of cases of arachnodactyly, Arch. Ophthal. **17**:69, 1937.
218. Lloyd, R. I.: Clinical course of the ocular complications of Marfan's syndrome, Arch. Ophthal. **40**:558, 1948.
219. Loughridge, L. W.: Renal abnormalities in the Marfan syndrome, Quart. J. Med. **28**:531, 1959.
220. Loveman, A. B., Gordon, A. M., and Fliegelman, M. T.: Marfan's syndrome. Some cutaneous aspects, Arch. Derm. (Chicago) **87**:428, 1963.
221. Low, A.: Measurements of infants at birth, Ann. Eugen. **15**:210, 1950.
222. Lowe, R. C.: Polycythemia vera (erythremia). Arachnodactyly with congenital defect of vertebral column, and familial muscular dystrophy in Negroes; case reports, Tri-State Med. J. **13**:2679, 1941.
223. Lutman, F. C., and Neel, J. V.: Inheritance of arachnodactyly, ectopia lentis and other congenital anomalies (Marfan's syndrome) in the E. family, Arch. Ophthal. **41**:276, 1949.
224. Lynas, M. A.: Marfan's syndrome in northern Ireland; an account of thirteen families, Ann. Hum. Genet. **22**:289, 1958.
225. Lynas, M. A.: Unpublished observations referred to in reference 358.
226. Lynas, M. A., and Merrett, J. D.: Data on linkage in man; Marfan's syndrome in northern Ireland, Ann. Hum. Genet. **22**:310, 1958.
227. MacCallum, W. G.: Dissecting aneurysm, Bull. Hopkins Hosp. **20**:9, 1909.
228. McCann, J. S., and Porter, D. C.: Calcification of the aorta as an aid to the diagnosis of syphilis, Brit. Med. J. **1**:826, 1956.
229. McKeown, F.: Dissecting aneurysm of the coronary artery in arachnodactyly, Brit. Heart J. **22**:434, 1960.
230. McKusick, V. A.: Primordial dwarfism and ectopia lentis, Amer. J. Hum. Genet. **7**:187, 1955.
231. McKusick, V. A.: The cardiovascular aspects of Marfan's syndrome, Circulation **11**:321, 1955.
232. McKusick, V. A.: Cardiovascular sound in health and disease, Baltimore, 1958, Williams & Wilkins Co.
233. McKusick, V. A.: The genetic aspects of cardiovascular diseases, Ann. Intern. Med. **49**:556, 1958.
234. McKusick, V. A.: Hereditary disorders of connective tissue, Bull. N.Y. Acad. Med. **35**:143, 1959.
235. McKusick, V. A.: Chromosomes in Marfan's disease (letter), Lancet **1**:1194, 1960.
236. McKusick, V. A.: Unpublished observations.
237. McKusick, V. A., Hahn, D. P., Brayshaw, J. R., and Humphries, J. O'N.: Some hemodynamic effects of the Hufnagel operation for aortic regurgitation. Studies in models and a patient, Bull. Hopkins Hosp. **95**:322, 1954.
238. McKusick, V. A., Murray, G. E., Peeler, R. G., and Webb, G. N.: Musical murmurs, Bull. Hopkins Hosp. **97**:136, 1955.
239. MacLeod, M., and Williams, W. A.: The cardiovascular lesions in Marfan's syndrome, Arch. Path. **61**:143, 1956.
240. McSherry, B. J., Ferguson, A. E., and Ballantyne, J.: Dissecting aneurysm in turkeys, J. Amer. Vet. Med. Ass. **124**:279, 1954.
241. Maier, C., Rubli, J. M., Schaub, F., and Hedinger, C.: Kardiale Störungen beim Marfanschen Syndrom, Cardiologia **24**:106, 1954.
242. Mamou, H., and Hérault, P.: Maladie de Marfan et maladie de Scheuermann, Sem. Hôp. Paris **27**:3071, 1951.
243. Mandel, W., Evans, E. W., and Walford, R. L.: Dissecting aortic aneurysm during pregnancy, New Eng. J. Med. **251**:1059, 1954.
244. Marchesani, O.: Brachydaktylie und angeborene Kugellinse als Systemerkrankung, Klin. Mbl. Augenheilk. **103**:392, 1939.
245. Marchesani, O.: Jubilee Volume for Prof. Vogt, part II, Basle, 1939, Benno Schwage & Co., p. 32.
246. Marfan, A. B.: Un cas de déformation congénitale des quatre membres plus prononcée aux extrémités charactérisée par l'allongement des os avec un certain degré d'amincissement, Bull. Mém. Soc. Méd. Hôp. Paris **13**:220, 1896.
247. Marfan, A. B.: Sur la ponction du péricarde et en particulier sur la ponction par voie épigastrique sous-xiphoidienne, Arch. Mal. Coeur **29**:153, 1936.

248. Marks, J., and Gerson, K. L.: Importance of autopsies—an illustrative case, J.A.M.A. **168**:1450, 1958.
249. Martin, R.: Lehrbuch der Anthropologie, Jena, 1928, Gustav Fischer.
250. Martin, V. A. F., and Cowan, E. C.: Bilateral secondary glaucoma and systemic hypertension in Marfan's syndrome, Brit. J. Ophthal. **44**:123, 1960.
251. Marvel, R. J., and Genovese, P. D.: Cardiovascular disease in Marfan's syndrome, Amer. Heart J. **42**:814, 1951.
252. Master, A. M., and Stone, J.: The heart in funnel-shaped and flat chests, Amer. J. Med. Sci. **217**:392, 1949.
253. Maxwell, G. M.: Chest deformity in children with congenital heart disease, Amer. Heart J. **54**:368, 1957.
254. Meara, R. A.: Ehlers-Danlos syndrome and ?elastoma verruciforme perforans (Miescher), Trans. St. Johns Hosp. Derm. Soc. (London) **40**:72, 1958.
255. Medawar, P. B.: The future of man, New York, 1960, Basic Books, Inc., Publishers, p. 72.
256. Meilman, E., Urivetsky, M. M., and Rapoport, C. M.: Urinary hydroxyproline peptides, J. Clin. Invest. **42**:40, 1963.
257. Méry, H., and Babonneix, L.: Un cas de déformation congénitale des quatre membres: hyperchondroplasie, Bull. Mém. Soc. Méd. Hôp. Paris **19**:671, 1902.
258. Meyer, K. (New York City): Personal communication.
259. Meyer, S. J., and Holstein, T.: Spherophakia with glaucoma and brachydactyly, Amer. J. Ophthal. **24**:247, 1941.
260. Millant, R.: Les eunques à travers les ages, Paris, 1908, Vigot Frères.
261. Miller, R., Jr., and Pearson, R. J., Jr.: Mitral insufficiency simulating aortic stenosis. Report of an unusual manifestation of Marfan's syndrome, New Eng. J. Med. **260**:1210, 1959.
262. Moretti, G., LeCoulant, P., Staeffen, J., Catanzano, G., and Bronstet, A.: La peau dans le syndrome de Marfan, Presse Méd. **72**:2985, 1964.
263. Moretti, G. F., Staeffen, J., Bertrand, E., and Bronstet, A.: Bloc auriculo-ventriculaire complet dans le syndrome de Marfan, Presse Med. **72**:605, 1964.
264. Moses, M. F.: Aortic aneurysm associated with arachnodactyly, Brit. Med. J. **2**:81, 1951.
265. Mouquin, M., and colleagues: Les dissections aortiques du syndrome du Marfan, Arch. Mal. Coeur **54**:141, 1961.
266. Muller, W. H., Damman, J. F., and Warren, W. D.: Surgical correction of the cardiovascular deformities in Marfan's syndrome, Ann. Surg. **152**:506, 1960.
267. Neilson, G. H., and Sullivan, J. J.: Dissecting aneurysm of the aorta associated with Marfan's syndrome, Med. J. Aust. **1**:925, 1956.
268. Nelson, J. D.: The Marfan syndrome, with special reference to congenital enlargement of the spinal canal, Brit. J. Radiol. **31**:561, 1958.
269. Nemoto, H., and Yanai, N.: Marfan's syndrome, a family report, Jap. J. Hum. Genet. **5**:199, 1961.
270. Nodes, J. D. S., and Henes, F.: Total rupture of an aneurysm of the splenic artery immediately after labor, Trans. Obstet. Soc. London **42**:305, 1900.
271. Norcross, J. R.: Arachnodactylia—a report of three cases, J. Bone Joint Surg. **20**:757, 1938.
272. Novell, H. A., Asher, L. A., Jr., and Lev, M.: Marfan's syndrome associated with pregnancy, Amer. J. Obstet. Gynec. **75**:802, 1958.
273. Olcott, C. T.: Arachnodactyly (Marfan's syndrome) with severe anemia, Amer. J. Dis. Child. **60**:660, 1940.
274. Ollier, L. X. E. L.: Traité expérimental et clinique de la régénération des os et production artificielle du tissu osseux, Paris, 1867, Masson & Cie.
275. Oram, S., and East, T.: Rupture of aneurysm of aortic sinus (of Valsalva) into the right side of the heart, Brit. Heart J. **17**:541, 1955.
276. Ormond, A. W.: The etiology of arachnodactyly, Guy's Hosp. Rep. **80**:68, 1930.
277. Oswald, N., and Parkinson, T.: Honeycomb lungs, Quart. J. Med. **18**:1, 1949.
278. Pahwa, J. M., and Cupta, D. P.: Marfan's syndrome, Brit. J. Ophthal. **46**:105, 1962.
279. Papaioannou, A. C., Agustsson, M. H., and Gasul, B. M.: Early manifestations of the cardiovascular disorders in the Marfan syndrome, Pediatrics **27**:255, 1961.
280. Pappas, E. G., Mason, D., and Denton, C.: Marfan's syndrome: a report of three patients with aneurysms of the aorta, Amer. J. Med. **23**:426, 1957.

281. Parish, J. G., Calnan, C. D., and Lawrence, J. S.: Heritable disorders of connective tissue, Proc. Roy. Soc. Med. **53**:515, 1960.
282. Parker, A. S., Jr., and Hare, H. F.: Arachnodactyly, Radiology **45**:220, 1945.
283. Pasachoff, H. D., Madonick, M. J., and Drayer, C.: Arachnodactyly in four siblings with pneumoencephalographic observations of two, Amer. J. Dis. Child. **67**:201, 1944.
284. Peiper, A.: Ueber die Erblichkeit der Trichterbrust, Klin. Wschr. **1**:1647, 1922.
285. Perl, E., and Catchpole, H. R.: Changes induced in the connective tissue of the pubic symphysis of the guinea pig with estrogen and relaxin, Arch. Path. **50**:233, 1950.
286. Pierce, R. E.: Traumatic dissecting aneurysms of the thoracic aorta, U. S. Armed Forces Med. J. **5**:1588, 1954.
287. Pino, R. H., Cooper, E. L., and Van Wien, S.: Arachnodactyly and status dysraphicus; a review, Ann. Intern. Med. **10**:1130, 1937.
288. Piper, R. K., and Irvine-Jones, E.: Arachnodactylia and its association with congenital heart disease; report of a case and review of the literature, Amer. J. Dis. Child. **31**:832, 1926.
289. Pirie, A.: The vitreous body. In Davson, H., editor: The eye, New York, 1962, Academic Press, Inc.
290. Pommerenke, W. T.: Experimental ligamentous relaxation in guinea pig pelvis, Amer. J. Obstet. Gynec. **27**:708, 1934.
291. Ponseti, I. V., and Baird, W. A.: Scoliosis and dissecting aneurysm of the aorta in rats fed with lathyrus odoratus seeds, Amer. J. Path. **28**:1059, 1952.
292. Ponseti, I. V., and Shepard, R. S.: Lesions of the skeleton and of other mesodermal tissues in rats fed sweet-pea (Lathyrus odoratus) seeds, J. Bone Joint Surg. **36-A**:1031, 1954.
293. Poynton, F. J., and Maurice, W. B.: Arachnodactyly with organic heart disease, Trans. Clin. Soc. London **75**:21, 1923.
294. Prockop, D. J., and Sjoerdsma, A.: Significance of urinary hydroxyproline in man, J. Clin. Invest. **40**:843, 1961.
295. Pygott, F.: Arachnodactyly (Marfan's syndrome) with a report of two cases, Brit. J. Radiol. **28**:26, 1955.
296. Rados, A.: Marfan's syndrome, Arch. Ophthal. **27**:477, 1942.
297. Rambar, A. C., and Denenholz, E. J.: Arachnodactyly, J. Pediat. **15**:844, 1939.
298. Ravitch, M.: Pectus excavatum and heart failure, Surgery **30**:178, 1951.
299. Read, R. C., Thal, A. P., and Wendt, V. E.: Symptomatic valvular myxomatous transformation (the floppy valve syndrome): a possible *forme fruste* of Marfan's disease, Circulation. In press.
300. Reeh, M. J., and Lehman, W. L.: Marfan's syndrome (arachnodactyly) with ectopia lentis, Trans. Amer. Acad. Ophthal. **58**:212, 1954.
301. Reeve, R., Silver, H. K., and Ferrier, P.: Marfan's syndrome (arachnodactyly) with arthrogryposis (amyloplasia congenita), Am. J. Dis. Child. **99**:101, 1960.
302. Reeves, J. E., and Irwin, H. R.: Marfan's syndrome. Report of a probable case, Calif. Med. **86**:183, 1957.
303. Reis, R. A., Baer, J. L., Arens, R. A., and Stewart, E.: Traumatic separation of symphysis pubis during spontaneous labor with clinical and x-ray study of normal symphysis pubis during pregnancy and puerperium, Surg. Gynec. Obstet. **55**:336, 1932.
304. Resnik, W. H., and Keefer, C. S.: Dissecting aneurysm with signs of aortic insufficiency, J.A.M.A. **85**:422, 1925.
305. Reynolds, G.: The heart in arachnodactyly, Guy's Hosp. Rep. **99**:178, 1950.
306. Reynolds, S. R. M., Light, F. W., Sr., Ardran, G. M., and Prichard, M. M. L.: Qualitative nature of pulsatile flow in umbilical blood vessels with observations on flow in the aorta, Bull. Hopkins Hosp. **91**:83, 1952.
307. Rich, A. R., and Oppenheimer, E. (Baltimore): Personal communication.
308. Risser, J. C.: Clinical evaluation of scoliosis, J.A.M.A. **164**:134, 1957.
309. Roark, J. W.: Marfan's syndrome. Report of one case with autopsy, special histological study and review of the literature, Arch. Intern. Med. **103**:123, 1959.
310. Ross, J. K., and Gerbode, F.: The Marfan syndrome associated with an unusual interventricular septal defect, J. Thorac. Surg. **39**:746, 1960.
311. Ross, L. J.: Arachnodactyly: review of recent literature and report of case with cleft palate, Amer. J. Dis. Child. **78**:417, 1949.

312. Rottino, A.: Medical degeneration in a non-ruptured aorta appearing syphilitic macroscopically, Arch. Path. **27**:320, 1939.
313. Rubin, E. H.: Diseases of the chest, Philadelphia, 1947, W. B. Saunders Co.
314. Rutherford, W. J.: Hereditary scoliosis, Brit. Med. J. **2**:87, 1934.
315. Rywlin, A.: Medionecrosis idiopathica cystica unter dem Bilde des diffusen Aortenaneurysmas. Beziehungen zur Marfanschen Syndrom, Frankfort Z. Path. **63**:187, 1952.
316. Sainsbury, H. S. K.: Congenital funnel chest, Lancet **2**:615, 1947.
317. Salle, V.: Ueber einen Fall von angeborener abnormen Grosse der Extremitaten mit einen an Akronemegalia erinnerden Symptomenkomplex, Jahrb. Kinderheilk. **75**:540, 1912.
318. Sando, D. E., and Helm, S.: Acquired coarctation in new channel of healed dissecting aneurysm, Ann. Intern. Med. **37**:793, 1952.
319. Sautter, H.: Aplasie des Dilatator pupillae beim Marfanschen Symptomenkomplex, Klin. Mbl. Augenheilk. **114**:449, 1949.
320. Schilling, E. D., and Strong, F. M.: Isolation, structure and synthesis of a lathyrus factor from L. odoratus, J. Amer. Chem. Soc. **76**:2848, 1954.
321. Schilling, V.: Striae distensae als hypophysäres Symptom bei basophilem Vorderlappenadenom (Cushingschem Syndrom) und bei Arachnodaktylie (Marfanschem Symptomenkomplex) mit Hypophysentumor, Med. Welt. **10**:183, 1936.
322. Schneider, W. F.: Arachnodactyly; unusual complication following skull injury, J. Pediat. **27**:583, 1945.
323. Schnitker, M. A., and Bayer, C. A.: Dissecting aneurysm of the aorta in young individuals, particularly in association with pregnancy, with report of case, Ann. Intern. Med. **20**:486, 1944.
324. Schorr, S., Braun, K., and Wildman, J.: Congenital aneurysmal dilatation of the ascending aorta associated with arachnodactylia; angiocardiographic study, Amer. Heart J. **42**:610, 1951.
325. Schwartz, H.: Abraham Lincoln and the Marfan syndrome, J.A.M.A. **187**:473, 1964.
326. Segal, B., Kasparian, H., and Likoff, W.: Mitral regurgitation in a patient with the Marfan syndrome, Dis. Chest **41**:457, 1962.
327. Segal, B. L., and Likoff, W.: Late systolic murmur of mitral regurgitation, Amer. Heart J. **67**:757, 1964.
328. Segal, B. L., Tabesh, E., Imbriglia, J. E., and Likoff, W.: The Marfan syndrome. Necropsy findings in three patients with a review of the cardiovascular complications, Angiology **13**:444, 1962.
329. Sheehan, H. L.: The pathology of obstetric shock, J. Obst. Gynaec. Brit. Comm. **16**:218, 1939.
330. Sheehan, H. L., and Falkiner, N. M.: Splenic aneurysm and splenic enlargement in pregnancy, Brit. Med. J. **2**:1105, 1948.
331. Sheldon, W. H.: Atlas of men. A guide for somatotyping the adult male at all ages, New York, 1954, Gramercy Publishing Co., p. 338.
332. Shields, G. S., Coulson, W. F., Kimball, D. A., Carnes, W. H., Cartwright, G. E., and Wintrobe, M. M.: Studies on copper metabolism. XXXII. Cardiovascular lesions in copper-deficient swine, Amer. J. Path. **41**:603, 1962.
333. Siegenthaler, W.: Die kardio-vaskulären Veränderungen beim Marfan-Syndrom (Arachnodatylie), Cardiologia **28**:135, 1956.
334. Sinclair, R. J. G.: The Marfan syndrome, Bull. Rheum. Dis. **8**:153, 1958.
335. Sinclair, R. J. G., Kitchin, A. H., and Turner, R. W. D.: The Marfan syndrome, Quart J. Med. **29**:19, 1960.
336. Sinha, K. P., and Goldberg, H: Marfan's syndrome: a case with complete dissection of the aorta, Amer. Heart J. **36**:890, 1958.
337. Sjoerdsma, A. (Bethesda): Personal communication.
338. Sjoerdsma, A., Davidson, J. D., Udenfriend, S., and Mitoma, C.: Increased excretion of hydroxyproline in Marfan's syndrome, Lancet **2**:994, 1958.
339. Skyring, A.: Personal communication.
340. Slack, H. G. B.: Metabolism of elastin in the adult rat, Nature **174**:512, 1955.
341. Sloper, J. C., and Storey, G.: Aneurysms of the ascending aorta due to medial degeneration associated with arachnodactyly (Marfan's disease), J. Clin. Path. **6**:299, 1953.

342. Smiley, J. D., and Ziff, M.: Urinary hydroxyproline excretion and growth, Physiol. Rev. **44**:30, 1964.
343. Snyder, L. H., and Curtis, G. M.: An inherited "hollow chest," koilosternia, a new character dependent upon a dominant autosomal gene, J. Hered. **25**:445, 1934.
344. Sosman, M. C.: Xanthomatosis, J.A.M.A. **98**:110, 1932.
345. Soulié, P., and colleagues: Les manifestations cardiovasculaires de la maladie de Marfan (a propos de 8 observations personnelles), Arch. Mal. Coeur **54**:121, 1961.
346. Spencer, F. C., and Blake, H.: A report of the successful surgical treatment of aortic regurgitation from a dissecting aortic aneurysm in a patient with the Marfan syndrome, J. Thorac. Cardiov. Surg. **44**:238, 1962.
347. Spenser, J. T.: Post-mortem caesarian delivery after rupture of dissecting aortic aneurysm, Lancet **2**:565, 1952.
348. Spickard, W. B.: Arachnodactyly, description of the clinical characteristics with report of autopsied case, Stanford Med. Bull. **6**:422, 1948.
349. Starke, H.: Zur Pathogenese des Marfan-Syndroms, Von Gräfe's Arch. Ophthal. **151**:384, 1951.
350. Steinberg, I.: Aneurysm of the aortic sinuses with pseudo-coarctation of the aorta, Brit. Heart J. **18**:85, 1956.
351. Steinberg, I.: Dilatation of the aortic sinuses in the Marfan syndrome, Amer. J. Roentgen. **83**:320, 1960.
352. Steinberg, I., and Finby, N.: Clinical manifestations of the unperforated aortic sinus aneurysm, Circulation **14**:115, 1956.
353. Steinberg, I., and Geller, W.: Aneurysmal dilatation of aortic sinuses in arachnodactyly: diagnosis during life in three cases, Ann. Intern. Med. **43**:120, 1955.
354. Steinberg, I., Mangiardi, J. L., and Noble, W. J.: Aneurysmal dilatation of the aortic sinuses in Marfan's syndrome; angiocardiographic and cardiac catheterization studies in identical twins, Circulation **16**:368, 1957.
355. Stephens, F. E.: Inheritance of diseases primary in the muscles, Amer. J. Med. **15**:558, 1953.
356. Stephenson, W. V.: Anterior megalophthalmos and arachnodactyly, Amer. J. Ophthal. **28**:315, 1954.
357. Stettner, E.: Wachstum und Wachstumsstorungen, Mschr. Kinderheilk. **80**:387, 1937.
358. Stevenson, A. C.: Comparisons of mutation rates at single loci in man. In Effects of radiation on human heredity, Geneva, 1957, World Health Organization, p. 125.
359. Stevenson, A. C.: Personal communication.
360. Stewart, R. M.: A case of arachnodactyly, Arch. Dis. Child. **14**:64, 1939.
361. Stoddard, S. E.: The inheritance of "hollow chest." Cobbler's chest due to heredity—not an occupational deformity, J. Hered. **30**:139, 1939.
362. Stolz, H. R., and Stolz, L. M.: Somatic development of adolescent boys. A study of the growth of boys during the second decade of life, New York, 1951, The Macmillan Co.
363. Stonesifer, G. L., Jr.: Emergency correction of ascending aortic dissecting aneurysms, Surgery **56**:594, 1964.
364. Storck, H.: Ein Fall von Arachnodaktylie (Dystrophia mesodermalis congenita), Typus Marfan, Dermatologica **104**:321, 1952.
365. Stratz, C. H.: Der Körper des Kindes, Stuttgart, 1902, Ferdinand Enke.
366. Straub, H.: Die elastischen Fasern in den Bändern des menschlichen Fusses, Acta Anat. **11**:268, 1950.
367. Strayhorn, D., and Wells, E. B.: Arachnodactylia with aneurysmal dilatation of the aorta, Trans. Amer. Clin & Climat. Ass. **59**:205, 1947.
368. Sutton, G. E. F.: Cardiac anomalies associated with funnel chest, Bristol M. Clin. J. **64**:45, 1947.
369. Sweet, R. H.: Pectus excavatum. Report of two cases successfully operated upon, Ann. Surg. **119**:922, 1944.
370. Talbot, N. B., Sobel E. H., McArthur, J. W., and Crawford, J. D.: Functional endocrinology, Cambridge, Mass., 1952, Harvard University Press.
371. Tatoń, J.: Zagadnienie zespou Marfana w świetle wasnych spostrzezeń (Problem of Marfan's syndrome in the light of personal observations), Pol. Arch. Med. Wewnet. **30**:1111, 1960.
372. Theobald, G.: Histologic eye findings in arachnodactyly, Amer. J. Ophthal. **24**:1132, 1941.

373. Thomas, J., Brothers, G. B., Anderson, R. S., and Cuff, J. R.: Marfan syndrome. A report of three cases with aneurysm of the aorta, Amer. J. Med. **12**:613, 1952.
374. Thursfield, H.: Arachnodactyly, St. Bartholomew's Hosp. Rep. **53**:35, 1917-1918.
375. Tjio, J. H., Puck, T. T., and Robinson, A.: The human chromosomal satellites in normal persons and in two patients with Marfan's syndrome, Proc. Nat. Acad. Sci. USA **46**:532, 1960.
376. Tobin, J. R., Jr., Bay, E. B., and Humphries, E. M.: Marfan's syndrome in the adult dissecting aneurysm of the aorta associated with arachnodactyly, Arch. Intern. Med. **80**:475, 1947.
377. Toes, N. A.: Ruptured splenic artery aneurysm during parturition, Brit. Med. J. **1**:495, 1956.
378. Tolbert, L. E., Jr., and Birchall, R. B.: Marfan's syndrome with interventricular septal defect found at autopsy, Ochsner Clin. Rep. **2**:48, 1956.
379. Tourniaire, A., Deyerieux, F., and Bastien, P.: Dilatation du segment initial de l'aorte: gigantisms de l'appareil valvulaire aortique, Arch. Mal. Coeur **44**:153, 1951.
380. Traisman, H. S., and Johnson, F. R.: Arachnodactyly associated with aneurysm of the aorta, Amer. J. Dis. Child. **87**:156, 1954.
381. Traub, E.: Epiphyseal necrosis in pituitary gigantism, Arch. Dis. Child. **14**:203, 1939.
382. Troxler, E. R., and Niemetz, D.: Generalized xanthomatosis with pulmonary, skeletal and cerebral manifestations: report of a case, Ann. Intern. Med. **25**:960, 1946.
383. Troy, J. M.: Marfan's disease complicated by hemothorax, J. Indiana Med. Ass. **48**:488, 1955.
384. Trüb, C. L. P.: Aortenwanderkrankung (Medianecrosis aortae idiopathica), Aortenzerreissung und Arbeitsunfall, Mschr. Unfallheilk. **54**:321, 1951.
385. Tuna, N., and Thal, A. P.: Some unusual features of the Marfan syndrome, report of 4 cases, Circulation **24**:1154, 1961.
386. Tung, H. L., and Liebow, A. A.: Marfan's syndrome. Observations at necropsy with special reference to medio-necrosis of the great vessels, Lab. Invest. **1**:382, 1952.
387. Usher, C. H.: A pedigree of congenital dislocation of the lenses, Biometrika **16**:273, 1924.
388. Uyeyama, H., Kondo, B., and Kamins, M.: Arachnodactylia and cardiovascular disease, Amer. Heart J. **34**:580, 1947.
389. Van Buchem, F. S. P.: Cardiovascular disease in arachnodactyly, Acta Med. Scand. **161**:197, 1958.
390. Van der Hyde, M. N., and Zwaveling, A.: Resection of an abdominal aneurysm in a patient with Marfan's syndrome, J. Cardiov. Surg. **2**:359, 1961.
391. Varga, B.: The type of inheritance in Marfan's syndrome, Orv. Hetil. **103**:438, 1962.
392. Vejdonsky, V.: Marfan's syndrome, Lek. Listy. **1**:539, 1946.
393. Vesely, D. G., Bray, C. B., and Bryant, V. M.: Arachnodactyly, a case report, J. Med. Ass. Alabama **24**:276, 1955.
394. Viva-Salas, E., and Sanson, R. E.: Sindrome d Marfan, sin cardiopatia congenita y con endocarditis lenta conformada por la autopsia, Arch. Inst. Cardiol. México **18**:217, 1948.
395. Von Meyenburg, H.: Ueber spontane Aortenrupture bei zwei Brudern, Schweiz. Med. Wschr. **20**:976, 1939.
396. Von Noorden, G. K., and Schultz, R. O.: A gonioscopic study of the chamber angle in Marfan's syndrome, Arch. Ophthal. **64**:929, 1960.
397. Wachtel, F. M., Ravitch, M. M., and Grisham, A.: The relation of pectus excavatum to heart disease, Amer. Heart J. **52**:121, 1956.
398. Wagenwoort, C. A., Neufeld, H. N., and Edwards, J. E.: Cardiovascular system in Marfan's syndrome and in idiopathic dilatation of the ascending aorta, Amer. J. Cardiol. **9**:496, 1962.
399. Wajda, I., Lehr, D., and Krukowski, M.: Sex difference in aortic rupture induced by lathyrus odoratus in immature rats, Fed. Proc. **16**:343, 1957.
400. Warwick, W. T., and Wiles, P.: The growth of periosteum in long bones, Brit. J. Surg. **22**:169, 1934.
401. Wawzonek, S., Ponseti, I. V., Shepard, R. S., and Wiedenmann, L. G.: Epiphyseal plate lesions, degenerative arthritis, and dissecting aneurysm of the aorta produced by aminonitriles, Science **121**:63, 1955.
402. Weber, F. P.: Familial asthenia ("paralytic") type of thorax with congenital ectopia of lenses, a condition allied to arachnodactyly, Lancet **2**:1472, 1933.
403. Webster, B., Rich, C., Densen, P. M., Moore, J. E., Nicol, C. S., and Padget, P.: Studies in

cardiovascular syphilis. III. The natural history of syphilitic aortic insufficiency, Amer. Heart J. **46:**117, 1953.

404. Weill, G.: Ectopie du cristallin et malformations générales, Ann. Ocul. **169:**21, 1932.
405. Weissman, N., Shields, G. S., and Carnes, W. H.: Cardiovascular studies on copper-deficient swine, J. Biol. Chem. **238:**3115, 1963.
406. West, L. S.: Two pedigrees showing inherited predisposition to hernia, J. Hered. **27:**449, 1939.
407. Weve, H.: Ueber Arachnodaktylie (Dystrophia mesodermalis congenita, typus Marfanis), Arch. Augenheilk. **104:**1, 1931.
408. Weyers, H.: Zur Kenntnis der Arachnodaktylie und ihrer Beziehungen zu anderen mesodermalen Konstitutionsanomalien, Z. Kinderheilk. **67:**308, 1949.
409. White, P. D.: Personal communication.
410. Whitfield, A. G. W., Arnott, W. M., and Stafford, J. S.: "Myocarditis" and aortic hypoplasia in arachnodactylia, Lancet **1:**1387, 1951.
411. Whittaker, S. R. F., and Sheehan, J. D.: Dissecting aortic aneurysm in Marfan's syndrome, Lancet **2:**791, 1954.
412. Wilkins, L.: The diagnosis and treatment of endocrine disorders in childhood and adolescence, Springfield, Ill., 1950, Charles C Thomas, Publisher.
413. Wilkinson, K. D.: Aneurysmal dilatation of the pulmonary artery, Brit. Heart J. **2:**255, 1940.
414. Williams, E.: Rare cases, with practical remarks, Trans. Amer. Ophthal. Soc. **2:**291, 1873-1879.
415. Wilner, H. I., and Finby, N.: Skeletal manifestations in the Marfan syndrome, J.A.M.A. **187:**490, 1964.
416. Wilson, R.: Marfan's syndrome: description of a family, Amer. J. Med. **23:**434, 1957.
417. Witkin, M.: Arachnodactyly in a Bantu child, S. Afr. Med. J. **32:**45, 1958.
418. Wolff, K.: Unbekannte Erkrankung der Säuglingsaorta mit Schwund des elastischen Gewebes, Virchow Arch. Path. Anat. **285:**369, 1932.
419. Wolff, K.: Ueber die Ursachen der sogenannten spontanen Aortenzerreissungen, Virchow Arch. Path. Anat. **289:**1, 1933.
420. Wong, F. L., Friedman, S., and Yakovac, W.: Cardiac complications of Marfan's syndrome in a child. Report of a case with rapidly progressive course terminating with rupture of dissecting aneurysm, Amer. J. Dis. Child. **107:**404, 1964.
421. Wunsch, M. C., Steinmetz, E. F., and Fisch, C.: Marfan's syndrome and subacute bacterial endocarditis, Amer. J. Cardiol. **15:**102, 1965.
422. Yettra, M., and Laski, S. L.: Aneurysmal dilatation of the aorta associated with cystic medial necrosis, Amer. Heart J. **33:**516, 1947.
423. Young, J.: Relaxation of pelvic joints in pregnancy: pelvic arthropathy of pregnancy, J. Obstet. Gynaec. Brit. Comm. **47:**493, 1940.
424. Young, M. L.: Arachnodactyly, Arch. Dis. Child. **4:**190, 1929.
425. Zabriskie, J., and Reisman, M.: Marchesani syndrome, J. Pediat. **52:**158, 1958.
426. Zaidi, Z. H.: Bilateral ectopia lentis in Marfan's syndrome: review of features with report of two cases, Canad. Med. Ass. J. **82:**265, 1960.
427. Zanchi, M.: Medionecrosis idiopathica cystica dell'aorta ed aneurisma fusiforme puro giovanile in soggetto Basedowiano, Folio Hered. Path. (Milano) **7:**287, 1958.

4

Homocystinuria

Historical note

The discovery of an inborn error of metabolism reflected by the presence of homocystine in the urine and associated with systemic abnormalities of connective tissue is so recent that it can barely be considered history. In the course of a survey of mentally retarded persons in northern Ireland, using urine chromatography, Carson and Neill[5] detected several instances of homocystinuria and noted the occurrence of ectopia lentis.[3] Simultaneously and independently, Waisman and colleagues[12,13] in Madison, Wisconsin, discovered the same metabolic defect. The occurrence of vascular lesions soon became evident and the confusion with the Marfan syndrome was pointed out on the basis of restudy of cases previously reported as instances of Marfan's syndrome.[15] Mudd and coworkers[30] demonstrated that the specific enzyme defect involves cystathionine synthetase. The prevalence of the disorder, the range of its clinical manifestations, such as the absence of mental changes in some cases, the pathogenesis of the phenotypic feature, and dietary therapy are currently under active study.

Clinical manifestations

Changes in the central nervous system, eye, cardiovascular system, and skeletal system are reflected in clinical manifestations.

Subjects in the initially described cases were mentally retarded, having been detected in the course of screening a mentally retarded group. In most of the subsequently detected cases there has also been retardation in some degree, but as families have been investigated and other categories of cases, such a those with ectopia lentis, have been surveyed, affected persons with normal or near-normal intelligence have been discovered.[11,24,35] In our own series of thirty-eight patients, at least sixteen are of normal intelligence. Five attended college. (As experience with phenylketonuria and galactosemia increases it is discovered that homozygotes with normal or little-impaired intelligence occur in those conditions also.)

Patients of teen age and older have often been highly nervous, and a diagnosis of schizophrenia has been made in some. A striking family history of schizophrenia was noted in one instance.[4] Seizures have occurred in some patients.[4] The electroencephalogram was abnormal in all eight patients tested, including two with normal intelligence. The patient of Gerritsen and Waisman[6,14] had extreme spasticity and hyperreflexia and died at 1 year of age.

Localizing neurologic signs are attributable to intracranial arterial and/or venous thrombosis. Acute hemiplegia occurred in an 8-year-old child.[35] Early intracranial thrombosis led to the nonspecific diagnosis of cerebral palsy in one patient who died at 3 years of age.[35]

Ectopia lentis of a type apparently indistinguishable from that of the Marfan syndrome has been present in all cases in which it was sought. It is possible, of course, and indeed likely, that some cases will lack this feature. In one patient (Case 4) dislocation of the lenses is minimal and was detected only by repeat examinations after the diagnosis of homocystinuria was established. In several patients there is evidence that the displacement of the lens has been progressive, suggesting that ectopia lentis may not be present in young patients. Possibly, downward displacement of the lens is more frequent in homocystinuria than in the Marfan syndrome. Zonular cataracts and cystic degeneration of the retina have been reported.[4,13,24] Myopia and optic atrophy have been observed.[38] Retinal detachment was observed in some.[4] In some cases acute glaucoma develops[4,24] secondary to lens dislocation with pupillary block. One child developed buphthalmos by this mechanism.[4]

The cardiovascular lesions of homocystinuria consist mainly of thrombosis in arteries of intermediate size, particularly the coronary arteries, renal arteries, and main branches of the aorta supplying the extremities and the brain, as well as smaller cerebral vessels. Venous thrombosis and pulmonary embolism have been noted. Hypertension, myocardial infarction, stroke, intermittent claudication, bruits over the femoral, subclavian, and other arteries, and acute gangrene of the extremities are among the clinical manifestations resulting from arterial thrombosis. Death from acute coronary occlusion occurred in a 20-year-old female (Case 2) and from internal carotid thrombosis in an 18-year-old male (Case 1). Anteroseptal myocardial infarction occurred at age 31 in another female. Damage to blood vessels, as in venipuncture, arterial puncture, or arteriography, may precipitate thrombosis. Arterial and venous thrombosis seems to occur frequently after surgical procedures.[4] Insofar as possible, surgery and arteriography should probably be avoided in homocystinurics. Gastrointestinal bleeding, either massive or occult, may occur in older homocystinuric patients and is probably related to the vascular disease.

The cardiac findings are mainly those of coronary occlusive disease: symptoms and electrocardiographic changes of coronary insufficiency or myocardial infarction. A 44-year-old patient has atrial fibrillation. Auscultatory signs of valvular involvement are usually absent. A mitral opening snap and a mid-diastolic apical murmur have been heard in some cases (e.g. Cases 2 and 3) and may be related to endocardial elastosis observed in the left atrium at autopsy. Definite aortic regurgitation has not been noted, although a short early diastolic murmur of possible aortic valve origin was heard in Case 2. One patient with normal findings of right heart catheterization (Case 4) has idiopathic dilatation of the pulmonary artery. Aortic aneurysm was found in none of the twenty-three patients I have personally studied. Thrombosis of the abdominal aorta occurred in one patient who died at age 28 from portal vein thrombosis with infarction of the bowel.

Joint laxity, genu valgum, kyphoscoliosis, pigeon breast deformity, and excessively long extremities have been features in some cases. Many of the patients walk with the feet everted in a flat-footed "Chaplin" gait. Loose-jointedness is a less striking feature than in the Marfan syndrome. The hands in homocystinurics tend to have a "tight feel" of restricted joint mobility in the fingers. Contracture of the fingers[4] has been observed. Radiologic study shows generalized osteoporosis in most cases. Codfish vertebrae and/or some degree of collapse of vertebral bodies has been present in all older patients. Fractures occur with increased frequency. Most of the patients are unusually tall and the upper segment–lower segment ratio (US/LS) is unusually low, falling in the range of values shown by Marfan patients. Osteoporosis with vertebral collapse undoubtedly contributes to the low US/LS value.

Bilateral inguinal hernias[13] have been observed, and a large omphalocele was present in one case in our series.

Unlike cystinuria and cystinosis, in homocystinuria renal calculi and tissue deposits have not been observed.

In addition to the above features most homocystinurics have a characteristic malar flush. Most patients develop intense flushing of the face with exertion in hot weather, and a violaceous flush of the face is likely to develop when the patient is recumbent. In one of the oldest of our patients (Case 7) the face is intensely flushed. The skin elsewhere may be blotchy red, or show livedo reticularis.[4] The skin of the face is coarse and large-pored in older patients. The

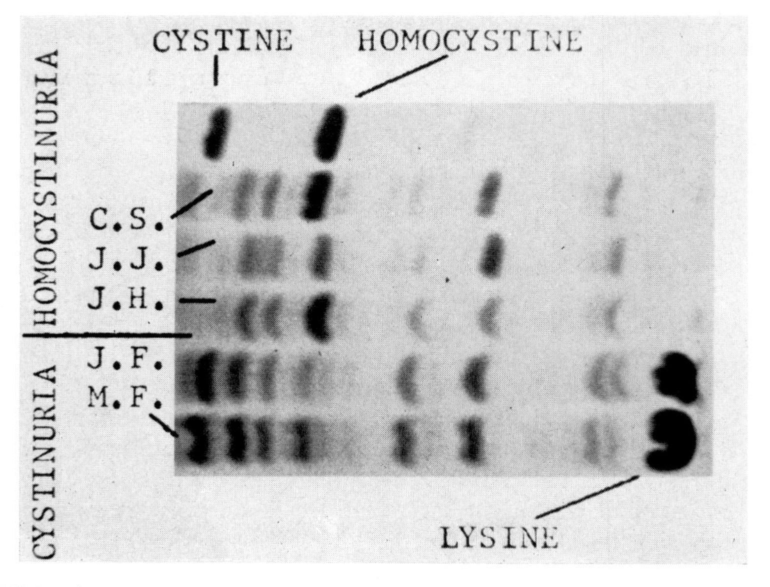

Fig. 4-1. High-voltage paper electrophoresis of urine from three patients with homocystinuria and two with cystinuria. For comparison, a mixture of cystine and homocystine is shown in the top run. The large amount of lysine in the cystinurics is another feature distinguishng homocystinuria from cystinuria.

hair is fine, sparse, and blond in some cases. The teeth are usually crowded and irregularly aligned.

Severely affected infants show poor growth and "failure to thrive." Hepatomegaly is often present. Serum isocitric dehydrogenase level was elevated in six patients tested by Carson and colleagues,[4] who attributed the finding to hepatic dysfunction.

Diagnosis

The specific diagnosis is made by demonstration of homocystine in the urine. The cyanide nitroprusside test used in the diagnosis of cystinuria is positive also in homocystinuria. The test is performed as follows: a mixture of 5 ml. of urine and 2 ml. of a 5% solution of NaCN is left to react at room temperature for 10 minutes. On addition of 2 to 4 drops of a 5% sodium nitroprusside solution a beet-red color develops in the presence of cysteine or homocysteine. (NaCN reduces cystine and homocystine to cysteine and homocysteine.)

Cystine and homocystine give a spot at the same location on paper chromatography. They can be distinguished, however, by high-voltage electrophoresis or by specific assay by means of the Stein-Moore column chromatographic automatic amino acid analyzer.

Homocystinuria is probably present from birth and constant thereafter. However, under some circumstances, such as large urine volume and perhaps low protein intake, the qualitative cyanide nitroprusside test may be negative.

Prognosis

Patients dying at ages 1,[14] 2,[41] 3,[35] 7,[41] 8,[41] 9,[35] 9½,[4] 11,[34] 13,[34] 14,[34] 15,[34] 18,[35] 20,[35] and 28[4,35] years have been reported. On the other hand, seven patients in our series (Table 4) are living and reasonably well at the age of 40 or over, and eight others are alive at the age of 22 years or more. The full range of severity of homocystinuria is yet to be determined. Occlusive vascular disease is the principal cause of death.

Pathology

The most distinctive lesions are those of the arteries.[15] Usually many arteries show evidence of partial luminal obstruction, apparently due to episodic thrombosis followed by fibroelastic organization. The media of these vessels shows drastic changes. The artery is dilated with thinning out of muscular elements that became separated by a ground substance whose nature has not been determined.

The elastic weave of the aortic media, i.e. the array of elastic lamellae, is abnormal in some cases. Aneurysmal dilatation of the aorta is not a conspicuous feature, however, and dissecting aneurysm has not been observed. Peculiar transverse intimal striations were noted in the descending aorta in one case,[4] and areas of disruption of elastic fibers in the media underlay the intimal striations. Thrombosis of the abdominal aorta occurred in a 28-year-old man. Fibroelastic thickening of the endocardium of the left atrium has been found in most cases.

The brain shows focal necrosis and gliosis.[4] Degenerative changes were described in the zonular fibers of the lens by light and electron microscopy. Chou and Waisman[6] described severe spongy degeneration of the brain together with micropolygyria and hypoplasia of the corpus callosum in a child who died at 1 year of age. Although the changes in some ways resembled those of van Bogaert-Bertrand spongy degeneration,[44] it was thought that they were probably different.

The first case of Gerritsen and Waisman[13] showed multiple pulmonary emboli, the patient having died at 1 year of age. Two 9-year-old patients of Brenton and associates[2] died of pulmonary embolus after eye surgery. Thrombosis of the portal vein was the cause of death in one patient of our series (Case 8).

Fatty liver has been found in several cases and is correlated with hepatomegaly observed clinically. A twofold increase in the neutral lipids of liver was measured by Carson and colleagues.[4]

Basic defect and pathogenesis

Deficient activity of the enzyme cystathionine synthetase (or synthase) has been demonstrated in the liver[30] and brain[29] of affected persons. Affected persons have less than 5% of normal activity. (The enzyme is normally absent from erythrocytes, leukocytes, platelets, skin, and intestinal mucosa.) Although threonine deaminase[17] and serine deaminase[36] activities are demonstrated by cystathionine synthetase of the rat, threonine deaminase activity was found[31] to be normal in a homocystinuric.

Reasoning from the elevation of homocystine and methionine in the blood and the position of cystathionine synthetase in the metabolic chain leading from methionine to cystine (Fig. 4-2), one is forced to conclude that homocystinuria is not due to a renal tubular defect, as exists in cystinuria, but is a variety of overflow aminoaciduria consequent to a specific Garrodian inborn error of metabolism. (Actually there is no renal threshold for homocystine.)

The conversion of methionine to cystine has been shown to proceed as outlined in abbreviated form in Fig. 4-2. (See reference 28.) Homocystinurics fail to demonstrate the normal increase in urinary inorganic sulfate when a methio-

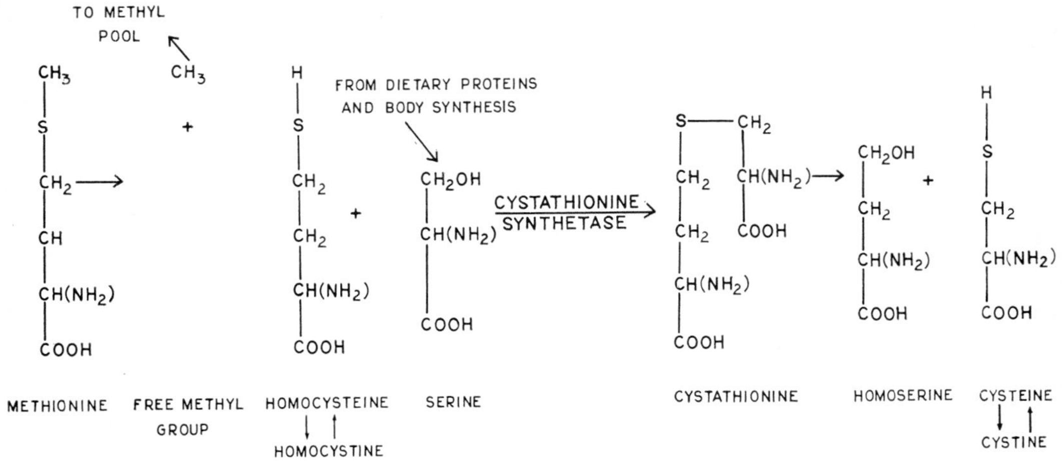

TO METHYL POOL

FROM DIETARY PROTEINS AND BODY SYNTHESIS

CYSTATHIONINE SYNTHETASE

METHIONINE: CH_3–S–CH_2–CH–$CH(NH_2)$–COOH

FREE METHYL GROUP: CH_3

HOMOCYSTEINE: H–S–CH_2–CH_2–$CH(NH_2)$–COOH ⇅ HOMOCYSTINE

SERINE: CH_2OH–$CH(NH_2)$–COOH

CYSTATHIONINE: S–CH_2–CH_2–$CH(NH_2)$–COOH; S–CH_2–$CH(NH_2)$–COOH

HOMOSERINE: CH_2OH–CH_2–$CH(NH_2)$–COOH

CYSTEINE: H–S–CH_2–$CH(NH_2)$–COOH ⇅ CYSTINE

Fig. 4-2. Abbreviated schema of the metabolic pathway from methionine to cystine. Cystathionine synthetase activity in liver is very low in patients with homocystinuria.

nine load is administered.[23] With cystine-loading, however, urinary inorganic sulfate rises in a normal manner. Peptide-bound methionine is increased in the urine to levels actually exceeding that of homocystine.[23] The accumulation of homocystine is probably partially counteracted by transmethylation of homocysteine back to methionine, since Brenton and co-workers[2] found that the activities of betaine-homocysteine transmethylase and of thetin methyl transferase are normal in homocystinuric liver.

As in most inborn errors of metabolism, two main alternatives exist as to origin of pathologic changes: (1) deficiency of substances distal to the block may result in pathologic manifestations or (2) substances accumulating proximal to the block may have toxic effects. The two possibilities are, of course, not mutually exclusive.

Only limited information is available on pathologic effects of increased concentrations of homocystine[21] or other metabolites of methionine.

Cystathionine is normally found in brain tissue, in relatively abundant amounts,[19,39] and is absent from the brain of the homocystinuric.[2,13] In fact its concentration is normally higher in the brain than in other tissues and higher in the brain of man than of other species.[39] Cystathionine synthetase is normally present in the brain but was absent in one case of homocystinuria studied by Mudd.[29] Whether the deficiency of cystathionine is itself responsible for the mental retardation and psychic changes in homocystinuria is unknown. It is also useless to speculate about the reason for the variation in degree of mental retardation, from none to very severe. Whereas most of the homocystinurics studied have essentially no cystathionine synthetase activity in the liver, a 24-year-old patient with homocystine in the urine, who had normal mentality and had no other clinical features of homocystinuria, showed about 12% residual activity.[11] The interpretation of this puzzling case, in a patient who had a relative with typical features, remains in doubt.

Preliminary studies of homocystinurics using S^{35}-labelled methionine suggest that little if any radioactivity appears in cystine.[2] Absence of cystathionine synthetase might make the affected person dependent on absorbable dietary cystine for protein synthesis. Unfortunately, the disulfide cystine is relatively insoluble and therefore not well absorbed. During periods of rapid growth, dietary cystine might be insufficient for anabolic requirements. It has been suggested[3] that affected infants receiving cow's milk in the first weeks of life may be less adequately nourished than those breast-fed, since cow's milk is a much poorer source of cystine.[37]

Are the changes in connective tissue elements of the eye, skeleton, and arteries due to a relative deficiency of cysteine and cystine? Since collagen is notably deficient in sulfur-containing amino acids,[4] a deficiency in an amino acid building block for collagen is not likely to be responsible for the connective tissue changes. (Deasy[9] found homocystine or homocysteine in steerhide corium and kangaroo rat tendon.) It is possible that the metabolism of acid mucopolysaccharides suffers from a deficiency of sulfate donor and that as a secondary result collagen synthesis, in which mucopolysaccharide plays a role (p. 387), suffers. Since glutathione contains cystine, it is also possible that glutathione-dependent reactions are retarded. Interference with collagen crosslinking by homocysteine is yet another possibility.

Ectopia lentis might be the consequence of cystine deficiency. Normally, rapid increases in beta crystallin of the lens, which has a high cystine content,[32] occurs in early embryonic growth.[33] Furthermore, the lens becomes isolated early in embryonic life and is dependent upon its own enzymes for synthesis of necessary protein constituents. Dardenne and Kirsten[8] found that the lens has the capacity to convert methionine to cystine by the pathway shown in Fig. 4-2. They stated that ". . . the autonomy of the metabolism of the sulfur-containing amino acids is a consequence of the ontogenetically very early separation of the lens. In the human embryo of 12 mm. length, the lens is already completely separated from surrounding tissue."*

Another possible connection between cysteine deficiency and ectopia lentis is suggested by the lens's high content,[6,20,32] especially in its cortex, of glutathione, a tripeptide containing cysteine as one of its three constituent amino acids.

Clinically there is no evidence of abnormality of insulin or posterior pituitary hormone, proteins with high cystine content. The hair changes described above may reflect an abnormality of keratin, which also has a high cystine content.

Many of the clinical and anatomic changes are the result of arterial stenosis or occlusion. McDonald and colleagues[27] claimed that platelet adhesiveness is increased in homocystinuria. Using a different method, we demonstrated no abnormality of platelet adhesiveness in patients in our series. The drastic changes in vessel wall may be adequate explanation for the thrombotic changes. Microscopic cracks in the intima might, for example, create foci[43] for aggregation of platelets, initating thrombosis. The clinical course in several patients suggests that hypertension accelerates the thrombotic process, probably through increased dilatation of the defective vessels.

Prevalence and inheritance

Cases of homocystinuria will probably prove to be rather frequent. It is likely that the closest estimate of frequency will be provided by the screening of ectopia lentis cases, now in progress. Homocystinuria may compete with galactosemia for second position in frequency, next to phenylketonuria, among those inborn errors of metabolism which have thus far been identified and which lead to mental retardation. Probably about 5% of patients with nontraumatic ectopia lentis have homocystinuria. Probably a similar proportion of persons with "Marfan's syndrome" have homocystinuria.

With the exception of a reported American Negro family[18] and three of Jewish extraction in our series,[34] all affected families have been of northern European origin—Irish, Scottish, English, Dutch, German, Swedish. The patient of Mudd and colleagues[30] was of Lithuanian origin. One sibship[34] is of mixed southern Italian and Irish-Lithuanian parentage. None of Oriental extraction has been identified, but experience is, of course, still limited.

Like other inborn errors of metabolism, homocystinuria is inherited as a recessive. It is determined by an autosomal gene in homozygous state.[34] The autosomal recessive inheritance is supported by the finding that males and females are affected with about equal frequency (Table 4) and that both parents of a patient with homocystinuria have about half the normal level of hepatic cystathionine synthetase activity. No reliable method for identifying the heterozygote, short of enzyme assays of liver biopsy material, has been devised.

*From Dardenne, V., and Kirsten, G.: Exp. Eye Res. 1:415, 1962.

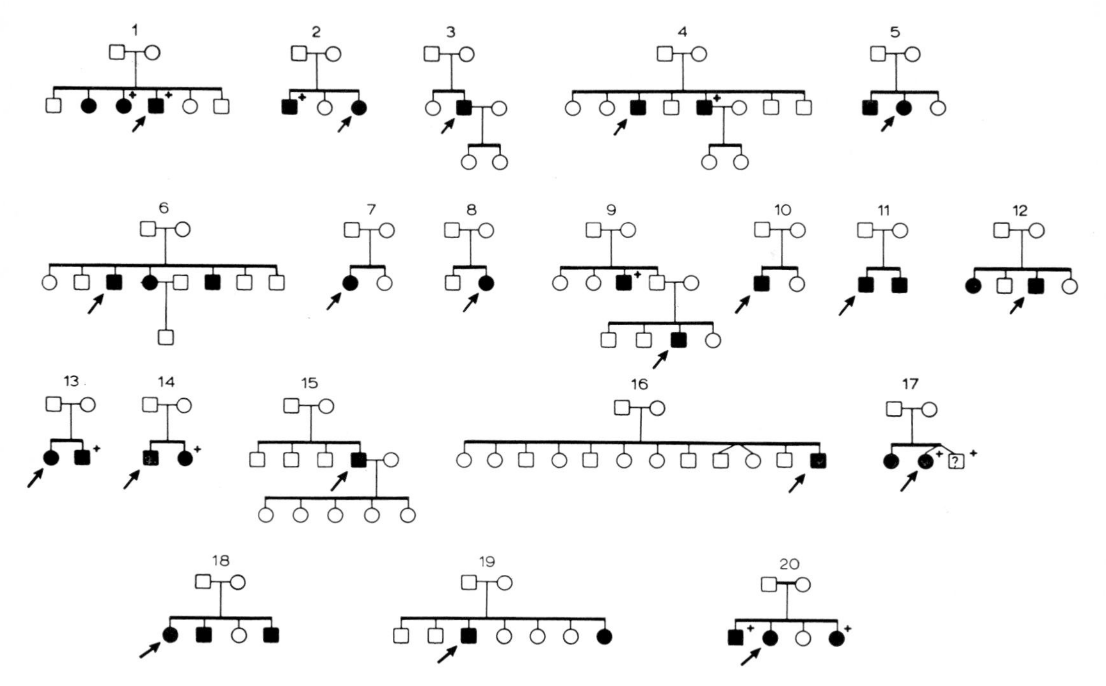

Fig. 4-3. Fragment pedigrees of twenty personally studied kindreds with one or more homocystinuric. The parents were closely related (first cousins) only in Family 20.

Segregation analysis by the Lenz-Hogben method in our series of twenty families containing twenty-one affected sibships (Fig. 4-3) shows an excess of affected sibs, compared with the number predicted by the recessive hypothesis. However, this method of analysis assumes that the probability of ascertainment of a given family is unrelated to the number of affected persons in the family, whereas the ascertainment is in fact probably influenced by this factor. Indeed, when the method of analysis appropriate to so-called single ascertainment is used, that is, when the proband is removed from each sibship, the proportion of remaining sibs who are affected is very nearly 25%.

Four affected adults in our series are married to unaffected and unrelated spouses and have in all ten children, all unaffected.

In twenty personally studied families, one instance of parental consanguinity (first cousins) was found. Consanguinity was suspected in three other instances; in two, both parents were of Jewish extraction, and in the third both parents were born in the Dalarne area of Sweden.

One patient with normal mentality and no other clinical signs of homocystinuria, the cousin of a "typical" case, had a lesser degree of homocystinuria and enzyme activity about 12% of normal.[11] The genetic basis of this difference is unclear.

Other considerations

Differentiation from the Marfan syndrome is summarized in Table 5. Patients with homocystinuria have been reported as instances of the Marfan syndrome.[25,26] All the patients described in detail below were considered at one time to have the Marfan syndrome. Family A, reported by Lynas[26] as showing the Marfan syndrome, has been found to have homocystinuria. One can speculate about the diagnosis in other reported cases, e.g. the patient with presumed Marfan syndrome and thrombotic occlusion of the aorta described by Dexter and associates.[10] The parents were related but unaffected. Follow-up in 1964 showed* that the patient died in 1962 at the age of 42 years of acute myocardial infarction and hypertension; autopsy was not performed.

Rational therapy must await clearer understanding of pathogenetic mechanisms. It is quite credible that methods can be devised for preventing some aspects of the pathologic picture, including the vascular ones that mainly endanger life. A low methionine–high cysteine diet will be worthy of further trial, although results to date[4,34] have been disappointing. It may be necessary to institute treatment earlier than has thus for been possible. Supplementary cystathionine may be necessary, but it is unknown to what extent factors such as intestinal absorption, the lack of renal threshold, and the "blood-brain barrier" may limit the effectiveness of oral administration.

CASE REPORTS

Mainly by screening for homocystine the urine of patients having ectopia lentis and those with presumed Marfan syndrome, twenty families containing thirty-eight affected persons have thus far (June 1, 1965) been identified.[34] Some aspects are summarized in Table 4. The following are descriptions of these thirty-eight cases.

Family 1

Case 1. D. Ho. (B.C.H. 328838), an 18-year-old white male, was in good health until ten days before death. (Ectopia lentis had been noted, and mild mental retardation was evident from his school record.) Following physical exertion he noted the onset of weakness and numbness of the right arm and leg. Examination at that time showed the blood pressure to be 180/120 mm. Hg; no abnormal neurologic signs were detected. One week later he was admitted to the hospital for investigation of hypertension.

Physical examination showed a healthy appearing, normally developed, and well-nourished young man. The blood pressure was 180/110 mm. Hg in both arms. Bilateral subluxation of the lenses was detected. A grade II systolic mumur was heard at the left sternal border and was not transmitted into the neck. Wide variability in intensity and some variability in quality of this murmur were noted. Pulsation was thought to be diminished in the left common carotid artery and both femoral arteries, and a loud bruit was audible over the bifurcation of the abdominal aorta and both femoral triangles. No pulses were palpable in the feet. The only abnormal neurologic finding was weakness of the right trapezius muscle.

On the day after admission to the hospital, the patient noted the sudden onset of weakness of the right arm and hand. This progressed to involve the right side of the face and Babinski's sign was noted on the right. Retrograde aortogram demonstrated no abnormality of the major branches of the aortic arch. The right hemiparesis increased, and the patient became unresponsive to all except painful stimuli. Ophthalmodynamometry showed marked depression of arterial pressure in the left eye. A left common carotid arteriogram showed obstruction of the internal carotid artery immediately above the bifurcation. At this time cyanotic discoloration and a lack of pulsations in the right upper extremity were noted.

Surgical exploration of the left common carotid artery was performed on the fourth hospital day. A thrombus was removed from the left internal carotid for a distance of about 3 cm. beyond

*Follow-up information courtesy Dr. Lyman O. Warren, Bay Pines, Fla.

Table 4. Personal series of homocystinurics

Case	*Patient*	*Sex*	*Age presently or at death*	*Alive or dead*	*Intelligence*
1	D. Ho.	M	18	Dead	Retarded
2	E. Ho.	F	20	Dead	Retarded
3	J. Ho.	F	25	Alive	Retarded
4	J. Har.	F	11	Alive	Retarded
5	S. Har.	M	3	Dead	Retarded
6	C. So.	M	44	Alive	Normal
7	J. Je.	M	40	Alive	Normal
8	W. Je.	M	28	Dead	Normal
9	L. Br.	M	24	Alive	Normal
10	K. Br.	F	22	Alive	Retarded
11	D. Ap.	M	25	Alive	Normal
12	J. A. Mc.	F	23	Alive	Normal
13	C. Ap.	M	19	Alive	Normal
14	T. Bu.	F	8	Alive	Retarded
15	M. Ba.	F	12	Alive	Retarded
16	S. Bo.	M	11	Alive	Retarded
17	F. Bo.	M	9	Dead	Retarded
18	A. Wz.	M	6	Alive	Retarded
19	R. Hd.	M	9	Alive	Retarded
20	D. Hd.	M	8	Alive	Retarded
21	J. Gil.	M	15	Alive	Retarded
22	S. Gil.	F	22	Alive	Retarded
23	J. Te.	F	45	Alive	Normal
24	C. Te.	M	18	Dead	Normal
25	M. St.	M	17	Alive	Normal
26	N. St.	F	11	Dead	Normal
27	I. MacD.	M	45	Alive	Normal
28	S. Han.	M	11	Alive	Retarded
29	J. Mat.	F	22	Alive	Retarded
30	M. Mat.	F	13	Dead	Retarded
31	P. Tu.	F	44	Alive	Normal
32	C. Tu.	M	31	Alive	Normal
33	W. Tu.	M	43	Alive	Normal
34	D. How.	M	16	Alive	Retarded
35	De. How.	F	10	Alive	Retarded
36	J. S.	F	45	Alive	Retarded
37	P. S.	M	14	Dead	Normal
38	A. S.	F	15	Dead	Retarded
		22 of 38 male	3 to 45 years	28 of 38 alive	16 of 38 normal

the bifurcation, but adequate backflow was not achieved. The patient died about twenty-four hours after operation.

Autopsy. Both internal carotid arteries were completely occluded proximal to the circle of Willis. On the left the thrombosis was old and organized, and on the right there was evidence of both old and recent thrombosis. Both femoral arteries and the right brachial and the right coronary artery ostia were partly occluded. The aorta showed only scattered atheromata, and no aneurysm was found in any vessel. Histologically, all large vessels showed peculiar dis-organization of the medial elastic fibers but no medial necrosis. There was marked endocardial

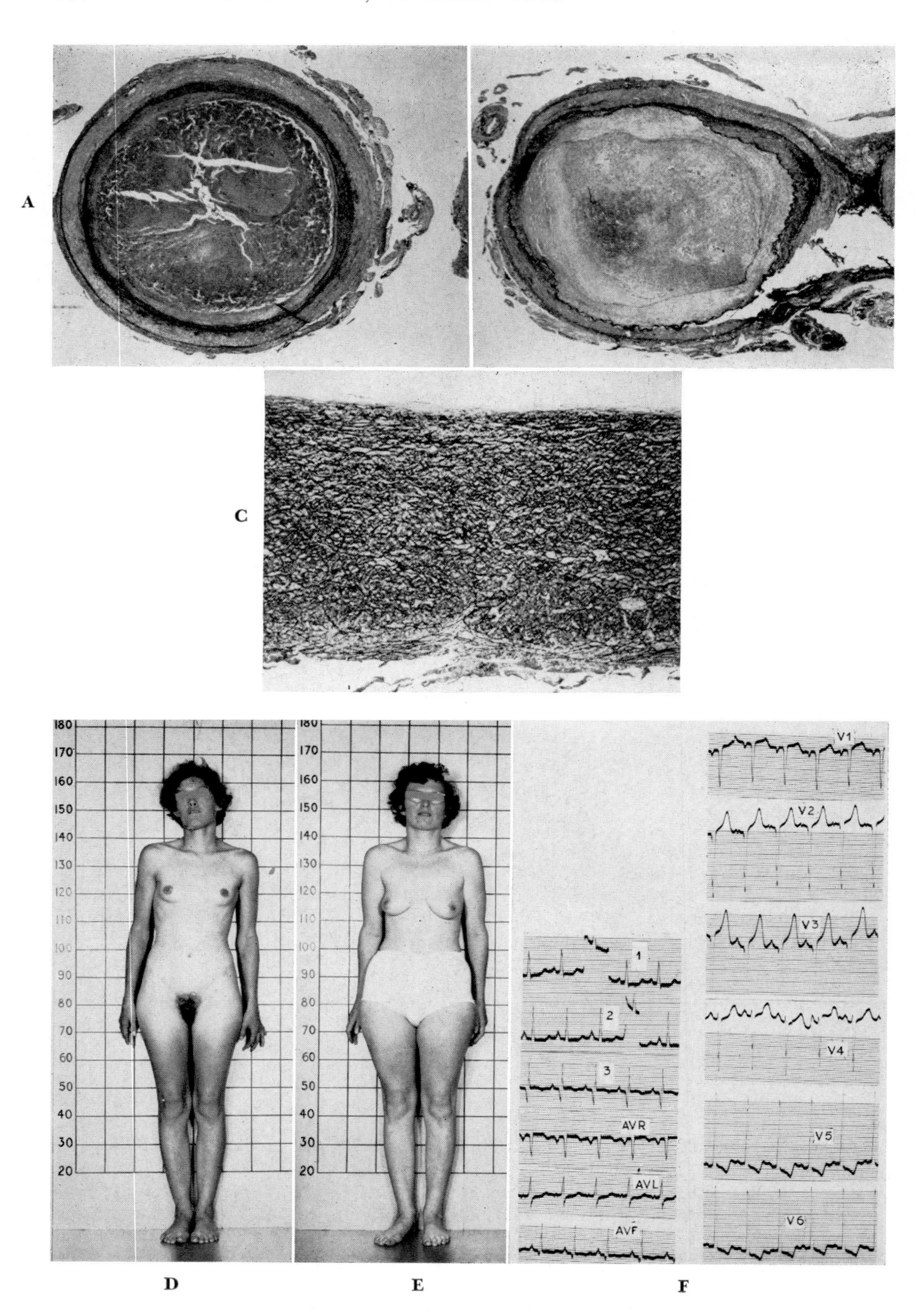

Fig. 4-4. For legend see opposite page.

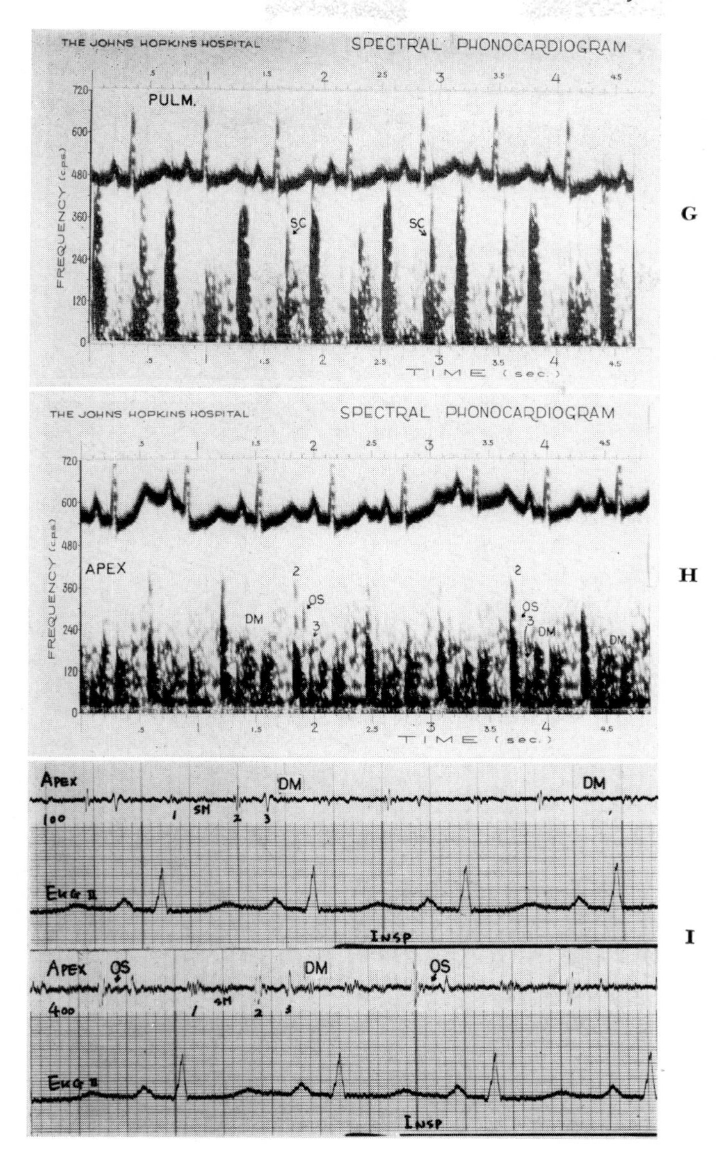

Fig. 4-4. Data on three homocystinuric sibs (Family 1, p. 158). **A,** Thrombosed right internal carotid artery in D. Ho., Case 1. Note thinning of media with dilatation of artery. **B,** Thrombosed left internal carotid artery in same patient. Thrombosis has occurred episodically with formation of new internal elastic lamellae. **C,** An abnormal elastic weave of the aortic media was demonstrated by both longitudinal and transverse section. **D,** Body habitus in E. Ho., Case 2, age 20 years. **E,** Body habitus in J. Ho., Case 3, age 22 years. **F,** Electrocardiogram in E. Ho., Case 2, age 20 years, indicating old posterior myocardial infarction. **G** to **I,** Spectral phonocardiograms demonstrate a conspicuous systolic ejection click in the pulmonary area, **G,** and a mitral opening snap, third heart sound, and mid-diastolic murmur at the apex, **H.** The findings at the apex are confirmed by the oscillographic phonocardiogram shown in **I. J** and **K,** Coronary artery in E. Ho., Case 2. The media is markedly thickened. The branch is spared. The dark-staining muscle fibers of the media are separated by a ground substance. **L,** Face showing coarse wide-pored skin in J. Ho., Case 3. **M,** Spine showing osteoporosis in J. Ho., Case 3. **N,** Skull showing osteoporosis and large sinuses in J. Ho., Case 3.

Continued.

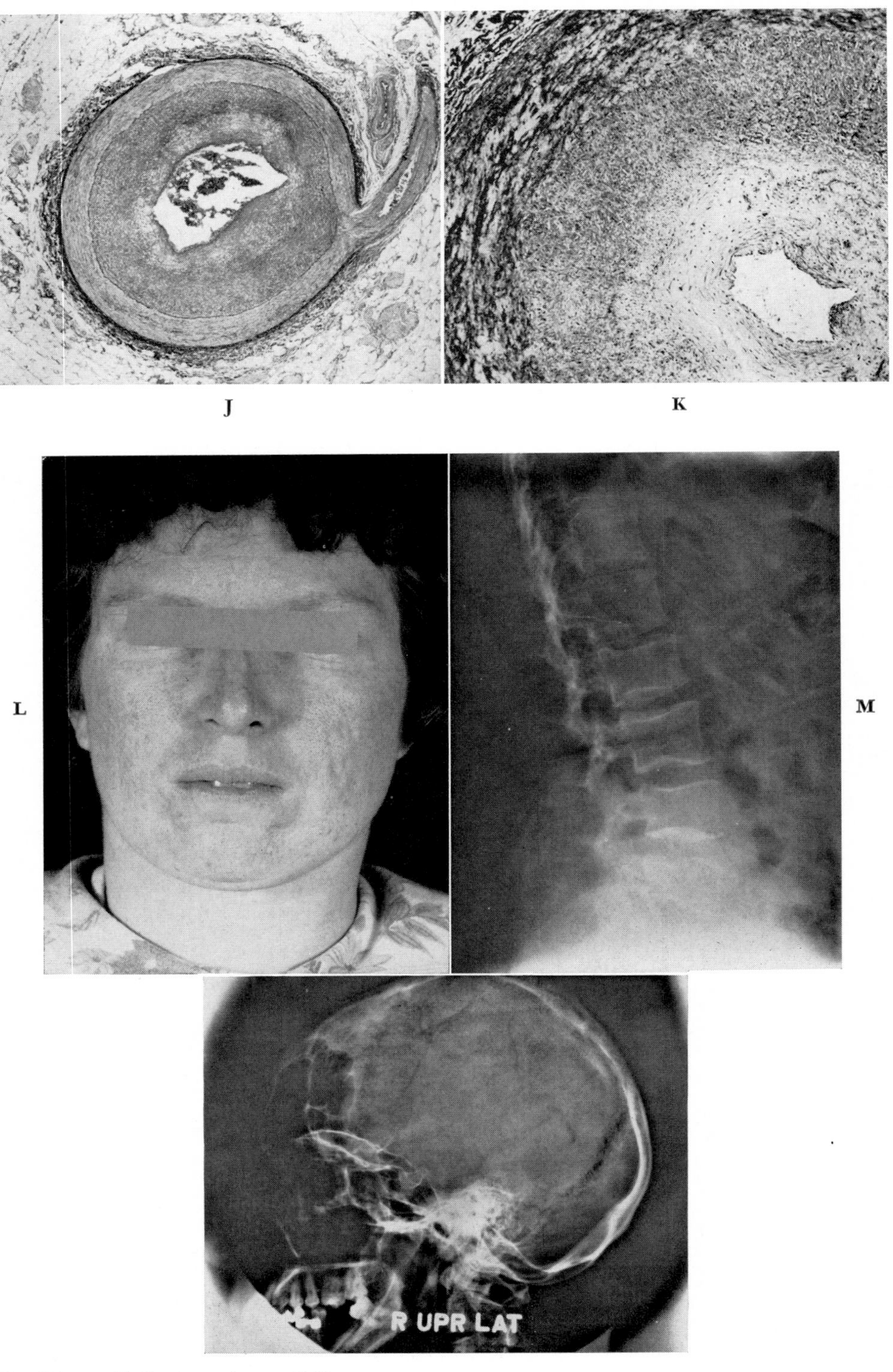

Fig. 4-4, cont'd. For legend see p. 161.

elastosis of the left atrium. The right kidney weighed 150 grams and the left kidney, 230 grams. Hypertrophy of the left ventricle suggested rather long-standing hypertension.

Comment. The hypertension is adequately accounted for by the smallness of the right kidney.

Case 2. E. Ho. (J.H.H. 1037640), the 20-year-old sister of D. Ho. (Case 1), was examined after her brother's death. She was a nervous, emotionally unstable girl. She described breathlessness and "jabby" sensations around the left breast about the time of menstruation and said she felt tired all the time. She had suffered three fractures. Her academic record in school was poor, but she completed high school at 19 years 9 months of age. Bilateral lens extraction was performed at age 17 years. Her blood pressure was 120/70 mm. Hg. She was 65½ inches tall with upper segment–lower segment ratio of 1.01. Except for bilateral surgical aphakia and tachycardia no abnormality was detected on physical examination. On a later examination, the patient complained of an ache below the left breast which occurred intermittently with either rest or exercise. The heart rate was 100 per minute. Third and fourth heart sound gallops were easily heard at the apex. A short musical early diastolic murmur was audible in the third left interspace close to the sternum.

An electrocardiogram showed changes interpreted as left ventricular hypertrophy and an old posterior myocardial infarction.

Six months after the first examination the patient suddenly developed chest pain and was dead on arrival at the hospital.

Autopsy (Medical examiner). All major coronary arteries showed moderately severe atherosclerosis. Old scarring was present in the anterior part of the interventricular septum and the anterior wall of the left ventricle. Close histologic study of the coronary arteries showed the same type of change as was seen in Case 1.

Comment. If the patient had the same type of change in the left atrial endocardium as did her brother, the mitral opening snap may be no surprise. The origin of the presumed early diastolic murmur in Erb's area is not clear.

Case 3. J. Ho. (J.H.H. 1037641), the only surviving affected sib of Cases 1 and 2, was born in 1940. In 1961 she had hematemesis for which investigations uncovered no satisfactory explanation. She had always stuttered somewhat, but this became more pronounced after her hematemesis. Because of backache, intravenous pyelography was performed in 1956 and 1958, with demonstration of a bifid collecting system on the left. She also complained of ache in the left arm, unrelated to exertion. Weakness in the left leg and pain in both legs were likewise noted.

Examination in 1962 showed height of 64 inches with upper segment–lower segment ratio of 0.94. The lenses had been removed. All deep tendon reflexes were hyperactive, especially in the left leg, where ankle clonus and Babinski's sign were demonstrated.

Because of increasing nervousness and peculiar behavior, psychiatric care was required, with apparent improvement. Pain in the region of the left breast has been a frequent complaint. A fracture of the left wrist occurred with adequate trauma and healed satisfactorily. On another occasion, fracture of the coccyx resulted from slipping on the ice. Bilateral partial detachment of the retina was detected in 1964.

Her left leg becomes cyanotic if she crosses her legs for any length of time, and it becomes stiff if she is nervous or walks a long distance. Occasionally she has numbness without tingling, beginning in the fingers of the left hand and slowly progressing to involve her face. The episodes last about ten minutes. Difficulty in picking up small objects with the left hand has been noted.

Blood pressure, normal during the early part of the period of observation, was about 155/100 in both arms on recent examinations. Furthermore, pulses are weak in the left carotid, radial, femoral, dorsalis pedis, and posterior tibial arteries. A faint early or mid-diastolic murmur is audible at the apex. The left leg is weak and she walks with a limp. The toenails are smaller on the left foot than on the right, and the left thumbnail is somewhat smaller than the right one. Hypalgesia of the entire left side is inconsistently present.

Laboratory evaluation showed normal hematologic studies, fasting and postprandial glucose, serum cholesterol, total serum lipids, serum electrolytes, liver function studies, urinalysis, protein-bound iodine, serum proteins, and electrocardiogram. The electroencephalogram (EEG) was abnormal, demonstrating diffuse disorganization without localization or lateralization. There were no seizure potentials. Intermittent photic stimulation did not cause activation. Hyper-

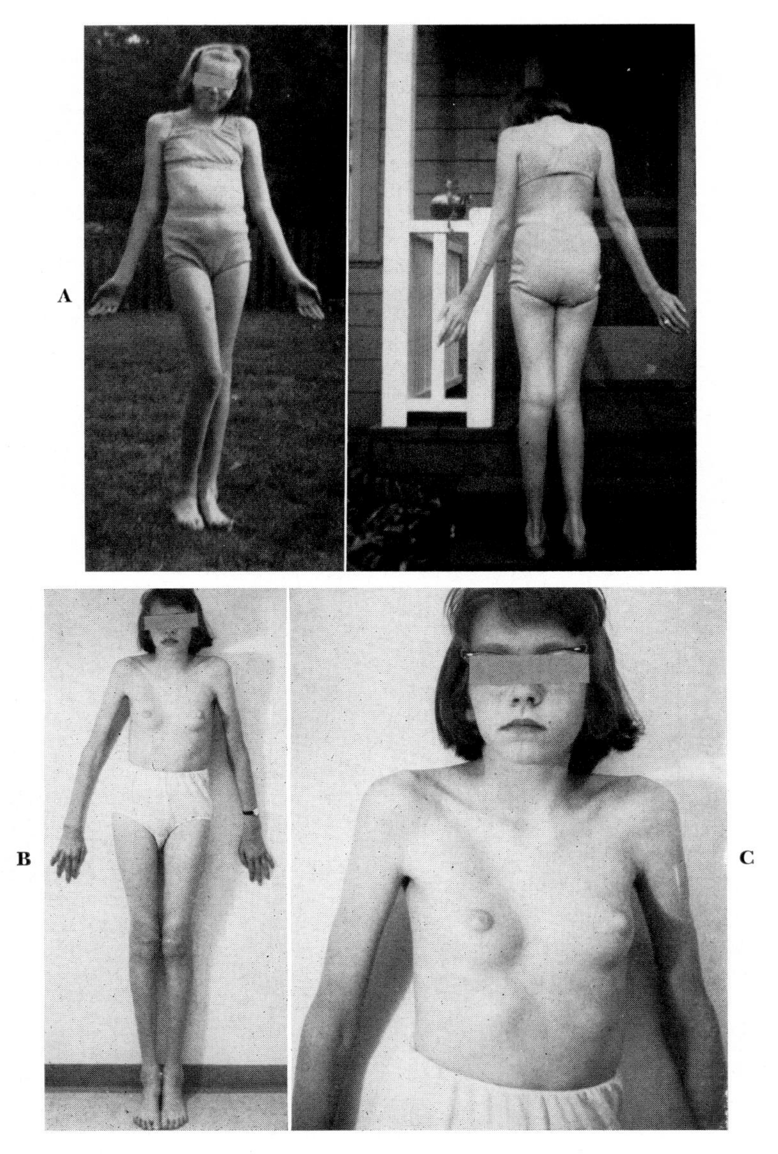

Fig. 4-5. Homocystinuria simulating the Marfan syndrome in J. Har. (Case 4, p. 166). **A,** Marfan-like skeletal features at age 9¾ years. **B,** Same at age 11½ years. Height 68½ inches. **C,** Pectus excavatum. **D,** Hands showing contracture of the fifth fingers, which become irregularly white on forced extension. **E,** Long narrow feet. **F** and **G,** X-ray films at age 7 years. Dilatation of the pulmonary artery and reduced anteroposterior dimension are demonstrated.

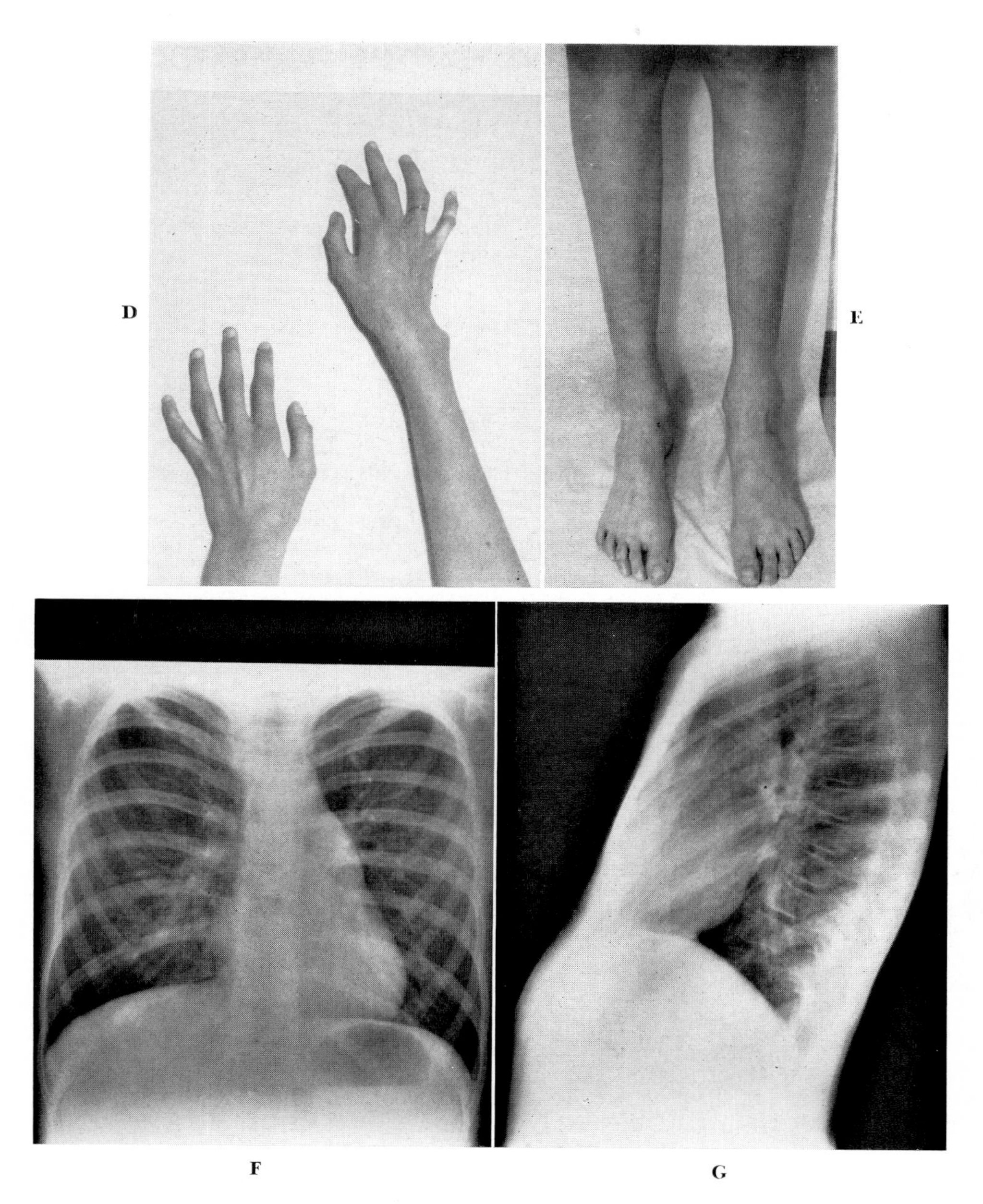

Fig. 4-5, cont'd. For legend see opposite page.

ventilation gave rise to only a minimal increase in slowing but no abnormal discharges. The EEG pattern was essentially unchanged two hours after a methionine load.

Coagulation studies were performed both before and 90 minutes after an oral methionine load. They showed clotting times of 11.13 and 9.12 minutes (glass) and were essentially unchanged in silicone. Prothrombin time was 25 and 23 seconds and bleeding time was 2½ and 4½ minutes, before and after methionine. Platelets were 250,000 and 183,000 per cubic millimeter, and partial thromboplastin time was 75 and 85 seconds. Fibrinogen was 210 mg.% and did not change. Euglobulin clot lysis time was normal both before and after methionine. None of these values or changes therein were significant. Platelet adhesiveness was considered to be within normal limits. Platelet survival was also normal.*

Chest x-ray results were normal except for some scoliosis of the thoracic spine. Skeletal x-ray films demonstrated generalized osteoporosis with early "cod-fish" changes in the lumbar vertebrae. There was rarefaction of the skull bones, and the frontal and ethmoidal sinuses were unusually large.

Family 2

Cases 4 and 5. J. Har. (Case 4), a white female born in November, 1953, first came to specific medical attention in 1959 because of a heart murmur. Chest x-ray films in 1960 showed dilatation of the pulmonary artery (Fig. 4-5*F* and *G*). At that time the diagnosis of Marfan's syndrome was suggested because of striking skeletal features (Fig. 4-5*A*). Right heart catheterization, performed without complication in 1964, showed normal pressures and no evidence of intracardiac shunt.

The patient has worn glasses for high-grade myopia since 1960. Repeated eye examinations in 1965 after the diagnosis of homocystinuria was established showed minimal but definite dislocation of the lenses.

Spinal curvature has developed in recent years. Loose-jointedness has never been conspicuous. The fifth fingers of both hands cannot be fully extended.

The parents have observed her "high coloration" and a tendency to become unusually flushed with exertion in hot weather. The hair and complexion are appreciably lighter than those of both parents and the surviving unaffected sib. Orthodontal correction of malaligned front teeth was necessary in recent years. Despite numerous traumata, she has sustained no fracture. Menarche occurred at age 11.

The patient is definitely retarded in her learning ability. Coordination of brain and body seem poor. She has never learned, for example, to use scissors. She learns by rote reasonably well, and through patient instruction she has learned to read and spell well. In school, "social studies" and arithmetic are more difficult for her.

Examination in 1965 showed mild upper malar flush. At 11 years 6 months of age she was 69½ inches tall with a US/LS ratio of 0.72. The palate was abnormally high. The hands and feet were cold, but the pulses were normal. The hands had a "tight feel"—probable reduced joint mobility; both fifth fingers were mildly incurved and could not be fully extended. Pectus excavatum was striking, and considerable scoliosis was present.

The parents are not related, and the ancestry of both originated in the British Isles. The mother had had three pregnancies: (1) A male, born in 1950, died in 1953. He had "cerebral palsy" and never learned to walk, although he could sit. At birth a large omphalocele requiring surgical repair was present. Autopsy showed "fatty metamorphosis of the liver." It is suspected that he had homocystinuria (Case 5 of this series) and that intracranial thromboses were responsible for the cerebral palsy. (2) A female, born in 1952, is normal in every respect. (3) The proband was born in 1953.

Family 3

Case 6. C. S., a white male farmer born in 1921, was reasonably well, except for ectopia lentis, until early 1965. The left lens was extracted in 1945 with complications leading to residual corneal opacification. Right inguinal herniorrhaphy was performed in 1947. The right lens was extracted in 1952. About 1959 he suffered from rightsided "sciatica." Manipulations

*Determination, courtesy Dr. N. Raphael Shulman, National Institutes of Health, Bethesda, Md.

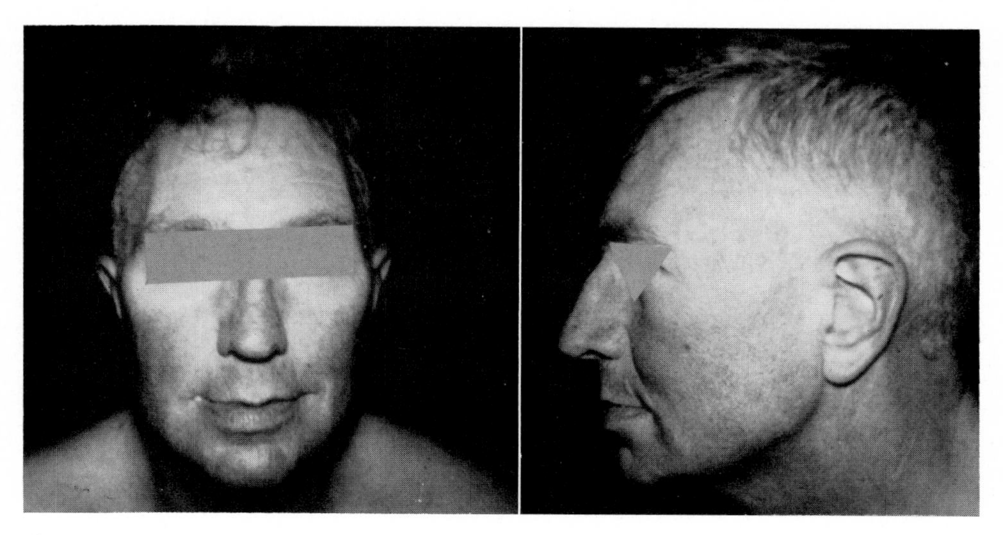

Fig. 4-6. Telangiectatic facial flush in C. S. (Case 6, p. 166).

by a chiropractor afforded relief. About 1963 he was refused insurance because of albuminuria and hypertension.

In January, 1965, the patient developed weakness and palpitations without pain and was thought to have had a heart attack. The electrocardiogram showed atrial fibrillation, probable old myocardial infarction, and unifocal ventricular premature contractures.

Examination in 1965 showed intense violaceous flushing of the face and most of the body. The trunk and proximal portions of the extremities showed livedo reticularis, and with brief dependency the feet became purple. The nose, lips, buccal mucosa, and hands showed deep purple cyanosis.

The height was 73½ inches with a US/LS value of 0.98. The chest showed a combination of pectus excavatum and carinatum, and mild scoliosis was present. A grade III/IV systolic ejection murmur was heard over the precordium. Blood pressure was 220/110 mm. Hg (sitting) in the right arm and 190/100 in the left arm. The liver was enlarged, 2 to 3 finger-breadths below the right costal margin. Intelligence seemed to be normal. Hemoglobin was 17.7 gm.%; hematocrit, 51 vol.%; red blood cell count, 4.9 million.

The parents were not known to be related. However, both came from the Dalarne region of Sweden. The proband was an only child.

Family 4

Case 7. J. Je. (1153704), a white male truck driver born in 1925, had had hypertension since at least age 18, when it was first discovered during a Selective Service examination. An ocular defect was also discovered at that time. The left lens was extracted in 1956. In 1957 acute glaucoma developed in the right eye and because of a delay in medical attention total loss of vision in that eye resulted. He was otherwise asymptomatic, however, until 1959 when he developed pneumonia necessitating hospitalization. Shortly thereafter, apparently related to the death of his brother, W. Je., (Case 8), J. Je. suffered a "nervous breakdown." He recovered without specific psychiatric therapy. During a hospitalization during the same period, an abnormal substance, presumably homocystine, was revealed in the urine by paper chromatography but was not identified. About 1963 he suffered a brief episode of blindness and weakness while driving. This cleared spontaneously and did not recur. He was told in 1959 that pulses were absent in the left leg, but no symptoms were attributable thereto. He had been aware of tachycardia for at least twenty years. He did heavy work as a furniture truck driver and denied claudication and impotence.

In February of 1965 he injured his remaining (left) eye on a car mirror, producing retinal detachment for which surgery was performed.

The parents were healthy and were not related. The ancestry was English and Irish. Of seven sibs, the patient and brother W. Je. (Case 8) have homocystinuria. The other five sibs are apparently healthy.

Examination in 1965 showed a well-developed, alert, cooperative man of normal intelligence. The face showed malar flush with coarse large-pored skin. The skeletal findings were in no way remarkable. The heart showed persistent tachycardia and grade II (out of 6) systolic ejection murmur at the left sternal border. Blood pressure was 180/110 in both arms, standing and recumbent. A large varicocele was present on the left. Both femoral pulses were decreased, the left being almost absent. A loud bruit was heard over the right femoral triangle and a softer one on the left. The left foot was cooler than the right. The neurologic findings were within normal limits.

Case 8. W. Je., the brother of J. Je. (Case 7), had bilateral ectopia lentis and long-standing hypertension. He died at age 28 following surgery for infarction of the bowel. For several months he had been markedly nervous with recurring attacks of abdominal pain and backache. At operation the arterial supply to the bowel seemed adequate, whereas extensive venous thrombosis was present. Autopsy showed thrombosis of the portal vein, thrombosis in the terminal aorta, occlusion of the left iliac artery, and multiple small infarctions of the myocardium and kidneys.

Family 5

Cases 9 and 10. L. Br., a white male born in 1941, and his sister, K. Br., born in 1943, were first examined in 1954 when they sought treatment for ectopia lentis. At that time the Marfan syndrome was diagnosed. The skeletal features were more suggestive in the brother than in the sister (Fig. 4-7*A* and *B*).

L. Br. developed weakness in the left leg in 1951 and a diagnosis of poliomyelitis was rendered. Function returned to normal in the following few years. In 1957 he sustained a fracture of the right tibia and fibula, which required open reduction with application of a plate. A few weeks later admission to hospital was required because of the development of acute respiratory symptoms. X-ray studies showed "segmental type pneumonia" with pleural effusion on the right. (Pulmonary embolism seems likely.)

Ectopia lentis was first noted at age 6 years and glasses were worn from that age, but no surgery has been performed. Despite school absences necessitated by the neurologic episode in 1951 and the fracture and its complications in 1957, the patient graduated from a state teachers college in 1965 and plans to teach at the high school level. He was active in intramural athletics. He has always been of nervous inclination.

Examination in 1965 showed a height of 72 inches and a US/LS value of 0.84. The feet and hands were long. He wore a size 12D shoe. He had high color of the cheeks and coarse wide-pored facial skin. Pectus excavatum was present. Deep tendon reflexes were hyperactive but symmetric. The intelligence quotient (IQ) was estimated to be between 105 and 110. Platelets were normal in number, morphology, and adhesiveness.

K. Br. was noted to have ectopia lentis at age 3 years. At age 11, the right lens was removed. The lenses were described as somewhat globular and dislocated downward and nasally. She did poorly in school and at the age of 21 had not yet succeeded in completing requirements for graduation from high school. Menarche occurred at age 11.

Examination in 1965 showed a height of 65 inches with a US/LS value of 0.88. As indicated by the measurements and by the photographs (Fig. 4-7*C*), her body habitus was much less suggestive of the Marfan syndrome than the brother's. The patient "toed out" and the feet were flat and everted. An ejection pulmonary systolic murmur was present when the patient was recumbent. The intelligence quotient was estimated to be about 80.

The parents are not related. The father and mother are 68 and 66 inches tall, respectively. The father is of Dutch extraction, and the mother German. A third child, a female born in 1947, is normal.

Family 6

Case 11. D. Ap. (1153651), a white male born in 1940, had normal birth and development and finished two years of college, being forced to stop because of failing vision. In 1961 and 1963 lenses were extracted without complication. At age 17 years he developed recurrent thrombo-

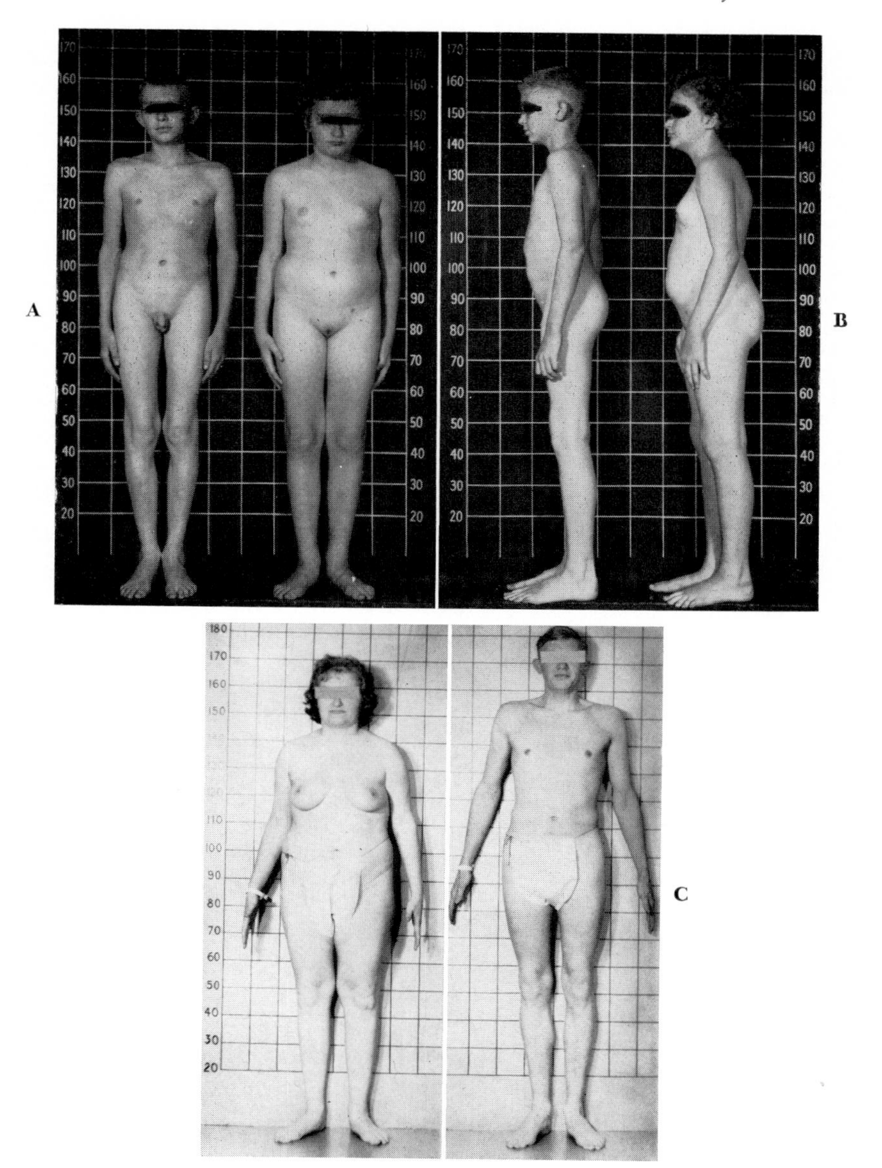

Fig. 4-7. Homocystinuria in brother and sister (Cases 9 and 10, p. 168). **A** and **B,** L. Br. (left), age 13½ years; K. Br. (right), age 10¾ years. Long everted feet and mild scoliosis and pectus excavatum are demonstrated. **C,** K. Br., age 22 years (left), and L. Br., age 25 years (right).

phlebitis and varicosities in the left leg. Traumatic fracture of the right femur has been sustained. He has his own insurance business.

The parents, of English-Irish-German extraction, are well and are not known to be related. Of their seven children, three (Cases 11, 12, and 13) have homocystinuria.

Examination showed normal blood pressure, prominent malar flush with coarse, wide-pored skin of the face, fine blond hair, and moderately high palate. The height was 71 inches and US/LS about 1.0. The left leg showed stasis dermatitis and venous varicosities. The left foot was red-blue on dependency with thick nails. All pulses were adequate and no arterial bruits were heard. Intelligence is apparently normal and he has a pleasing personality.

X-ray films showed calcification of the left femoral artery (and/or vein), over an extended segment, and generalized osteoporosis.

Case 12. Mrs. J. A. McC. (1153679), a sister of D. Ap. (Case 11), born in 1942, quit school in grade 11 presumably because of visual difficulties. Upper canine teeth were removed because of crowding. She is married and has one child, age 4 years.

Examination in 1965 showed normal blood pressure, height 68 inches, US/LS about 1.0, thin blond hair, high color of the cheeks, bilateral dislocation of the lenses with iridodonesis, and high arched palate. She is probably mildly retarded, and by x-ray examination she is shown to have generalized osteoporosis.

Case 13. C. Ap., born in 1946, a brother of the last two patients, has ectopia lentis. Although he has not thus far been examined by us, he has been found to have homocystinuria. He is thought to be of normal intelligence.

Family 7

Case 14. T. Bu., a female born July 15, 1957, sat at 6 months and walked at 14 months, although she was noted to be clumsy, She first wore glasses at 3 years 6 months of age, when her parents were told she had dislocated lenses. During the following three years progressive downward dislocation of the lenses took place. She was always a "slow learner" and was placed in a special school. In November, 1963, she developed acute glaucoma in the left eye. Surgery was not done. In February, 1964, acute glaucoma occurred in the right eye. Following needling, the lens fell back into position.

Examination in 1965 showed a cooperative child with short attention span. The IQ was estimated to be below 70. Malar flush was striking and livedo reticularis mild. The eyes showed obvious iridodonesis, displaced lenses, and high-grade myopia. Lumbar lordosis was exaggerated, with protuberant abdomen and mild scoliosis. Genu valgum was noted. The hair is blonder than that of any other member of the family.

The parents are well and are not known to be related. Both are of Irish extraction. One sib of the proband, 5 years old, is normal.

Family 8

Case 15. M. Ba., a female born in May, 1953, was ascertained through a urine screening of patients with ectopia lentis. Birth weight was 7 pounds 8 ounces, and except for vomiting in the neonatal period no abnormality was noted early in life. She was always irritable, and in hot weather her face became beet-red. She was noted to have myopic astigmatism from the age of about 4 years. Although she was seen by several compenent ophthalmologists, ectopia lentis was not detected until 1964, suggesting that the dislocation may have been progressive. Several teeth were removed because of crowding.

Examination in 1965 showed crowded teeth, venous flush of the face when recumbent, dry skin, and thick nails. The lenses were dislocated downward bilaterally. She walked with exaggerated lumbar lordosis attributable to spondylolisthesis demonstrated by x-ray study. Her height was 54 inches with US/LS ratio of 0.76. IQ was estimated to be less than 70.

X-ray films showed generalized demineralization of the lumbar vertebrae with some flattening of the vertebral bodies. Calcification was visualized in the lateral occipital ligaments. Spina bifida occulta and spondylolisthesis were present in the lumbar spine. The electroencephalogram was considered abnormal because of an unusual amount of slow activity and bioccipital slowing and sharp wave activity more on the left side.

The parents are not known to be related. Both are of Russian-Jewish extraction. Both are well. The mother and maternal grandfather have von Recklinghausen's neurofibromatosis. The mother is only 59 inches tall, and the father 65 inches tall. A brother of the proband is unusually intelligent at age 16 years.

Family 9

Case 16. S. Bo. (1152914), a white male born Aug. 1, 1954, was noted to have "flickering of the iris" when as a baby he would sit on his mother's lap. Furthermore he held his picture books close to his eyes. Because of ectopia lentis in this patient's paternal uncle, his parents were alert to the possibility of ectopia lentis. Glasses were worn from the age of 5 years. The diagnosis of Marfan syndrome was made soon thereafter.

The boy has been a " slow learner." He repeated the first grade and at age 10 entered the fourth grade of a special class. He is hyperkinetic, strongly motivated to learn, enjoys reading, learns well by rote, and does well in spelling but poorly in "social studies," apparently because of difficulties in reasoning.

The parents are well. Both are of German extraction. Three sibs, two older brothers and a younger sister, are well.

Examination revealed bilateral ectopia lentis with iridodonesis, malaligned teeth undergoing orthodontic correction, a late systolic murmur introduced by a click, and mild pectus excavatum. Genu valgum and mild livedo reticularis and malar flush were noted. The IQ was estimated as less than 70.

Case 17. F. Bo., the paternal uncle of S. Bo. (Case 16), had bilateral ectopia lentis and had lens extraction. Always sickly and retarded in mental development he died in 1927 at the age of 9, of scarlet fever. The diagnosis of homocystinuria is considered quite certain.

Family 10

Case 18. A. Wz. (1155861), born July 30, 1959, was first seen by me in March, 1961, when the diagnosis of Marfan syndrome had been made because of the finding of ectopia lentis, high arched palate, and long hands and feet. Physical and intellectual development had been retarded. He did not yet walk or sit unaided. Prominent veins over the forehead and anterior upper chest were noted. Height was 33¾ inches and the head, which seemed relatively large, measured 20¼ inches. The hair was blond and the eyes blue. Muscular hypotonia was striking. On x-ray study the thoracolumbar spine was considered normal at age 1 year 6 months.

The child began to walk when about 3 years of age. Mental retardation was evident throughout. Dislocation of the lenses may have progressed. In May, 1965, examination revealed an unusually tall boy, measuring 52½ inches, with long, narrow feet and hands, narrow high-arched palate, and crowded front teeth. Iridodonesis, dilated veins over the chest, pulmonary systolic ejection murmur when recumbent, and lumbar kyphos in sitting were also noted. The hands, specifically the fingers, had a "tight feel."

The parents are not related and are apparently healthy. The mother has severe myopia. They are of old American stock—English, French, and Irish. A younger female sib of the proband is healthy. A maternal first cousin of the proband, age 24, is institutionalized for a psychiatric disorder and a brother of this first cousin, age 19, is mentally retarded, requiring attendance at a special school. A maternal second cousin of the proband, age 22, is also mentally retarded and attends a "farm school." A first cousin of the proband's mother, age 43 years, is mentally retarded. On the paternal side, a cousin has had detached retina from an early age. In several of these relatives, screening tests show no homocystine in the urine.

Family 11

Case 19. R. Hd. (994522), a white male born in 1956, crawled at 7 months, walked at 17 months, and talked at 2 years 6 months. He always seemed backward mentally. The mother noted dislocation of his left lens at age 5. Both lenses were extracted in 1961. At 3 or 4 months of age he had left-sided seizures. At age 7 six teeth were extracted to relieve crowding. On several occasions the mother was told he had a heart murmur. He does very poorly in school.

Examination in 1965 showed a slender, blond-haired, obviously retarded boy. The skin was pale and unusually transparent but showed no flushing or livedo reticularis. The front teeth were prominent. Other findings included pigeon breast, systolic ejection pulmonary murmur, and genu valgum.

The parents, of English and Irish extraction, were healthy and were not related. This boy and D. Hd. (Case 20) were the only children.

Case 20. D. Hd. (1154438), the brother of R. Hd., born in 1957, developed pneumonia at age 11 months and shortly thereafter began to have seizures and left-sided paresis. Seizures were reasonably well controlled with phenobarbital and by 19 months he was walking. At age 4 he developed severe seizures with a period of coma and right-sided paresis. About the same time, aseptic necrosis of the right femoral head, necessitating traction for fourteen months, was discovered. Bilateral lens extractions were performed at age 5. By age 6 he was able to play actively with little evident incapacity. At age 7 he again had pneumonia with uneventful recovery. About four months later his right leg became blue and swollen. Following, about three weeks later, was the same phenomenon in the left leg. He also had prolapse of the rectum, and the physician told the mother he had a "clot in the bowels." The veins of the anterior abdominal wall became prominent. In March, 1965, he developed fever leading to coma. The right arm became blue and swollen.

Examination in April, 1965, showed an emaciated, obtunded boy who responded only to painful stimuli. The only satisfactory pulse was the left radial. Others were absent or only very weakly palpable. The front teeth were protruding, with malocclusion and high palate. The hair was blond and the skin transparent. Prominent venous collaterals on the anterior surface of the trunk filled from below, becoming particularly prominent when he cried. All four extremities were cold. Deep tendon reflexes were essentially unobtainable.

Both brothers showed generalized osteoporosis of moderately severe degree. The skull had a granular or finely reticular appearance.

Family 12

Case 21. J. Gil., born in 1950, had breath-holding attacks as an infant. Physical and mental development was at all stages retarded. Bilateral ectopia lentis was detected at an early age.

Examination at age 15 showed a boy who looked old for his age. The eyes were sunken. He was nervous and apprehensive and, obviously, severely retarded. The face and trunk developed a venous flush when he was supine. The skin of the face was coarse and large pored. The

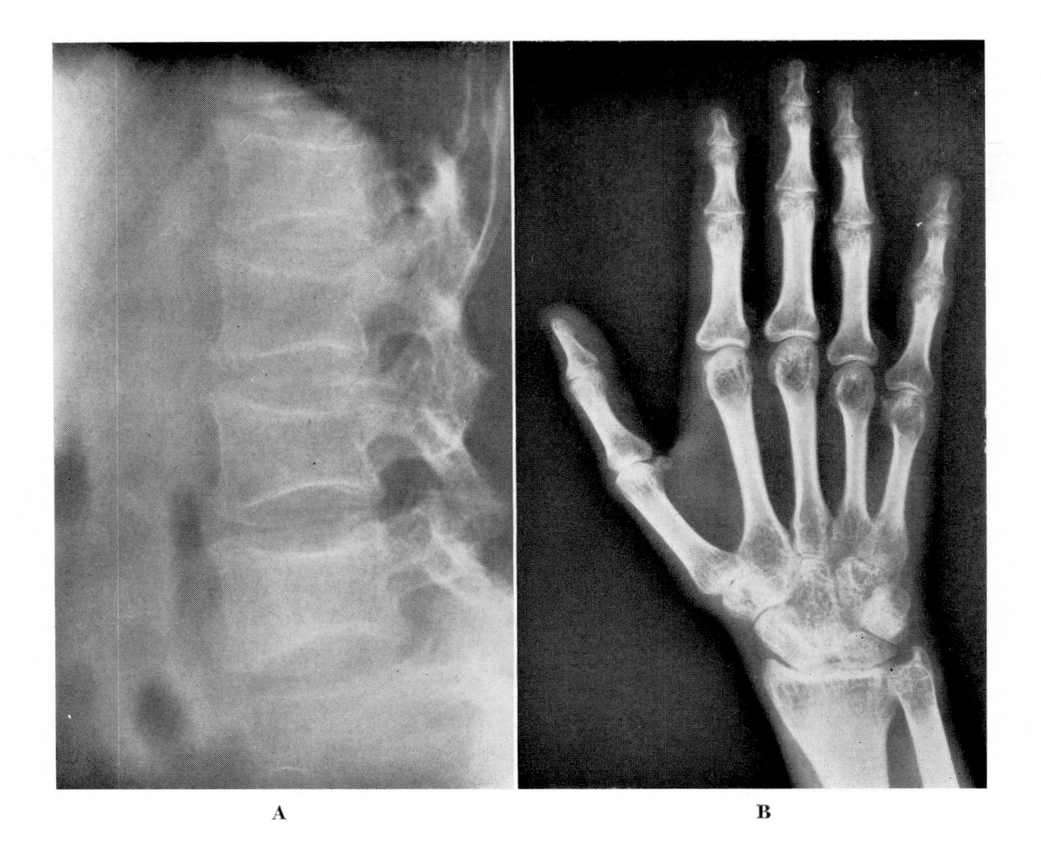

A B

Fig. 4-8. Severe osteoporosis of spine, **A**, and hand, **B**, in 22-year-old homocystinuric (Case 22, p. 173).

blood pressure was 160/80 mm. Hg and labile. Tachycardia and an ejection pulmonary systolic murmur in recumbency were present. The liver was not enlarged. Pectus carinatum was present. An unusually wide space separated the first and second toes. The foot showed a striking pes cavus deformity. (Fracture had been sustained in the right foot.) Varicose veins were present. The liver was not enlarged. There were no localizing neurologic signs.

Case 22. S. Gil., a sister of J. Gil (Case 21), born in 1943, had breath-holding attacks in infancy. She also is severely retarded, although somewhat less so than her brother, and is nervous and apprehensive. Examination in 1965 showed crowded teeth, dilated venules over the legs, especially the ankles, a flaring of the lower ribs but no sternal deformity, and pulmonary ejection systolic murmur in the recumbent position. There were no localizing neurologic signs.

Marked osteoporosis of the spine, skull, and hands was demonstrated radiologically in both sibs. The electrocardiogram was normal in both.

Both parents, of Irish extraction, are well and are not known to be related. The sibship of the above patients contains two other children, who are normal, a boy 19 years of age and a girl 14 years.

Family 13

Case 23. J. Te. (764615), a white female office worker born July 28, 1920, has suffered all her life from eye abnormalities consisting of myopia, ectopia lentis, and retinal detachment; she had a well-documented anteroseptal myocardial infarction at age 31 years. During hospitalization for this, intermittent arterial spasm in the left foot was noted. At age 42 the patient was hospitalized for arterial occlusion in the right arm. Despite these handicaps she attended college for three years and has worked as a civilian employee for a defense agency of the government since May, 1942. Palpitations due to extrasystoles (present since age 18) and intermittent angina pectoris have been the main nonocular symptoms.

Examination in 1965 showed an alert, intelligent, emotionally stable woman with excellent recall. Habitus is dumpy, with fat hips and a height of 66 inches. The skeletal features are not remarkable. The heart is moderately enlarged, with auscultatory and electrocardiographic signs of right bundle branch block.

The patronymic was derived from a French ancestor who settled in New Haarlem in 1652. The mother came from a well-known family, of Irish origin, which settled in Maryland before 1700. The parents were not related. A brother (Case 24) is thought to have died of the complications of homocystinuria at age 18 years. Another brother died at a few weeks of age, presumably of meningitis.

Case 24. C. Te., the brother of J. Te. (Case 23), had "bad eyes" and was 76 inches tall. At age 18 he was seized with severe chest pain while doing farm chores and died one week later following recurrence of the pain. He had graduated from high school a few months previously. Death was certified as due to "coronary occlusion due to vascular spasm."

Family 14

Case 25. M. St., a white male born Sept. 10, 1947, is 73½ inches tall and in the tenth grade of school. He may be normally intelligent but "has had many emotional problems all his life." His school standing suggests retardation. He has bilateral ectopia lentis. The left lens was needled in 1961. Glaucoma on the right occurred in 1964 and a cataractous dislocated lens was extracted. At age 15, spontaneous pneumothorax occurred. He had suffered from bronchial asthma for several years. The left testis was removed following trauma.

The parents of this patient, of Jewish extraction, were not known to be related. Both are now dead, the father having died in an airplane accident and the mother died of breast cancer. The only sib is Case 26.

Case 26. N. St., a white female, died in September, 1964, at age 11 years 9 months, while a patient in the Neurologic Institute at Columbia. She had had bilateral ectopia lentis, the right lens being dislocated up and out and the left lens nasally displaced. The left lens was needled in 1960; a cataractous right lens was extracted in 1962. At the time of the terminal admission in 1964, recurrent leg fractures, gigantism, and decreased strength in the left arm were noted. Since childhood, she had had difficulty in walking. A limp "favoring" the left leg was attributed to previous fractures. The child had complained of numbness in the left hand, for six to eight weeks, with difficulty in use of the left hand for one week. Left central facial weakness and weakness of the left arm and leg were present. In the last twelve days of life, she developed hypertension (blood pressure 210/130 mm. Hg) and evidence of thrombosis in the carotid arteries, lower aorta, common iliacs, femoral and subclavian arteries. A brachial arteriogram for demonstration of the aortic arch and cranial vessels showed "essentially complete obstuction of the right internal carotid artery near its origin." Left carotid arteriogram showed the left internal carotid artery to be very small through its entire course. The electroencephalogram was strikingly abnormal.

Family 15

Case 27. I. MacD., a white male born in 1920, had a history of visual difficulties from the age of about 20 years. Subluxated lenses were detected in 1945. In 1964 the right lens was found to be dislocated infranasally and the left lens, nasally. The fundi were normal. The left lens was extracted in 1964. At that time blood pressure, electrocardiogram, and chest x-ray films were normal.

This man got a B.S. degree in chemistry before World War II and a B.S. in chemical technology after World War II. He now works as a food technologist. During that war he served as captain in an airborne division in France. In 1942 he fractured a tibia in a jump. Shortly after an automobile accident in 1944 he noted swelling behind the knees, and possible inferior vena caval thrombosis was subsequently diagnosed. Venous stripping was performed bilaterally in 1954. The patient, who is 74 inches tall and wears a 12B shoe, is of Scottish-English-Irish descent. Three male sibs are well. He has five children, all well.

Family 16

Case 28. S. Ham., a white male born Aug. 14, 1954, was slow in physical and mental development from the first. He did not walk until age 4. An eye problem was not noted until age 7, when acute glaucoma developed. Asthmatic attacks occurred on several occasions. Beginning in 1963 he has had multiple "spells" consisting of stiffening of the left side without loss of consciousness. He appears to be intolerant to sun, developing facial swelling on exposure but no blisters or red urine.

Physical examination in 1965 showed a hyperactive boy with dull expressionless face. The teeth were carious and crowded. Corneal edema suggested chronic glaucoma. Other features were pectus carinatum, genu valgum, height of 57 inches, long narrow toes, and everted feet with thick calluses on the inner aspect of both insteps.

The proband is the youngest of twelve children of a Jewish father and Irish mother. The ages of the other children range from 32 to 12. Four of them are married, with children. None has homocystinuria, by screening test, and none has symptoms suggesting this disorder.

Family 17

Case 29. J. Mat., a white female born March 14, 1943, was found to have ectopia lentis in 1949, at which time the left lens was extracted. The right lens was needled in 1955. In 1959 she was admitted to hospital because of thrombophlebitis in the right leg. In May, 1960, thrombophlebitis in the left leg, probably secondary to trauma and accompanied by pulmonary embolus, again prompted hospitalization. In November, 1960, superficial thrombophlebitis occurred in the left leg. Her IQ was estimated to be 74. (She eventually completed the tenth grade.) Psychiatric consultation was sought because of a possible schizophrenia, but no evidence to support that diagnosis was found. In June, 1962, another pulmonary embolus occurred and inferior vena caval ligation was performed. In December, 1962, the patient was complaining of "pins and needles" in the feet. No pulses were felt in either leg below the popliteals. Arteriograms showed complete occlusion of the right superficial femoral artery with a "rippled appearance of fibromuscular hyperplasia" in patent portions of the arterial tree. Multiple areas of narrowing and dilation were present bilaterally, more on the right side than the left.

In 1965 at the age of 22 years the patient showed blood pressure of 160/110 (both arms); height, 69 inches; obesity; prognathism; faint malar flush; high palate; chronic ulcer of right heel; edema of both legs; livedo reticularis of arms, with cool hands.

Case 30. M. Mat., a female born Oct. 7, 1947, died Oct. 1, 1960, of massive venous thromboses and pulmonary emboli. She had had recurrent convulsions. Autopsy* showed height 70

*Courtesy Dr. Joseph Spellman, Chief Medical Examiner, City of Philadelphia.

inches and weight 189 pounds. The arms were long and tapering, with long thin tapering fingers. The legs were thick and stocky. Superficial veins formed a prominent network over the anterior thorax centrally and over the left hip anteriorly. Thrombi were palpable in the superficial saphenous veins. The inferior vena cava and both iliac and both femoral veins contained organizing thrombi. No changes in the vein wall were described. Old and recent pulmonary emboli and a large thrombus in the main pulmonary artery were also found. The heart showed "interstitial collagenosis," the muscle fibers being separated by wide collagenous areas. Parenchymal cells of the liver (which weighed 2,760 grams) showed large lipid vacuoles; fatty liver, type undetermined, was diagnosed.

Family 18

Case 31. P. Tu., a white female born March 25, 1921, has bilateral ectopia lentis and skeletal features suggesting the Marfan syndrome. Congestive heart failure and renal insufficiency have been problems in the last few years. Blood pressure is normal. She has had asthma since childhood. Adrenocortical steroid given for asthma probably aggravated congestive heart failure. She is 67 inches tall and weighs 125 pounds. Intelligence is apparently normal. The patient enjoys opera and good books. She completed high school. She is of high-strung and dominating temperament, in the view of her brothers.

The parents were of English stock and were not related. One unaffected sib was born Sept. 16, 1929. No sibs are dead.

Case 32. C. Tu., a white male born in June, 1934, has bilateral ectopia lentis and skeletal features suggesting the Marfan syndrome. He completed high school. He has a "ruddy complexion" and dry skin. He is considered the "black sheep" of the family and is an alcoholic and a sociopsychopath. He completed high school and is considered to have normal intelligence.

Case 33. W. Tu., a white male born April 14, 1922, has bilateral ectopia lentis and skeletal features suggesting the Marfan syndrome. He is 69 inches tall and weighs 160 pounds. Both lenses have been removed. The right eye is sightless as a result of detached retina. He has a "ruddy complexion" that has often been commented on by friends. Dry skin with abundant flaking has been present most of his life. He has had no fractures. He graduated from college and is a kitchen employee of a Veterans Administration hospital.

Family 19

Case 34. D. How., a white male born Feb. 15, 1949, has bilateral ectopia lentis. At age 16 he is 75 inches tall and weighs 211 pounds. Because of mental retardation he attends a special school and is in the third grade. The patronym is the same as that of Family 1. It has been impossible to establish a connection between Families 1 and 19; on the other hand, a connection has not been disproved, but if present must be remote.

Case 35. De. How., sister of Case 34, born Sept. 9, 1955, is 57 inches tall and weighs 100 pounds. She has ectopia lentis and is mentally retarded.

Family 20

Case 36. J. S. (160377), born Aug. 24, 1920, is of Jewish extraction. The parents are first cousins. Ectopia lentis was first detected in 1928. Bilateral lens extraction was performed in 1939, prompted by acute secondary glaucoma in the right eye. Both lenses had been dislocated, first nasally and later downward. Severe myopia was also present. When seen in 1955 she displayed on the right exotropia, scarring of the cornea, and phthisis of the globe. The left eye was normal.

The patient was recognized to be slow in mental development from the beginning. In 1929 she was diagnosed as having encephalitis. The family impressed physicians as highly neurotic, and in addition to mental retardation there seemed to be a psychiatric problem.

In 1938 "slight athetosis" and a "systolic cardiac blow" were described. Asymmetry of the face with flattening of the right labial folds suggested seventh nerve abnormality.

Case 37. P. S. (Sinai 55812, 13540), born in 1916, was admitted in 1930 for repair of right inguinal hernia and hydrocele. He was noted to have high-grade myopia with "cloudy lenses," ane "extremely" long extremities leading to a diagnosis of gigantism. Because of malocclusion, the mouth was usually half open. The chest showed marked xiphisternal despression. Seventeen days after operation he developed tachycardia, fever, and severe headaches followed by Jacksonian seizures and showed a positive Babinski bilaterally, with inequality of the pupils. The spinal fluid was negative. He died twenty-two days after operation. The final diagnosis was encephalitis. Autopsy was not performed. Extensive intracranial thrombosis is likely.

Case 38. A. S. (Sinai 7320-3) was born Feb. 7, 1932, and died Nov. 10, 1947. Harelip was present at birth. She walked at 2 years 6 months but had poor coordination. All her education was done at home. She learned very little reading and could not write well. In 1947 a few weeks before death she showed positive Babinski's signs bilaterally, chorioathetosis, and a short pulmonary systolic murmur. In 1938 she had sustained fractures of the humerus and of the neck of the right femur. At that time she had an expressionless facies, was uncooperative, and uttered only a few indistinct words. Four weeks before the terminal admission abdominal pain, vomiting, pallor, and polyuria developed. Jaundice also appeared. Multiple skeletal deformities, particularly scoliosis and pectus excavatum, were present. The blood urea nitrogen was found to be 280 mg.%. Autopsy was not performed.

Intra-abdominal arterial and/or venous thromboses seem likely.

SUMMARY

Homocystinuria is an inborn error of metabolism simulating the Marfan syndrome in many respects. Ectopia lentis, disruption of the arterial media, and skeletal changes are connective tissue disorders secondary to the metabolic defect. The precise mechanisms of the connective tissue changes are not known. Table 5 summarizes the differences between the Marfan syndrome and homocystinuria.

Table 5. Comparison of homocystinuria with the Marfan syndrome

	Homocystinuria	*Marfan syndrome*
Inheritance	Recessive	Dominant
Skeletal abnormality	Osteoporosis, fractures, occasional arachnodactyly	Arachnodactyly and loose-jointedness more striking
Pectus excavatum or carinatum	Frequent	Frequent
Ectopia lentis	Present	Present
Vascular disease	Dilatation with thrombosis in medium-sized arteries and veins	Dilatation and/or dissection of aorta
Skin	Malar flush, livedo reticularis	Striae distensae
Mental retardation	Frequent	Absent

REFERENCES

1. Arnott, E. J., and Greaves, D. P.: Ocular involvement in homocystinuria, Brit. J. Ophthal. **48**:688, 1964.
2. Brenton, D. P., Cusworth, D. C., and Gaull, C. E.: Homocystinuria. Biochemical studies of tissues, Pediatrics **35**:50, 1965.
3. Carson, N. A. J., Cusworth, D. C., Dent, C. E., Field, C. M. B., Neill, D. W., and Westall, R. D.: Homocystinuria: a new inborn error of metabolism associated with mental deficiency, Arch. Dis. Child. **39**:425, 1963.
4. Carson, N. A. J., Dent, C. E., Field, C. M. B., and Gaull, C. E.: Homocystinuria: clinical and pathological review of ten cases, J. Pediat. **66**:565, 1965.
5. Carson, N. A. J., and Neill, D. W.: Metabolic abnormalities detected in a survey of mentally backward individuals in northern Ireland, Arch. Dis. Child. **37**:505, 1962.
6. Chou, S.-M., and Waisman, H. A.: Spongy degeneration of the central nervous system. Case of homocystinuria, Arch. Path. **79**:357, 1965.
7. Daisley, K. W.: Synthesis of glutathione by normal and x-irradiated lens, Biochem. J. **60**:x1, 1955.
8. Dardenne, V., and Kirsten, G.: Presence and metabolism of amino acids in young and old lenses, Exp. Eye Res. **1**:415, 1962.

9. Deasy, C.: Evidence for the existence of homocystine (or homocysteine) in steerhide corium and in kangaroo tail tendon, J. Amer. Leather Chem. Ass. **59**:691, 1964.
10. Dexter, M. W., Lawton, A. H., and Warren, L. O.: Marfan's syndrome with aortic thrombosis, Arch. Intern. Med. **99**:485, 1957.
11. Finkelstein, J. D., Mudd, S. H., Irreverre, F., and Laster, L.: Homocystinuria due to cystathionine synthetase deficiency: the mode of inheritance, Science **146**:785, 1964.
12. Gerritsen, T., Vaughn, J. G., and Waisman, H. A.: The identification of homocystine in the urine, Biochem. Biophys. Res. Commun. **9**:493, 1962.
13. Gerritsen, T., and Waisman, H. A.: Homocystinuria: absence of cystathionine in the brain, Science **145**:588, 1964.
14. Gerritsen, T., and Waisman, H. A.: Homocystinuria, an error in the metabolism of methionine, Pediatrics **33**:413, 1964.
15. Gibson, J. B., Carson, N. A. J., and Neill, D. W.: Pathologic findings in homocystinuria, J. Clin. Path. **17**:427, 1964.
16. Glynn, M. F., Movat, H. Z., Murphy, E. A., and Mustard, J. F.: Study of platelet adhesiveness and aggregation, with latex particles, J. Lab. Clin. Med. **65**:179, 1965.
17. Greenberg, D. M., and Nagabhushanam, A.: Isolation and properties of a homogeneous preparation of cystathionine synthetase-serine and threonine dehydratase, 1964, Proceeding 6th International Congress of Biochemistry, Moscow, (abstract 461) p. 310.
18. Hall, W. K., Coryell, M. E., Hollowell, J. G., Jr., and Thevaos, T. G.: A metabolic study of homocystinuria (abstract), Fed. Proc. **24**:470, 1965.
19. Hope, D. B.: Cystathionine accumulation in brains of pyridoxine-deficient rats, J. Neurochem. **11**:327, 1964.
20. Kinsey, V. E., and Merriam, F. C.: Studies on the crystalline lens. II. Synthesis of glutathione in the normal and cataractous lens, Arch. Ophthal. **44**:370, 1950.
21. Klavins, J. V.: Pathology of amino acid excess. I. Effects of administration of excessive amounts of sulphur containing amino acids: homocystinuria, Brit. J. Exp. Path. **44**:507, 1963.
22. Komrower, G. M., and Wilson, V. K.: Homocystinuria, Proc. Roy, Soc. Med. **56**:996, 1964.
23. Laster, L. (Bethesda, Md.): Personal communication.
24. Lieberman, T. W., Podos, S. M., and Hartstein, J.: Acute glaucoma, ectopia lentis, and homocystinuria. In press.
25. Loughridge, L. W.: Renal abnormalities in the Marfan syndrome, Quart. J. Med. **28**:531, 1959.
26. Lynas, M. A.: Marfan's syndrome in northern Ireland; an account of thirteen families, Ann. Hum. Genet. **22**:289, 1958.
27. McDonald, L., Bray, C., Field, C., Love, F., and Davies, B.: Homocystinuria, thrombosis and the blood platelets, Lancet **1**:745, 1964.
28. Meister, A.: Methionine and cysteine. In Biochemistry of the amino acids, vol. 2, ed. 2, New York, 1965, Academic Press, Inc., pp. 757-818.
29. Mudd, S. H. (Bethesda, Md.): Personal communication.
30. Mudd, S. H., Finkelstein, J. D., Irreverre, F., and Laster, L.: Homocystinuria: an enzymatic defect, Science **143**:1443, 1964.
31. Mudd, S. H., Finkelstein, J. D., Irreverre, F., and Laster, L.: Threonine dehydratase activity in humans lacking cystathionine synthase, Biochem. Biophys. Res. Commun. 1965.
32. Pirie, A., and van Heyningen, R.: Biochemistry of the eye, Springfield, Ill., 1956, Charles C Thomas, Publisher, pp. 12-31, 19-22, 60-63.
33. Sauer, F. C.: Development of beta crystallin in the pig and prenatal weight of the lens, Growth **3**:381, 1939.
34. Schimke, R. N., McKusick, V. A., Huang, T., and Pollack, A. D.: Homocystinuria, a study of 38 cases in 20 families, J.A.M.A. **193**:711, 1965.
35. Schimke, R. N., McKusick, V. A., and Pollack, A. D.: Homocystinuria simulating Marfan's syndrome, Trans. Ass. Amer. Phys. **78**:60, 1965.
36. Selim, A. S. M., and Greenberg, D. M.: An enzyme that synthesizes cystathionine and deaminates L-serine, J. Biol. Chem. **234**:1474, 1959.
37. Soupart, P., Moore, S., and Bigwood, E. J.: Amino acid composition of human milk, J. Biol. Chem. **206**:699, 1954.
38. Spaeth, G. L., and Barber, G. W.: Homocystinuria: a new syndrome. Presented to Amer. Acad. Ophthal. Otolar., October, 1964.

39. Tallan, H. H., Moore, S., and Stein, W. H.: L-cystathionine in human brain, J. Biol. Chem. **230:**707, 1958.
40. Tristarn, G. R., and Smith, R. H.: The amino acid composition of some purified proteins, Advances Protein Chem. **18:**227, 1963.
41. White, H. H., Thompson, H. L., Rowland, L. P., Cowen, D., and Araki, S.: Homocystinuria, Trans. Amer. Neurol. Ass. **89:**24, 1964.
42. Wright, L. D.: An inborn error of metabolism associated with deficiency of enzyme cystathionine synthetase leading to homocystinuria, New York J. Med. **65:**559, 1965.
43. Zucker, M. B., and Borrelli, J.: Platelet clumping produced by connective tissue suspensions and by collagen, Proc. Soc. Exp. Biol. Med. **109:**779, 1962.
44. Zu Rhein, G. M., Eichman, P. L., and Puletti, F.: Familial idiocy with spongy degeneration of central nervous system of van Bogaert-Bertrand type, Neurology **10:**998, 1960.

5

The Ehlers-Danlos syndrome

Historical note

None of the hereditary disorders of connective tissue, except possibly osteogenesis imperfecta, has as ancient a history as does the Ehlers-Danlos syndrome. The first definitive case* of this syndrome seems to have been described in 1682[171] by Job van Meekeren, a surgeon of Amsterdam. In Fig. 5-1 is presented van Meekeren's illustration of the "extraordinary dilatability of the skin" in a 23-year-old Spaniard who could pull the right pectoral skin to the left ear, the skin under the chin up over the head like a beard, and the skin of the knee area out about one-half yard. On being released, the skin retracted promptly to fit snugly over the underlying structures. This phenomenon was limited to the skin of the right side of the body.

Various dermatologists, including Kopp[87] and Williams,[183] published scattered references to this condition, which was usually observed as a curiosity in "India rubber men" of side shows. Kopp's report in 1888 is particularly noteworthy, since he described the condition in father and son. Gould and Pyle[65] published the photograph made in Budapest in 1888 of an exhibitionist named Felix Wehrle, "who besides having the power to stretch his skin could readily bend his fingers backward and forward." Du Mesnil[45] in 1890, Williams[183] in 1892, working in Unna's laboratory in Hamburg, and Unna[170] himself in 1894 reported

*In *Airs, Waters and Places* Hippocrates,[99] in the fourth century B.C., described the Scythians as having markedly lax joints. "I will give you a strong proof of the humidity (laxity?) of their constitutions. You will find the greater part of the Scythians, and all the Nomades, with marks of the cautery on their shoulders, arms, wrists, breasts, hip-joints, and loins, and that for no other reason but the humidity and flabbiness of their constitution, for they can neither strain with their bows, nor launch the javelin from their shoulder owing to their humidity and atony: but when they are burnt, much of the humidity in their joints is dried up, and they become braced, better fed, and their joints get into a more suitable condition." Is it possible that the cigarette paper scars of the Ehlers-Danlos syndrome were misinterpreted? Against this suggestion is the fact that burning the skin around joints became an established treatment for dislocation of joints, in the ancient world. Another statement is of much interest: "... they afterwards became lame and stiff at the hip-joint, such of them, at least, as are severely attacked with it." (From Adams, F.: The Genuine Works of Hippocrates, New York, 1891, William Wood & Co.)

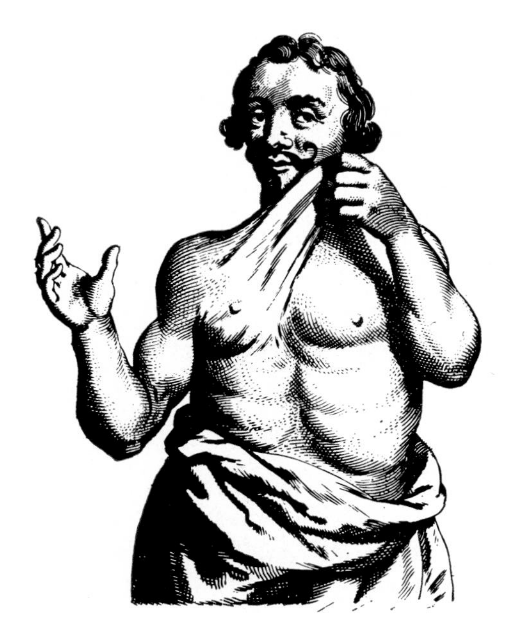

Fig. 5-1. Job van Meekeren's case of "extraordinary dilatability of the skin."

"In the year 1657, in the presence of the very distinguished John van Horne and Francis Sylvius, professors of medicine in the famous academy of Leyden, as well as of William Piso and Francis vander Schagen, practitioners of Amsterdam, we saw in our hospital a certain young Spaniard, 23 years of age, by the name of George Albes, who with his left hand grasped the skin over his humerus and right breast and stretched it till it was quite close to his mouth. With each hand he first pulled the skin of his chin downward like a beard to his chest, hence he lifted it upwards to the vertex of his head so as to cover each eye with it. As soon as he removed his hand the skin contracted to reassume its proper smoothness. In the same way he pulled the skin of his right knee upwards or downwards, to the length of half an ell; then it easily returned to its natural position. It was worthwhile noting that the skin which covered the forementioned parts on the left side could not be extended since it firmly adhered to them. It has, thus far, not been possible to learn the cause [of this anomaly?]."—Translated from original Latin by Dr. Owsei Temkin.

on histologic studies. In general, these authors were puzzled by the absence of more specific changes and encountered difficulties in the interpretation of what they did find. The contribution in 1901 by Ehlers[47] of Denmark[35] consisted of pointing out the associated loose-jointedness and the subcutaneous hemorrhages that are prone to occur. Danlos[34] in 1908 rounded out the clinical description with inclusion of the tumors that may develop at subcutaneous sites.

With considerable justification Jansen[74] argues that Tschernogobow[165,166] is most deserving of credit for the first detailed clinical description of this syndrome. In 1891 he presented to the Moscow Dermatologic and Venereologic Society two cases of the syndrome. He described the fragility as well as the hyperelasticity of the skin, the failure of the skin to hold sutures, the hypermobility and luxation of joints, and the molluscoid pseudotumors of the knees, elbows, and other areas. Most important, he tied all these features together as manifestations of a fundamental and generalized inadequacy of connective tissue; "Erschlaffung des Bindegewebes" were his words.

One of Tschernogobow's patients[165] was a 17-year-old epileptic male who, in falling frequently on his face, had left there and elsewhere broad fissures running in all directions. The skin of the knees, elbows, and wrists was unusually spongy and loose, suggesting elephantiasis mollis or fibroma molluscum. Joint changes were especially pronounced on the left side, where dislocations of the elbow and hip, dating from childhood, were present. In the second patient,[166] a 50-year-old woman, "tumors" were present not only on the elbows and knees but also on the buttocks, presumably in the vicinity of the ischial tuberosities. When one of these "tumors" was removed, it was discovered that sutures did not hold well and dehiscence of the wound occurred in a couple of days.

Many terms have been used for this syndrome or more often for its individual features. As in the case of the Marfan syndrome, the eponymic designation seems preferable, since it does not convey any connotations of the invariable occurrence of an individual manifestation or any ill-founded notion of the nature of the basic defect. "E-D" is the abbreviated label that will be used frequently in this presentation.

This survey of E-D is based on a personal study of over thirty kinships, each with at least one quite unequivocally affected person. Comparison of the findings with those reported in the literature is made.

Clinical manifestations[88,160]

The manifestations of the Ehlers-Danlos syndrome can conveniently be discussed under these headings: cutaneous, skeletal, ocular, and internal.

The skin.[7,19,85,133,142] Characteristically, the skin in E-D is velvety in appearance and feel. It may also resemble wet chamois in feel. In the infant, it may be impressively white. It is hyperextensible, yet not lax (Fig. 5-2*A*).

The term *cutis laxa* is inappropriate in the typical case in young persons. Except as noted below, the skin is truly hyperelastic.* Cutis laxa is a term properly reserved for a separate genetically determined entity.[37,135] (See p. 218.)

In addition, the skin is fragile and brittle. Minor trauma may produce gaping, fish-mouth wounds. One of my patients was for a time a professional boxer, a mutilating occupation for one with this disorder. Another, 16 years old at the

---

*There is so much confusion in the biologic literature with reference to the term *elasticity* that some care must be exercised. Burton writes as follows:

> Elasticity is properly defined as the property of materials which enables them to resist deformation by the development of a resisting force or "tension." All coefficients of elasticity are defined as the ratio of this resisting force (which at equilibrium is equal to the applied deforming force, or "load") to the measure of deformation produced. Thus, by the physical definition, a material of "high elasticity" resists deformation, e.g., stretching, by a large force; so that it takes a large force to produce a given deformation. A material of "low elasticity" cannot resist deformation so well, and it takes only a small force to produce the same degree of deformation. Thus glass or steel has a much higher elasticity than does rubber.
>
> Most unfortunately, popular usage of the adjective "elastic" connotes the opposite. If a material like rubber is easily stretched, it is is popularly said to be "elastic" and glass is "not so elastic" as rubber. (From Burton, A. C.: Physiol. Rev. **34**:619, 1954.)

As used in this discussion of E-D, *elasticity* refers to physical properties like those of rubber, specifically stretchability, and restoration after deformation.

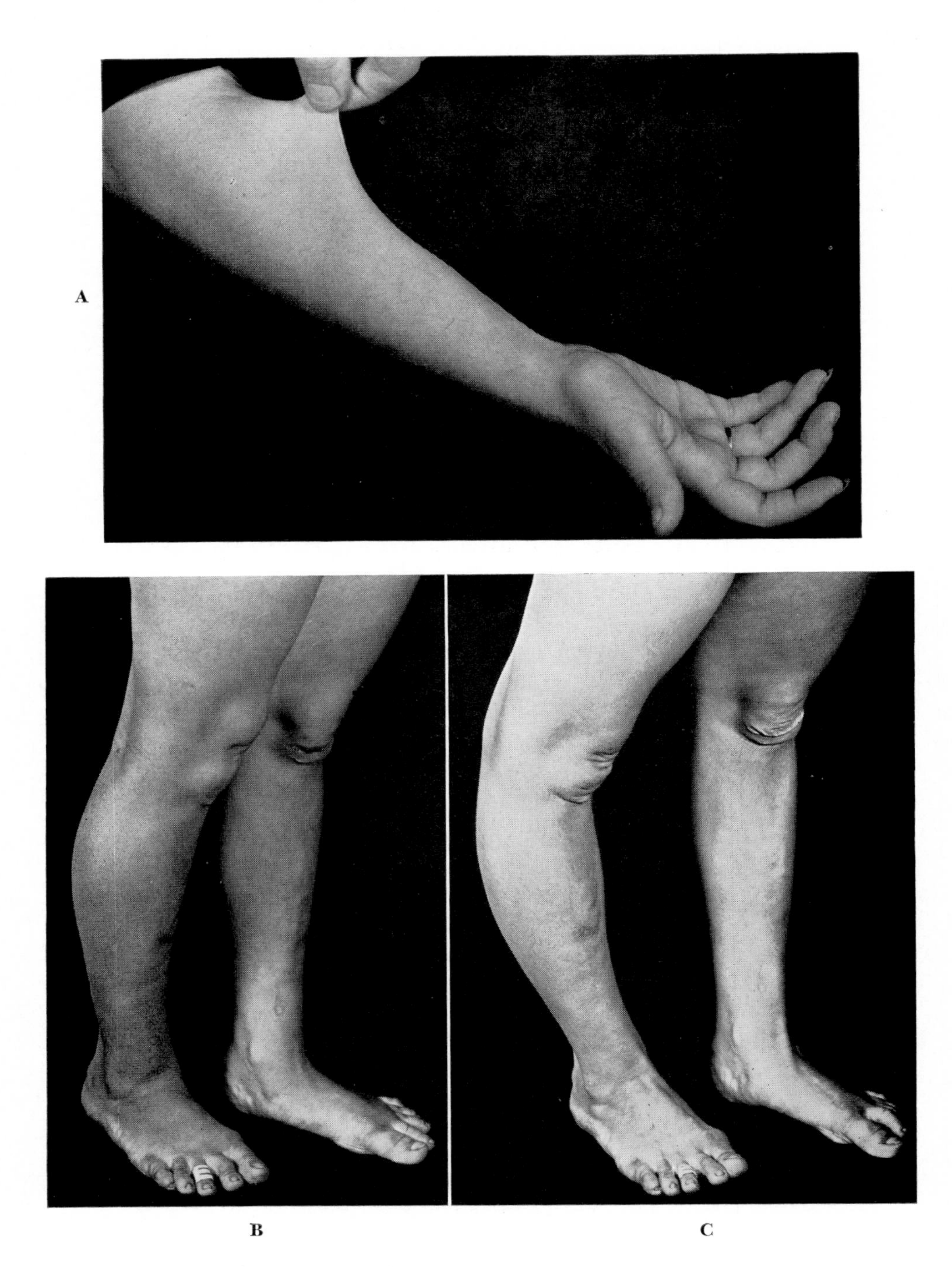

Fig. 5-2. Changes in skin and joints of 16-year-old girl, D. V. (A41965). **A,** Cutaneous hyperelasticity. **B,** Normal position of knees. Note papyraceous scars over the knees and flat feet. **C,** Genu recurvatum, more on the right. **D,** Hyperextensibility of fifth finger. **E,** Hyperextensibility of thumb. Note, in the left hand, the hyperextension of the index finger and the abnormal separation of the knuckles. **F,** Hyperextensibility of fingers. **G,** Unusual mobility of hip and knee joints.

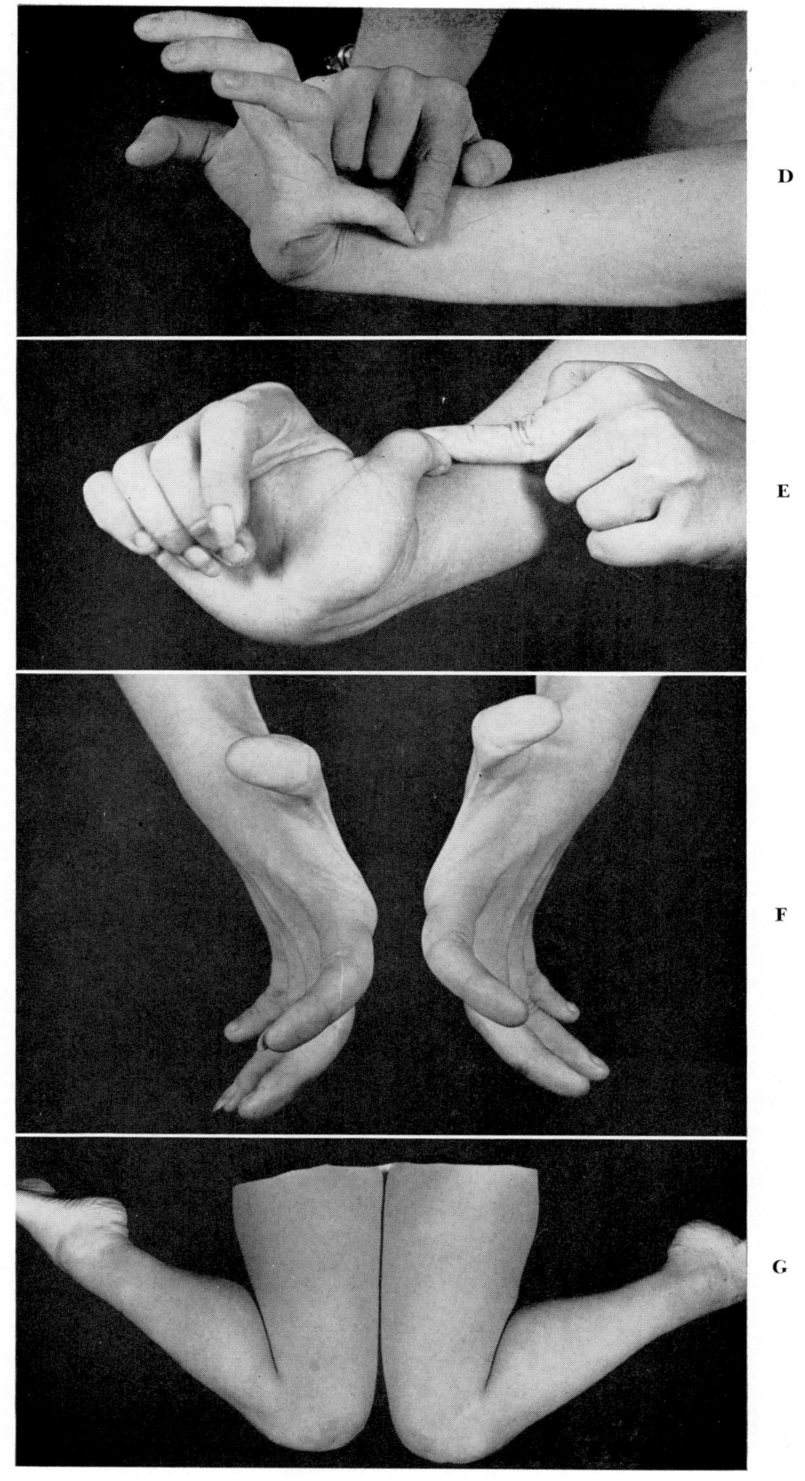

Fig. 5-2, cont'd. For legend see opposite page.

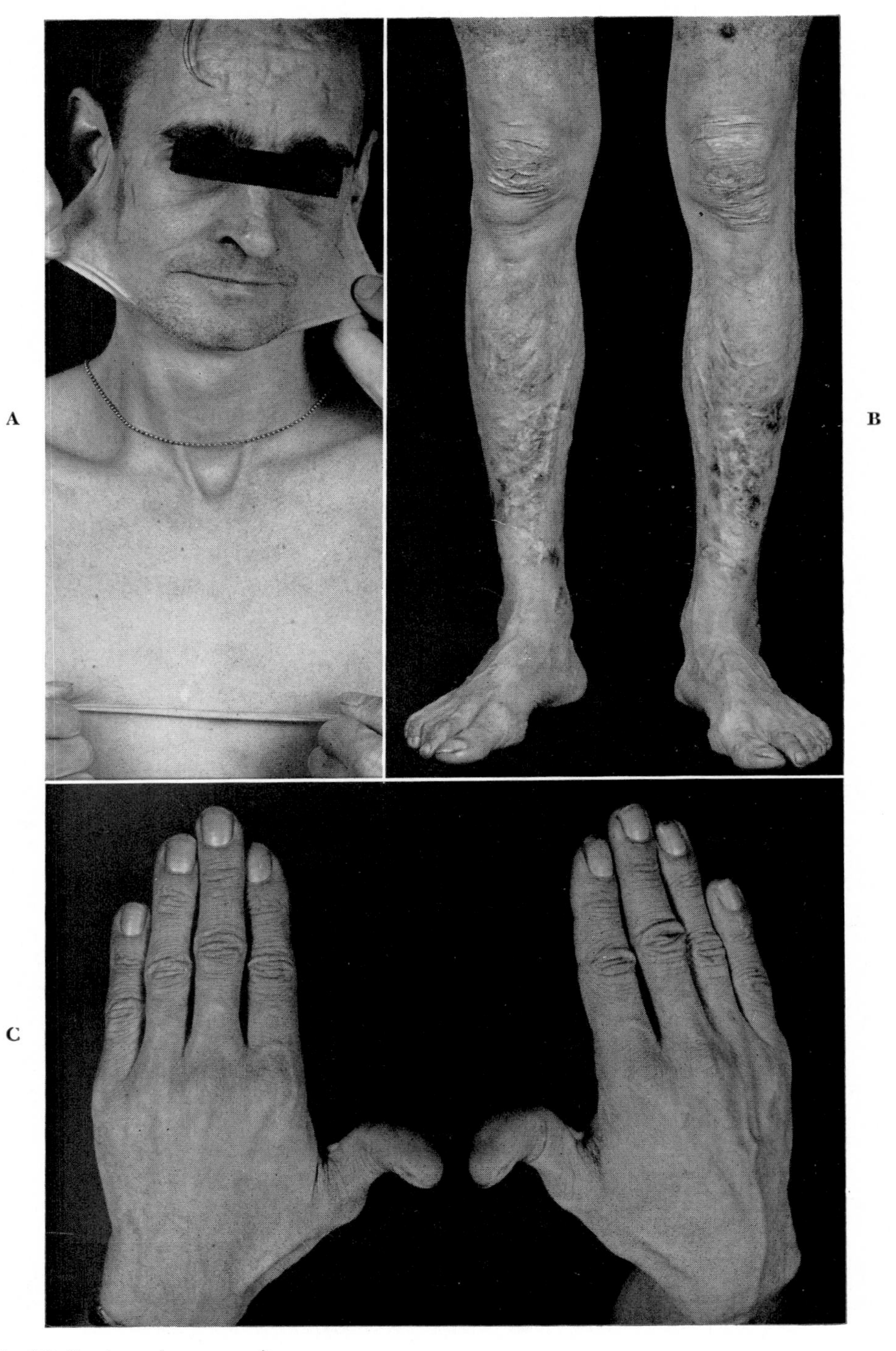

Fig. 5-3. For legend see opposite page.

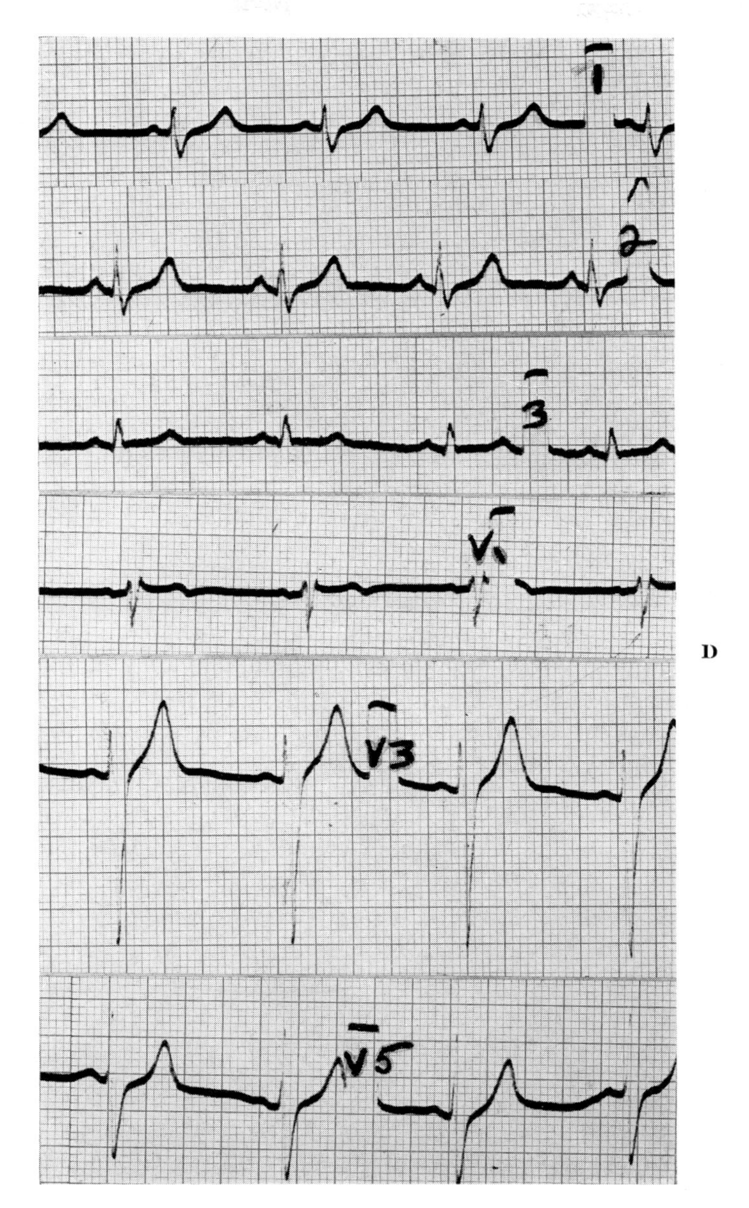

Fig. 5-3. Patient 35 years of age (a son has the E-D syndrome). **A,** Note scars of forehead and hyperextensibility of the skin. The patient was a professional boxer for a time. **B,** Note the spherical tumor in the skin of the anterior aspect of the left thigh. **C,** Ability to hyperextend the thumb occurs frequently as an isolated, inherited characteristic.[60,180] **D,** Incomplete right bundle branch block present since at least the age of 19 years and almost certainly all of life. No other cardiovascular or internal medical disorder was demonstrable.

time of study (Fig. 5-2), had had a total of 148 cutaneous stitches taken during her lifetime. Often stitches hold poorly in the skin,[80,140] and the patients and physicians resort to the use of adhesive tape. In the patient of Brown and Stock,[16] 282 stitches had been taken before count was stopped. Thomas and associates[161] described slow healing of a skin biopsy site and dehiscence of an ocular incision for removal of an ectopic lens. Packer and Blades[122] observed disruption of an appendectomy scar four times in thirty months. In one of my cases, a surgeon described the tissue at laparotomy as being like wet blotting paper. The tissues at autopsy are likely to be abnormally friable *(v. seq.)*.

Very little bleeding occurs from the skin wounds. On the other hand, easy bruisability is the rule and, together with other hemorrhagic phenomena, frequently leads these patients to consult hematologists. The subsequent organization and calcification of the hematomas at times result in one type of pseudotumor.

So-called molluscoid pseudotumors[124,129] develop at pressure points—heels, knees, elbows, etc. These were the basis for the misconceived term of Hallopeau and Mace de Lépinay[34,68]: "juvenile pseudodiabetic xanthomatosis." Another type of tumor, small to be sure, seen in these cases is the so-called spherule, which is usually pea-sized or smaller and slips about under the skin an inch or more without causing the patient any discomfort. These are small fat-containing cysts that may become calcareous.[175] They are most frequently the basis for subcutaneous calcifications that may be demonstrable radiologically,[11,70] another basis being calcified hematomas as noted above. Congenital lipomatosis has been described in association with Ehlers-Danlos syndrome by Tobias.[164] It is entirely possible, however, that the fatty tumors in his case were an integral part of the connective tissue disease. At times actual ossification occurs.[83] The subcutaneous calcifications are characteristically ovoid in shape and 2 to 8 mm. in largest dimensions. They occur principally on the legs and, to a lesser extent, on the arms. Radiologically they display a diffuse inner calcification with a more dense surrounding shell. They are not laminated like phleboliths. These characteristics, together with the facts that they are not in muscle (as are calcified parasitic cysts) and are too widely distributed to be phleboliths, should permit the radiologist to make the diagnosis of E-D.[91]

Easily recognized changes develop in the skin overlying the knees, shins, and elbows; it becomes shiny, parchment-thin, and hyperpigmented (Figs. 5-2*B* and 5-3*B*). Resulting are the so-called "cigarette paper" or "papyraceous" scars. Telangiectases sometimes develop in the region of these atrophic scars. The skin changes may suggest those produced by exposure to x-rays.

Bleeding may occur from the gums with brushing of the teeth, from tooth sockets after dental extractions, from the pharynx after tonsillectomy, and at the site of operations on the joints.[173] Petechiae in late pregnancy and prolonged postpartum hemorrhage have been described.[146] Gastrointestinal bleeding occurs in some patients.[72,146] Recurrent hemoptysis has been described.[136] Contrariwise, in one of my patients it is difficult to get blood for cell counts by finger puncture, and venipunctures are also difficult, seemingly because of very small and collapsed superficial veins. In another of my patients (Fig. 5-4), a strain of the tendons of the hamstring muscles at the knee resulted in the subcutaneous dissection of blood down to the ankle. E-D must be included in the differential diagnosis of

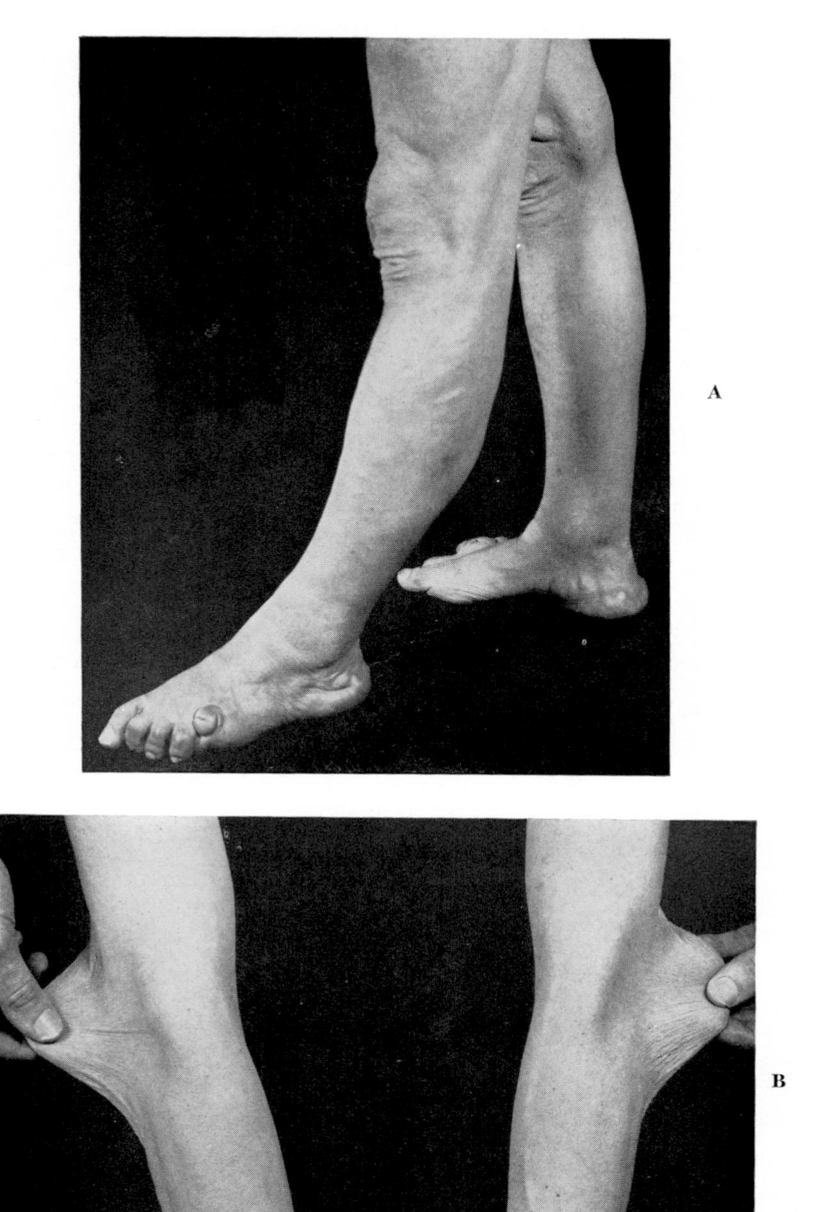

Fig. 5-4. K. W. (667280), 48-year-old man. **A,** Note deformity of feet, molluscoid tumors around heels (seen less distinctly in Fig. 5-2*B*). The soles appeared to be loose-fitting and like moccasins. There are cigarette paper scars over the knees. **B,** Dewlaps of both elbows.

Continued.

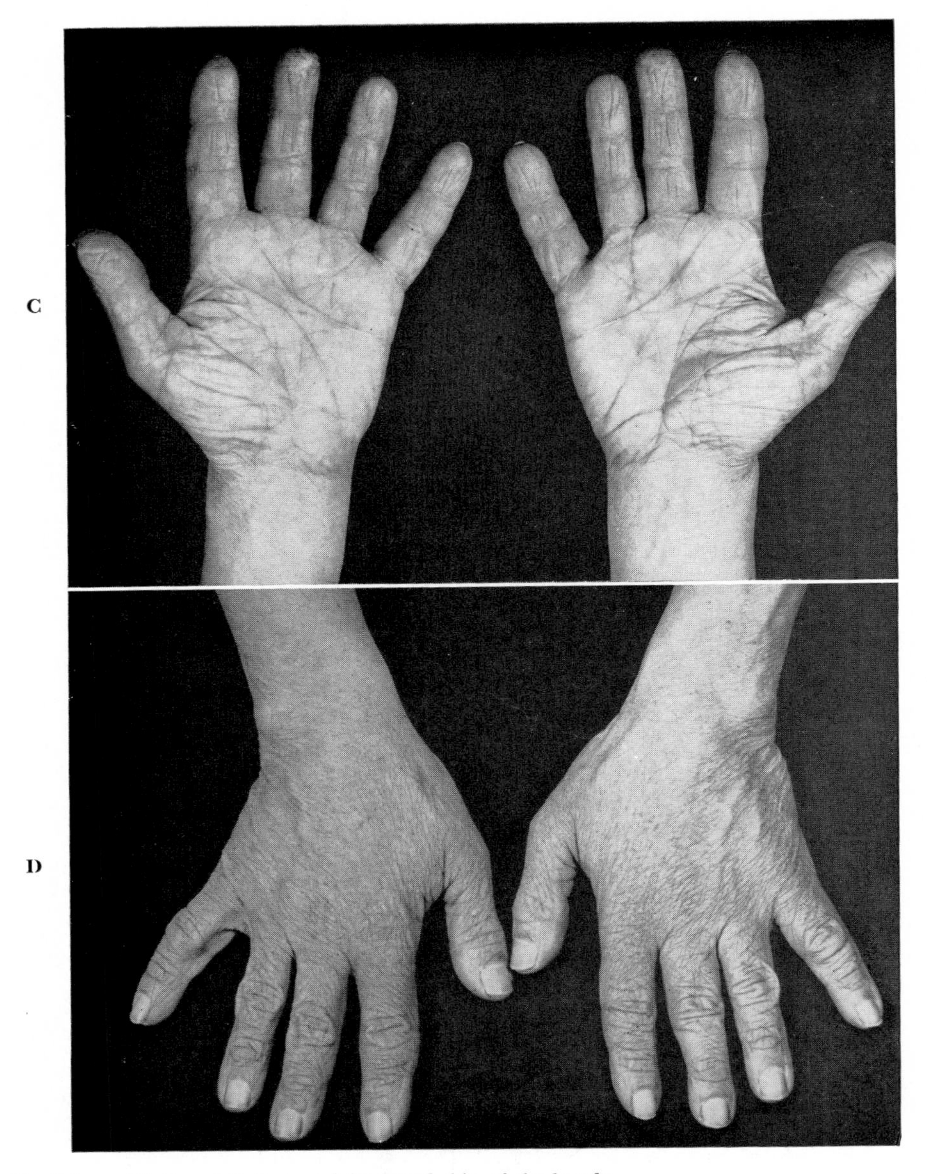

Fig. 5-4, cont'd. C and **D,** Lax and furrowed skin of the hands.

familial hemophilia-like state. All tests of coagulation are usually normal[17,72,158,167] except that the Rumpel-Leede test may be positive.[54,122,123,144,146,169] In a family with E-D transmitted through four generations, a mother and daughter studied by Lisker and associates[98] showed deficiency of plasma thromboplastin component (Christmas factor, factor IX). A deficiency of Hageman factor was described by Fantl.[50] Goodman and co-workers[61] found defective platelet thromboplastic function and clot retraction, as well as a vascular defect. On the other hand, Day and Zarafonetis[36] and Wigzell and Ogston,[182] like others referred to

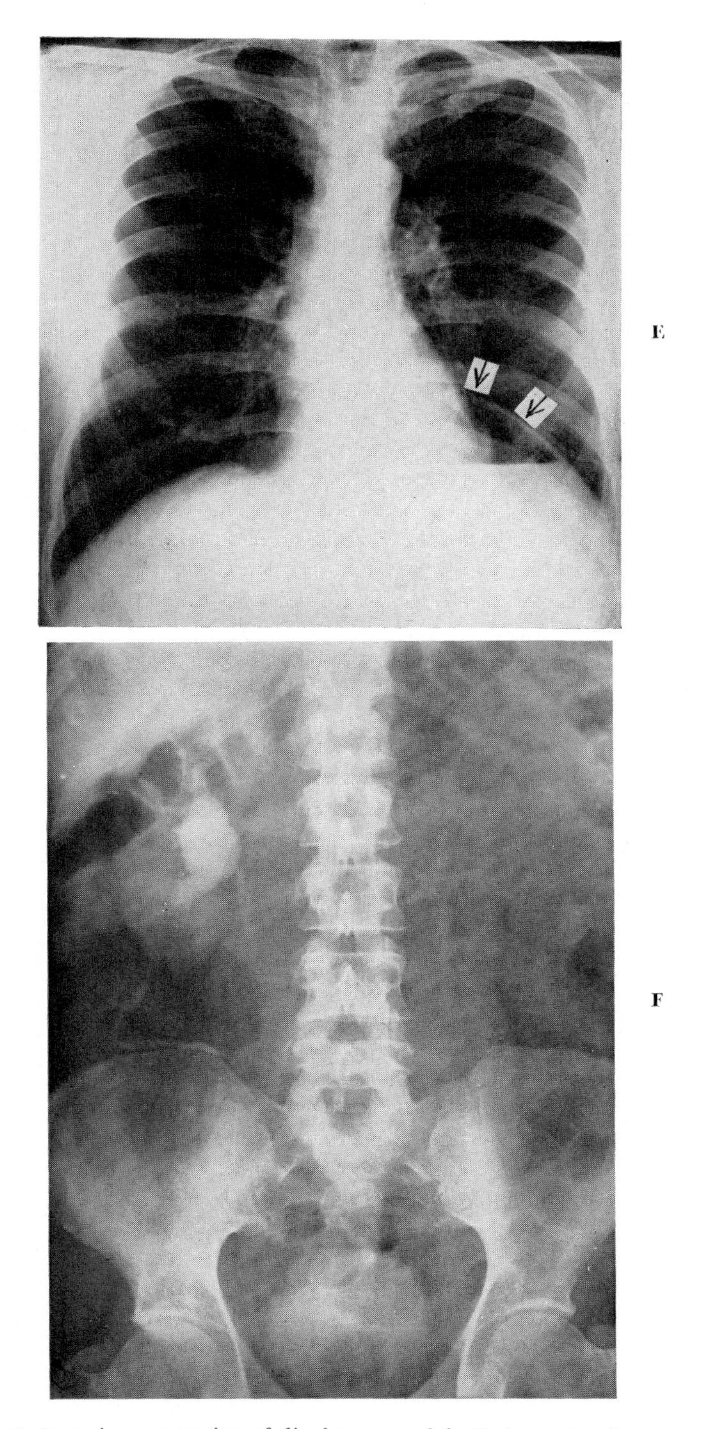

Fig. 5-4, cont'd. E, Posterior eventration of diaphragm on left. **F,** Anomaly of ureteropelvic junction, bilaterally. Nonfunctioning kidney on left.

above, found normal tests of coagulation in patients with the syndrome and concluded that the subcutaneous bleeding is the result of some defect other than one of platelets or plasma clotting factors. They expressed the opinion that reported clotting defects in E-D are coincidental associations—a conclusion I am inclined to agree with. Dr. Dudley P. Jackson has been unable to demonstrate a coagulation defect in several of my patients.

Blisterlike lesions may develop, suggesting epidermolysis bullosa (see Weber's interpretation of Burrows' case[18]).

The limitation of the cutaneous changes, particularly hyperelasticity, to one side of the body, as recounted by van Meekeren[171] in 1682, is almost completely incredible but is probably possible *(v. infra)*. Limitation of integumental hyperelasticity to the mucous membranes, specifically those of the mouth and tongue, has been described,[43] and many patients show evidences of changes (hyperelasticity and/or fragility) at these sites.[43,55,97,163,178] It is said that affected women do not get striae gravidarum.[80]

The skin of the hands and the soles of the feet tends to be redundant (unlike most of the skin elsewhere, which fits snugly); with pressure it flattens out like a loose glove or moccasin (Fig. 5-4*A*, *C*, and *D*). A comparable change may develop in later years at the elbows, where the skin may hang lax like a dewlap (Fig. 5-4*B*). In general, late cases tend to show cutis laxa more than cutis hyperelastica, whereas, as emphasized above, cutis laxa is not an accurate designation in the typical case in young persons.

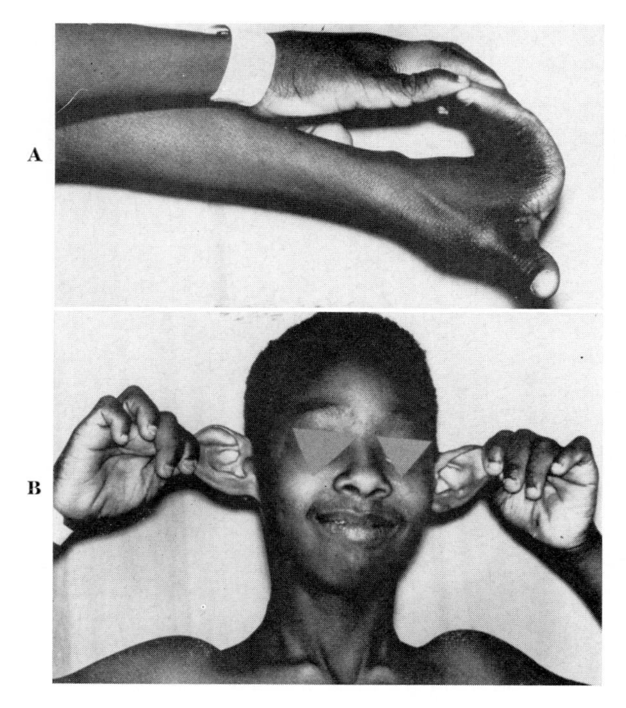

Fig. 5-5. Negro boy, age 12 years, with typical features of E-D, including hyperextensible joints, **A,** and stretchable ears, **B.** The skin was unusually stretchable, but fragility and bruisability were not present. (Courtesy Dr. Glenn R. Stoutt, Louisville, Ky.)

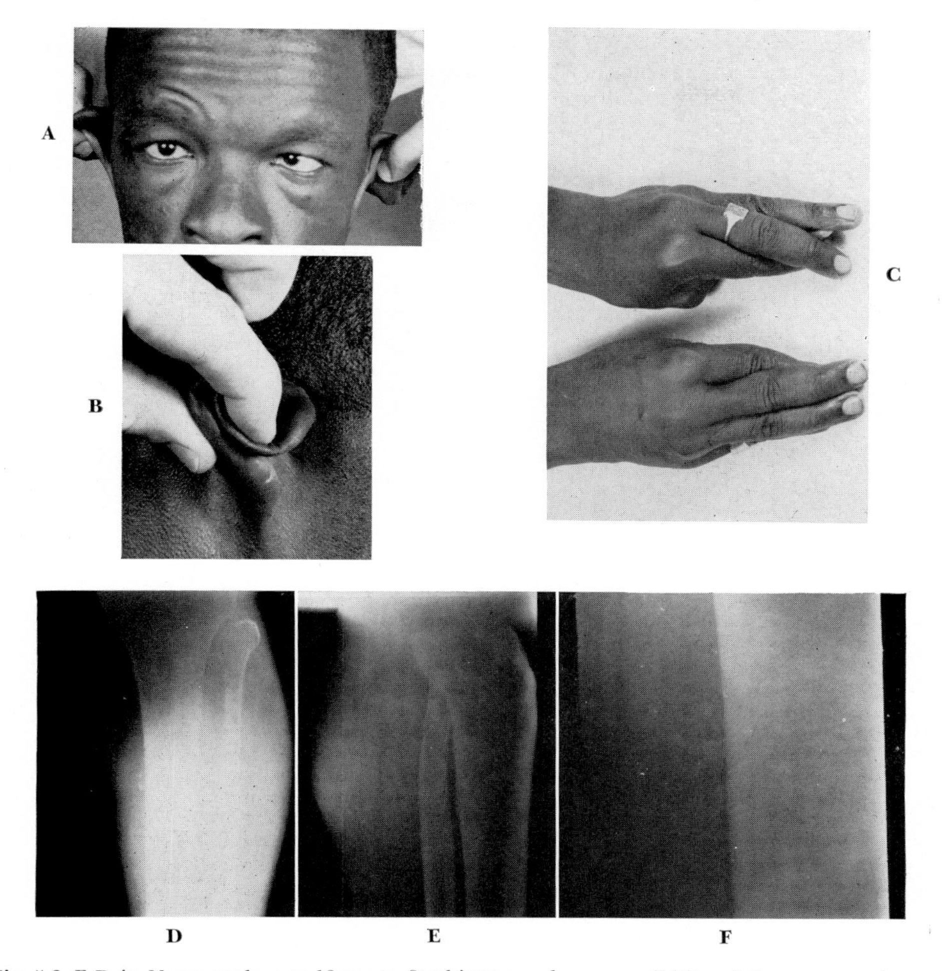

Fig. 5-6. E-D in Negro male, age 12 years. Strabismus and compressibility of the ears are demonstrated in **A** and **B.** The ease of folding the hand is shown in **C.** X-ray films demonstrated soft tissue calcifications, or spherules, **D, E,** and **F.**

"Lop ears," ears which project farther than normally from the head and tend to face downward to some extent, occur commonly in E-D and occur also as an isolated heritable anomaly[100] (Fig. 5-17*A*). Normally the ear makes a 30-degree angle with the head.[101] The ears are, furthermore, unusually stretchable (Fig. 5-5*B*) and can be folded into a ball-like mass (Fig. 5-6*B*). Gorlin[64] points out that many E-D patients display unusual ease in touching the tip of the nose with the tip of the tongue (Fig. 5-7*B*).

Acrocyanosis and chilblains have been described as a seemingly integral component, by French authors in particular,[53,59,83,112,118,131,151] but by others,[16,26,142,169] as well. There seem to be few American reports of this complaint. In general, chilblains are much less common in this country than in Europe, possibly because of our more universal use of central heating. E-D is at least one basis for acrocyanosis that "runs in a family." It may be the presenting complaint in

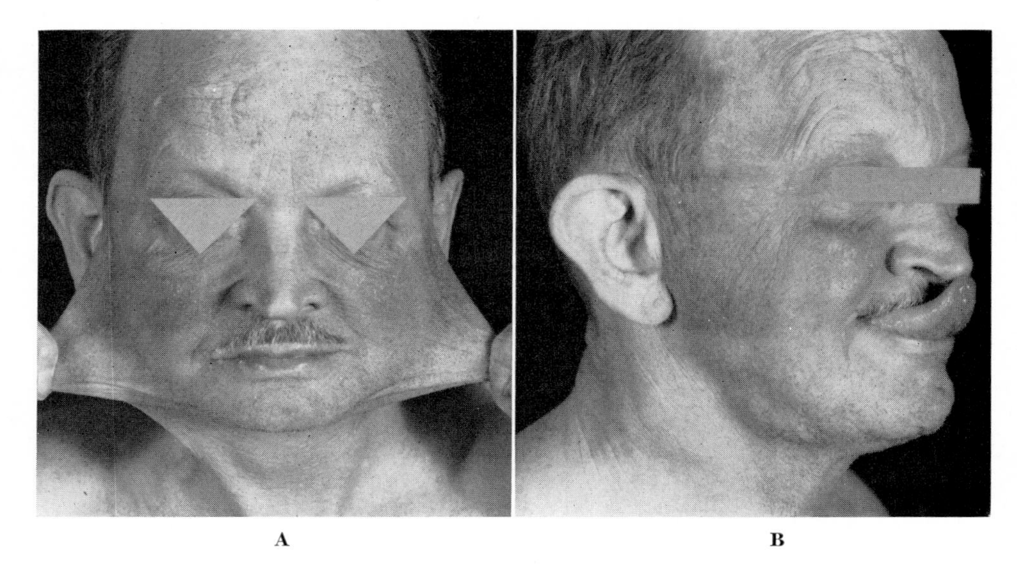

Fig. 5-7. R. A. (911928), age 60 years, has all the typical features of E-D. He subsequently died of metastatic squamous cell carcinoma of the nasopharynx. No other member of his family is known to be affected. **A,** Excessively stretchable skin and scars of the forehead are demonstrated. **B,** Gorlin's sign, unusual facility in touching the tip of the nose with the tip of the tongue, is demonstrated.

E-D. For example, Gilbert and associates[59] described a 22-year-old man who had had cyanosis of the hands, feet, and ears from birth and displayed the other characteristic features of E-D. In the patient's family there were several other cases of "cyanosed limbs and ulcerated chilblains" in association with E-D. Burrows[18] provided an excellent photograph of the hand of one of these patients, showing both joint hyperextensibility and cyanosis of the fingers. I have seen two patients (A. H., 796695; Mrs. R., P3479), both women, in whom acrocyanosis was a striking feature. They suffered severely from cold and displayed the Raynaud phenomenon.

Conceivably the abnormality with hyperelasticity, either of the supporting tissues about the arterioles or of the connective tissue in the vessel wall itself, interferes with blood flow. My observations of difficulties in obtaining blood by finger puncture or venipuncture, mentioned above, are significant in this connection.

Associated neurofibromatosis has been reported in at least three instances.[33,61,169] The association is probably coincidental.

The musculoskeletal system. Hyperextensibility of the joints is characteristic (Figs. 5-2*D* to *E*, 5-3*C*, and 5-8*A* and *B*). This and the corresponding change in the skin make the victims of advanced forms of this disease the "India rubber men," "human pretzels," and contortionists of side shows. The hyperextensibility tends to become less marked as the patient becomes older. Frequently the patients have joint effusions, especially in the knees, because of traumatization as a result of the joint instability. Hemarthroses also occur.[113] Flat feet occur commonly (Fig. 5-3*B*). Clubfoot is described.[12] The foot deformity is often a particularly

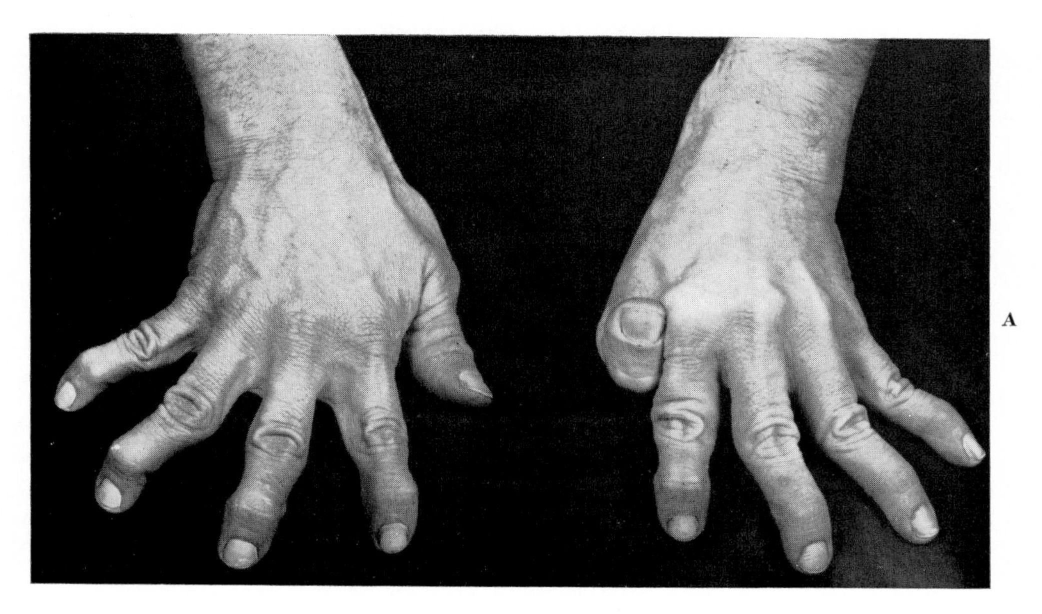

A

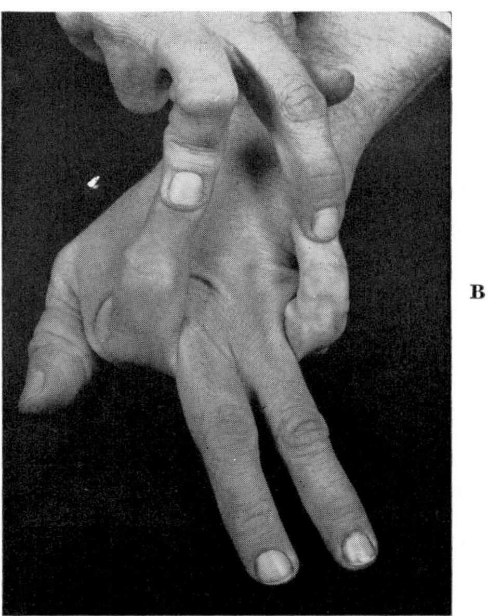

B

Fig. 5-8. C. G. (287731), 47 years old. Long history of "congenital dislocation of right hip," treated with a spica at the age of 2 years and with several operations in his twenties. Bilateral inguinal hernias repaired. Hiatal hernia is apparently responsible for epigastric and substernal pressure, which occurs especially in the recumbent position and is relieved by belching. Dehiscence followed attempts at surgical repair of the hiatal hernia. Two operations on knee for presumed trauma of automobile accident. At the age of 27 years, "relaxation of right radiocarpal joint" necessitated application of a cast. Hyperelasticity of the skin, although present, was a subsidiary feature in this patient.

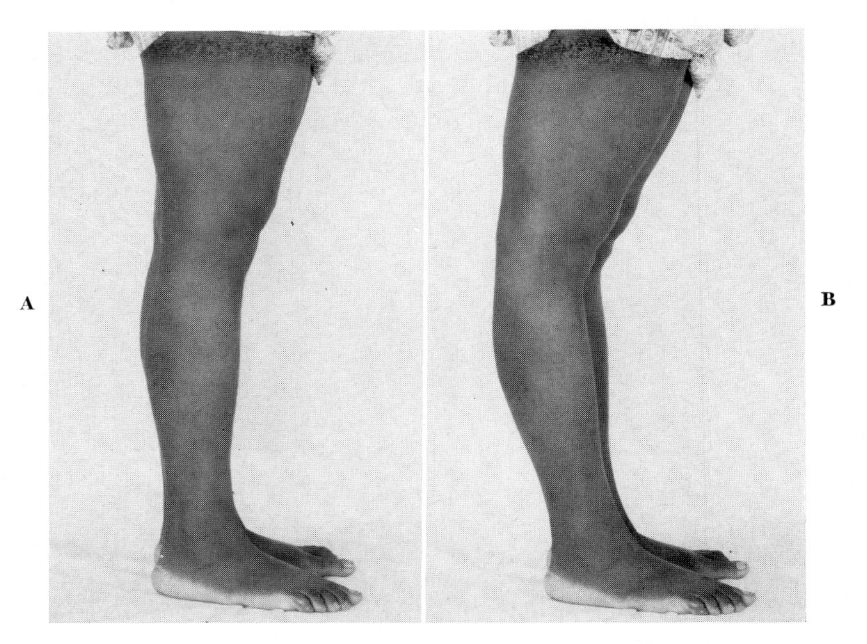

Fig. 5-9. H. L. W. (395947), an example of "simple" joint hypermobility. Seemingly no similar disorder in family. Although the knees and feet are most markedly affected, with genu recurvatum and pes planus, all joints of the body are more mobile than the average. The pes planus is of the dynamic type; the arch of the foot appears fairly normal except during weight bearing. The joint instability at the knees resulted in recurrent hydrarthroses. The patient has worn knee braces with benefit. There are no associated cutaneous or internal manifestations to suggest E-D. The patient did have strabismus (intermittent exotropia) for which resection and advancement of left medial rectus muscle was performed. This case illustrates how difficult it is to be sure of the proper diagnostic classification in a patient with manifestations that may represent an incomplete form of the E-D syndrome, especially when there is in the family no more full-blown example of the disorder. **A,** Position of rest. **B,** Forced backward displacement of knees to demonstrate genu recurvatum. In addition to flat feet, a few scars were suggestively papyraceous.

troublesome feature (see patients shown in Figs. 5-9 and 5-10). The loose-jointedness, in the knees in particular, may result in a gait and stance suggesting tabes dorsalis[84] (Figs. 5-2*C* and 5-4*A*). Habitual dislocation of the hip,[24,34,116,123,177] patellae[22,23,44,116] (Fig. 5-11*E*), shoulder,[23,125] radii,[84] clavicle,[65] and other joints is a frequent feature. As in Marfan's syndrome, the sternal ends of the clavicle may be very loose.[84] There is likely to be genu recurvatum[177] (Fig. 5-2*C*). The patients are often able to pull their fingers out longitudinally for an appreciable distance, even to almost twice their length,[123] and allow them to snap back into place on release. The loose-jointed hand is evident in the handshake. Indeed, the limp feel has been compared to that of a fine foam-rubber sponge.[94] The hand can be folded up as shown in Fig. 5-12. Some patients may show restricted motion in joints such as the elbows and hips.[102] Radioulnar synostosis[95] has been said[145] to occur. Posterior dislocation of the radial heads[28] may be a feature. Kyphoscoliosis is likely to develop,[38,84,116,139,149,159,169,179] Coventry[32] observed thoracolumbar kyphoscoliosis with anterior wedging of several vertebrae,

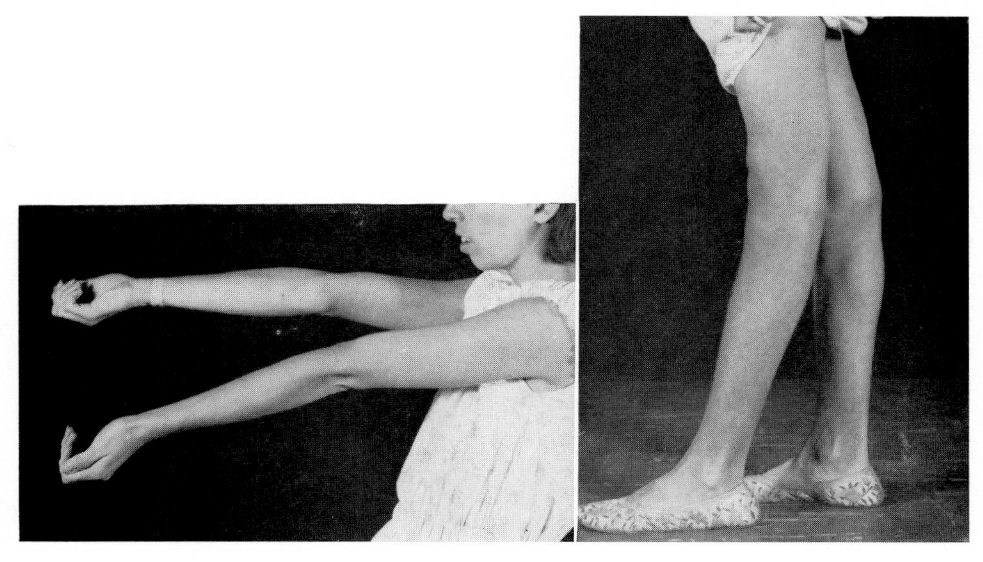

Fig. 5-10. M. W. (688052), 28-year-old female, is another example of "simple" joint hypermobility. Loose-jointedness is most striking in the knees and elbows, as shown. Unusual stretchability, bruisability, fragility, and scarring of the skin were not present. The mother and at least one sib and one offspring are similarly affected.

long, giraffelike neck, downward curvature of the upper ribs, and a tendency to reversal of the normal spinal curves. Spondylolisthesis has been a troublesome problem in at least two of my patients (R. W., 709823; L. S., 1117754) (Fig. 5-13). Spina bifida occulta is described[86] and also wedge-shaped deformity of vertebral bodies.[102] Dental deformities are frequent,[53,84,114] and Gothic palate may be present.[82] Muscular hypotonicity and underdevelopment seem to exist in these patients. In one of my cases, a 4-year-old child, amyotonia congenita of Oppenheim was the initial diagnosis. Smith[151] describes a similar experience. Hernias occur frequently.[175] In some, repair of an umbilical hernia at a young age is necessary.

Ectopic bone formation with formation of osseous bridges between the acetabula and the femoral trochanters has been described by Katz and Steiner.[83] The pathogenesis may have involved hemorrhage from increased joint mobility.

Short stature has been a feature of some cases.

Severe leg cramps, occurring at night and at other times, such as while watching television, have been a major problem over a period of many years in one patient (Fig. 5-3). Quinine and quinidine afford relief. The cramps may result indirectly from the loose-jointedness. Individuals with flat feet or disorders of the low back are prone to night cramps.

The eye. Changes have been described in the ocular adnexa, the cornea, the sclera, the suspensory mechanism of the lens, and the fundus.

The skin about the eyes often lies in redundant folds and can be pulled out to a considerable distance, like the skin elsewhere. Epicanthal folds are frequent[3,7,58,80,115,130,147,150] (Fig. 5-14*C*); at least three of our patients showed them. (Epicanthal folds occur, of course, in mongolism; they are also part of the facies

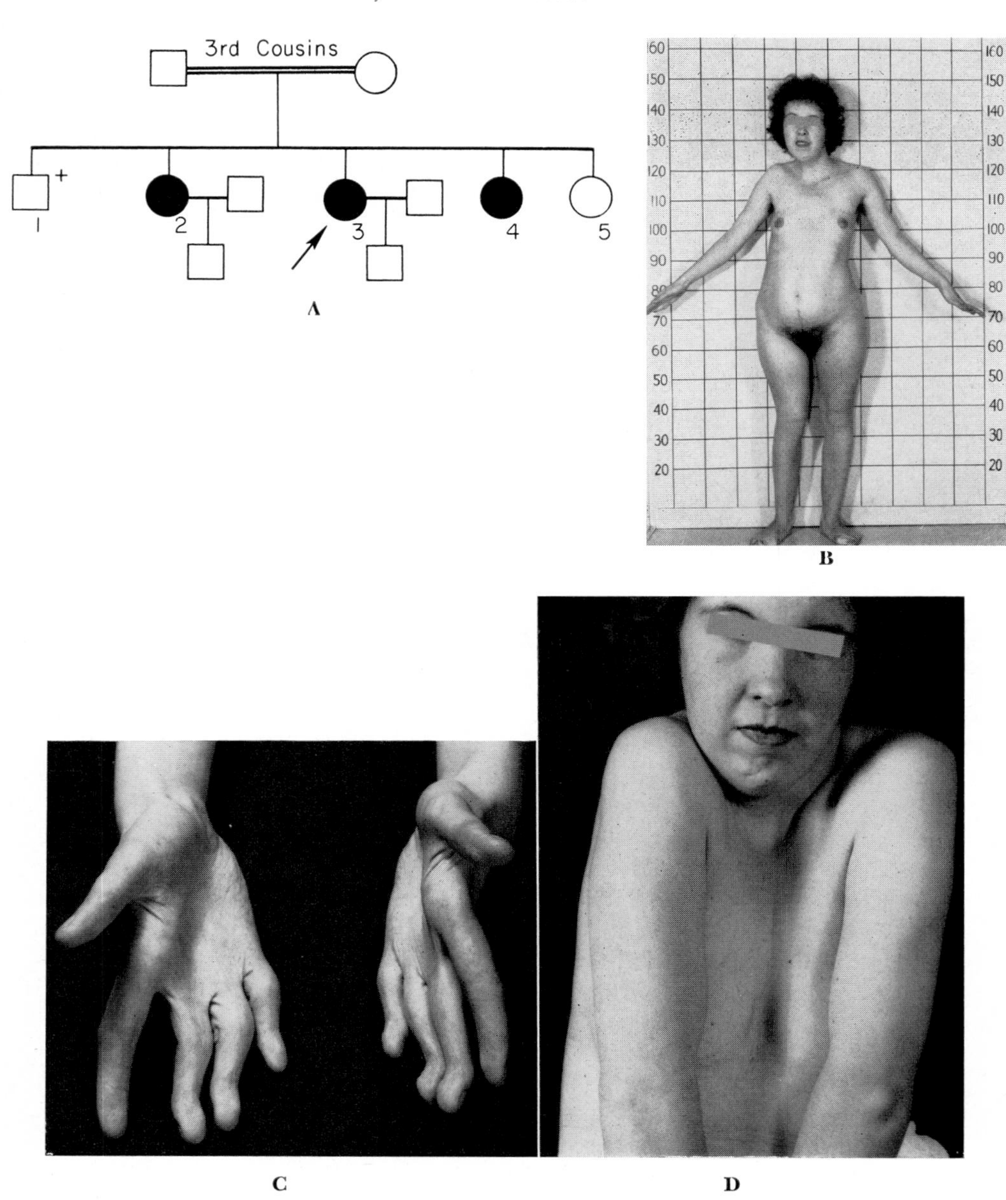

Fig. 5-11. Marked loose-jointedness. ?Inherited as an autosomal recessive. E. D. (970801), indicated by arrow in pedigree, **A,** and age 25 years at the time of study, has marked hyperextensibility of many joints, especially those of the hands, feet, shoulders, and spine. Dislocations at both hips and both elbows have resulted in limitation of motion in these joints. The bridge of the nose is broad, and she has myopia, microphthalmia, and intermittent exotropia. She is 58 inches tall. The fingers are somewhat webbed. The skin is not excessively stretchable or fragile, but there is some increased bruisability. There are no "cigarette-paper scars"; no striae resulted from pregnancy. No chromosomal abnormality could be identified. A sister (2 in the pedigree) has had dislocation of the knees about twenty-five times, beginning at age 6 years. She also has bilateral dislocation of the patella and scoliosis. A young sister (II-4) also has habitual dislocation of the patellae. Neither parent shows any abnormality resembling those in the children,

Legend continued on opposite page.

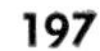

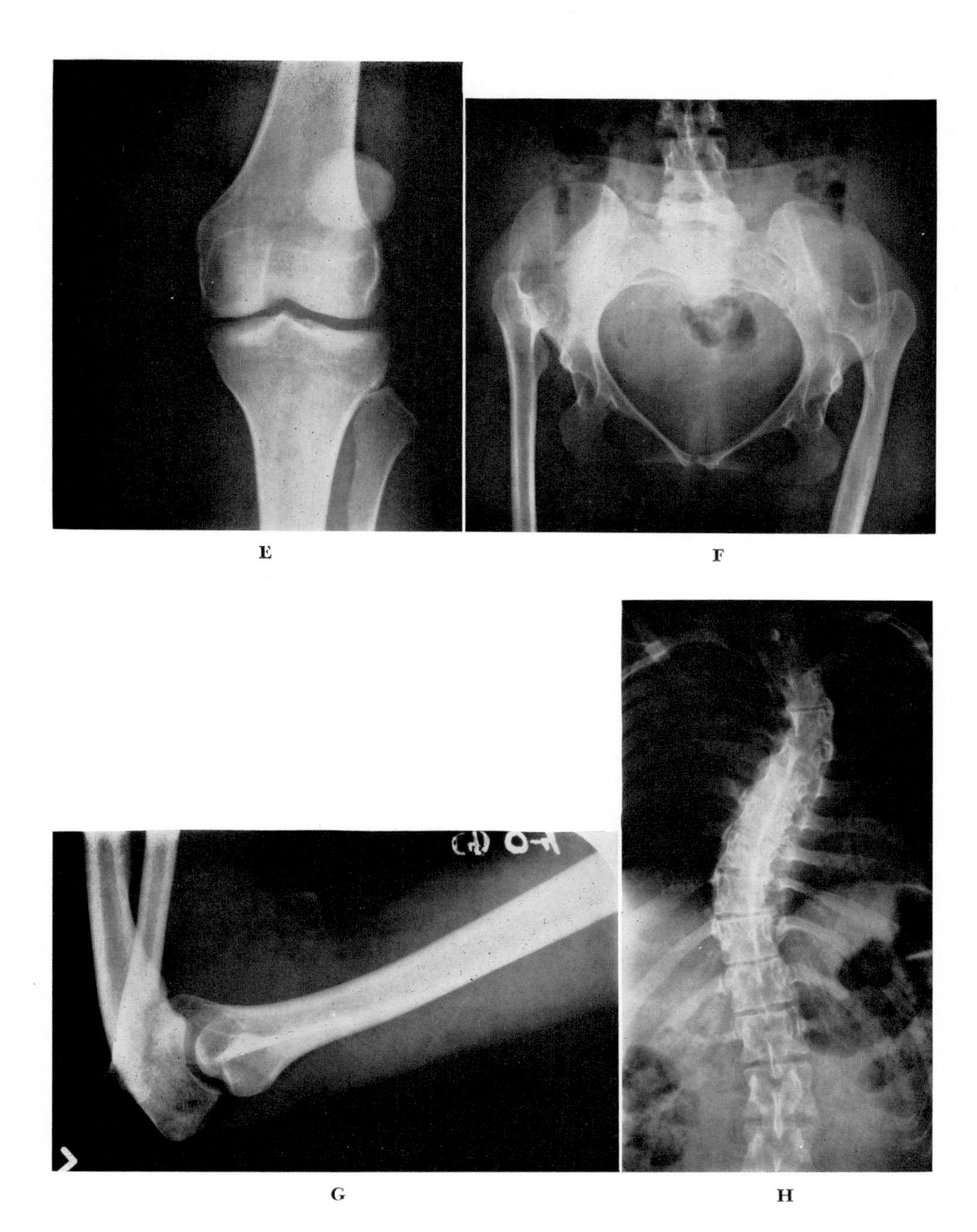

E F

G H

and the two offspring of affected sibs show no abnormality. In **B, C,** and **D** are demonstrated general features and the loose-jointedness. Acrocyanosis is suggested in **C. E** to **H** show the radiologic features of the proband. Both patellae, **E,** both hips, **F,** and the head of each radius, **G,** are dislocated. Scoliosis is marked, **H.** It is suggested that a form of severe loose-jointedness behaving as an autosomal recessive is present in this family. (Family studied by Dr. R. M. Goodman and Dr. Yves Duchastel.)

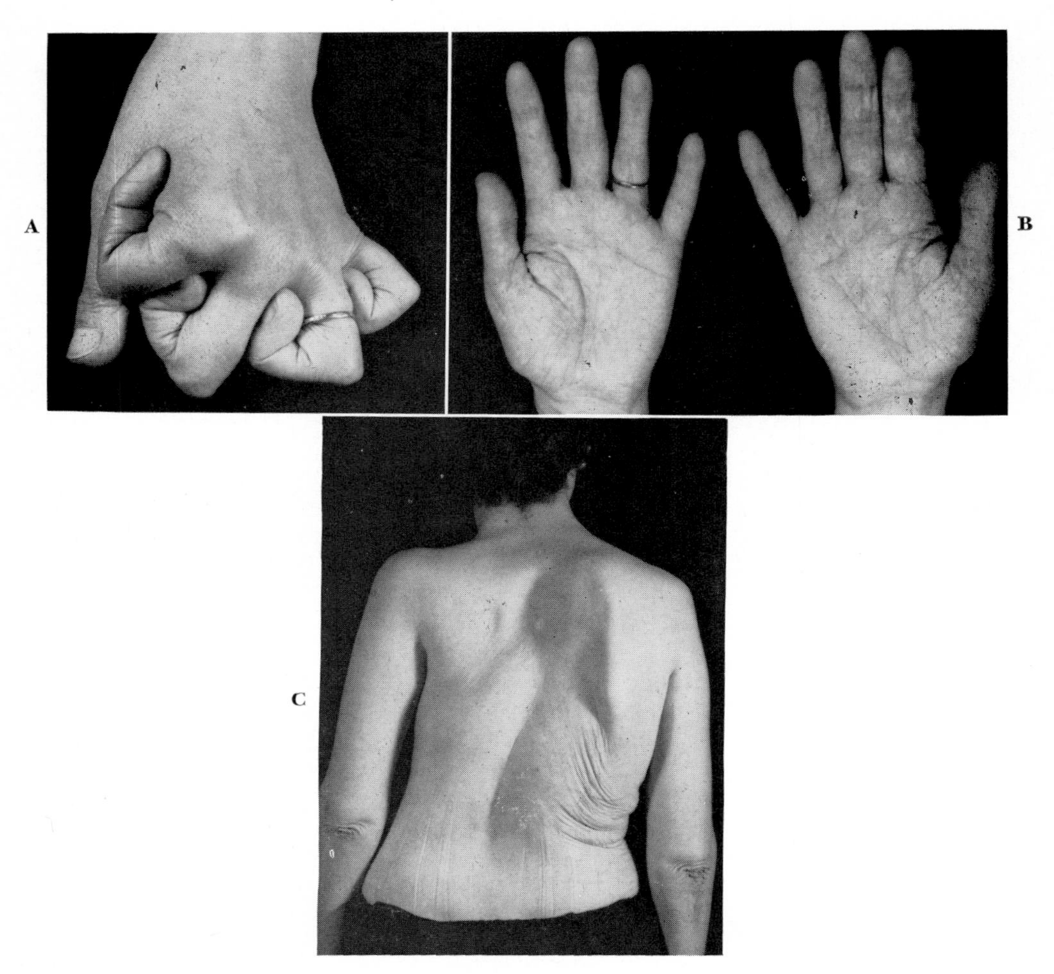

Fig. 5-12. Severe scoliosis and acrocyanosis in E-D. I. B. (983764), 37-year-old white female, has had loose-jointedness, **A,** stretchable and fragile skin, and acrocyanosis, **B,** all her life. She spent several months in an orthopedic hospital at age of 12 for treatment of "clubfoot" and again at age 15 for treatment of scoliosis, **C.** Ocular complications also were present. From the age of 6 years she wore spectacles for myopia. Microcornea, blue sclerae, and glaucoma were noted at age 27 and were described in brief by Durham.[46] Between ages 35 and 37 years complete detachment, first of the left and then of the right retina, occurred. A brother and one of his sons are known to have E-D also.

characteristic of thalassemia; in other instances, they are inherited as a trait with no syndromal significance.) Méténier[108] has lent his name to a frequent phenomenon, namely, unusual ease in everting the upper lid. Strabismus has been encountered frequently.[5,30,31,74,150]

Blue sclerotics have been described commonly.[13,46,162] Microcornea with associated glaucoma was described in one patient[46] in whom the small size of the cornea was thought to be responsible, at least indirectly, for an impediment to ocular drainage. Microcornea and myopia were present in Schaper's first patient.[147] Keratoconus is also described.[162]

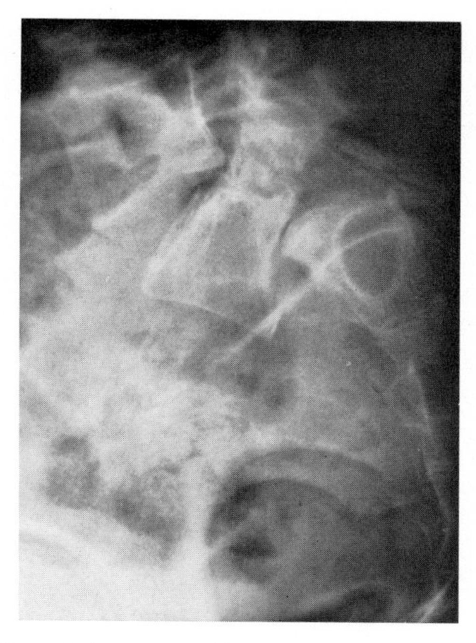

Fig. 5-13. Severe spondylolisthesis in L. S. (1117734), 17-year-old white girl with all the cardinal features of E-D. The fifth lumbar vertebra has almost slipped off the first sacral vertebra.

Ectopia lentis occurred in at least one twice-reported patient.[161,162]

In one patient, the author[12] described and illustrated changes in the fundus, consisting of retinitis proliferans, pigment spots that were interpreted as residua of microhemorrhages, and detachment of the retina of secondary type (no retinal tear was detected). Retinal detachment occurred bilaterally in the patient shown in Fig. 5-12.

Internal ramifications. The internal manifestations of E-D have not been investigated to any significant extent. Those manifestations which have been identified include (1) diaphragmatic hernia, (2) ectasia of portions of the alimentary and respiratory tracts, (3) spontaneous rupture of the lung, (4) dissecting aneurysm of the aorta, and (5) certain congenital malformations of more conventional type.

One of my patients has eventration of the left leaf of the diaphragm (Fig. 5-4*E*). Differentation from a large posterior diaphragmatic hernia is uncertain. We have observed *hiatal hernia* in a second patient, of whom other illustrations are shown in Fig. 5-8. Brombart and associates[14] described a patient in whom hiatal hernia, diverticulum of the stomach, duodenal diverticulum, and colonic diverticulosis occurred in association with E-D. *Gastrointesinal diverticula* were present in patient 4 (see below) and are demonstrated in Fig. 5-15*F* to *H*. Megaesophagus, megatrachea, and megacolon were described in another case.[112] Bladder diverticulum is described,[157] as are also ptosis viscerum[2,121] and gastric atony.[142]

In one reported patient,[122] repeated episodes of mediastinal and subcutaneous emphysema occurred, and I have observed spontaneous pneumothorax in one patient. It is to be noted that in the first case of dissecting aneurysm described

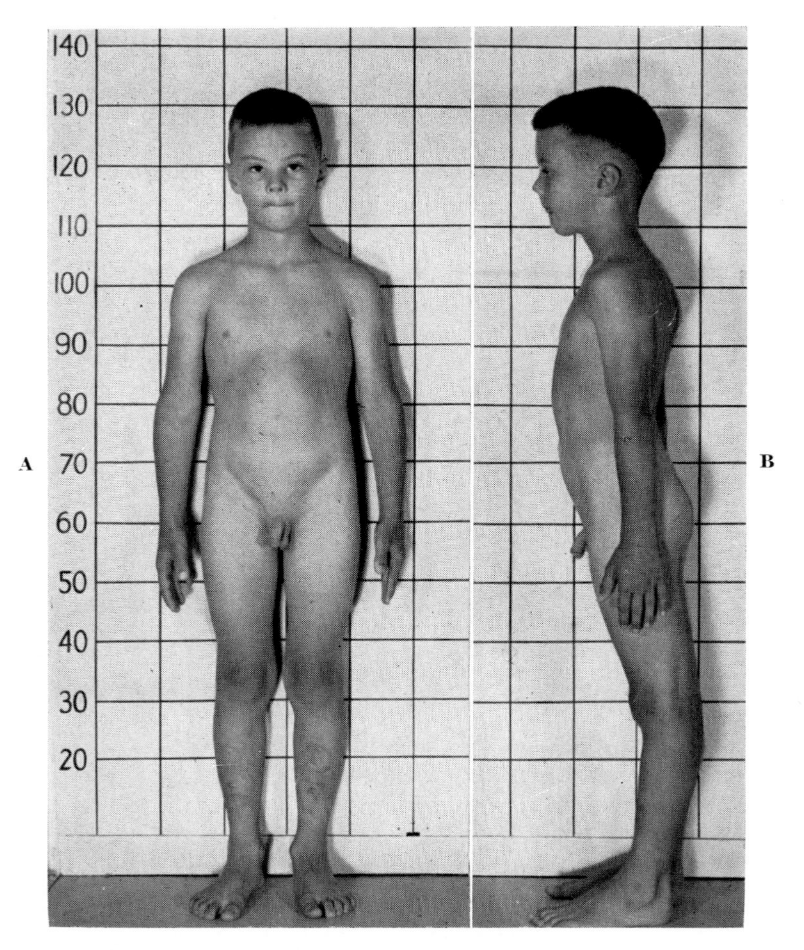

Fig. 5-14. R. R. (B53739), 8¾ years of age, shows characteristic pretibial scarring, mild genu recurvatum, flat feet, and looseness of the soles. The skin generally is abnormally stretchable and the joints hypermobile. Easy bruisability was the presenting complaint. An epicanthal fold, **C,** which is not present in unaffected members of his family, is a frequent finding in this syndrome, as is also mild retardation of growth. The characteristic scars are evident also on the forehead and right side of the face. Bilateral inguinal hernias and an umbilical hernia were repaired at the age of 2 years. No other members of the family are definitely affected. The patient has four brothers and no sisters. One brother had pectus excavatum severe enough to warrant surgical repair, and a second brother has mild pectus excavatum. (From McKusick, V. A.: Bull. N. Y. Acad. Med. **35:**143, 1959.)

below, the lungs revealed subpleural blebs, and subcutaneous emphysema was present.

Known to me are three cases of *dissecting aneurysm of the aorta,* patients in whom the diagnosis of E-D is distinctly possible. In a fourth patient, uncontrollable bleeding from a large artery was the cause of death. Interestingly, the histologic changes in the aorta in at least one of these were those of Erdheim's cystic medial necrosis and indistinguishable from those discovered in some cases of the Marfan syndrome. Abstracts of these cases follow.

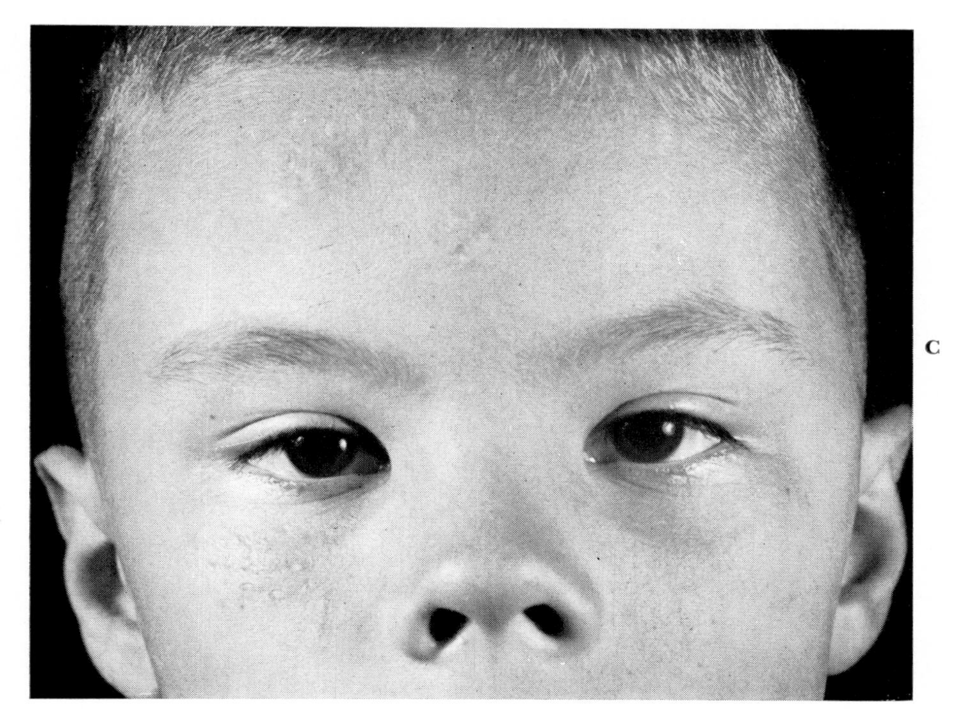

Fig. 5-14, cont'd. For legend see opposite page.

Case 1. H. L. R.,* a 15-year-old Negro student, with a history of always having been sickly, was thrown forcibly to the ground by a schoolmate. He complained immediately of pain in the chest extending down the right arm and soon developed signs and symptoms of circulatory collapse. He was taken to the neighboring office of a physician, where he died within ten minutes.

Autopsy revealed an adequately developed and nourished Negro male weighing 140 pounds and measuring 5 feet 6 inches in height. The skin showed many scars; some resembled burn scars. One on the right thigh was covered with thin epidermis and measured 15 by 3.8 cm. An ulcer with hemorrhagic base, 25 mm. in diameter, was located on the medial aspect of the left ankle. There was considerable subcutaneous emphysema below the right rib margin.

During the dissection, the connective tissues were found to be very friable. They tore easily, and even the skeletal muscles pulled apart with incredible ease. (The autopsy was performed only a few hours after death. The tissue was not autolyzed histologically. Dr. Thoma, the prosector, had never encountered such fragility of tissues and considered it highly significant.) Fourteen hundred milliliters of blood were found in the right hemithorax. The mediastinal structures were infiltrated with blood, which also had dissected along the fascial planes of the neck. The lungs showed multiple large emphysematous subpleural bullae and were easily torn. The heart weighed 300 grams. The gastrointestinal tract tore easily.

Histologic studies, including stains by the periodic acid-Schiff method and elastic tissue stains, were unrevealing of definite abnormality.

Further investigation of the boy's previous health and of his family revealed that he had always been sickly, did not play as actively as his contemporaries, and often complained of severe headache. He "cut" his skin easily and healed poorly. At the age of 11 years he had sprained his ankle; x-ray films of the injured part were not considered abnormal on review.

*For calling this case to my attention I am indebted to Robert K. Osborne, then a fourth-year student, Medical College of Virginia. For much information bearing on the case I am indebted to Dr. George W. Thoma, formerly Assistant Chief Medical Examiner, Commonwealth of Virginia.

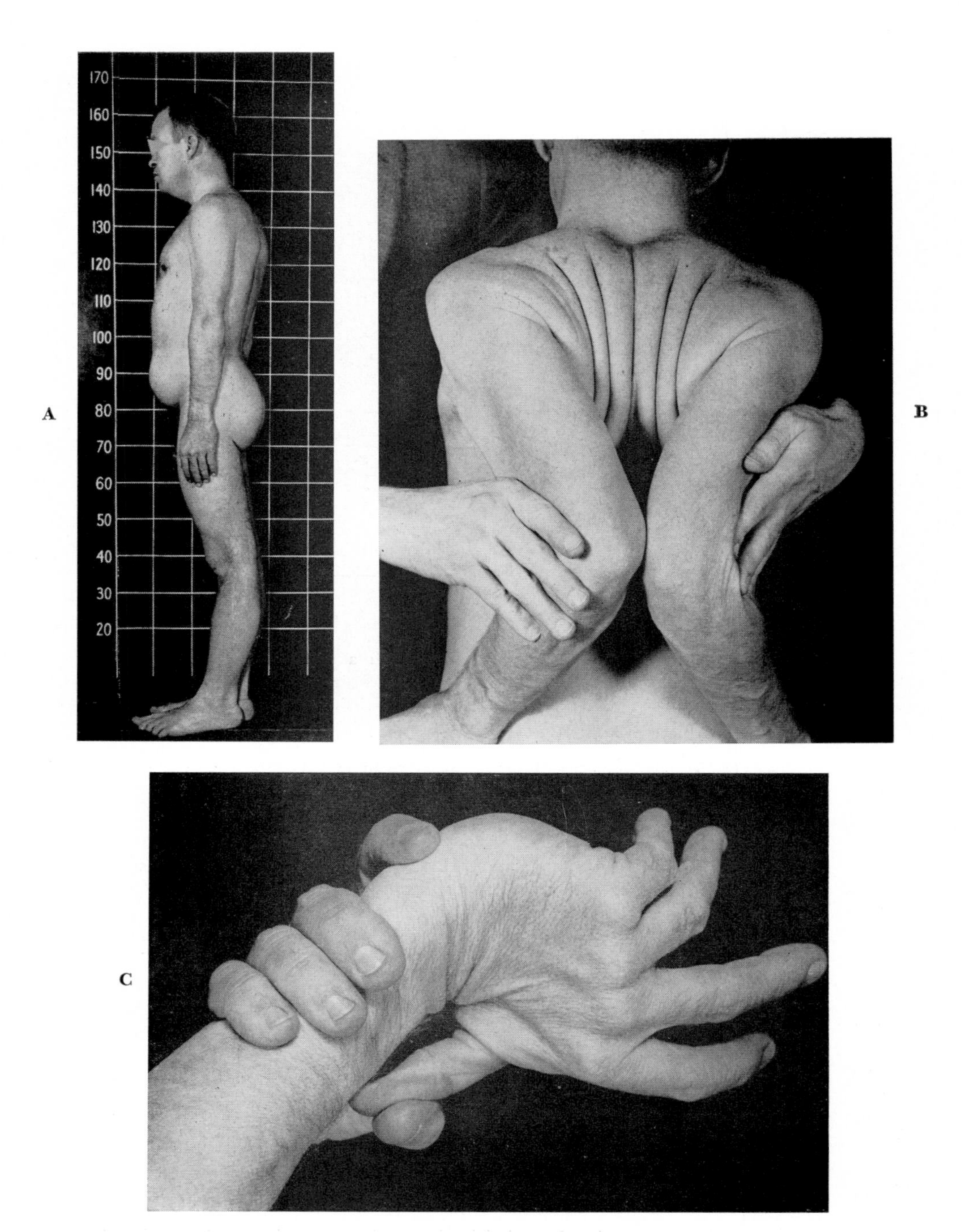

Fig. 5-15. Case 3. **A,** Lateral view. Note genu recurvatum and short stature. **B,** Hyperextensibility of the shoulders. **C,** Joint hypermobility. Note also the loose coarse-grained appearance of the skin resembling that in the patient shown in Fig. 5-4.

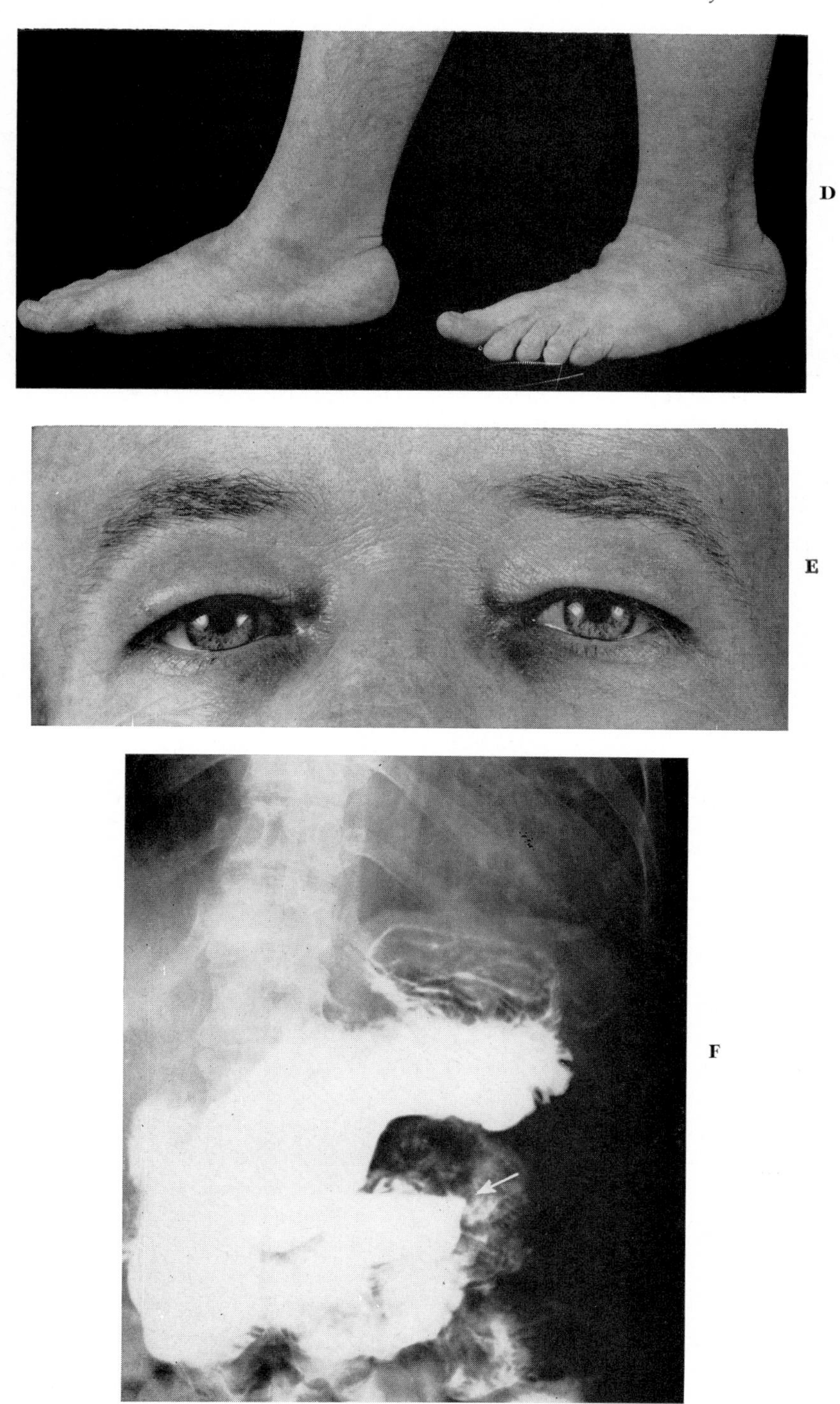

Fig 5-15, cont'd. D, Flat feet; lose, redundant soles. **E,** Redundant skin of lids. **F,** Film from gastroduodenal series to show large duodenal diverticulum arising in region of ligament of Treitz and extending up behind the stomach.

Continued.

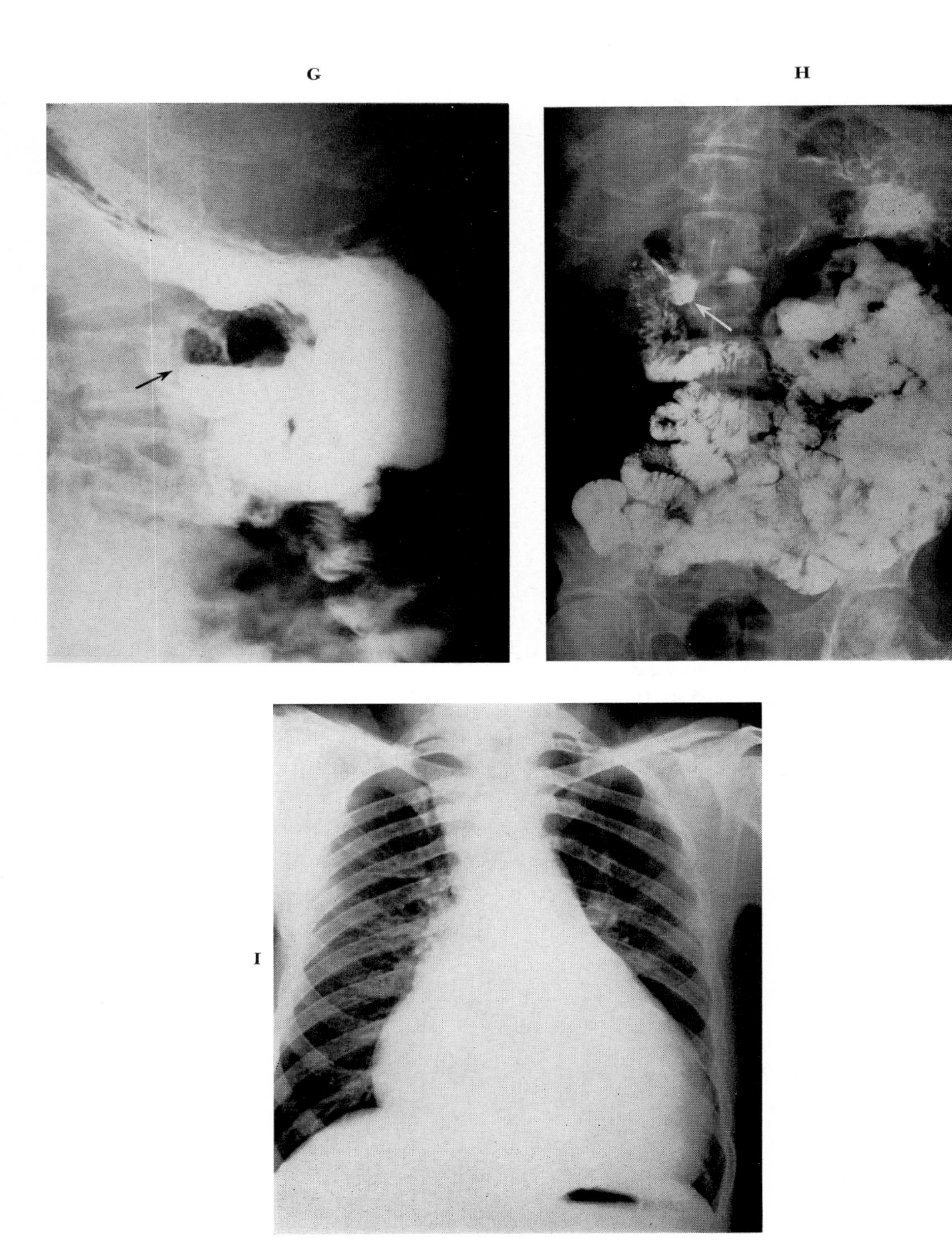

Fig. 5-15. cont'd. G, Same as **F,** lateral view. **H,** Gastrointestinal x-ray film showing diverticulum of second part of duodenum (arrow). **I,** Chest x-ray film to show general cardiomegaly.

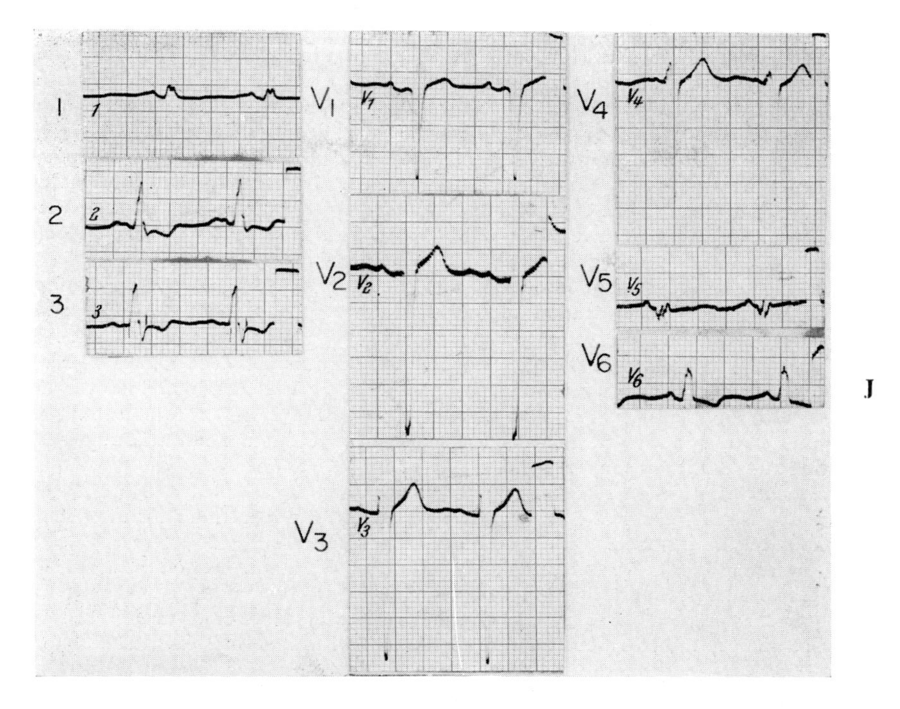

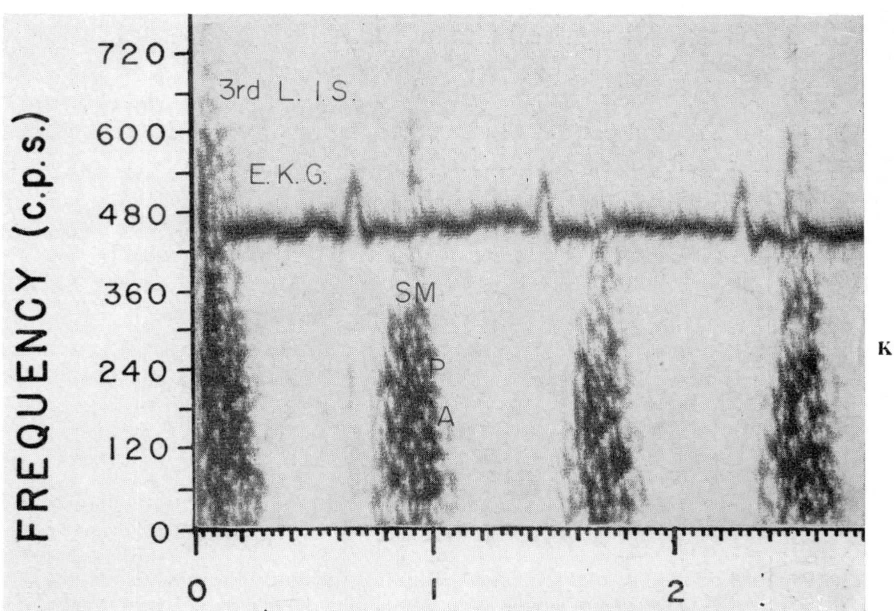

Fig. 5-15, cont'd. J, Electrocardiogram. Left bundle branch block; broad, notched P waves. **K,** Spectral phonocardiogram, aortic area. The systolic murmur is consistent with aortic stenosis. There may be paradoxical splitting of S_2. The systolic murmur may extend to the pulmonary component (which is first) but not to the aortic. Recordings at the third left interspace and in the left mid-precordial area showed a diastolic murmur of arterial type, probably indicative of aortic regurgitation.

The father of the patient died at the age of 21 or 22 years, of asthma. The mother died at the age of 22 years after a twenty-four-hour illness beginning with abdominal pain, nausea, and vomiting, and characterized by progressive circulatory failure. Autopsy was not performed but the diagnosis given on the death certificate was "internal hemorrhage of unknown cause." There were no siblings of the propositus.

Case 2. J. M. M.,* a 24-year-old white man, was well until 6 A.M. on the morning of Dec. 31, 1946, when he awoke with a vague discomfort in the abdomen. In the course of two hours this developed into pain in the right flank and lower quadrant of the abdomen. By the time he was admitted to the hospital, a few hours after onset, he was in profound shock. The administration of fluids intravenously raised the blood pressure from an indeterminably low level to 90/60 mm. Hg. The white count was 25,000 and 28,000 per cubic millimeter on two determinations. The hemoglobin concentration fell from 82 to 69% of normal during the afternoon. By 3 P.M. the patient was complaining of pain in the region of the right shoulder. Abdominal exploration was undertaken at 5 P.M. The abdomen contained blood-stained fluid. A large retroperitoneal hematoma involved the right kidney. There was dissection into the mesentery, which was torn in several places. The surgeon compared the tissues to wet blotting paper. Bleeding and clotting times determined postoperatively were 1 and 4 minutes, respectively. The patient died at 4:15 A.M. on Jan. 1, 1947.

Subsequent investigation revealed that the patient had always bled and bruised easily. He also had sustained a number of fractures. The possibility of minor trauma during the previous evening could not be excluded.

Autopsy revealed a body measuring only 62 inches in length. Despite this, arachnodactyly was thought to be very impressive. The prosector may have been unduly impressed because of the recognized association of arachnodactyly and dissecting aneurysm. During the opening of the chest at autopsy the ribs were thought to fracture with abnormal ease. The abdomen contained 500 ml. of bloody fluid. The aorta and the renal and iliac arteries were described as hypoplastic. A dissection of the right renal artery with infarction of the kidney was discovered. Histologically the media of the aorta was thin, with numerous areas of "myxomatous degeneration" and basophilically staining material. There was some fragmentation of the elastic fibers, which seemed to be normally abundant but morphologically abnormal. The renal artery showed marked fragmentation of elastic fibers.

Although the second patient was included as an instance of arachnodactyly in reports[62,63] of a series of cases of dissecting aneurysm, the short stature, the easy bruisability, and the friability of the tissues at operation and at autopsy suggest E-D. The case of MacFarlane at the Radcliffe Infirmary, Oxford (described by Mories[110,111]), has parallels to these two cases. A 15-year-old white boy, the elder of twins, developed a swelling in the right groin after falling from his bicycle. Trueta attempted to stop the bleeding, which was obviously the cause of the inguinal swelling, by ligature. However, all the vessels were so extremely friable that hemostasis was impossible. At autopsy, all tissues, especially muscle and fascia, were very friable and the abdominal aorta tore readily. Histologically there was said to be an increase in the elastica of the aorta, with degeneration and hyalinization of the collagenous elements.

Dr. S. Miles Bouton, Jr., of Lynchburg, Va., has informed me of yet another case:

The boy died at the age of 14 years, of dissecting aneurysm of the aorta. At the age of 7 years spontaneous rupture of the outer two coats of the sigmoid colon, with intra-abdominal bleeding, produced severe pain in the left lower abdomen and required surgical exploration. Two weeks after operation symptoms of partial obstruction of the large bowel appeared but were resolved with conservative measures. Six months later partial bowel obstruction necessi-

*I am indebted to Dr. John F. Brownsberger of Takoma Park, Md., for much information on this patient.

tated surgical release of adhesions. Less than four weeks later, the child was sitting in school when he was seized with left upper quadrant pain radiating to the shoulder, which doubled him up. Operation revealed peritonitis secondary to perforation of the splenic flexure of the colon. About three years later, at the age of 10 years, perforation of the sigmoid colon and pelvic abscess again required operation.

It was noted repeatedly that lacerations of the knees, legs, and scalp occurred unusually readily. Healing of the skin occurred normally, however. The boy tended to constipation.

Later, at the age of 11 years, the boy again suffered a perforation of the colon; the transverse and descending portions of the colon were removed. Four months later the monotonous accident was repeated; the ascending colon ruptured spontaneously; the remainder of the colon was resected and the ileum was anastomosed to the rectum. In the postoperative period there was intra-abdominal hemorrhage with shock, and drainage of a subdiaphragmatic hematoma was necessary.

Three years after the last surgical episode, at the age of 14 years, this apparently healthy boy, who did, however, get skin lacerations at slight provocation, went to summer camp. One night, while in bed, he suffered the onset of severe pain in the back and abdomen. He died on the way to his home.

Autopsy revealed two transverse intimal tears, one in the descending portion of the arch and the other just proximal to the renal arteries. A large volume of blood occupied the left pleural cavity. The entire aorta and its branches appeared to be unusually delicate. Dissection extended from the reflection of the pericardial sac to the bifuraction of the aorta and into the right iliac artery.

Histologically the bowel removed at surgery revealed disarrangement, irregular development, and, in places, marked hypoplasia of the smooth muscle elements.

McFarland and Fuller[103] described two patients who died of spontaneous rupture of large arteries. One was a 12-year-old boy who suffered rupture of the right popliteal artery that apparently occurred spontaneously during sleep. Trauma at play during the previous day could not be excluded. The second was a 17-year-old boy who died of rupture of the right subclavian artery, which occurred during the course of strenuous cheering at a basketball tournament.

Rubinstein and Cohen[144] described a 47-year-old white female with typical E-D and multiple intracranial aneurysms. (A brother also had E-D. One of her children died at the age of 1 month of massive ectasia of the gastrointestinal tract through the abdominal wall. Another child, who had hyperelastic skin, died at the age of 2 years, of a congenital cardiac defect.) François and colleagues[52] observed a case with an intracranial arteriovenous aneurysm. I have observed a 30-year-old woman with E-D subarachnoid hemorrhage, presumably from an intracranial aneurysm (Fig. 5-16).

There is in the literature at least one other case of abnormal friability of the intestine and uncontrollable internal hemorrhage in E-D. Jacobs,[72] in describing a case of E-D, stated that a brother, during appendectomy at the age of 37 years, was found to have very friable bowel which was covered with numerous hemorrhages. In the postoperative period wound disruption occurred and the patient died of uncontrolled gastrointestinal hemorrhage. *Spontaneous perforation of the bowel,* as discussed by Robertson and associates,[134] probably has multiple predisposing causes. The Ehlers-Danlos syndrome is sometimes one.

In one patient, an 11-year-old girl, Bell's palsy followed a large subgaleal hematoma that was produced by a fall, with blow to the occiput.[158]

In the *heart* one reported patient had interatrial septal defect[53]; another had tetralogy of Fallot[174] One patient had partial persistent atrioventricular canal[50]

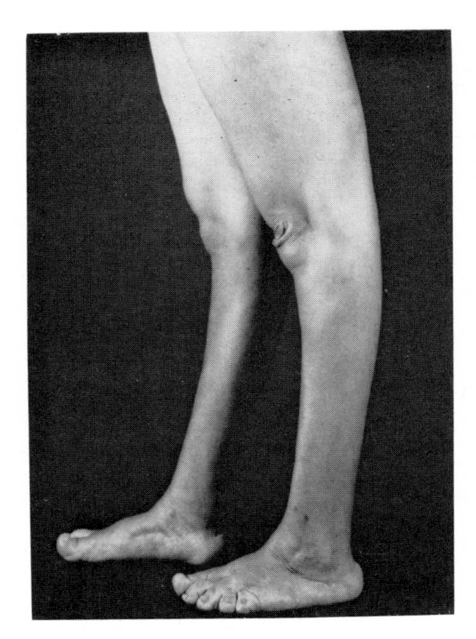

Fig. 5-16. Deformed foot in L.D.P. (1121524), 30-year-old schoolteacher. Several operations for "clubfoot" were performed in childhood. Other cardinal features of E-D are present. Dislocation of the shoulder and of the patella has occurred on several occasions. Intracranial hemorrhage, presumably from berry aneurysm, occurred in this patient.

and another had aneurysm of a sinus of Valsalva and other abnormal cardiac findings on physical examination, without more definitive diagnosis of the defect.[167] One patient had a bicuspid right atrioventricular valve.[103] One patient in the series reported by Sestak[148] had atrial septal defect. Madison and coworkers[105] described a 17-year-old Negro patient with features of E-D and intractable heart failure from mitral and tricuspid regurgitation. Autopsy findings seemed to exclude rheumatic heart disease and showed redundant chordae tendineae and valve cusps considered compatible with the same defect as in other connective tissue structures. A loud systolic murmur in the pulmonary area, audible also in the left interscapular area of the back, was described in one patient.[106] One of my patients has demonstrated for many years, probably all his life, the electrocardiographic pattern of incomplete right bundle branch block without subjective or other objective cardiovascular manifestations (Fig. 5-3*D*). Sestak[148] also observed incomplete right bundle branch block in two patients, in one of whom atrial septal defect was present.

The chordae tendineae of the atrioventricular valves are indeed tendons, and the cusps themselves and fibrous skeleton of the heart are largely collagenous. Possibly the marvel is that serious cardiac difficulties occur so relatively uncommonly in these patients. It is likely that as more experience and, especially, more pathologic information accumulate the cardiovascular involvement in E-D will fit into a definite pattern, just as it does in the Marfan syndrome. Case 3 described below represents a case of grave cardiac abnormality in association with E-D. The precise nature of the cardiac abnormality is not known.

Case 3. W. E. W.* (765864), a white male born in 1917, was referred to Dr. Helen B. Taussig and Dr. Richard S. Ross, for study of his heart condition.

To the patient's knowledge, no condition similar to his existed in his family. The father died of cerebral hemorrhage at 54 years. The mother, who had diabetes, died in childbirth at age 37 years. Six brothers, 20 to 44 years of age, were living and well and six sisters were likewise well. Part of the siblings were half-brothers and half-sisters. The patient had no children.

He was the shortest member of his family. He had always had unusually soft, smooth, elastic skin, with abnormal hyperextensibility of all joints. Both the joints and the skin had tended to become less elastic as he grew older. At no time was there any bleeding tendency, fragility of the skin, or unusual scarring over exposed areas. The patient had had prolapse of the rectum on several occasions.

Shortly after birth a murmur was discovered and it was described on each of many examinations as he was growing up. He was rejected for Armed Service in World War II because of the murmur. In 1948 his physician described a harsh systolic murmur, loudest at the apex but audible over the entire heart, with no diastolic murmur. By x-ray examination there was left ventricular enlargement. In 1955 the first signs of congestive heart failure appeared. Left bundle branch block was discovered; how long it has been present is unknown.

Early in 1957 the patient had the onset of abdominal pain. Gastrointestinal x-ray films showed redundancy of the colon, a small diverticulum in the second portion of the duodenum, and a huge diverticulum at the ligament of Treitz.

Physical examination revealed an intelligent, moderately deaf, rather short man (Fig. 5-15*A*), who appeared to be about his stated age of 40 years. The head was short and round. The skin was smooth, velvety, and loose, with redundant skin of the upper lid. When stretched, the skin returned promptly to its normal position on release. All joints displayed hyperextensibility. There was pes planus, genu recurvatum, and ability to hold a pencil between the knuckles. The hands could be folded together transversely, with opposition of the thenar and hypothenar portions. Audiogram showed impairment of all tones bilaterally. (The patient was aware of impairment of hearing only in the left ear. This had begun following a purulent discharge at the age of 18 years.) The hard palate was unusually high arched.

The heart was massively enlarged (Fig. 5-15*I*), with a localized point of maximum impulse in the seventh interspace, just outside the anterior axillary line. At the base a grade III harsh systolic murmur was transmitted into the neck. At the apex a higher-pitched systolic murmur was of approximately grade II intensity (on a base of six). A soft, decrescendo, diastolic murmur was audible down the left sternal border. The liver edge was two fingerbreadths below the costal margin. Blood pressure was 100/70 mm. Hg.

The left testis was undescended.

Serum cholesterol was 217 mg.%. X-ray films revealed great enlargement of the heart, involving all chambers. Right heart catheterization showed no evidence of shunt. Pressure in the right ventricle was 56/2/5 mm. Hg.

It was concluded that aortic stenosis and/or mitral regurgitation would best account for the physical findings.

Fig. 5-15 demonstrates the photographs, electrocardiograms, phonocardiograms, and x-ray films in this patient. Although no special search for calcified subcutaneous spherules typical of E-D was made by x-ray, one such body, oval in shape, was visible on chest x-ray examination in the skin of the left upper arm.

The patient died suddenly at home about five months after these studies. Autopsy was not performed.

Another of my patients has a bilateral congenital anomaly of the ureteropelvic junction (Fig. 5-4*F*). In the case of Marfan's syndrome it was pointed out that there are a number of manifestations which are congenital malformations in the conventional sense and which occur often enough to be considered bona fide components of the syndrome. It was proposed that these are secondary mani-

---

*I am indebted to Dr. John G. Smith of Rocky Mount, N. C. for making the diagnosis of the Ehlers-Danlos syndrome and referring the patient to the Johns Hopkins Hospital.

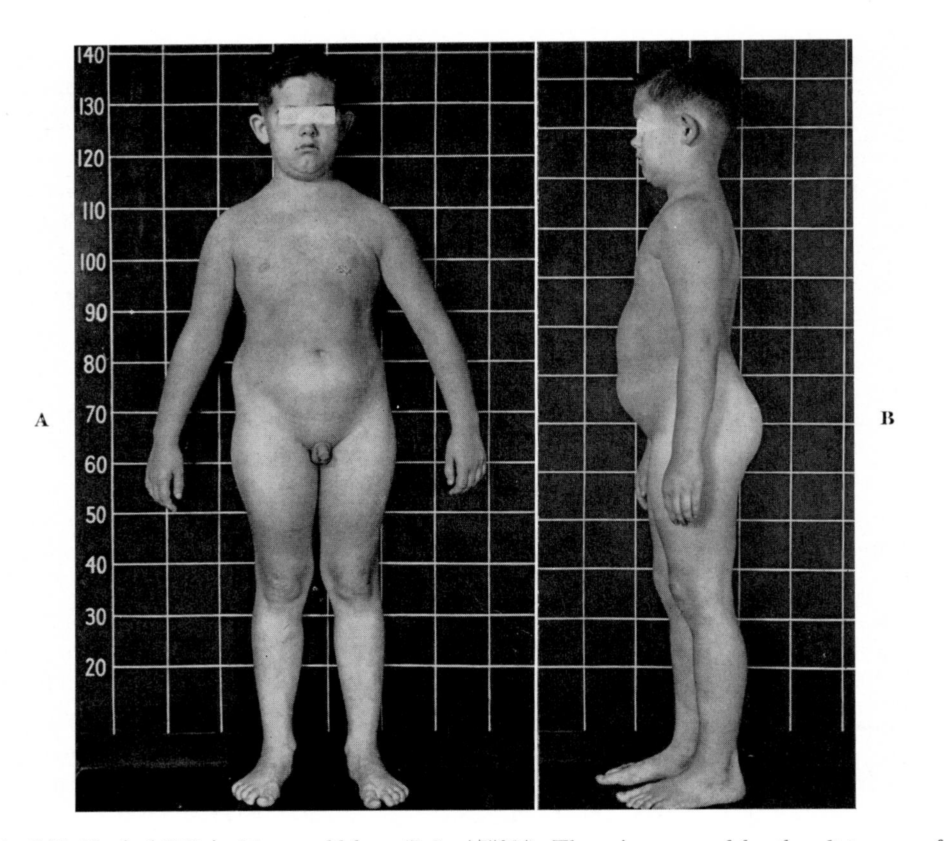

Fig. 5-17. Typical E-D in 10-year-old boy (J. I., A75064). There is a normal brother $1\frac{1}{2}$ years of age. The mother and father are unaffected and no similar cases are identified in the family of either parent. There is striking fragility of the skin as evidenced by many scars, e.g. of the knees, forehead, and shins. The wounds, of which dozens have occurred, are almost round, and subcutaneous areolar tissue herniates up through the break in the epidermis. The joints are strikingly hyperextensile. When not bearing weight, the pedal arches appear higher than normal, but with bearing weight the feet become strikingly flat. There is knobby redundancy of the skin of soles, especially around the heels. The fragility and hyperelasticity extend to the buccal and lingual mucosa (at one time stitches had to be taken in a cut in the tongue) and possibly to the pharyngeal and laryngeal areas, where redundancy of the mucosal lining appears to be responsible for a chronic cough, especially during the winter months. The ears are large and "floppy," with less prominent landmarks than is normally the case. There is bilaterally an epicanthal fold. The skin under the chin is loose and redundant. Bilateral cervical ribs are present; members of the father's family show this anomaly. Easy bruising has been a striking feature. The patient is less active than normal because of voluntary restriction and has become somewhat obese as a result. The regular use of bandages of the legs has helped avoid much trouble with cuts on the shins. Biopsy of skin and skeletal muscle in the left pectoral area revealed increase in the number of elastic fibers in the corium and in the perimyal areas. Some of the arteries showed what appeared to be anomalous elastic fibers. **A,** Front view. **B,** Lateral view. Note the scars of the face and knees, the knobby appearance of the soles, the flat feet, the peculiarly shaped pinnae, and the epicanthal folds. **C,** Loose collagen meshwork and unusually abundant elastic fibers (stained black) in the subcutaneous area overlying pectoral muscle (Verhoeff-van Giesen stain; ×200; reduced 3/7). **D,** Increased elastic fibers in small artery in pectoral muscle (Verhoeff-van Giesen stain; ×200; reduced 3/7).

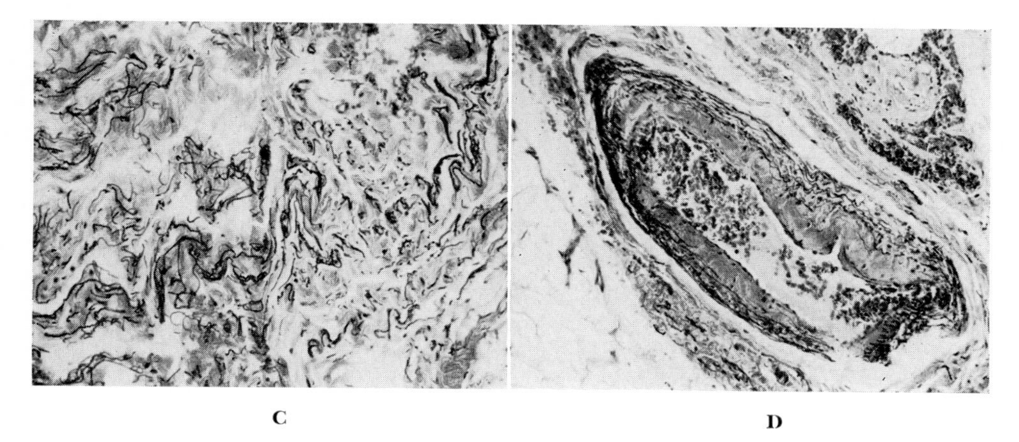

Fig. 5-17, cont'd. For legend see opposite page.

festations, that the hereditary disorder of connective tissue creates an ontogenetic setting in which certain predictable congenital anomalies occur with increased frequency. In E-D, ureteropelvic anomaly, tetralogy of Fallot, and interatrial defect may fall into this category of secondary manifestations. However, since, to my knowledge, each has been described in only one patient, it is equally reasonable to suspect that these manifestations may have occurred by coincidence.

Spina bifida occulta has been described fairly frequently.[74,108,115] Furthermore, the dental anomalies may be interpreted as falling into this category of malformations that are secondary manifestations of the basic connective tissue defect. The teeth may be irregularly formed,[93] irregularly positioned,[59,88,147] abnormally small,[92,106,129] or even absent. Crenation of the incisors has been noted.[97,106]

As a rule, mental retardation is not a feature of this syndrome. However, occasionally patients show it, probably as a coincidentally associated finding.[92,97] Severe essential hypertension occurred in one patient as a probable incidental finding.[83]

Pathology

In none of the seven main disorders of connective tissue discussed in this series is the microscopic anatomy in such a disputed state as in E-D.[88]

Increase in elastic tissue of the corium has been described by many writers.[5,13,80,108,109,130,131,140,153,161,164] Some of these described morphologic abnormalities of the elastic fibers, as did Smith[151] and Pittinos,[128] who, however, did not consider the elastic fibers to be more numerous than normal. Williams[183] and Pautrier[124] found the elastic fibers *normal,* and Brown and Stock[16] believed them to be *decreased.*

Diminution and morphologic abnormalities of collagen fibers have been described.[120,151,164] Katz and Steiner[83] report histochemical studies that they interpret as indicating increase of mucopolysaccharide of corium.

Studying skin biopsies from three cases of E-D, Wechsler and Fisher[176] confirmed a relative decrease in collagen and increase in elastic tissue. Other histochemical stains, enzyme studies (with elastase and pepsin), and electron microscopic studies of collagen periodicity showed no differences from the normal.

Jansen[76] points out, with excellent illustrations, that "in normal skin, a system of robust, well directed, crossing and tightly interlacing collagen fibre bundles is present. The whorled disorderly structure in hyperelastic (E-D) skin is remarkable; the collagen bundles seem to have been insufficiently united." By electron microscopy collagen and elastin were morphologically normal. This corroborates the finding of Tunbridge and collaborators,[168] but Jansen was unable to agree that there was an absolute increase in the number of elastic fibers.

Collections of giant cells are sometimes found.[139] The subcutaneous nodules or spherules are apparently fat-containing cysts.[175] They frequently become calcified. It seems likely that they are related to minor traumata and to the general fragility of the connective tissue in which the fat deposits normally exist. Molluscoid pseudotumors that develop at pressure points are characterized by cyst formation.[74]

How much of the bleeding is due to a defect in the supporting tissues and how much due to weakness of the vessel walls themselves is not clarified by histologic studies. Abnormal, dilated, weak-appearing vessels have been described by Tobias[164] and by others.[97] An abnormality (Fig. 5-17*D*) of the connective tissue of the wall of small arteries was demonstrated in one of my cases, and similar changes are seen in Fig. 21 of Jansen's report.[74]

Unfortunately, studies of tissues other than skin have not been reported, with the exception of an autopsy case described by Leinhart,[97] one by Nicod,[115] two by McFarland and Fuller[103] and, of course, the cases of dissecting aneurysm described above. In Leinhart's patient, a 22-year-old woman who died of pulmonary tuberculosis, no internal abnormality referable to the connective tissue defect was discovered. Nicod[115] studied bone and cartilage and could detect no abnormality.

Behar and Rachmilewitz[6] described arterial changes in a 32-year-old male with E-D. Since the patient died of chronic glomerulonephritis, the changes may have been exaggerated by the accompanying hypertension. The findings consisted of hypoplasia and aplasia of the internal elastic lamina, multiple dissections of the aorta, pulmonary artery, and atrial endocardium, and Erdheim's cystic medial necrosis of the aorta.

The basic defect

Superficial consideration of the clinical manifestations of E-D might suggest an abnormality of elastic tissue as the fundamental defect, probably a superabundance of elastic fibers in the skin and joint capsules. However, the histologic studies by no means afford unequivocal substantiation of this theory. Brown and Stock[16] suggested and others (notably, and most recently, Jansen[76]) maintain[57] that the defect may reside in the collagen fibers which, because of lack of normal tensile strength, permit the skin, joint capsules, ligaments, and so forth to be stretched beyond the normal limits. The elastic fibers may function in connection with the process of restoration to normal configuration of these tissues. According to the "collagen theory," the histologic changes, both quantitative and qualitative, are interpretable as secondary effects of the abnormality of collagen. I am

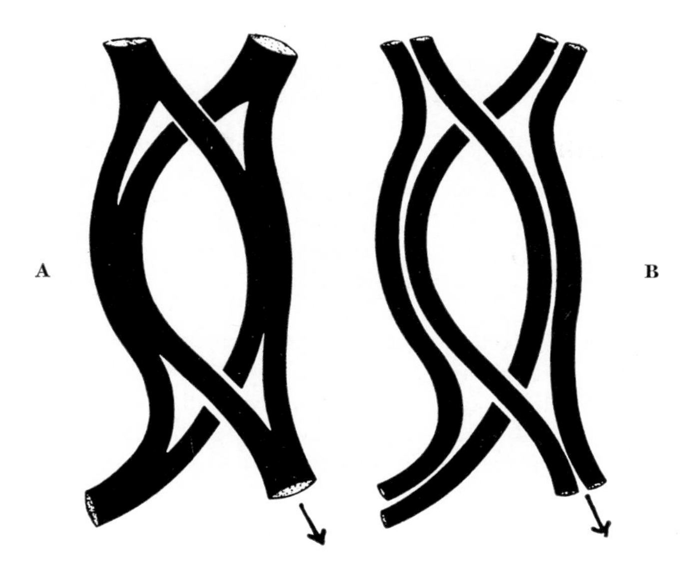

Fig. 5-18. Jansen's schematic representation of the postulated defect in collagen fasciculation in E-D. **A,** Normal. **B,** E-D syndrome. (From Jansen, L. H.: Dermatologica **110:**108, 1955.)

inclined to favor the view that the Ehlers-Danlos syndrome is another heritable disorder of collagen, biochemically, morphologically, clinically, and, of course, genetically distinct from the others which are under discussion in this book.

The comparative inextensibility of normal collagen may depend upon some specific molecular or intermolecular structure which is altered in E-D, with resulting increase in extensibility. This is assumed to be the case in the theory of Brown and Stock and has been explicitly stated by Froelich[56] and by others. Jansen[76] has recently advanced a related theory, incriminating collagen but placing the defect at a higher level of organization of collagen—that E-D is a disorder of the organization of collagen fibrils into bundles and of the bundles into a strong network. He refers to the disease as one of a "defective wicker-work" of collagen. The evidence he assembles (see discussion of pathology) and the clinical aspects of the disease outlined here make Jansen's version of the "collagen theory" highly probable.

It is possible that, in some patients and at some subcutaneous and articular locations, production of an excessive number of elastic fibers is stimulated by the repeated and excessive stretching. In tissue culture, Maximow[107] and Bloom[10] thought the tugging of contractile myocardial cells was a factor in the formation of elastic fibers.

The changes that occur in the skin of the feet and hands and at the elbows of older patients fit in well with the view that the primary defect resides in the collagen fibers: the normal elastic tissue may, with the passage of time, "wear out" from excessive stress imposed upon it, and the cutis laxa (as opposed to cutis hyperelastica) of late cases become evident.

In Hungary, Banga and Baló,[4] who discovered the elastolytic enzyme in pancreas, also demonstrated that normal serum contains an elastase inhibitor. In Tunbridge's department in Leeds, Hall and Saxl[67] found in two patients with

E-D a concentration of elastase inhibitor in the blood that was "between 50 and 100 times as great as that in pooled normal serum." Carter and Walford[25] could, however, demonstrate no increase in elastase inhibitor in seven patients.

Prevalence and inheritance

Thus far, this syndrome has been described principally in Europeans and persons of European extraction. There is one report from India[26] of the disease in a 12-year-old Hindu girl. The disorder has been seen in Japan.[121] In addition to those reported here, a number of Negro cases of E-D have been reported.[17,36,105]

Schaper[147] stated in 1952 that only ninety-three cases of this syndrome had been reported. Although the number is now probably well in excess of 150, it is possible that fewer of these cases have been reported than of any of the other syndromes discussed in this series. This is, in part, the result of greater difficulties of recognizing the syndrome, since cutaneous and articular hyperelasticity is a graded trait. I hazard to say, however, that in actuality this is one of the most frequent of the heritable disorders of connective tissue. My photographer, in the course of the study of other patients with E-D, recalled that his brother-in-law could do contortionist tricks with his hands. On investigation this individual was found to have had congenital dislocation of the right hip, bilateral inguinal hernias, diaphragmatic hernia, and trouble with one knee and the right wrist (Fig. 5-8). Although these had all been considered unrelated, the diagnosis of the Ehlers-Danlos syndrome is quite certain and all these manifestations are clearly part of the syndrome. This patient illustrates how easy it is to overlook the generalized disorder.

In a majority of the kindreds I have studied, now numbering over thirty, multiple members are affected and, in most, affected persons were found in successive generations. Since mild manifestations tend to be overlooked by laymen and since only the propositus was examined in several instances, the above evidence can be taken only as a rough indication of autosomal dominant inheritance.

In 1949 Johnson and Falls[80] reviewed sixteen families reported in the literature as having more than one affected member.[65,86] In these families, a total of eighty affected individuals had been identified, of whom exactly half were male. Brown[15] found nineteen affected members in a family numbering forty-seven individuals. Johnson and Falls[80] studied the pattern of inheritance in detail and concluded that the disorder is inherited as a dominant. Two sisters with an unusually severe form of the disease were children of cousins, each with a mild form of the disease; this suggested to the authors that the trait might have occurred in homozygous state in these girls. Consanguinity was thought to be a factor in the cases observed by Ronchese[140] and by Weber and Aitken.[175] For an extensive review of most of the published pedigrees, see Jansen.[74,75]

Although the survey of the literature by Johnson and Falls[80] indicated a sex ratio of one, in the kindred they studied personally there were twenty-one affected males and eleven affected females. Furthermore, Jansen,[75] on the basis of a more extensive survey, concluded that the incidence of this disorder is consistently higher in males.

Coe and Silver[29] and Ormsby and Tobin[120] presented illustrations of members of three generations displaying the E-D syndrome; Stuart,[154] Mories,[110] and Husebye[71] traced it through four generations; the largest pedigree is that of Johnson and Falls,[80] with six generations affected. Here there was again clear evidence of dominant inheritance. The disease has been described in one of twins who were probably fraternal.[42]

Penetrance in this disease is probably considerably lower than in Marfan's disease, for example. This, however, is merely the result of the greater difficulty of recognizing mild and graded abnormality of the joints and skin as opposed to less equivocal manifestations, e.g. ectopia lentis, in Marfan's syndrome.

As always, the possibility of the existence of more than one genotype in this disease must be kept prominently in mind. Some minor phenotypic differences—for example, the lack of skin fragility in cases such as that shown in Fig. 5-15—suggest this possibility but are not sufficiently clear-cut to make one certain. Somatic mutation is a possible explanation for unilateral involvement, as in the famous case of van Meekeren. However, there are no clearly described similarly unilateral cases reported in recent times. That of Du Bois[44] is too sketchily reported to permit analysis.

Miscellaneous considerations

"Simple" hypermobility of joints, known also as congenital laxity of ligaments, may occur as an isolated finding,[23,32,84,137,156] with a genetic background distinct from that in E-D. For example, in Key's family[84] sex-linked inheritance was mistakenly suggested; the disorder occurred only in males, but male-to-male transmission was observed. Loose-jointedness occurs also in the Marfan syndrome and with osteogenesis imperfecta, whereas reduced joint mobility is characteristic of the Hurler syndrome. In the differential diagnosis of loose-jointedness, especially in children, cerebrocortical degeneration or malformation, mongolism, cretinism, rickets, and nonspecific cachexia must be kept in mind. Carter and Wilkinson[24] emphasized the importance of persistent joint laxity in the occurrence of congenital dislocation of the hip.

Hass and Hass[69] suggest that there is a distinct entity of loose-jointedness or, as they term it, *arthrochalasis multiplex congenita,* which is a "constitutional dyscrasia of mesenchyme," has wide variability and severity, and may occur with or without skin changes. In this view E-D is apparently construed as merely those cases of arthrochalasis multiplex congenita in which skin involvement happens to be present. It seems more likely, however, that there are a number of genetic causes of loose-jointedness, and that although E-D may occur without much or any skin change, most cases do show changes in both the skin and joints.

Ellis and Bundick[48] have measured joint mobility in 500 subjects, about half male, half female, spanning eight decades of age. The gauge of mobility was extensibility of the fifth finger as shown in Fig. 5-19*A*. The subject placed his extended hand on a flat surface with the forearm parallel to the examining surface. The examiner then extended the fifth finger as far as comfortably possible and measured the angle made by the proximal phalanx with the flat surface with a protractor to the closest multiple of 15 degrees. The results are charted in Fig. 5-19*B* and *C*. Most children have a high degree of mobility. Between ages 15 and 50 years a high degree of mobility is considerably more frequent in female subjects than in males. Although no quantitative study of the subject has been

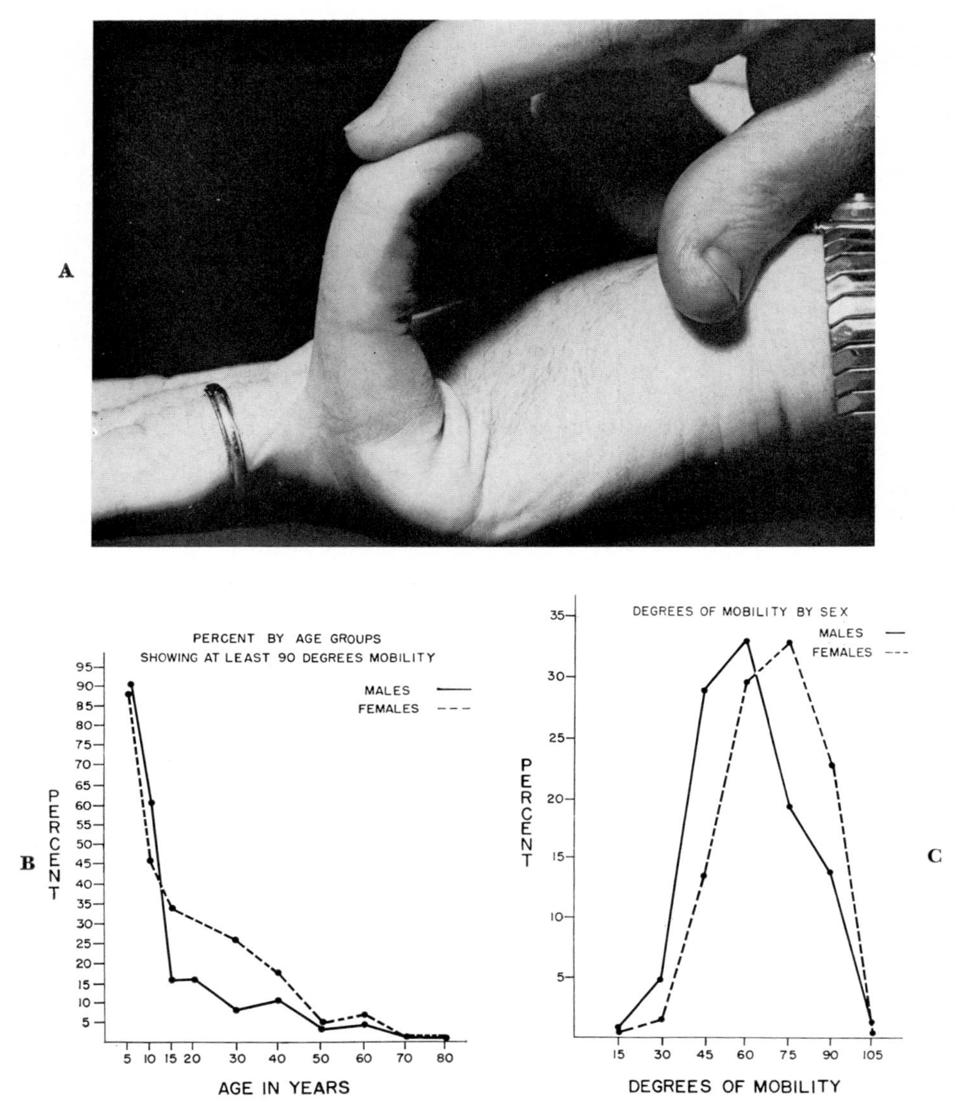

Fig. 5-19. A, The Ellis-Bundick method for quantifying joint mobility. **B** and **C,** Joint mobility by age and sex, as determined by the Ellis-Bundick method in 500 subjects. **B,** Most young children under 5 years of age show at least 90-degree mobility. In the groups of intermediate age the incidence is appreciably greater in women. **C,** Female subjects show higher grades of mobility. (**B** and **C** from Ellis, F. A., and Bundick, W. R.: Arch. Derm. **74:**22, 1956.)

made, there is a clinical impression that Negroes are more loose-jointed than whites.

Measures of joint elasticity and other characteristics such as plasticity and viscosity will be valuable in the study of E-D. Promising progress in the quantitation of loose-jointedness and delineation of the components of joint stiffness has been made by Wright and Johns.[78,79,184]

Interesting physiologic studies of skin elasticity and tensile strength have been done in recent years.[40,41,77,86,118,139,179] Skin elasticity can be measured with the "pinchmeter" of Olmsted and associates[117] or the elastometer of Schade or by the simple although subjective method of Ellis and Bundick.[48] In this last technique, the skin of the dorsum of the wrist is elevated between the forefinger and thumb and relative elasticity estimated. Normal elasticity is indicated by 2+, reduced elasticity by 1+, and increased elasticity by 3+. Scleroderma on this scale is 0 and full-blown E-D, 4+. Rollhäuser[139] found least tensile strength in the skin of infants under 3 months (about 0.25 kg. per square millimeter); more in adults (about 1.6 kg. per square millimeter); and yet more in aged individuals (over 2 kg. per square millimeter). With aging, furthermore, skin became progressively less extensible. These observations may explain the tendency for the cutaneous fragility and extensibility in E-D to become less striking as the affected individual ages. Rollhäuser[139] studied the skin tensile strength of a 35-year-old man with E-D and found it to be very low (0.34 kg. per square millimeter). It is of interest that this worker found parallel changes in the tensile strength and extensibility of tendons, suggesting that the properties measured in the skin may be constitutional and generalized. Wenzel[179] found lesser tensile strength in female skin and made important observations indicating reduction in the strength of the skin in normal pregnancy and in Cushing's syndrome. In connection with the latter condition, it is noteworthy that the fragility of the skin and easy bruisability are rather similar in E-D and in Cushing's syndrome.[89] However, in all likelihood, the similarity is only superficial.

Blue sclerae are not uncommon in E-D,[13,46] and presence of this feature cannot be taken as evidence of associated osteogenesis imperfecta. Biering and Iversen[9] have reported a more convincing case of association of the two connective tissue disorders. There was no familial history of manifestations of osteogenesis imperfecta, but in the father's line there was joint and skin hyperextensibility. The description[75,97,138] of associated dolichostenomelia (long, thin extremities as in the Marfan syndrome) cannot be taken as evidence that E-D and the Marfan syndrome coincided in those patients, since no ectopia lentis was detected and no unequivocal cases of the Marfan disease in other members of the family were described.

At least three seemingly bona fide instances of coincident E-D and pseudoxanthoma elasticum have been described.[31,116,125] In Cottini's patient[31] there were angioid streaks, and lesions of the skin of the neck characteristic of pseudoxanthoma elasticum (Chapter 8); in addition there were cigarette paper scars of the elbows and knees and hyperextensible skin and joints characteristic of E-D. The pseudoxanthoma elasticum, which appears to be a recessive trait, was not transmitted to a daughter who suffered from acrocyanosis or to a son who had hyperextensible skin and joints, hernia, and varices of the leg veins. The 22-year-old woman described by Pelbois and Rollier[125] consulted them because of the cosmetically undesirable lesions of pseudoxanthoma elasticum involving the skin of the neck and other areas of flexure. As well as angioid streaks of the fundus (characteristic of pseudoxanthoma), the patient had multiple cicatrices indicative of cutaneous fragility, striking cutaneous hyperelasticity, and articular hypermobility. The parents were first cousins, a fact significant in the appearance of the recessive trait, pseudoxanthoma. The parents were themselves unaffected by pseudoxanthoma, although a maternal aunt of the patient was affected. As for E-D, the patient's mother displayed features of this syndrome and had probably transmitted it as a dominant trait to her daughter. These are, then, examples of accidental coincidence of the two syndromes, one behaving as a dominant and one as a recessive trait.

There is a distinct, although less well defined, entity to which the name *cutis laxa* can be specifically applied.[135] The unusual patient described by Rossbach in 1885[96] was probably in this category; in his discussion he also mentioned what was probably a true case of E-D and, in fact, the same case described later by Kopp.[87] In cutis laxa the skin hangs in inelastic folds (see references 48 and 135 for striking illustrations). Associated pulmonary emphysema, resulting in death, has been described in an infant with cutis laxa.[27] Some of the cases may be acquired, being secondary probably to inflammation, whereas other are congenital. Some of the latter group may have a genetic basis. Carney and Nomland[21] described a patient with pronounced looseness of the skin, prolapse of the uterus, relaxed abdomen, and such pronounced redundancy of the skin over the eyes that she had to suspend it with cellophane tape to see. The skin in pseudoxanthoma elasticum acquires the character of cutis laxa in extreme cases (Fig. 8-14, pp. 304 and 305). Cutis laxa (also called dermatochalasia and chalasoderma) in association with a form of dysostosis is discussed on p. 426.

In one patient, 61 years old,[114] E-D coexisted with muscular atrophy of the Aran-Duchenne type (amyotrophic lateral sclerosis). I find it impossible to agree with the authors[114] that an etiologic connection between the two conditions existed. In one of my cases, Oppenheim's disease (amyotonia congenita)[66] was the original diagnosis when the patient was first seen at the age of 4 years. Abnormality of creatine metabolism was reported in one patient,[128] and in another[126] there was coincident parathyroid tumor with osteitis fibrosa cystica. After correction of the hyperparathyroidism surgically, it appeared that the joint laxity, particularly the scoliosis, and the fragility of the skin decreased.

The Bonnevie-Ullrich-Turner syndrome[90] often has hyperelasticity of joints and skin as a feature. Furthermore, the skin of the hands may be loose and wrinkled as an aftermath of the lymphedema that is frequently present in the first year or so after birth. (More characteristic features are dwarfism, webbing of the neck, cubitus valgus, gonadal dysgenesis, and female phenotype with male sex chromatin pattern and usually XO sex chromosome constitution.) Rossi and colleagues[142,143] have emphasized the similar features. Rossi and Angst[142] write as follows: "The Ehlers-Danlos syndrome sufficiently closely resembles the pterygium syndrome that the former should be considered a forerunner of the latter." Although it is probably far-fetched to presume any fundamental relationship, the possibility of diagnostic confusion cannot be disputed.

In recent years a group of patients with what might be termed pseudo Turner's syndrome have been recognized. These are female patients with short stature, low-set ears, low posterior hairline, facial features reminiscent of the Turner syndrome, sometimes webbing of the neck, and short, square hands and feet with wrinkled skin of the palms and sole. Lymphedema of the feet may be present in early life or appear in the teens. However, secondary sex characters are normally developed, menstruation is normal, and sex chromatin and chromosomes are those of the normal female. Congenital malformation of the heart,

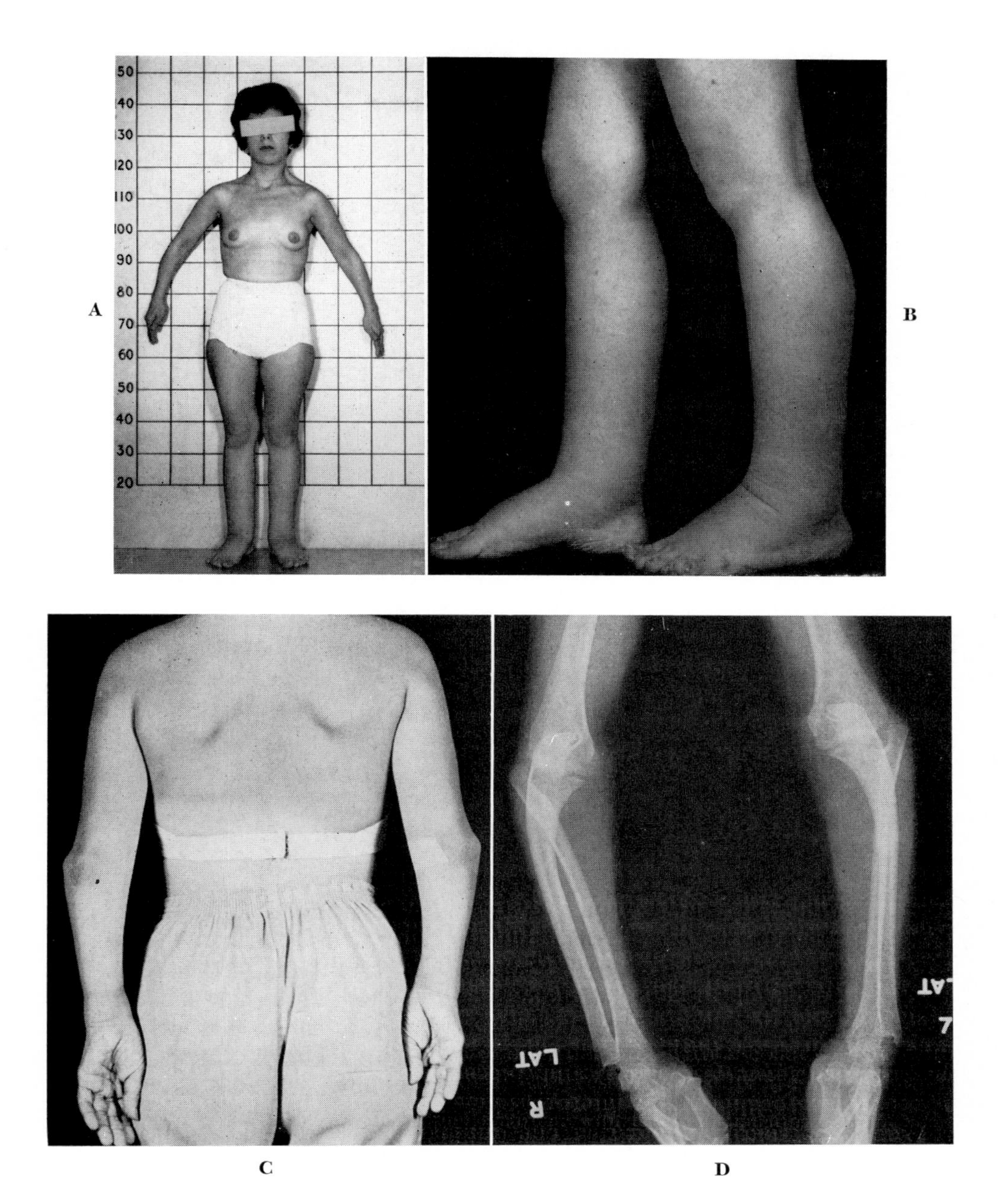

Fig. 5-20. Case of the female pseudo Turner syndrome with features simulating E-D. **A,** Short stature, low-set ears, and leg edema. **B,** Lymphedema shown here and in **A** probably is aggravated only to a minor extent by the heart disease. Secondary sexual characteristics are normally developed. **C,** Bilateral posterior dislocation of radial heads.[28] **D,** X-ray film of same. **E,** Hands. Note the loose, coarse-grained appearance of the skin. **F,** Feet. **G,** Chest x-ray film. Note cardiomegaly. **H,** Spectral phonocardiogram showing systolic and diastolic murmurs. The same auscultatory findings were present at the left lower sternal border and apex. **I,** Electrocardiogram.

Continued.

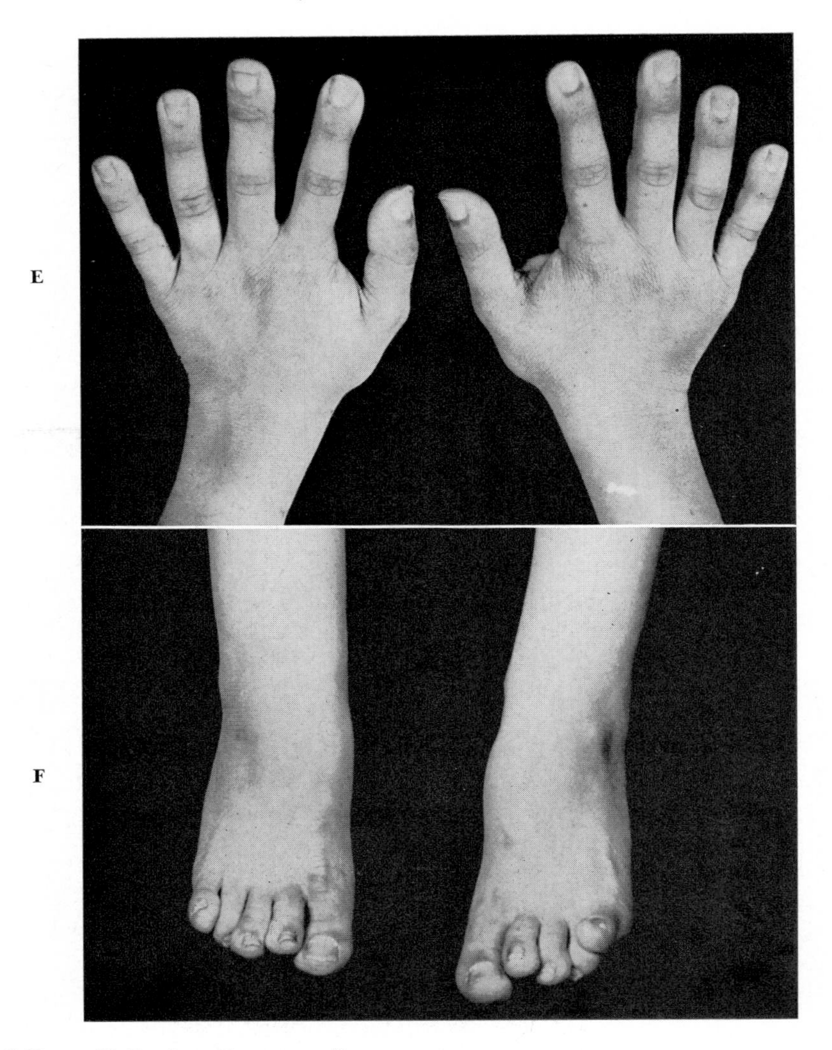

Fig. 5-20, cont'd. For legend see preceding page.

particularly pulmonary stenosis, is present in many. A similar syndrome occurs in males and is called the male Turner syndrome; in these cases the chromosomal findings have usually been those of a normal male.

Several of the features of the disorder suggest the Ehlers-Danlos syndrome. Patient C. E. (Fig. 5-20*A* to *I*), who was presented earlier (1960) as a case of E-D with cardiac malformation, is more likely an example of the pseudo Turner syndrome.

C. E. (B32309; 745114), a white female born in 1939, was first seen in this hospital in 1956 for opinion on her heart condition and for plastic surgery.

Apparently no other members of her family have skin, joint, or cardiac changes similar to hers. The parents and brother and sister are of average stature. Various members of the father's family were short. For example, the paternal grandfather was only five feet tall.

The patient was "very flabby" at birth. X-ray films were taken in the first days of life,

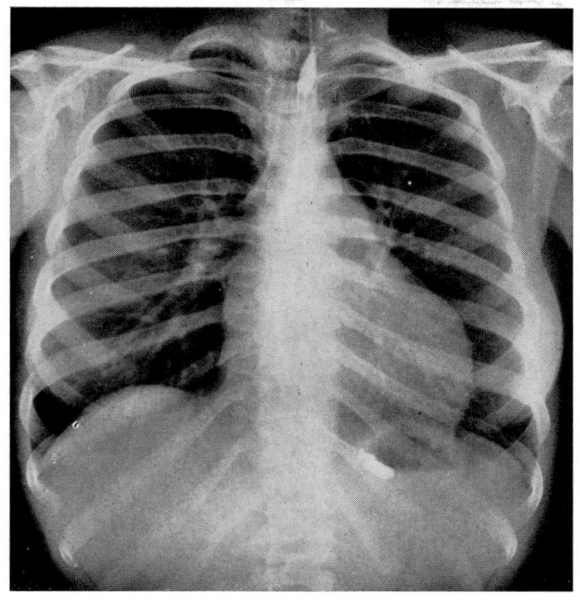

G

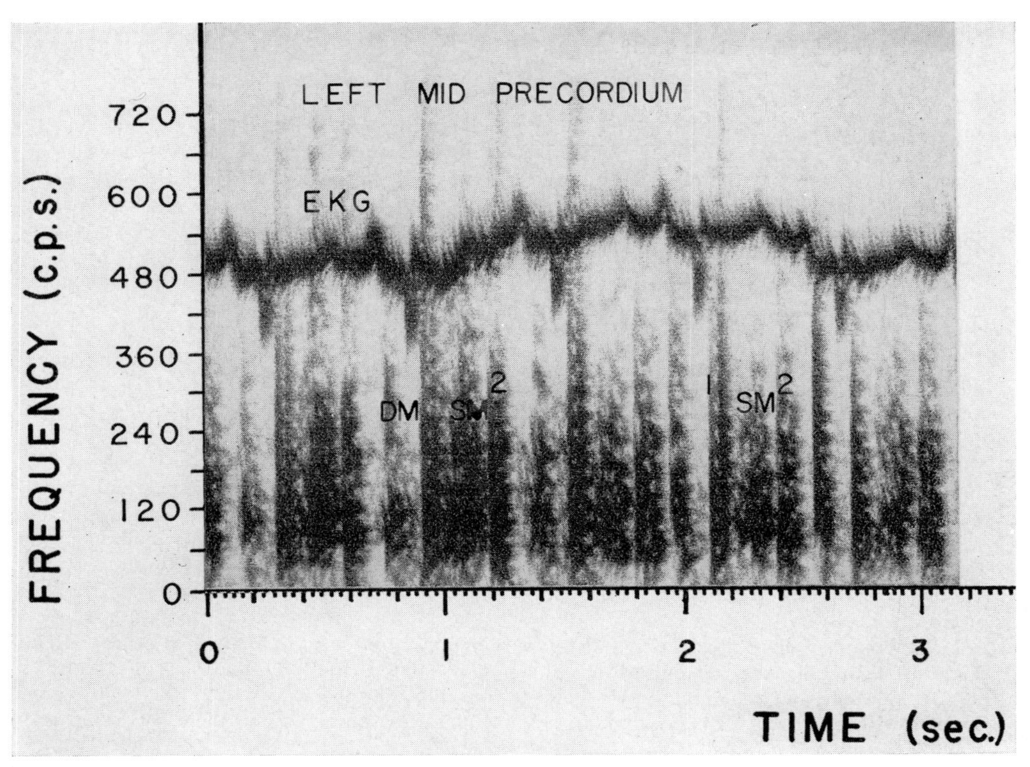

H

Fig. 5-20, cont'd. For legend see p. 219.

Continued.

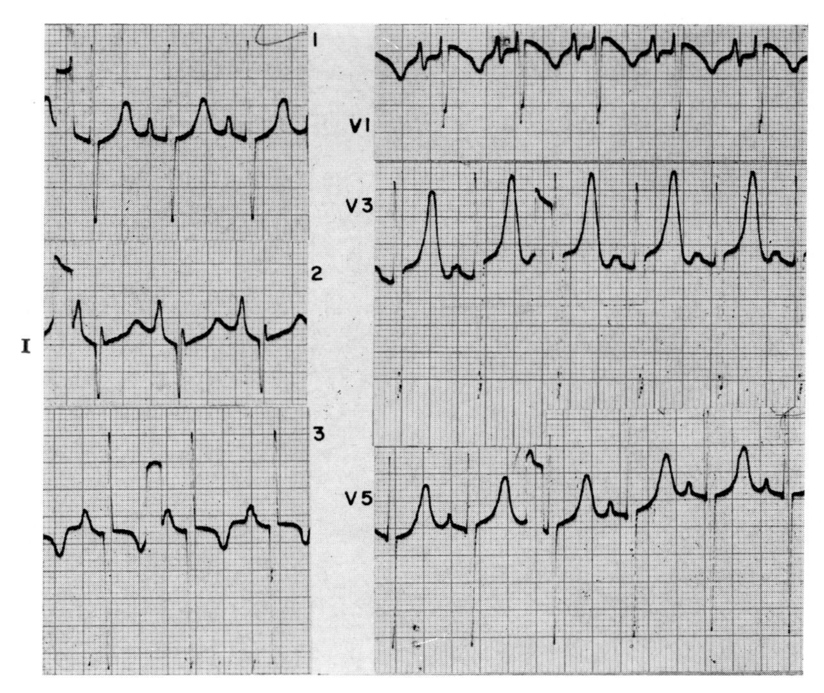

Fig 5-20, cont'd. For legend see p. 219.

probably because of dislocation of the elbows and possibly other joints (Fig. 5-20 *C* and *D*). No mention of a murmur or other sign of cardiac abnormality was made to the parents until the patient was 15 months old. At that time she was still flabby and did not stand or walk. The flabbiness was no longer apparent after the age of 9 or 10 years. An endocrinopathy, probably hypopituitarism, was suspected, mainly because of the short stature. However, sexual maturation occurred normally.

The patient lived a sheltered life. Palpitation was the only symptom definitely attributable to the heart. Both systolic and diastolic murmurs are known to have been present from the age of 10 years. At that time she weighed only 43 pounds and was 45 inches tall.

Physical examination in 1956 revealed an intelligent girl only 56 inches tall. There were generalized hypermobility of the joints and elasticity of the skin. The head of each radius was dislocated posteriorly. The patient could not extend the elbow beyond a point 18 degrees from full extension. Pronation of the wrists and forearms was moderately impaired.

The nose was hooked. Malocclusion with narrowing of the anterior vertical arch of the hard palate was present. The pinnae were also mildly deformed; they were low in position and rotated so that the lobule was located somewhat anteriorly to the external meatus and helix.

The heart was enlarged to the left anterior axillary line. The auscultatory findings were dominated by bizarre murmurs, in systole and diastole, of a scratchy quality, suggesting pericardial friction rub (Fig. 5-20 *H*). The murmurs were maximal at the apex and left midprecordium.

Photographs, electrocardiograms, phonocardiograms, and x-ray films are presented in Fig. 5-20 *C* to *I*. Angiocardiograms revealed dilatation of the entire right side of the heart.

Rhinoplasty and repair of both elbows by resection of the heads of the radii were performed with success. Healing after surgery was perfectly normal, and there were no late complications.

Surgery in the Ehlers-Danlos syndrome has often been accompanied by wound dehiscence[72,122] (Fig. 5-8). The tissues may be strikingly friable and hold sutures poorly. Hemostasis may be a problem. With particular care, Ricketson[132] was able to repair a large flaplike wound of the right shin; the scars of the other shin were removed and likewise replaced by a split-thickness graft with excellent results. Thoracoplasty was successfully performed in one patient with severe E-D.[141]

Almost always the skin and joint changes in E-D are evident from an early age. However, Jacobs[72] described a patient in whom the manifestations seemed quite clearly to appear first at the age of 29 years. Although the patient had been a pugilist, no friability of the skin had been noted earlier. A brother was also affected.

SUMMARY

The cardinal manifestations of the Ehlers-Danlos syndrome are loose-jointedness; hyperextensibility; fragility and bruisability of the skin, with "cigarette-paper" scarring; and generalized friability of tissues. Internal manifestations include rupture of great vessels; diaphragmatic and other hernias; gastrointestinal diverticula; friability of the bowel, leading to spontaneous rupture; and rupture of the lung with mediastinal emphysema and/or pneumothorax.

The basic defect is thought to concern the organization of collagen bundles into an intermeshing network.

The Ehlers-Danlos syndrome is inherited as an autosomal dominant trait.

REFERENCES

1. Adams, F.: The genuine works of Hippocrates, New York, 1891, William Wood & Co.; Airs, waters, and places, paragraphs 20 and 22, vol. 1, pp. 176-178.
2. Agostini, A.: Cited by Jansen.[74]
3. Angst, H.: Das Ehlers-Danlos Syndrom, Dissertation, Zürich, 1951. Cited by Jansen.[74]
4. Banga, I., and Baló, J.: Elastin and elastase, Nature (London) **171**:44, 1953.
5. Barber, H. S., Fiddes, J., and Benians, T. H. C.: The syndrome of Ehlers-Danlos, Brit. J. Derm. **53**:97, 1941.
6. Behar, A., and Rachmilewitz, E.: Ellis-van Creveld syndrome, Arch. Intern. Med. **113**:606 1964.
7. Benjamin, B., and Weiner, H.: Syndrome of cutaneous fragility and hyperelasticity and articular hyperlaxity, Amer. J. Dis. Child. **65**:247, 1943.
8. Bernard, J., Bassett, A., and Duperrat, B.: Syndrome de fragilité cutanée avec hémorragies multiples, Bull. Soc. Franc. Derm. Syph. **61**:486, 1954.
9. Biering, A., and Iversen, T.: Osteogenesis imperfecta associated with Ehlers-Danlos syndrome, Acta Paediat. **44**:279, 1955.
10. Bloom, W.: Studies on fibers in tissue culture. II. The development of elastic fibers in cultures of embryonic heart and aorta, Arch. Exp. Zellforsch. **9**:6, 1929.
11. Bolam, R. M.: A case of Ehlers-Danlos syndrome, Brit. J. Derm. **50**:174, 1938.
12. Bonnet, P.: Les manifestations oculaires de la maladie d'Ehlers-Danlos, Bull. Soc. Franc. Ophtal. **1**:211, 1953.
13. Bossu, A., and Lambrechts: Manifestations oculaires du syndrome d'Ehlers-Danlos, Ann. Oculist (Paris) **187**:227, 1954.
14. Brombart, M., Coupatez, G., and Laurent, Y.: Contribution à l'étude de l'étiologie de la hernie hiatale et de la diverticulose du tube digestif; un cas de maladie d'Ehlers-Danlos associée à une hernie hiatale, un diverticule de l'estomac, un diverticule duodénal, une diverticulose colique et une anémie sidéropénique, Arch. Mal. Appar. Dig. **41**:413, 1952.
15. Brown, A.: Ehlers-Danlos syndrome; description of 3 cases, Glasgow Med. J. **27**:7, 1946.
16. Brown, A., and Stock, V. F.: Dermatorrhexis; report of a case, Amer. J. Dis. Child. **54**:956, 1937.

17. Bruno, M. S., and Narashimhan, P.: The Ehlers-Danlos syndrome: a report of four cases in two generations of a Negro family, New Eng. J. Med. **264**:274, 1961.
18. Burrows, A.: Epidermolysis bullosa with cutis hyperelastica, Proc. Roy. Soc. Med. **25**:1319, 1932.
19. Burrows, A., and Turnbull, H. M.: Cutis hyperelastica (Ehlers-Danlos syndrome), Brit. J. Derm. **50**:648, 1938.
20. Burton, A. C.: Relation of structure to function of the tissues of the wall of blood vessels, Physiol. Rev. **34**:619, 1954.
21. Carney, R. G., and Nomland, R.: Acquired loose skin (chalazoderma): report of a case, Arch. Derm Syph. **56**:794, 1947.
22. Carter, C. O., and Sweetman, R.: Familial joint laxity and recurrent dislocation of the patella, J. Bone Joint Surg. **40-B**:664, 1958.
23. Carter, C. O., and Sweetman, R.: Recurrent dislocation of the patella and of the shoulder, J. Bone Joint Surg. **42-B**:721, 1960.
24. Carter, C. O., and Wilkinson, J.: Persistent joint laxity and congenital dislocation of the hip, J. Bone Joint Surg. **46-B**:40, 1964.
25. Carter P. K., and Walford, R. L.: Serum elastase inhibitor levels in Ehlers-Danlos syndrome, Ann. Rheum. Dis. **22**:198, 1963.
26. Chakraborty, A. N., Banerjee, A. K., and Ghosh, S.: Ehlers-Danlos syndrome (cutis hyperelastica), J. Indian Med. Ass. **23**:344, 1954.
27. Christiaens, L., Marchant-Alphant, A., and Fovet, A.: Emphysème congénital et cutis laxa, Presse Méd. **62**:1799, 1954.
28. Cockshott, W. P., and Omololu, A.: Familial congenital posterior dislocation of both radial heads, J. Bone Joint Surg. **40-B**:483, 1958.
29. Coe, M., and Silver, S. H.: Ehlers-Danlos syndrome (cutis hyperelastica), Amer. J. Dis. Child. **59**:129, 1940.
30. Corcelle and Fourcade: Maladie de Ehlers-Danlos et strabisme, Bull. Soc. Franc. Ophtal. **10**:931, 1956.
31. Cottini, G. B.: Association des syndromes de Groenblad-Strandberg et d'Ehlers-Danlos dans le même sujet, Acta Dermatovener. (Stockholm) **29**:544, 1949.
32. Coventry, M. B.: Some skeletal changes in the Ehlers-Danlos syndrome, J. Bone Joint Surg. **43-A**:855, 1961.
33. Crowe, J. F., Neel, J. V., and Schull, W. J.: A clinical and genetic study of multiple neurofibromatosis, Springfield, Ill., 1956, Charles C Thomas, Publisher, p. 112.
34. Danlos, M.: Un cas de cutis laxa avec tumeurs par contusion chronique des coudes et des genoux (xanthome juvenile pseudo-diabetique de M. M. Hallopeau et Mace de Lépinay), Bull. Soc. Franc. Derm. Syph. **19**:70, 1908.
35. Darier, M. J.: Notice nécrologiques sur M. Ehlers (1868-1937), Bull. Acad. Med. **117**:626, 1937.
36. Day, H. J., and Zarafonetis, C. J. D.: Coagulation studies in four patients with Ehlers-Danlos syndrome, Amer. J. Med. Sci. **242**:565, 1961.
37. Debré, R., Marie J., and Seringe, P.: "Cutis laxa" avec dystrophie osseuse, Bull. Soc. Méd. Hôp. Paris **61**:1038, 1937.
38. Debré, R., and Semelaigne, G.: A propos de la maladie d'Ehlers chez le nourrisson, Bull. Soc. Méd. Hôp. Paris **57**:849, 1936.
39. Dick, J. C.: Observations of the elastic tissue of the skin with a note on the reticular layer at the junction of the dermis and epidermis, J. Anat. **81**:201, 1947.
40. Dick, J. C.: The tension and resistance to stretching of human skin and other membranes, with results from a series of normal and edematous cases, J. Physiol. **112**:102, 1951.
41. Doerks, G.: Zur klinischen Prüfung der Hautdehnug, Arch. Kinderheilk. **136**:1, 1949.
42. Dorsch, H. H.: Ueber das Ehlers-Danlos-Syndrom, Veröffentlichung eines Falles bei einem Zwillingskind, Kinderaerztl. Prax. **21**:49, 1953.
43. Dreyfus, G., Weill, J., Martineau, J., and Mathivat, A.: Un cas de maladie d'Ehlers-Danlos, Bull. Soc. Méd. Hôp. Paris **52**:1463, 1936.
44. Du Bois: Cutis laxa (abstract), Zbl. f. Haut-u. Geschlkr. **35**:52, 1931.
45. Du Mesnil: Beitrag zur Anatomie und Aetiologie bestimmter Hautkrankheiten, Dissertation, Würzburg, 1880. Cited by Unna.[170]

46. Durham, D. G.: Cutis hyperelastica (Ehlers-Danlos syndrome) with blue scleras, microcornea, and glaucoma, Arch. Ophthal. **49**:220, 1953.
47. Ehlers, E.: Cutis laxa, Neigung zu Haemorrhagien in der Haut, Lockerung mehrerer Artikulationen, Derm. Zschr. **8**:173, 1901.
48. Ellis, F. A., and Bundick, W. R.: Cutaneous elasticity and hyperelasticity, Arch. Derm. **74**:22, 1956.
49. Ermert, W.: Das Ehlers-Danlos-Syndrom, Deutsch Med. Wschr. **85**:1386, 1960.
50. Fantl, P., Morris, K. N., and Sawers, R. J.: Repair of cardiac defect in patient with Ehlers-Danlos syndrome and deficiency of Hageman factor, Brit. Med. J. **1**:1202, 1961.
51. Flemming, J. W.: The Ehlers-Danlos syndrome, J. Florida Med. Ass. **42**:290, 1955.
52. François, P., Woillez, M., Warrot, and Maillet, P.: Maladie d'Ehlers-Danlos avec anévrysme artério-veineux intra-crânien. Bull. Soc. Franc. Ophtal. **5**:392, 1955.
53. Freeman, J. T.: Ehlers-Danlos syndrome, Amer. J. Dis. Child. **79**:1049, 1950.
54. Frick, P. G., and Krafchuk, J. D.: Studies of hemostasis in the Ehlers-Danlos syndrome, J. Invest. Derm. **26**:453, 1956.
55. Fritchey, J. A., and Greenbaum, S. S.: Two cases of Ehlers-Danlos syndrome, Arch. Derm. **42**:742, 1940.
56. Froelich, H.: Fibrodysplasia elastica generalisata (cutis laxa) und Nervensystem, Nervenarzt **20**:366, 1949.
57. Gadrat, J., and Bazex, A.: Sur le syndrome d'Ehlers-Danlos, Ann. Derm. Syph. **78**:430, 1951.
58. Geldmacher, M.: Ein Fall von Dystrophia adiposa generalisata mit Cutis laxa und hochgradiger Vulnerabilität der Haut, Inaugural Dissertation, Bonn, 1921. Cited by Jansen.[74]
59. Gilbert, A., Villaret, M., and Bosviel, G.: Sur un cas d'hyperélasticité congénitale des ligaments articularies et de la peau, Bull. Soc. Méd. Hôp. Paris **59**:303, 1925.
60. Glass, H. B.: Personal communication.
61. Goodman, R. M., Levitsky, J. M., and Friedman, I. A.: The Ehlers-Danlos syndrome and neurofibromatosis in a kindred of mixed derivation, with special emphasis on hemostasis in the Ehlers-Danlos syndrome, Amer. J. Med. **32**:976, 1962.
62. Gore, I.: Dissecting aneurysm of the aorta in persons under forty years of age. Arch. Path. **55**:1, 1953.
63. Gore, I., and Seiwert, V. S.: Dissecting aneurysm of the aorta; pathologic aspects; an analysis of 85 fatal cases, Arch. Path. **53**:121, 1952.
64. Gorlin, R. J., and Pindborg, J. J.: Syndromes of the head and neck, New York, 1964, McGraw-Hill Book Co., pp. 96-97.
65. Gould, G. M., and Pyle, W. L.: Anomalies and curiosities of medicine, Philadelphia, 1897, W. B. Saunders Co., p. 217.
66. Greenfield, J. G., Cornman, T., and Shy, G. M.: The prognostic value of the muscle biopsy in the "floppy child," Brain **81**:461, 1958.
67. Hall, D. A., Keech, M. K., Reed, R., Saxl, H., Tunbridge, R. E., and Wood, M. J.: Collagen and elastin in connective tissue, J. Geront. **10**:388, 1955.
68. Hallopeau and de Lépinay, M.: Sur un cas de xanthoma tubéreaux et de tumeurs juveniles offrant les charactères du xanthome diabetique, Bull. Soc. Franc. Derm. Syph. **17**:283, 1906.
69. Hass, J., and Hass, R.: Arthrochalasis multiplex congenita, J. Bone Joint Surg. **40-A**:663, 1958.
70. Holt, J. F.: The Ehlers-Danlos syndrome, Amer. J. Roentgen. **55**:420, 1946.
71. Husebye, K. C.: Tre familiäere tilfelle av Ehlers-Danlos syndrom, T. Norsk. Laegeforen, **72**:185, 1952.
72. Jacobs, P. H.: Ehlers-Danlos syndrome: report of a case with onset at age 29, Arch. Derm. **76**:460, 1957.
73. Jaeger, H.: Syndrome d'Ehlers-Danlos (deux cas familiaux), Dermatologica **100**:330, 1950.
74. Jansen, L. H.: De Ziekte van Ehlers en Danlos, Uitgeverij Excelsor's-Gravenhage, 1954.
75. Jansen, L. H.: Le mode de transmission de la maladie d'Ehlers-Danlos, J. Genet. Hum. **4**:204, 1955.
76. Jansen, L. H.: The structure of the connective tissue, an explanation of the symptoms of the Ehlers-Danlos syndrome, Dermatologica **110**:108, 1955.
77. Jochims, J.: Elastometrie an Kindern bei wechseln der Hautdehnung, Arch. Kinkerheilk. **135**:228, 1948.

78. Johns, R. J., and Wright, V.: Relative importance of various tissues in joint stiffness, J. Appl. Physiol. **17**:824, 1962.
79. Johns, R. J., and Wright, V.: An analytical description of joint stiffness, Biorheology **2**:87, 1964.
80. Johnson, S. A. M., and Falls, H. F.: Ehlers-Danlos syndrome; a clinical and genetic study, Arch. Derm. Syph. **60**:82, 1949.
81. Kalz, F.: Cutis laxa als Symptom allgemeiner Stützgewebsschwäche, Arch. Derm. u. Syph. **171**:155, 1935.
82. Kanof, A.: Ehlers-Danlos syndrome. Report of a case with suggestion of a possible causal mechanism, J. Dis. Child. **83**:197, 1952.
83. Katz, I., and Steiner, K.: Ehlers-Danlos syndrome with ectopic bone formation, Radiology **65**:352, 1955.
84. Key, J. A.: Hypermobility of joints as a sex-linked hereditary characteristic, J.A.M.A. **88**:1710, 1927.
85. King-Louis, F. J.: Two cases of Ehlers-Danlos syndrome, Proc. Roy. Soc. Med. **39**:135, 1946.
86. Kirk, E., and Kvorning, S. A.: Quantitative measurements of the elastic properties of the skin and subcutaneous tissue in young adults and old individuals, J. Geront. **4**:273, 1949.
87. Kopp: Demonstration zweier Fälle von "Cutis laxa." München Med. Wschr. **35**:259, 1888.
88. Korting, G. W., and Gottron, E.: Cutis laxa, Arch. Derm. u. Syph. **193**:14, 1951.
89. Laane, C. L.: Cushing's syndrome associated with obliterative arterial disease and multiple subcutaneous nodules (Ehlers-Danlos syndrome?), Acta Med. Scand. **148**:323, 1954.
90. Lamy, M., and Frézal, J.: Le syndrome de Bonnevie-Ullrich et ses rapports avec le syndrome de Turner, Analecta Genetica, vol. 6 (International Symposium, Turin, 1957).
91. Lapayowker, M. S.: Cutis hyperelastica: the Ehlers-Danlos syndrome, Amer. J. Roentgen. **84**:232, 1960.
92. Launay, C.: Syndrome d'Ehlers-Danlos chez un garcon de onze ans, associé à une arriération mentale, Bull. Soc. Méd. Hôp. Paris **56**:709, 1941.
93. Le Coulant, P.: Hyperelasticité cutanée et articulaire avec fragilité anormale de la peau et tumeurs molluscoides, chez un enfant de treize ans (syndrome d'Ehlers-Danlos), Gaz. Sci. Méd. Bordeaux **29**:1934.
94. Leider, M.: Forme fruste of Ehlers-Danlos syndrome, Urol. Cut. Rev. **53**:222, 1949.
95. Levy-Coblentz, G.: Radio-ulnar synostosis, Bull. Soc. Franc. Derm. Syph. **39**:1252, 1932.
96. Lewitus, Z.: Ehlers-Danlos syndrome; report of two cases with hypophyseal dysfunction, Arch. Derm. **73**:158, 1956.
97. Lienhart, O.: La maladie d'Ehlers-Danlos. Étude clinique, anatomo-pathologique et génetique, Thesis de Nancy, 1945 (No. 30).
98. Lisker, R., Noguerón, A., and Sánchez-Medal, L.: Plasma thromboplastin component deficiency in the Ehlers-Danlos syndrome, Ann. Intern. Med. **53**:388, 1960.
99. Littré, E.: Oeuvres complète d'Hippocrate, Paris, 1840, J. B. Baillière, vol. 2, pp. 67-83.
100. MacCollum, D. W.: The lop ear, J.A.M.A. **110**:1427, 1938.
101. McEvitt, W. G.: The problem of the protruding ear, Plast. Reconstr. Surg. **2**:480, 1947.
102. Macfarlane, I. L.: Ehlers-Danlos syndrome presenting certain unusual features, J. Bone Joint Surg. **41-B**:541, 1959.
103. McFarland, W., and Fuller, D. E.: Mortality in Ehlers-Danlos syndrome due to spontaneous rupture of large arteries, New Eng. J. Med. **271**:1309, 1964.
104. McKusick, V. A.: Hereditary disorders of connective tissue, Bull. N.Y. Acad. Med. **35**:143, 1959.
105. Madison, W. J., Jr., Bradley, E. J., and Castillo, A. J.: Ehlers-Danlos syndrome with cardiac involvement, Amer. J. Cardiol. **11**:689, 1963.
106. Margarot, J., Deneze, P., and Coll de Carrera: Hyperlaxité cutanée et articulaire (syndrome de Danlos) existant chez trois membres d'une même famille, Bull. Soc. Franc. Derm. Syph. **40**:277, 1933.
107. Maximow, A.: Development of argyrophile and collagenous fibers in tissue culture, Proc. Soc. Exp. Biol. Med. **25**:437, 1928.
108. Méténier, P.: A propos d'un cas familial de maladie d'Ehlers-Danlos, Thése d'Alger, 1939, No. 55.
109. Miguet, A.: Le syndrome d'Ehlers-Danlos, Thése, Paris, 1933, Louis Arnette.

110. Mories, A.: An investigation into the Ehlers-Danlos syndrome, Edinburgh Thesis, 1954.
111. Mories, A.: Ehlers-Danlos syndrome, with a report of a fatal case, Scot. Med. J. **5**:269, 1960.
112. Mounier-Kuhn, P., and Meyer, L.: Méga-organes (oesophage, trachée, colon), syndromes de Mickulicz et d'Ehlers-Danlos chez une hérédo-syphilitique, Bull. Soc. Méd. Hôp. Lyon, Nov. 9, 1943.
113. Murray, J. E., and Tyars, M. E.: A case of Ehlers-Danlos syndrome, Brit. Med. J. **1**:974, 1940.
114. Nicaud, P., Lafitte, A., and Buhot, S.: Syndrome d'Ehlers-Danlos fruste associé à une atrophie musculaire du type Aran-Duchenne, Bull. Soc. Méd. Hôp. Paris, Mar. 10, 1944.
115. Nicod, M.: Un cas de syndrome d'Ehlers-Danlos, Ann. Paediat. **167**:358, 1946.
116. Noto, P.: Cited by Pelbois and Rollier.[125]
117. Olmsted, F., Page, I. H., and Corcoran, A. C.: A device for objective clinical measurement of cutaneous elasticity; a "pinchmeter," Amer. J. Med. Sci. **222**:73, 1951.
118. Ona, C. K., and Cowdry, E. V.: Aging of elastic tissue in human skin, J. Geront. **5**:203, 1950.
119. Orlandi, O. V., and Rodrigues, Y. T.: Ehlers-Danlos syndrome; capillary microscopy in cases, Pediatria (Rio) **17**:189, 1952.
120. Ormsby, O. S., and Tobin, W. W.: Cutis hyperelastica; case report, Arch. Derm. Syph. **38**:828, 1938.
121. Ota, M., and Yasuda, T.: Erster Fall von "Syndrome d'Ehlers-Danlos" in Japan, Zbl. Haut. Geschlechtskr. **66**:120, 1941.
122. Packer, B. D., and Blades, J. F.: Dermatorrhexis; a case report; the so-called Ehlers-Danlos syndrome, Virginia Med. Monthly **81**:21, 1954.
123. Pascher, F.: Ehlers-Danlos syndrome, Arch. Derm. Syph. **67**:214, 1953.
124. Pautrier, M.: Note histologique sur un cas de cutis elastica, avec pesudotumeurs aux genoux et aux coudes, presenté par M. Danlos, Bull. Soc. Franc. Derm. Syph. **19**:72, 1908.
125. Pelbois, F., and Rollier, F.: Association d'un syndrome d'Ehlers-Danlos et d'un syndrome de Groenblad-Strandberg. Bull. Soc. Franc. Derm. Syph. **59**:141, 1952.
126. Perreau, P., Bangas, J., and Lecuit, P.: Osteitis fibro-kystique atypique et syndrome d'Ehlers-Danlos. Lesion parathyroidienne, Bull. Soc. méd. Hôp. Paris **57**:135, 1941
127. Péyri: Un cas de syndrome d'Ehlers-Danlos, probablement d'origine syphilitique, Bull. Soc. Franc. Derm. Syph. **44**:1744, 1937.
128. Pittinos, G. E.: Ehlers-Danlos syndrome with disturbance of creatine metabolism, J. Pediat. **19**:85, 1941.
129. Poumeau-Delille, G., and Soulié, P.: Un cas d'hyperlaxité cutanée et articulaire avec cicatrices atrophiques et pseudo-tumeurs molluscoides (syndrome d'Ehlers-Danlos), Bull. Soc. Méd. Hôp. Paris **50**:593, 1934.
130. Pray, L. G.: Cutis elastica (dermatorrhexis, Ehlers-Danlos syndrome), Amer. J. Dis. Child. **75**:702, 1948.
131. Raybaud, A., and Guidoni, P.: Hyperlaxité ligamentaire et cutanée; trouble du métabolisme calcique; maladie d'Ehlers-Danlos, Bull. Soc. Méd. Hôp. Paris **54**:738, 1938.
132. Ricketson, G.: The behavior of skin grafts and donor sites in a case of Ehlers-Danlos syndrome, Plast. Reconstr. Surg. **20**:32, 1957.
133. Ringrose, E. J., Nowlan, F. B., and Perry, H.: Ehlers-Danlos syndrome; report of a case, Arch. Derm. Syph. **62**:443, 1950.
134. Robertson, J. A., Eddy, W. A., and Vossler, A. J.: Spontaneous perforation of the cecum without mechanical obstruction; review of literature and case report, Amer. J. Surg. **96**:446, 1958.
135. Robinson, H. M., Jr., and Ellis, F. A.: Cutis laxa, Arch. Derm. **77**:656, 1958.
136. Robitaille, G. A.: Ehlers-Danlos syndrome and recurrent hemoptysis, Ann. Intern. Med. **61**:716, 1964.
137. Rocher, H. L.: Une nouvelle dysmorphose articulaire congénitale: laxité articulaire congénitale multiple. In Livre jubilarie d'Henri Hartmann, Paris, 1932, Masson et Cie.
138. Roederer, C.: Syndrome d'Ehlers-Danlos atypique coincidant avec une dolichosténomélie, Arch Franc. Pédiat. **8**:192, 1951.
139. Rollhäuser, H.: Die Zugfestigkeit der menschlichen Haut, Gegenbaur Morph. Jahrb. **90**:249, 1950.
140. Ronchese, F.: Dermatorrhexis with dermatochalasis and arthrochalasis (the so-called

Ehlers-Danlos syndrome); additional data on a case reported 12 years previously, Rhode Isl. Med. J. **32**:80, 1949
141. Ross, M., and Donneief, A. S.: Chest surgery in the presence of cutis hyperelastica (Ehlers-Danlos syndrome), New York J. Med. **57**:2256, 1957.
142. Rossi, E., and Angst, H.: Das Danlos-Ehlers Syndrome, Helv. Paediat. Acta **6**:245, 1951.
143. Rossi, E., and Caflisch, A.: Le syndrome du pterygium. Satus Bonnevie-Ullrich, dystrophia brevicolli congenita, syndrome de Turner et arthromyodysplasia congenita, Helv. Paediat. Acta **6**:119, 1951.
144. Rubenstein, M., and Cohen, N. H.: Ehlers-Danlos syndrome associated with multiple intracranial aneurysms, Neurology **14**:125, 1964.
145. Saemundsson, J.: Ehlers-Danlos syndrome; a congenital mesenchymal disorder, Acta Med. Scand. (supp. 312) **154**:399, 1956.
146. Samuel, M. A., Schwartz, M. L., and Meister, M. M.: The Ehlers-Danlos syndrome, U.S. Armed Forces Med. J. **4**:737, 1953.
147. Schaper, G.: Familiäres Vorkommen von Ehlers-Danlos Syndrome; ein Beitrag zur Klinik und Pathogenese, Zschr. Kinderheilk. **70**:504, 1952.
148. Sestak, Z.: Ehlers-Danlos syndrome and cutis laxa; an account of families in the Oxford area, Ann. Hum. Genet. **25**:313, 1962.
149. Shapiro, S. K.: A case of Meekrin-Ehlers-Danlos syndrome with neurologic manifestations, J. Nerv. Ment. Dis. **115**:64, 1952.
150. Shaw, A. B., and Hopkins, P.: A case of a boy, aged seven, showing (a) double-jointedness, (b) dermatolysis ("elastic skin") with great friability of the skin and excessive tendency to bruising, and (c) multiple subcutaneous tumours on the limbs (fibromata, neuronomata), Proc. Roy. Soc. Med. (Clin. Sec.) **6**:20, 1913.
151. Smith, C. H.: Dermatorrhexis (Ehlers-Danlos syndrome), J. Pediat. **14**:632, 1939.
152. Sodeman, W. A., and Burch, G. E.: Skin elasticity in scleroderma, Amer. Heart J. **17**:21, 1939.
153. Stillians, A. W., and Zakon, S. J.: Cutis laxa (Cutis hyperplastica), Arch. Derm. Syph. **35**:342, 1937.
154. Stuart, A. M.: Three cases exhibiting the Ehlers-Danlos syndrome, Proc. Roy. Soc. Med. **30**:984, 1937.
155. Stucke, K.: Ueber das elastische Verhalten der Achillessehne im Belastungsversuch, Arch. Klin. Chir. **265**:579, 1950.
156. Sturkie, P. D.: Hypermobile joints in all descendants for two generations, J. Hered. **32**:232, 1941.
157. Sullivan, J. D.: The Danlos-Ehlers syndrome; report of case with transient paralysis of vocal cord, Arch. Neur. Psychiat. **47**:316, 1942.
158. Summer, G. K.: The Ehlers-Danlos syndrome; a review of the literature and report of a case with a subgaleal hematoma and Bell's palsy, J. Dis. Child. **91**:419, 1956.
159. Sutro, C. J.: Hypermobility of bones due to "overlengthened" capsular and ligamentous tissues; cause for recurrent intra-articular effusions, Surgery **21**:67, 1947.
160. Taylor, F. R.: The Meekrin-Ehlers-Danlos syndrome, Urol. Cut. Rev. **47**:378, 1943.
161. Thomas, C., Cordier, J., and Algan, B.: Une étiologie nouvelle du syndrome de luxation spontanée des cristallins: la maladie d'Ehlers-Danlos, Bull. Soc. Belge Ophtal. **100**:375, 1952.
162. Thomas, C., Cordier, J., and Algan, B.: Les altérations oculaires de la maladie d'Ehlers-Danlos, Arch. Ophtal. (Paris) **14**:691, 1954.
163. Thurmon, F. M.: Ehlers-Danlos syndrome, Arch. Derm. **40**:120, 1939.
164. Tobias, N.: Danlos syndrome associated with congenital lipomatosis, Arch. Derm. Syph. **30**:540, 1934; ibid. **40**:135, 1939.
165. Tschernogobow, A.: Cutis laxa. (Presentation at first meeting of Moscow Dermatologic and Venereologic Society, Nov. 13, 1891), Mhft. Prakt. Derm. **14**:76, 1892.
166. Tschernogobow, A.: Ein Fall von Cutis laxa. Protokoly Moskowskawo wenerologitscheskawo i dermatologitscheskawo Obtschestwa, vol. 1, p. 23. Quoted in Jahresb. Ges. Med. **27**:562, 1892.
167. Tucker, D. H., Miller, D. E., and Jacoby, W. J., Jr.: Ehlers-Danlos syndrome with sinus of Valsalva aneurysm and aortic insufficiency simulating rheumatic heart disease, Amer. J. Med. **35**:715, 1963.

168. Tunbridge, R. E., Tattersall, R. N., Hall, D. A., Astbury, W. T., and Reed, R.: The fibrous structure of normal and abnormal human skin. Clin. Sci. **11**:315, 1952.
169. Turkington, R. W., and Grude, H. E.: Ehlers-Danlos syndrome and multiple neurofibromatosis, Ann. Intern. Med. **61**:549, 1964.
170. Unna, P. G.: The histopathology of the diseases of the skin. Translated from the German with the assistance of the author by N. Walker, New York, 1896, The Macmillan Co., pp. 984-988.
171. van Meekeren, J. A.: De dilatabilitate extraordinaria cutis, chap. 32, Observations medicochirugicae, Amsterdam, 1682.
172. Villegas, R., and Albornoz, R.: Posibles mecanismos causales del sindrome de Ehlers-Danlos, Acta Med. Venezolana **4**: 1956.
173. Vissian, L., and Rovinski, J.: Syndrome d'Ehlers-Danlos chez quatre membres d'une même famille, Bull. Soc. Franc. Derm. Syph. **62**:62, 1955.
174. Wallach, E. A., and Burkhart, E. F.: Ehlers-Danlos syndrome associated with tetralogy of Fallot, Arch. Derm. Syph. **61**:750, 1950.
175. Weber, F. P., and Aitken, J. K.: Nature of the subcutaneous spherules in some cases of Ehlers-Danlos syndrome, Lancet **1**:198, 1938.
176. Wechsler, H. L., and Fisher, E. R.: Ehlers-Danlos syndrome. Pathologic, histochemical, and electron microscopic observations, Arch. Path. **77**:613, 1964.
177. Weill, J., and Martineau, J.: A propos d'un cas de maladie d'Ehlers-Danlos. Étude anatomoclinique et biologique, Bull. Soc. Franc. Derm. Syph. **44**:99, 1937.
178. Weiss, R. S.: Danlos' syndrome, Arch. Derm. **40**:137, 1939.
179. Wenzel, H. G.: Untersuchungen über die Dehnbarkeit und Zerreissbarkeit der Haut, Zbl. Allg. Path. **85**:117, 1949.
180. Whitney, L. F.: Inheritance of double jointedness in thumb, J. Hered. **23**:425, 1932.
181. Wiener, K.: Gummihaut (cutis laxa) mit dominanter Vererbung, Arch. Derm. u. Syph. **148**:599, 1925.
182. Wigzell, F. W., and Ogston, D.: The bleeding tendency in Ehlers-Danlos syndrome, Ann. Phys. Med. **7**:55, 1963.
183. Williams, A. W.: Cutis laxa, Monatsschr. Prakt. Dermat. **14**:490, 1892.
184. Wright, V., and Johns, R. J.: The quantitative measurement of joint stiffness (abstract), J. Clin. Invest. **38**:1056, 1959.
185. Zaida, A. H.: Ehlers-Danlos syndrome with congenital herniae and pigeon breast, Brit. Med. J. **2**:175, 1959.

6

Osteogenesis imperfecta

Historical note

It has been suggested[114,210] that an early case of osteogenesis imperfecta was that of Ivar the Boneless, the mastermind behind the Scandinavian invasion of England in the last quarter of the ninth century. He is said to have had cartilage where bones should have been. He could not walk and was carried into battle on shields. Complete verification of the diagnosis is impossible because so much poetic glorification enshrouds any remaining records and Ivar's skeleton is no longer available for study, having been dug up and burned by William the Conqueror. A study of Ivar's descendants turned up no cases of osteogenesis imperfecta or other bone disease.

The recorded history of the development of knowledge of this disease is given in Table 6. Isolated cases were reported even before Ekman, from as early as 1678.[210]

The terms that have been applied to this syndrome are numerous and include, to mention a few, osteogenesis imperfecta (Vrolik[246]), mollities ossium (Ormerod[180]), fragilitas ossium (Gurlt[108]), and osteopsathyrosis idiopathica (Lobstein[155]). To complicate matters further, the disease is called *la maladie de Lobstein* in the French-speaking portion of the medical world. It is also known as Eddowes' syndrome (brittle bones and blue sclerae), van der Hoeve's syndrome (brittle bones, blue sclerae, and deafness), and Vrolik's disease (osteogenesis imperfecta congenita). Looser[156] suggested the terms osteogenesis imperfecta congenita (OIC) and osteogenesis imperfecta tarda (OIT).

The condition called periosteal dysplasia of Porak and Durante by French authors is probably the same as osteogenesis imperfecta congenita.

Clinical manifestations

Over one hundred kinships with at least one affected member have been identified in the records of the Johns Hopkins Hospital, the Children's Hospital School, and the Kernan Hospital for Crippled Children, Baltimore, Md.

The clinical aspects of osteogenesis imperfecta will be discussed under the

Table 6. Landmarks in the history of osteogenesis imperfecta

1788	O. J. Ekman.[72] In medical doctorate thesis at Uppsala, described "osteomalacia congenita" in three generations. (See Seedorff[210] for an extensive translation of Ekman's Latin thesis.)
1831	Edmund Axmann,[13] Wertheim, Germany. Described the disease in himself and his brothers, Paul and Anton. Made reference to the occurrence of articular dislocations and blue sclerotics. One of the brothers had been reported by Strack in 1807.[231]
1833	J. C. Lobstein (1777-1838), gynecologist and pathologist, Strasbourg. Wrote about adult form of the disease in his textbook of morbid anatomy.[155]
1849	Willem Vrolik (1801-1863), Dutch anatomist. Described disease in newborn infant.[246] See Fig. 6-1.
1859	Edward Latham Ormerod, Brighton, England. Early description of case of 68-year-old woman only 39½ inches tall. Disease was passed to a son and a daughter. The skeleton, in the Royal College of Surgeons, London, is reproduced in Bell's monograph.[22] Use of term "mollities ossium."
1862-1865	Ernest Julius Gurlt[108] (1825-1899), Professor of Surgery, Berlin. Use of term "fragilitas ossium."
1889	H. Stilling,[228] Strasbourg. Histologic studies.
1896	John Spurway,[223] Tring, England. Described blue sclerotics with fragility of bones.
1897	M. B. Schmidt,[203] Strasbourg. Proposed fundamental identity of the disease in adults and newborn infants.
1900	Alfred Eddowes,[71] London. Described blue sclerotics. Suggested that OI is generalized hypoplasia of mesenchyme.
1903	Leslie Buchanan,[42] Glasgow. Demonstrated that blue sclerotics are due to thinness of sclera. Fractures, deafness, or familial incidence not mentioned in his "A. M'C—, a girl aet. 9 years."
1906	E. Looser,[156] Heidelberg. Defended identity of disease in adult and newborn infant. Proposed terms osteogenesis imperfecta congenita (OIC) and osteogenesis imperfecta tarda (OIT).
1912	Charles A. Adair-Dighton,[1] Liverpool. Described deafness.
1918	J. van der Hoeve, Groningen, and A. de Kleyn, Utrecht.[240] Emphasized brittle bones, blue sclerae, and deafness as a syndrome.
1920	K. H. Bauer,[17,18] Breslau. Provided histologic support for view that OI is a "hypoplasia mesenchymialis." Described dental histology.
1919, 1922	E. Ruttin,[199,200] Vienna. Described otosclerotic nature of the deafness in OI.
1928	Julia Bell,[22] of the Galton Laboratory, London. Described dominant pattern of inheritance, especially of blue sclerotics, on basis of large number of pedigrees.

headings of skeletal, ocular, cutaneous, otologic, and internal. The osseous manifestations greatly outweigh the others in significance.

Clinically two varieties of OI have been distinguished. In so-called osteogenesis imperfecta congenita, the disease is so severe that the relatively minor traumata to which the fetus is exposed in utero produce numerous fractures. The victim is usually born dead or survives only a short time. The cranium is soft and membranous. Short clumsy extremities suggest achondroplasia (Fig. 6-2). In the second variety, so-called osteogenesis imperfecta tarda (or tardiva), the manifestations are so mild that blue sclerae may be the only manifestation, and fractures may occur only late in life or not at all. Seedorff[210] further divides osteogenesis imperfecta tarda into levis and gravis types. In the latter, the first fractures are likely to occur when the patient is an infant. In the former, the fractures occur only considerably later.

On the basis mainly of radiologic changes, Fairbank[77] distinguishes a "thick bone type," a "slender bone type," and a form he calls osteogenesis imperfecta cystica (Fig. 6-10). These, like the antenatal and postnatal distinction which he makes, probably have no basis so far as difference in the fundamental defect is concerned. During prepubertal years a patient may demonstrate an evolution from the "slender bone type" to the cystic type or the "thick bone type."

Experience with categories of genetic disease has repeatedly shown that what at first appears to be a single homogeneous entity is in fact several fundamentally distinct disorders. Examples are the cases of homocystinuria that have been classified as the Marfan syndrome in the past (p. 150 ff.) and the six distinct mucopolysaccharidoses (p. 389 ff.) that have at times been called Hurler's syndrome. A priori, therefore, heterogeneity in the category of osteogenesis imperfecta is almost a certainty. Later (p. 256), evidence will be reviewed that bears on the question of multiple distinct forms of osteogenesis imperfecta—the alternative being that the clinically somewhat different conditions are all the same entity, which has an exceedingly great range of clinical severity.

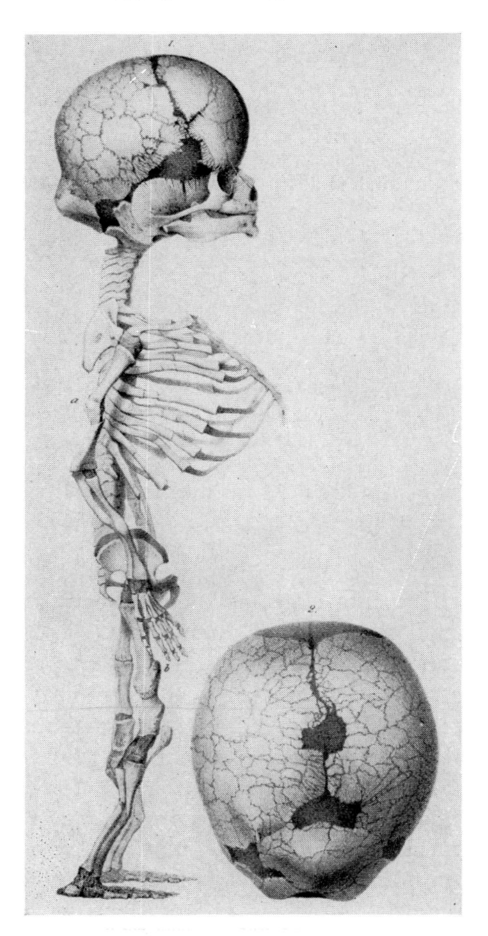

Fig. 6-1. Skeleton in osteogenesis imperfecta. Note the multiple Wormian bones of the caput membranaceum. (From Vrolik, W.: Tabulae ad illustrandam embryogenesim hominis et mammalium, tam naturalem quam abnormem, Amstelodami, 1849.)

The musculoskeletal system.[33] As will be seen later, osteogenesis imperfecta is a hereditary defect of the bone matrix. Calcification of whatever bone matrix is formed probably proceeds normally. Osteogenesis imperfecta is then a form of hereditary osteoporosis, inasmuch as osteoporosis is defined as a deficiency in the formation (or an acceleration of the breakdown) of bone matrix. This is an important consideration in the understanding of some of the clinical manifestations of the disease and in its rational therapy. For example, in later life, particularly if few fractures have occurred, the disease may masquerade as postmenopausal osteoporosis; immobilization is as bad for OI as it is for other forms of osteoporosis.

Caput membranaceum and micromelia ("tiny extremities") are the characteristics of OIC (Figs. 6-1 to 6-5). The limbs are described as bowed on the chest and abdomen at birth. If the patient survives, the bowing is likely to persist. Chondrodystrophia fetalis (achondroplasia) is often misdiagnosed. By x-ray examination (Fig. 6-3*B* and *C* and Fig. 6-4) the skull is likely to show a mosaic pattern as a result of the presence of numerous Wormian bones.[198] This mosaic phe-

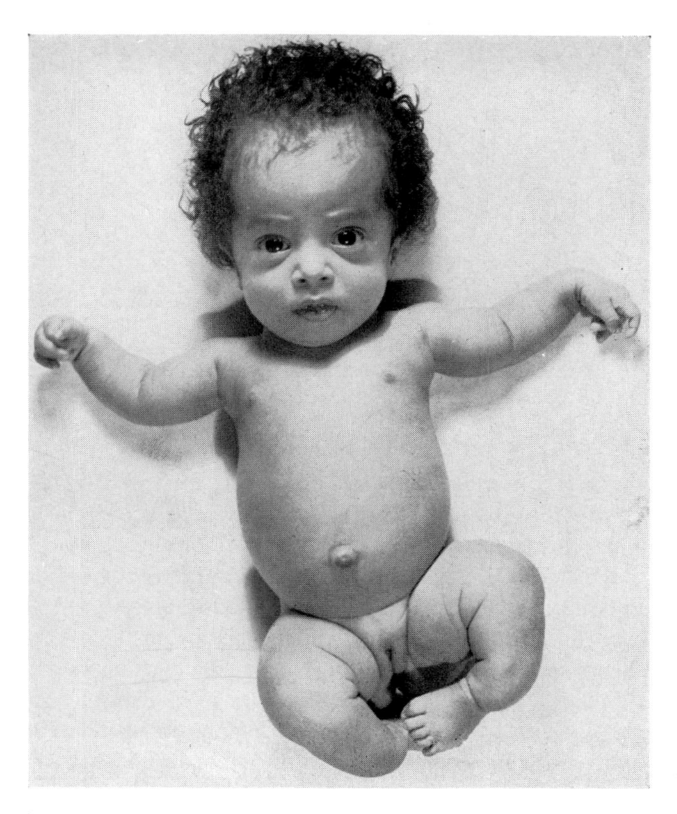

Fig. 6-2. P. D. (A42000), 3 months old, an instance of so-called osteogenesis imperfecta congenita. Micromelia is striking. The head appears disproportionately large. Numerous fractures were demonstrated immediately after birth. The patient was referred with the diagnosis of chondrodystrophia fetalis, however. The skull bones were described as "crumbly" on palpation. The parents and the parents' families were normal. By the age of 1 year there were evidences of well-advanced hydrocephalus. Death occurred at the age of 38 months.

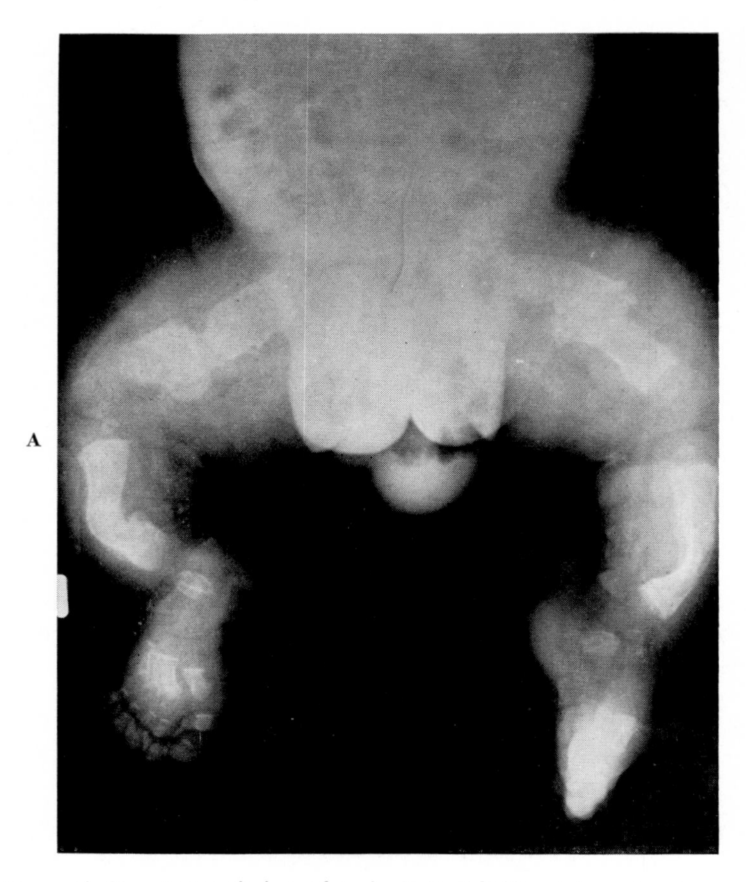

Fig. 6-3. "Congenital" osteogenesis imperfeta in K. K. (A95443), 2½ weeks of age. **A,** Multiple fractures, bowing of the extremities, and bilateral inguinal hernias are evident. **B** and **C,** Demonstration of multiple Wormian bones in the membranaceum. (**A** and **B** from McKusick, V. A.: Bull. N. Y. Acad. Med. **35:**143, 1959.)

nomenon was very striking in the case described and illustrated by Vrolik in 1849.[246] (See Fig. 6-1.) (This was the first case to which the name osteogenesis imperfecta was given.) Caffey states that the mosaic phenomenon occurs in only two conditions: osteogenesis imperfecta and cleidocranial dysostosis (see Fig. 43 of reference 44 and compare with Fig. 6-4 here). Pycnodysostosis,[161,163,164] a condition which in other ways simulates both osteogenesis imperfecta and cleidocranial dysostosis and from which Toulouse-Lautrec is now thought to have suffered (p. 261), should be added to the "causes" of multiple Wormian bones. The mosaic pattern persists throughout life. The patient whose skull was studied anatomically by Ruth[198] was variously estimated to be 46 to 55 years old. The diagnosis of OIC has been made at times in utero by means of x-ray films[67,85,97,107,166,184,201] (Fig. 6-5). In this form, OI is a lethal or sublethal trait. Death is usually the result of intracranial hemorrhage and other injury, since the calvarium offers little protection during delivery and later. Beading of the ribs by calluses is often misinterpreted as a rachitic rosary. Progressive hydrocephalus often occurs in OIC[84,201] (Figs. 6-2 and 6-5*B*). Hernia is frequent.[84]

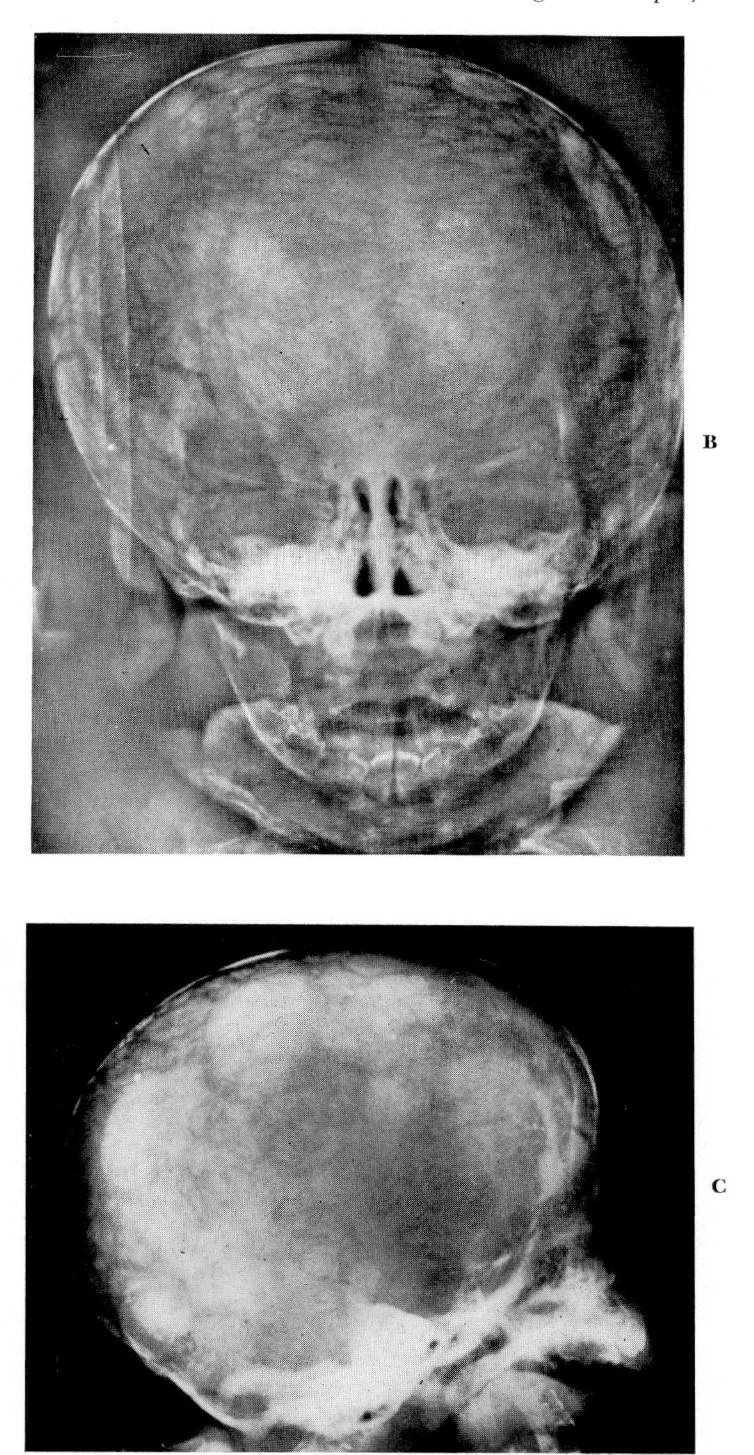

Fig. 6-3, cont'd. For legend see opposite page.

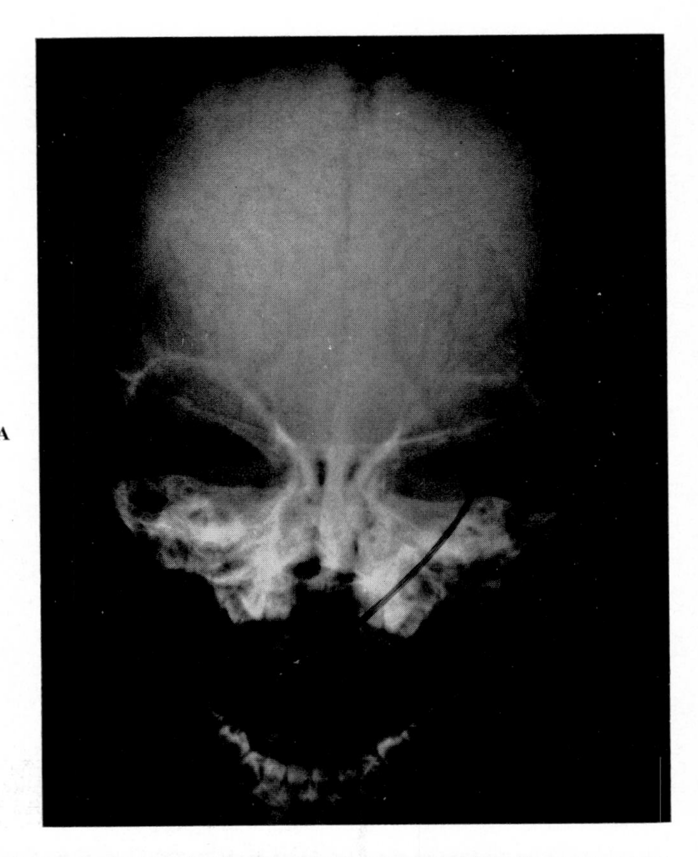

A

Fig. 6-4. W. B. (A79352), 2-month-old white male, radiographic views (**A** and **B**) of the skull in a case of osteogenesis imperfecta congenita, showing a mosaic of Wormian bones and the thin calvarium characteristic of so-called *caput membranaceum*.

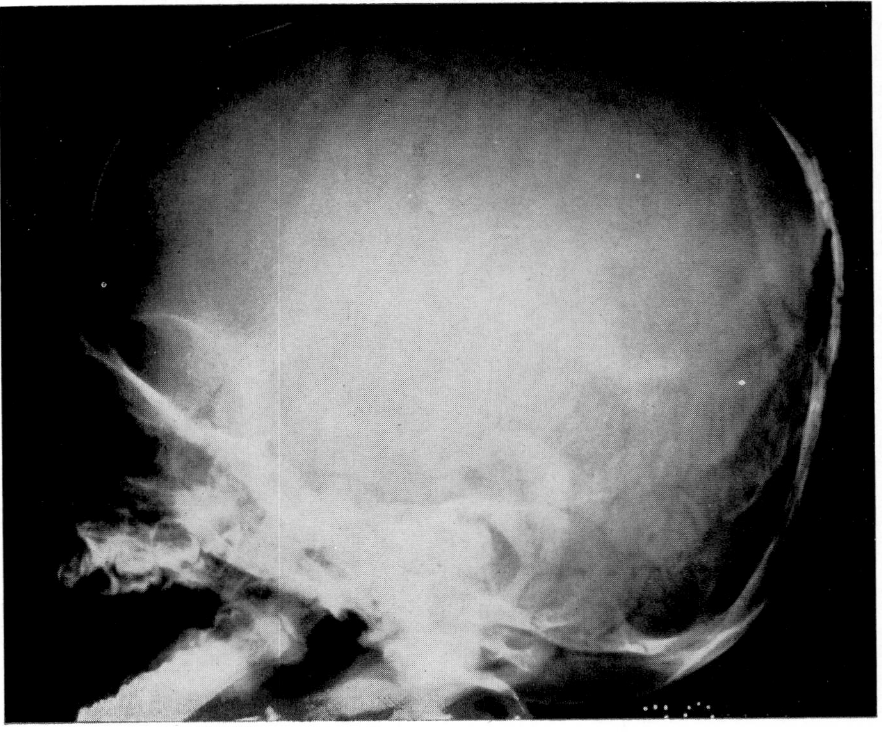

B

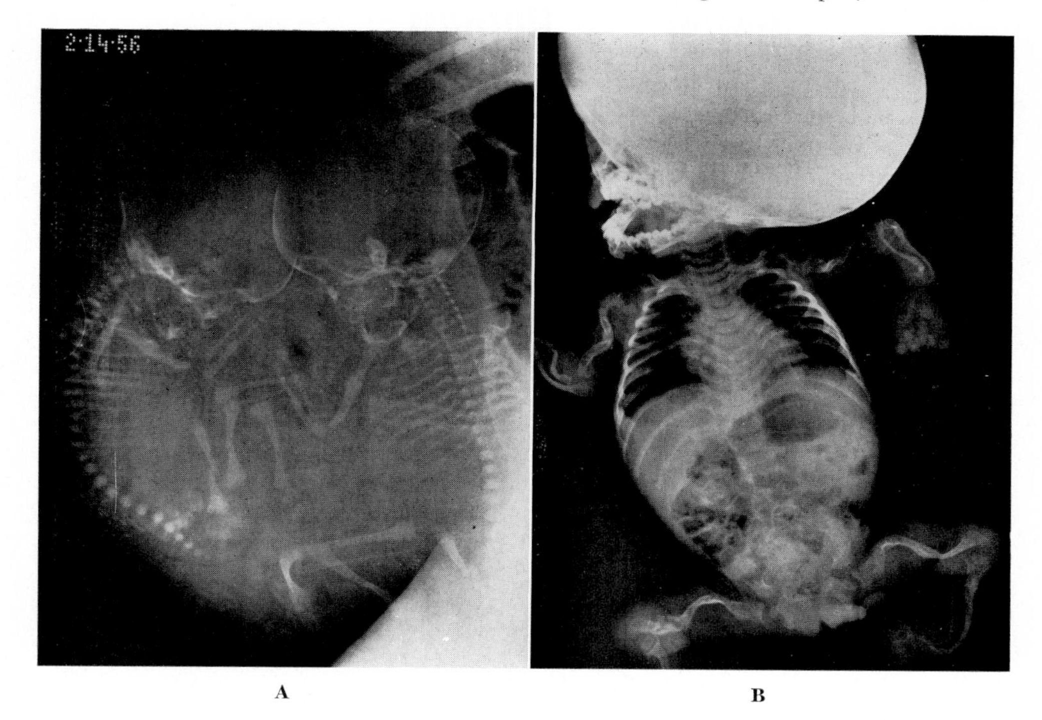

Fig. 6-5. Presumedly monozygotic twins with osteogenesis imperfecta congenita diagnosed in utero. The mother (M. B., B.C.H. 209850), father, and an only sibling show no stigmata of OI. The mother was admitted to the hospital on Feb. 13, 1956, because of irregular labor pains. The abdomen was very large and tense. **A,** X-ray film revealed twins in breech presentation, facing each other in boxing position. Both fetuses showed multiple fractures in various stages of healing. Delivery was spontaneous. The baby born second lived for thirty-three days. Autopsy revealed the characteristic changes of OI. There was a patent ductus arteriosus and mild hydrocephalus. The first-born twin lived for twenty-seven months. From the first the head was large and soft. Progressive enlargement occurred, so that the proportions indicated in **B** were attained. The sclerae were never impressively blue. Others[78,204,217,254] have described affected twins.

In OIT, the triviality of the trauma that may cause fracture is well known: fracture of the forearm in whittling or throwing a chip, of the phalanges in writing, of the femora when another person sits on the patient's lap[225] or when the patient stretches out in bed. Apert[8] called these patients "les hommes de verre." In one family severely affected children were referred to, appropriately, as "china dolls." (R. Y., B.C.H. 143029.)

Sudden muscle pulls may fracture bones: the olecranon, for instance, has been pulled off by the triceps muscle in swimming[1] or even less strenuous exercise. Relatively little pain tends to accompany the fracture, due probably to the facts that there is minimal soft tissue trauma and that the patients become accustomed to the frequent fractures. Occasionally they learn to set their own fractures.[243] The fractures appear to heal with normal speed, but occasionally the callus is so large (Fig. 6-10*A*) as to suggest osteosarcoma.[1,14,77,147,206,210,232] However, unlike Paget's disease, malignant degeneration is not recognized as a definite complication of this disease, although bone neoplasms have been described.[134,255] Patients

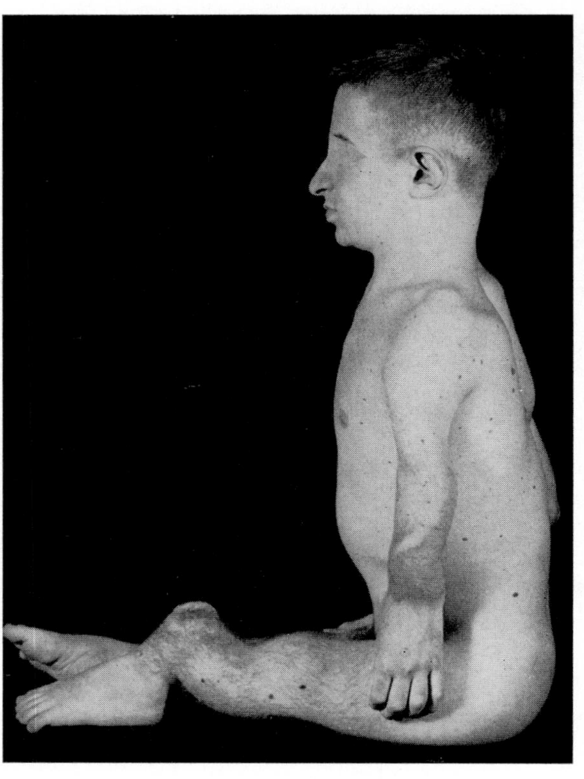

Fig. 6-6. Severely affected 14-year-old male (J. L., 757361). The family history reveals no similar manifestations. Two other children are normal. The father had cleft palate and harelip. The infant was born by vertex presentation. At birth the left thigh showed a swelling which was later found to be a fracture of the femur with callus formation. The mother estimated that about 107 fractures had occurred, all with minimal trauma at the most. The sclerae are not blue, and there is no deafness. The teeth are small and widely spaced, with translucent enamel. The entire body is covered with nevi, but there were no palpable subcutaneous neurofibromata and no definite café-au-lait spots. The skeletal deformity is adequately described by the photographs and the x-ray films. Calcium, phosphorus, and acid phosphatase of serum were normal. The alkaline phosphatase was 13.7 Bodansky units. Multiple osteotomies with stabilization by metal plates and medullary bars. **A,** General view. **B,** Anteroposterior view of both legs. **C,** Lateral view of both legs.

A

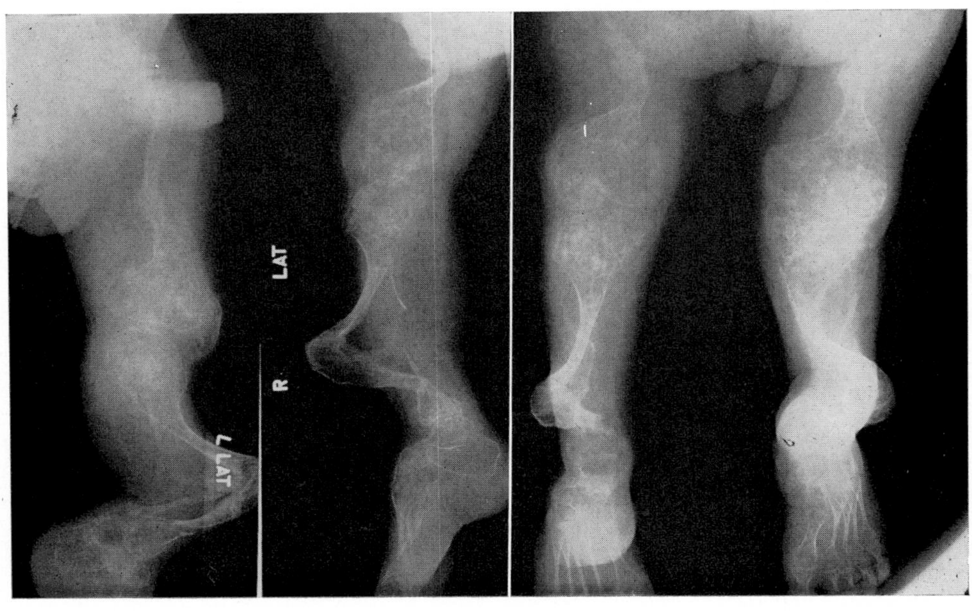

B C

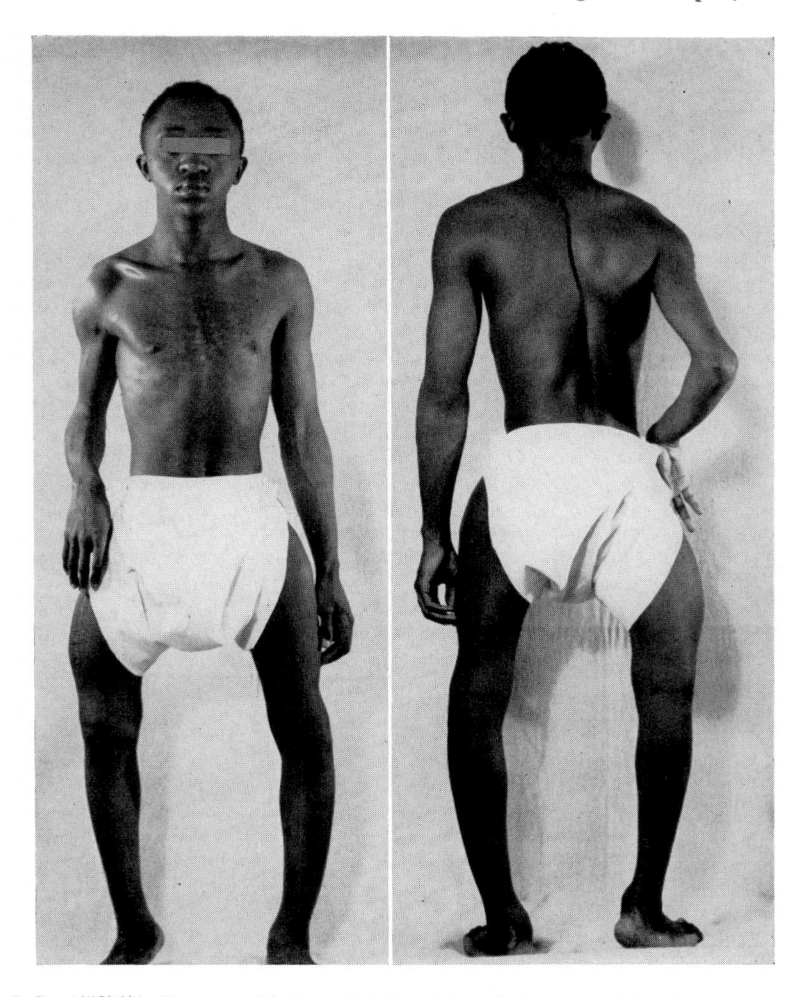

Fig. 6-7. J. B. (459707), 21 years old. Bowed deformities of the extremities, flat feet, and moderately bulging skull are evident. As a result of the bulging skull, the ears point forward and downward. Beginning at the age of 8 years the patient has had a total of approximately thirteen fractures with no decrease in the incidence of these at puberty. The sclerae are deeply blue.

(e.g. J. B. in Fig. 6-7) are sometimes operated upon for suspected osteosarcoma.[147] At times overgrowth of bone occurs without evident fracture, and exostosis-like abnormalities develop. (Wide hypertrophic scars occur at the sites of surgical operations such as laparotomy.[207] These may be fundamentally analogous to the hypertrophic callus formation.) Functionally awkward pseudoarthroses may develop. Pseudoarthrosis of the tibia or other bones may be the presenting manifestation[68,146] (S. E., H.L.H. A18674). (Neurofibromatosis[65] is another hereditary disorder in which pseudoarthrosis occurs.) The development of numerous Wormian bones in the occipital area of the skull[198] is a similar phenomenon seen particularly in the "congenital" form of the disease. In the series studied at this hospital, one cannot corroborate, in adults at least, the impression[16] that fracture of the neck of the femur is uncommon as compared with other types of osteo-

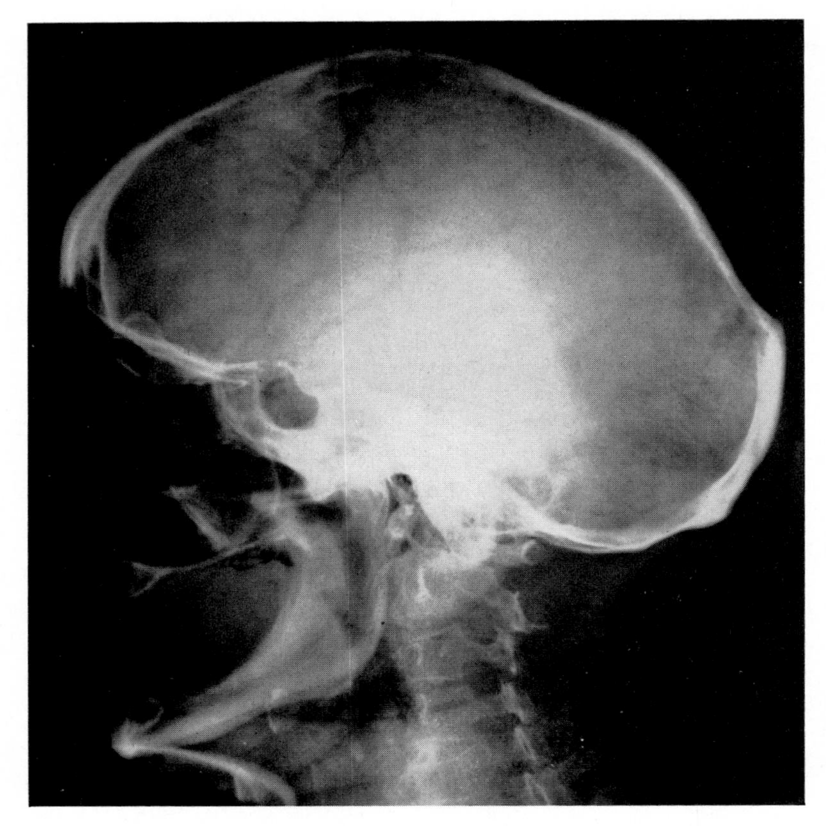

Fig. 6-8. "Overhanging occiput" with decrease in the vertical dimension is demonstrated by the skull of this 51-year-old patient (G. I., 587372). She is edentulous. Definite platybasia was judged to be present. The patient has deeply blue sclerae and has had a large number of fractures dating from birth and resulting in marked deformity. She is scarcely taller than a 3-year-old child. Deafness of conduction type dates from the age of 13 years following pertussis, and there has been intermittent tinnitus. She has had weakness of the left quadriceps muscle group, with absence of the left knee kick and anesthesia about the left knee, resulting presumably from a compression fracture of the lumbar spine.

porosis. (See, for example, patient G. I., Fig. 6-8.) There is no sex difference in the severity of the fragilitas ossium.

By x-ray examination all bones have thin cortices, and the long bones usually have a slender shaft with rather abrupt widening as the epiphysis is approached. There are instances, as Fairbank[76,77] has indicated, in which the shaft of the long bones is thick, and yet others in which a cystic appearance is presented on the x-ray film (Fig. 6-10*B*).

As in other types of osteoporosis, "codfish" or "hourglass" vertebrae develop as a result of the biconcave deformity produced by the pressure of the normally elastic nucleus pulposus on the abnormally soft bone of the vertebral body (Fig. 6-9). Furthermore, "schmorlsches Knötchen," actual herniations of the nucleus pulposus into the substance of the vertebral body, may occur. (Schmorl's nodes derive their eponym from G. Schmorl, who also did a classic study of Paget's disease of bone. See Chapter 10.)

Characteristically the adults have short legs as compared with the upper part of the body. The shortness of the lower extremities is due in part to bowing and to fractures in the shafts of the long bones but is also due in considerable degree to interference with growth by multiple microfractures at the epiphyseal ends of the bones. This feature may lead to the misdiagnosis of achondroplastic dwarfism. One patient (Fig. 6-8), now 56 years old, "is scarcely taller than a 3-year-old child." Marked bowing of the legs often results in a scissors-gait. On x-ray examination the femora often have a shepherd's-crook appearance.

Anterior bowing of the tibiae, producing saber shins, is a frequent occurrence. Gross deformities, which resemble somewhat those of Marfan's syndrome, such as kyphoscoliosis, koilosternia (pectus excavatum), and pigeon breast, are not uncommon. Arachnodactyly also has been described by several writers.[74,144,187,210] It must be remembered that arachnodactyly is a symptom, not a disease; that its presence does not indicate the coexistence of Marfan's disease. Unequivocal, or at least less equivocal, manifestations of the latter disease, such as ectopia lentis and involvement of the aortic media, have, with rare exceptions,[21] not been reported with osteogenesis imperfecta.

The back is usually round, and the thorax has a characteristic conic or beehive shape (see x-ray films). The face is usually triangular, due largely to the

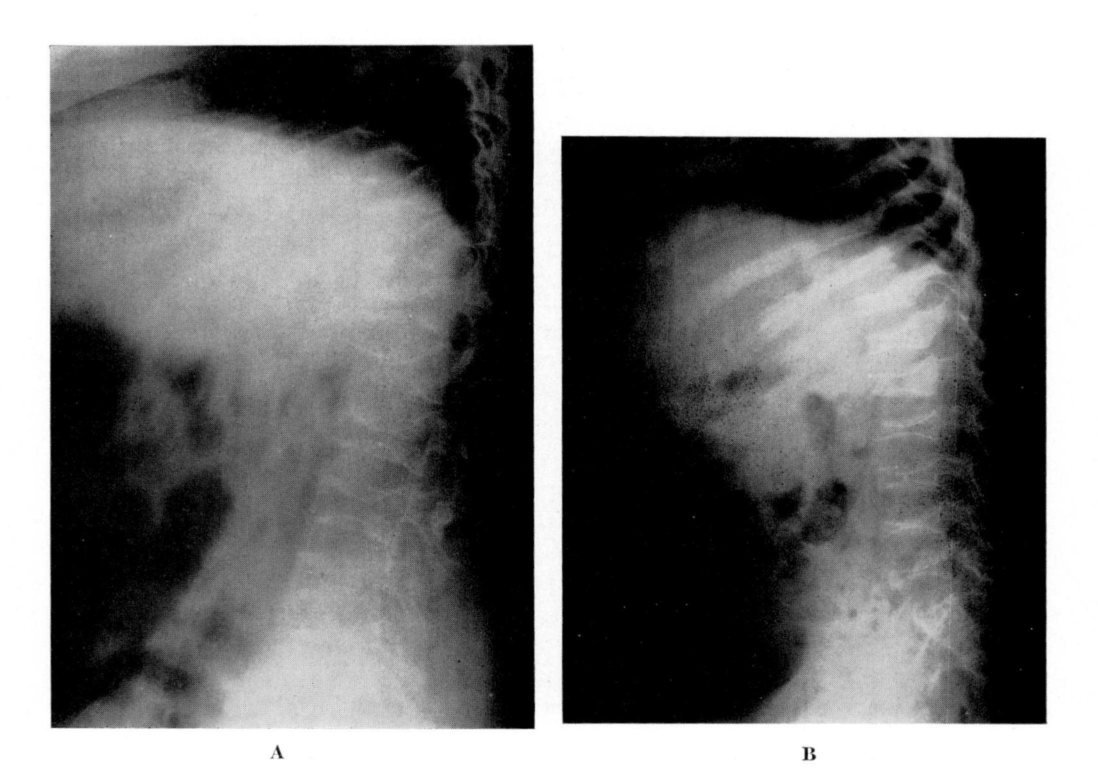

Fig. 6-9. Lateral views of the spine in two patients with codfish vertebrae. **A,** Patient J. L. L. (Children's Hosp. Sch.), 13 years of age. **B,** Patient H. R. (Children's Hosp. Sch.), 2 years of age. The marked change, called platyspondylisis,[265] is shown.

bulging calvarium and to faciocranial disproportion. The forehead is broad and domed and the temporal areas are overhanging. The "temporal bulge"[64] and the "overhanging occiput"[74] (Fig. 6-8) are characteristic. The victims have trouble getting hats large enough to fit them. As a result of the bulging calvarium, the ears tend to be displaced outward and to point downward. On skull x-ray film the inferosuperior dimension is reduced. This, together with the "occipital overhang," the frontal bossing, and the platybasia that may be present in severe cases, results in a mushroom appearance of the skull on lateral x-ray examination. Apert[8] referred to the skull as "crâne en rebord," and Nielsen[176] used the analogy "soldier's helmet," or "helmet head." In general, as with so many other hereditary disorders, victims of this disease tend to resemble each other closely, even though they are quite unrelated. The facies and skeletal proportions are so characteristic that one can usually recognize the victims from a photograph, a feature useful in pedigree investigations.[210]

Because of pelvic deformity, successful termination of pregnancy may be a serious problem.[137] Fracture of the rami of the pubis during delivery has been described.[23]

By x-ray the bones are more radiolucent than normal. If x-ray films are taken at times when no fractures are present, the skeleton may, at the most, be described as only very "porotic."[141] In fact, the x-ray films may show no definite abnormality, and it may be concluded that the findings do not justify the diagnosis of OI. In severe cases the cortex is thin, and gross deformities, such as are shown in Fig. 6-10, are demonstrated. Bone age is proportionate to chronologic age.

Because of hypercallosity at the site of fractures, osteogenic sarcoma has been suspected in some cases.[14,206] Actual sarcoma has not been described.

The teeth are particularly susceptible to caries, are easily broken (like the bones), hold fillings poorly, and, although normally shaped, may have an abnormal amber, yellowish brown, or translucent bluish gray coloration.[241] Both deciduous and permanent teeth may show this peculiarity. Witkop[261] states that the teeth which erupt first, e.g. the lower incisors, are the ones most affected. On x-ray examination the teeth are likely to show no pulp canal. Often during drilling, the patient feels no pain, only vibration. One patient (S. W., 782036) stated that although his teeth had always been embarrassingly yellow, they were unusually hard to drilling. Inspection revealed a good state of repair. Although most of each tooth was yellowish, the tip of each incisor was slightly translucent and blue. The lamina dura, as in acquired types of osteoporosis, remains intact. The enamel is thought to be fundamentally normal[20] and the abnormality is thought to reside in the dentine. This prompted Roberts and Schour[191] to suggest the name *dentinogenesis imperfecta** for the dental aspect of this disease rather than the terms *hereditary opalescent dentine* or *hereditary hypoplasia of the dentine,* which had been used before. Pedigrees in which this was presumably an isolated anomaly inherited as a dominant are described.[126,129,257] Some of these pedigrees[23,118,238] are undoubtedly instances of the generalized disease, osteogenesis imperfecta, in which the dental manifestations dominate overwhelm-

**Odontogenesis imperfecta* is a less specific term, inasmuch as the first portion refers to both enamel and dentine.

A

C

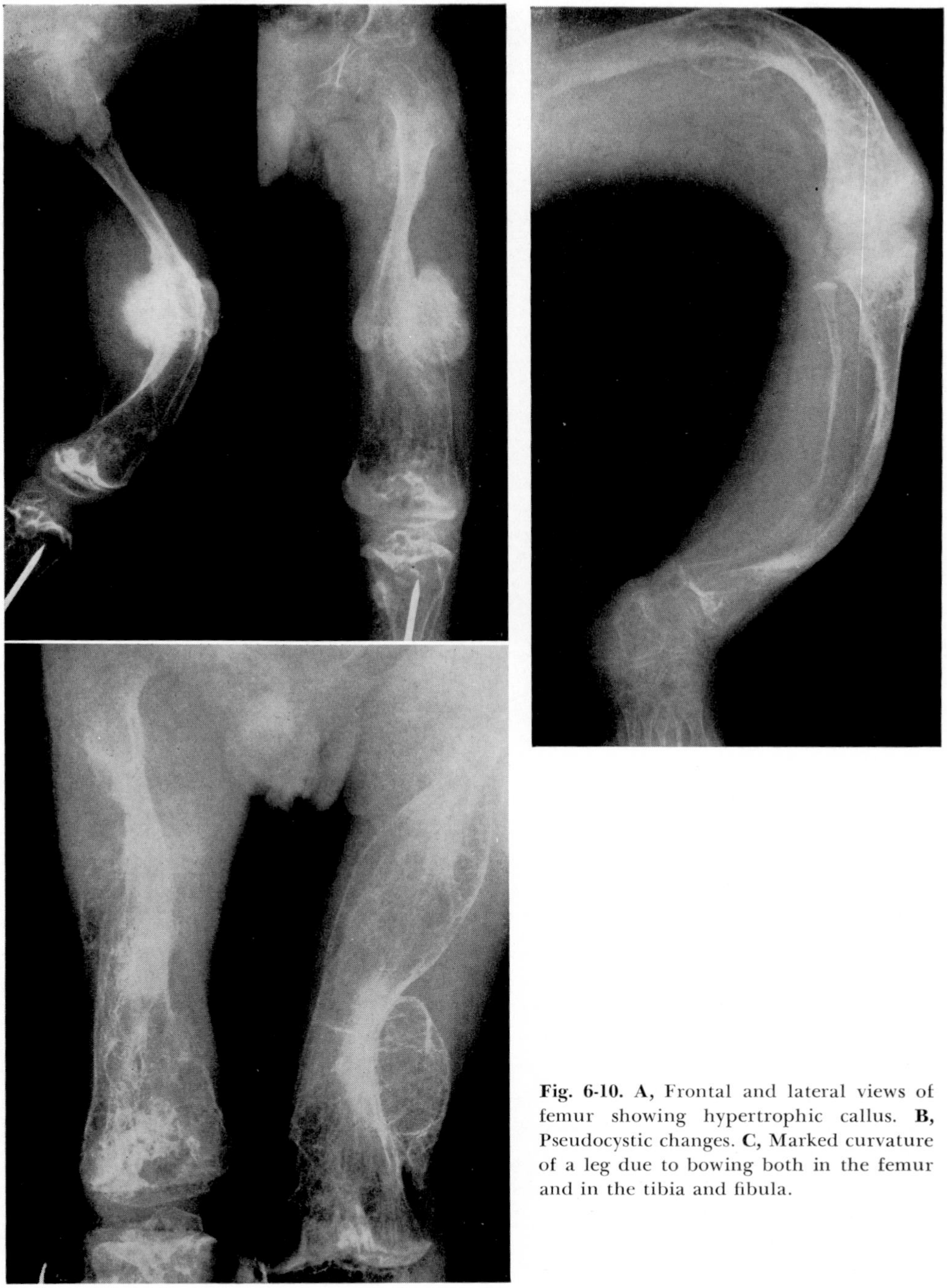

B

Fig. 6-10. A, Frontal and lateral views of femur showing hypertrophic callus. **B,** Pseudocystic changes. **C,** Marked curvature of a leg due to bowing both in the femur and in the tibia and fibula.

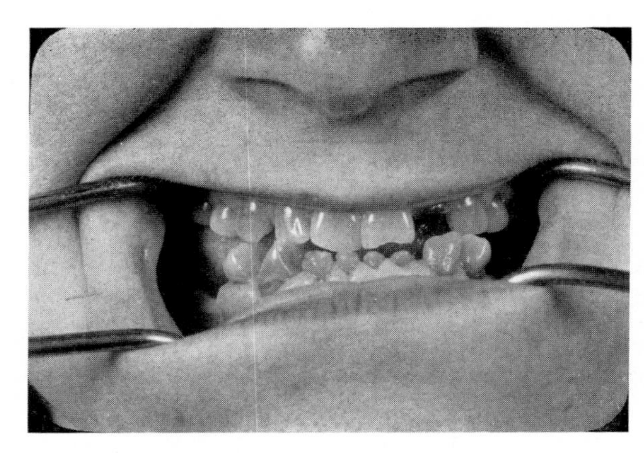

Fig. 6-11. Teeth in M. W., 32-year-old female with fragilitas ossium, blue sclerotics, and mild deafness. One of her two children (D. W., 736452) has OI. However, five siblings, both parents, and all other relatives are apparently unaffected. The stunting and discoloration of the lower incisor teeth are well demonstrated.

ingly. Roberts and Schour[191] were able to trace a family back five generations to 1763. The dental abnormality was very striking and was inherited as a strict dominant. Of forty-five individuals in five generations, twenty-two were affected. The authors made reference to other evidences of a mesenchymal defect. Wide variability in the manifestations of dentinogenesis imperfecta in individuals heterozygous for the dominant gene has been thought[148] to be responsible for several dentine dysplasias reported as separate clinical entities.

To be differentiated from odontogenesis imperfecta is the hereditary abnormality of enamel production that results in a discoloration of the teeth somewhat similar to that with OI. Known to me is a family in Maine with a characteristic of brown teeth traceable to a male ancestor who was born in 1805 and whose parents, of uncertain dental status, immigrated from England. A detailed investigation of this L. family was included in the report of Weinmann and associates.[253] Two types of hereditary abnormality of enamel formation (amyelogenesis imperfecta) are recognized: an inadequate production of enamel substrate and a subnormal calcification of enamel. Clinical points helpful in differentiating the two varieties have been outlined.[253]

The joints, typically, are excessively mobile[26,109,119,210] in this condition, just as in the Marfan syndrome and the Ehlers-Danlos syndrome. Both OI and E-D were thought to be present in one case.[28] It is said[210] that this characteristic is at times so striking that the subject can perform as a contortionist. The basis is in part the presence of weak, stretched tendons and joint capsules and in part the deformity and maladaptation of the bony surfaces of the joints. In one reported case,[34] the patient won prizes as a gymnast; his repertoire included the ability to put his feet into his trouser pockets. Pseudoarthroses may have been present. Key[145] described the Achilles tendon in one patient as, grossly, the "diameter of a lead pencil (0.6 cm.) and translucent in appearance, there being a striking absence of the dense white fibrous tissue usually seen." From the standpoint of histology and of pathologic involvement in a number of diseases, the sclera bears many resemblances to tendon.[88]

Rupture of the inferior patellar tendon may follow exertion with more forceful quadriceps activity than usual.[160,225] This accident occurred in at least four patients in our series (E. Z., H.L.H. 81588; K. Y., J.H.H. 594806; R. C., U.M.H. 40485; E. R., J.H.H. 602544). Habitual dislocation of joints,[15,21,40,125,227,236] or of the patella,[86] pes planus, and pseudoclubfoot[210] are frequent occurrences. In at least two patients (H.L.H. 19845; A94292) bilateral clubfoot was thought to be present at birth. The reason for confusion is evident from Fig. 6-2. The father of one of our patients (J. B., 541962), himself a victim of OI, has suffered from recurrent dislocation of the shoulder. The articular laxity probably exposes the victim to falls, which are so likely to result in fracture.

Wyllie and Schlesinger[263] reported two cases in children whose mothers consulted them because of the child's tardiness in walking. No fractures had oc-

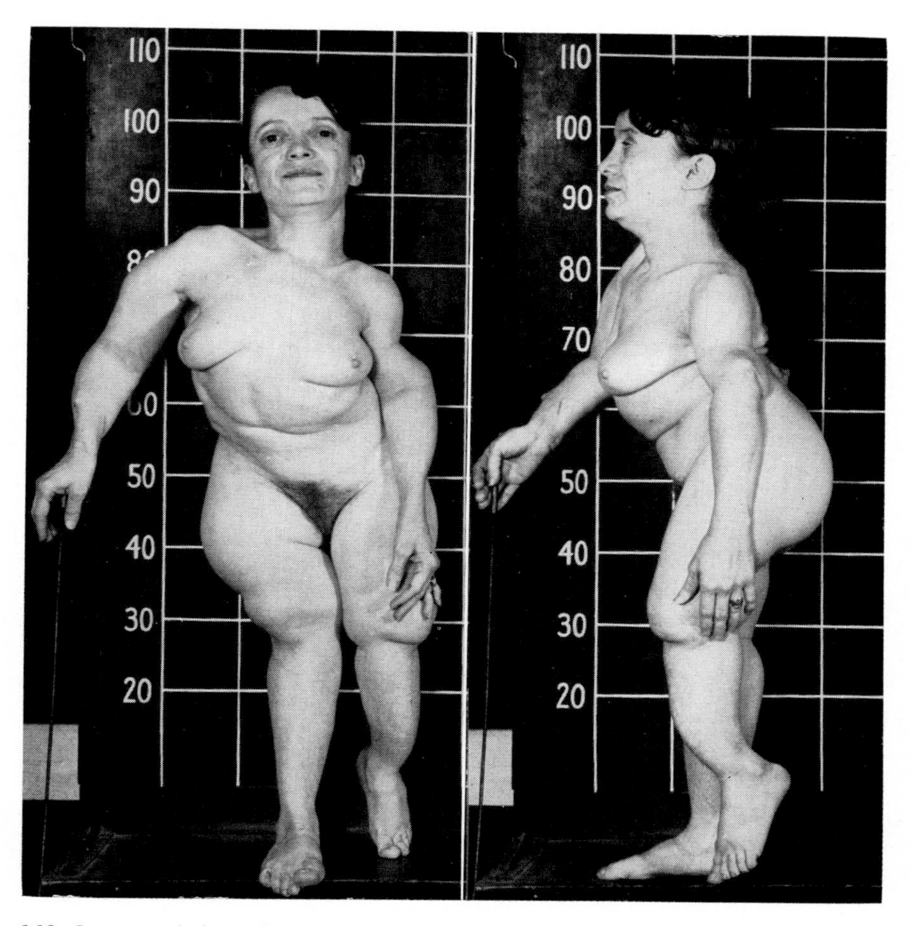

Fig. 6-12. Osteogenesis imperfecta in K. C. (673043), 35 years of age. Innumerable fractures have occurred, the first having been recognized at the age of 9 months. The sclerae are blue; hearing is intact. The patient is scarcely taller than a 4-year-old child. She has never walked and is carried about by a husky female friend. There are pseudoarthroses of the left humerus and left tibia. Of two pregnancies, one was terminated for therapeutic reasons and the other ended in spontaneous abortion. (From McKusick, V. A.: Bull. N. Y. Acad. Med. **35:**143, 1959.)

curred; at least none had been recognized. The presenting complaint, a not unusual one for OI, was apparently due to difficulty in fixing the joints for walking. The diagnosis of OI was based on the occurrence of clear cases in the family and of supporting radiologic changes in the patients. In one of our patients (R. F., J.H.H. 194765) there was such loose-jointedness and tardiness in walking and sitting that flaccid diplegia was suspected for a time.

Scoliosis may develop as a result of laxity of ligaments, as well as of vertebral osteoporosis (Fig. 6-12). The spinal deformity is often extreme. Pain in the back is frequent in these patients. As in the Marfan syndrome, muscular hypotonia and underdevelopment have been emphasized by several writers.[10,11,61] As in the Marfan syndrome, these features are quite clearly secondary to the anomalies of the tendons and joints and to general debility with reduced muscular activity. The fibrous skeleton of the muscles may be defective, but there is no evidence that the muscle cell itself is at fault. At times, in children (N. T., A46910), enlargement and weakness of the limbs have suggested pseudohypertrophic muscular dystrophy.

Hernia occurs with high incidence in these patients (see pedigree 603 in reference 22), as with most other hereditary connective tissue disorders under discussion, except pseudoxanthoma elasticum. The infant with OIC, shown in Fig. 6-3, clearly demonstrates the combination of multiple fractures and bilateral scrotal hernias. Cryptorchidism may occur in the males, in association with inguinal hernia (E. J. W., S.B.G. 6914).

The eye. Blue sclerotics constitute the ocular hallmark of this syndrome. The color of the sclera is described at times as robin's egg blue and at times as slate blue. "Wedgwood blue" is another vivid description. Of the manifestations of this disease, blue sclerotics are the most frequent. Occasionally they are absent in unmistakable instances of the syndrome. This is not surprising, since a high degree of variability in severity (expressivity) of this manifestation is to be expected and overlap with the curve of normal distribution is likely to occur. Impressively blue sclerae are not infrequently encountered in persons free from all other stigmata of this syndrome.

Often the part of the sclera immediately around the cornea is whiter, resulting in the so-called "Saturn's ring." There is probably some increased risk of traumatic perforation of the sclera, a complication that occurred in Buchanan's historic case.[42]

Embryotoxon, a congenital opacity in the periphery of the cornea, sometimes called arcus juvenilis, is very frequent.[38,183,193,239,260] By slit lamp the cornea is measurably thinner than normal.[260] Hypermetropia appears to be significantly frequent.[1,5,59,227,229] Chorioretinitis, probably on an independently inherited basis, was reported by Colden.[56]

Other clinical manifestations probably closely related to the same defect of scleral connective tissue are keratoconus[11,21,42,70] megalocornea,[70] and maculae corneae.[245] Keratoconus was present in one of our patients (E. Z., H.L.H. 81588). Behr's patient[21] had ectopia lentis. Premature arcus senilis is described.[245] However, this may have been merely the embryotoxon mentioned above. In two cases observed at this hospital[160] glaucoma has been present. In one, it was discovered soon after birth (R. F., 194765) and has been termed congenital; in the other (H. J., 428403), the right eye was rendered blind (phthisis bulbi), presumably by glaucoma, at the age of about 20 years, and the other eye later was affected by so-called chronic, wide-angle glaucoma. There are a few reports of associated glaucoma in the literature.[236,256]

The skin. The skin in this condition is characteristically thin and translucent. It may resemble prematurely the atrophic skin of the aged. Healing of skin wounds has been found, by study of surgical incisions in these patients, to result in wider scars than usual.[199] Subcutaneous hemorrhages* tend to occur after minor injuries,[48] and tests of capillary fragility may be positive.[210,214] Macular atrophy of the skin is described by Blegvad and Haxthausen.[32] This may be comparable to the spotty blueness of the sclera in some instances.[245]

Biebl and Streitmann[27] described elastosis perforans in a 16-year-old male with OI. Members of three generations of his family were affected. Reed and Pidgeon[186] also observed this skin change in OI. Elastosis perforans has been observed in the Marfan syndrome (p. 108), the Ehlers-Danlos syndrome, and pseudoxanthoma elasticum (p. 294), as well as in mongolism.

The ear.[36,38] Deafness is the least constant of the major features of OI.[47] Although the histologic patterns may be distinct, the clinical[30,33,40,54,83,199,229,236,240] pattern of the deafness which accompanies this syndrome differs in no respect from that of otosclerosis. Stenvers[226] demonstrated that characteristic sclerosis of the petrous portion of the temporal bone can be detected radiologically even before the impairment of hearing has its onset; and, of course, these changes may be present but not so located as to cause deafness. Deafness may have its onset in the teens; often it begins during pregnancy.[82,210] In Nager's patient,[173] hearing loss had its onset at the age of 9 years. As with otosclerosis of other origin, two types, a common stapes-ankylosing variety and a rarer cochlear type, have been described alone or in combination. Therefore, there may be either conduction or nerve type hearing loss.[87] Fenestration operation[133] has been performed in two patients with good results, by Shambaugh,[211] and in one, with indifferent results, by Watkyn-Thomas.[249] As with other types of otosclerosis, middle ear infection aggravates the hearing loss. There has been described[226] an interesting blueness of the tympanic membrane, analogous to the blue sclerotics as far as indicating thinness of the structure is concerned. The patient may complain of almost constant tinnitus for long periods and of attacks of vertigo. Labyrinthine disease uncomplicated by deafness has been described.[87,245] Leicher and Haas[152] described patients who had no dizziness and only mild difficulty walking in the dark, but little or no response to vestibule-stimulating maneuvers.

Internal manifestations. As for cardiovascular involvement, Sundberg[234] and Johansson[136] have described calcification of large peripheral arteries in victims of OIC. In one of our cases of OIC (557774; aut. 22803) in which there was neonatal death, necropsy revealed calcification of pulmonary and cerebral arteries. Arteries in the limbs were not studied histogically. Although Bauer[19] and Kaul[140] described changes in the connective tissue elements of the arterial wall, others have not been impressed with these. Lobeck,[154] Colden,[56] and Voorhoeve[245] described premature arteriosclerosis. Congenital heart disease was present in one patient.[245] Hass[113] described heart disease in several members of a kinship. From the descriptions of one of the members of that pedigree, rheumatic heart disease

*See discussion of hemorrhagic disease in OI, p. 249.

seems to have been present in that individual. In general, the heart disease was probably unrelated to the OI. Severe aortic regurgitation of obscure etiology was present in one patient with OI seen at the Johns Hopkins Hospital when he was 16 years old (G. S., J.H.H. U45942). Criscitiello and colleagues[62] described two OI patients, ages 43 and 47, with dilatation of the aortic root and aortic regurgitation. A third OI patient, age 50, had a bicuspid aortic valve, fenestration of the pulmonic valve, and an aneurysm of the anterior leaflet of the mitral valve.

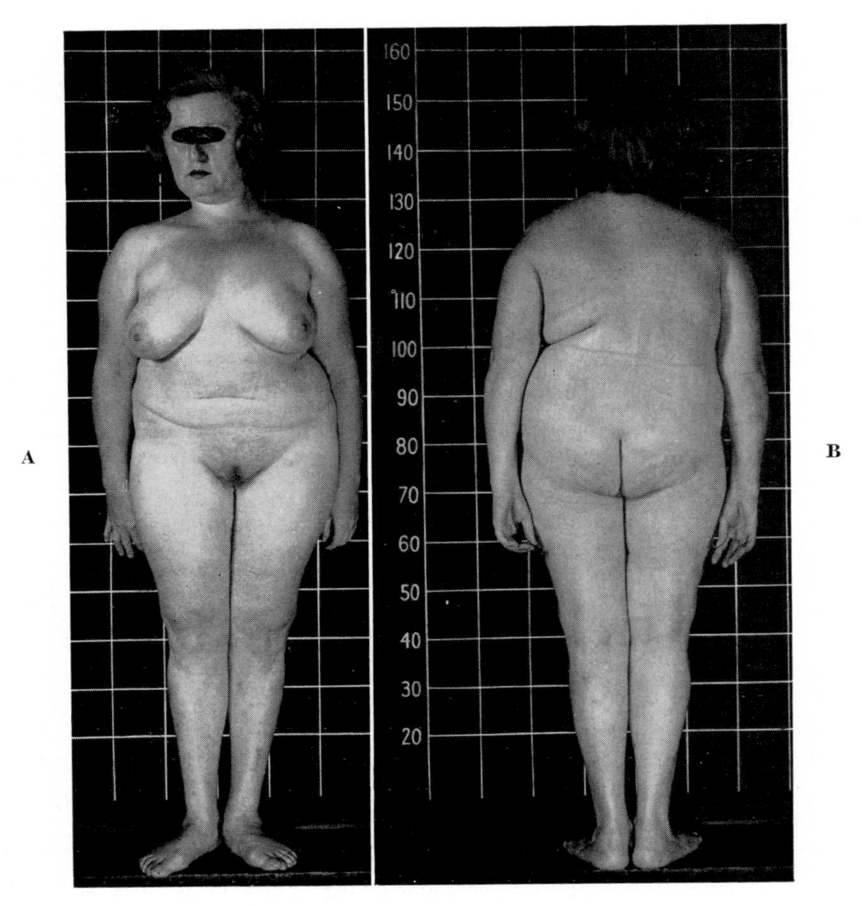

Fig. 6-13. J. G. (149692), 43 years old. In **A,** note the bulging calvarium with triangular facies. Flat feet and kyphoscoliosis are also evident in **A** and **B.** The x-ray film in **C** reveals the complex spinal deformity present in this patient. The bones are more radiolucent than is normal. The sclerae are deeply blue. Deafness has been present since at least the age of 25 years and tinnitus has often been distressing. Scoliosis was first noted at the age of 13 years, and since the age of 16 years back pain has been a major complaint. The patient is, in general, loose-jointed with flat feet; the head of the humerus was dislocated on one occasion when she was thrown from a bicycle at the age of 7 years. A ganglion on the right wrist was described at one time. X-ray film of the skull shows characteristic decrease in the vertical dimension. A diastolic murmur at the left sternal border remains unexplained. An amazing feature of this case of undoubted osteogenesis imperfecta is the fact that *no* fractures have occurred in spite of appreciable trauma on several occasions.

In one of my patients (J. G., 149692), with severe S-type rotary scoliosis (Fig. 6-13), a faint diastolic murmur has been heard to the left of the sternum, and there is a borderline increase in systemic arterial pulse pressure. Whether this sound represents regurgitation at the aortic or the pulmonic valve or possibly has an extracardiac origin is unclear. Severe spinal deformity may be followed by kyphoscoliotic cor pulmonale (e.g. C. B., 242806). Premature emphysema is frequent.

There are no pathognomonic chemical changes in the blood. Significant abnormalities of calcium and phosphorus do not occur. Alkaline phosphatase activity[221] is often increased as a result of multiple healing fractures. We have been unable to corroborate the report[95] that serum acid phosphatase activity is significantly increased in this disease. Jacobsen and colleagues[131] and Ginsberg[99] likewise found normal levels of serum acid phosphatase.

Siegel and co-workers[214] have described a 25-year-old man with OI and hemorrhagic diathesis manifested by epistaxes, hemoptyses, easy bruisability, and prolonged bleeding time. The Rumpel-Leede test was positive. A defect of the platelet was demonstrated by means of the thromboplastin generation test. There were multiple cases of OI in the family, but the only one available for study, a sister, did not show the abnormality. The authors suggested that the hemorrhagic diathesis was of the type described by Glanzmann[101] in 1918 as thrombasthenia. The cause of the capillary fragility was not clear. It was corrected

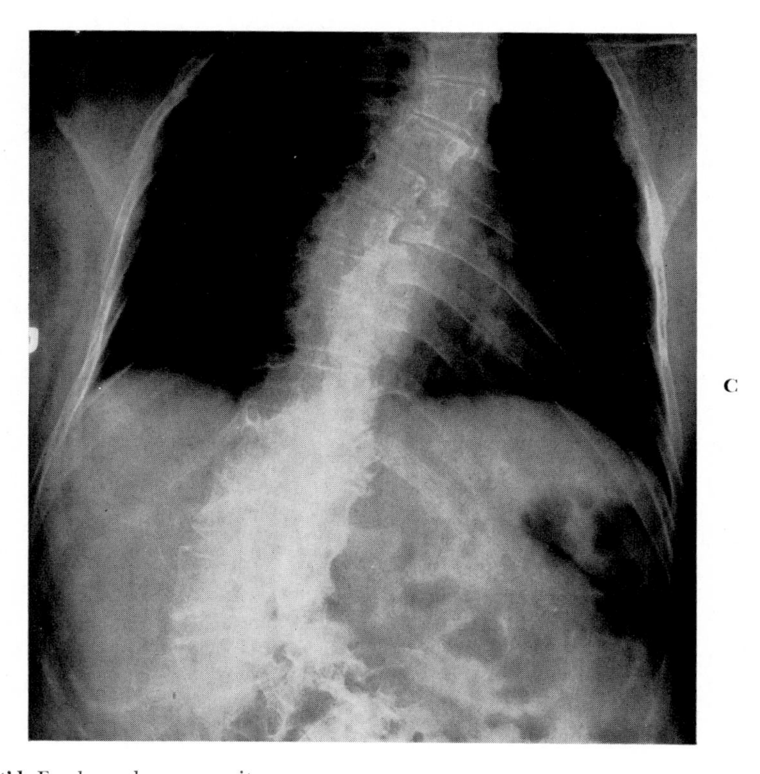

C

Fig. 6-13, cont'd. For legend see opposite page.

by cortisone; however, this can be a nonspecific effect. Gautier and Guinard-Daniol[94] described a 13½-month-old patient with OI in whom defective clot retraction was demonstrated. The mother had blue sclerae with bone disease, abnormal prothrombin consumption test, and impaired clot retraction. The last two tests showed impairment in the father, also. Siegel and co-workers[214] suggest that these two mesenchymal defects (OI and platelet defect) are related and not simply coincidental.

Neurologic symptoms, particularly those of platybasia and of spinal cord compression, occur occasionally but are usually submerged by the other types of incapacitation from which these patients suffer. Backache and leg pains, which may have an element of nerve root compression in their causation, are of frequent occurrence. Neurologic deficits attributable to this are less frequent. As with idiopathic varieties of platybasia (basilar impression), as well as that due to other bone-softening diseases such as Paget's disease, rickets, hyperparathyroidism, and sarcoid, four types of neurologic involvement should be sought[179]: (1) internal hydrocephalus; (2) bilateral, progressive cerebellar disturbance; (3) interference with the function of the lower cranial nerves; and (4) signs of spinal cord compression at the level of the foramen magnum. The impingement of the odontoid process of the axis on the brain stem is responsible for many of these manifestations. (Basilar impression in OI is discussed in references 127 and 235.)

Two methods are used to detect platybasia radiologically: Chamberlain's line (from the posterior end of the hard palate to the posterior lip of the foramen magnum) normally lies above the entirety of the cervical spine.[49] Such is not the case in platybasia. According to Bull's index,[43] the plane of the axis is normally parallel to that of the hard palate, whereas, in platybasia, the two planes make an acute angle with each other.

Bell[22] pictures the skeleton of a 12-year-old boy with marked skeletal changes of OI and with hydrocephalus. The skeleton is in the museum of the Royal College of Surgeons in London. Hydrocephalus developed in several of our patients with osteogenesis imperfecta congenita. (See Figs. 6-2 and 6-5*B*.)

Occasionally patients with OI have retarded intellect (e.g. S. V., H.L.H. 75237; R. F., 194765). Although arrested hydrocephalus may be the basis in some cases, others probably represent mere coincidence of OI and mental retardation on another basis.

The wide variability in severity of OI, permitting long survival in some cases, is well illustrated by the 95-year-old woman reported by Stool and Sullivan,[230] by the 58-year-old man shown in Fig. 6-14, and by the severely deformed 54-year-old man reported by Scherr.[202]

Summary of clinical manifestations. Bell[22] provides entirely credible figures for the incidence of the several manifestations: among adult individuals "with blue sclerotics approximately 60% have an associated liability to fracture, approximately 60% have an associated otosclerosis, and 44% suffer from all three defects." These values might be higher were it possible to eliminate those cases with hereditary blue sclerae on some other basis. It has not been established that blue sclerae can occur on an independent, genetically distinct basis and as an isolated anomaly. (They do occur with others of the hereditary disorders of connective tissue.) However, such seems likely from experience with similar situations.

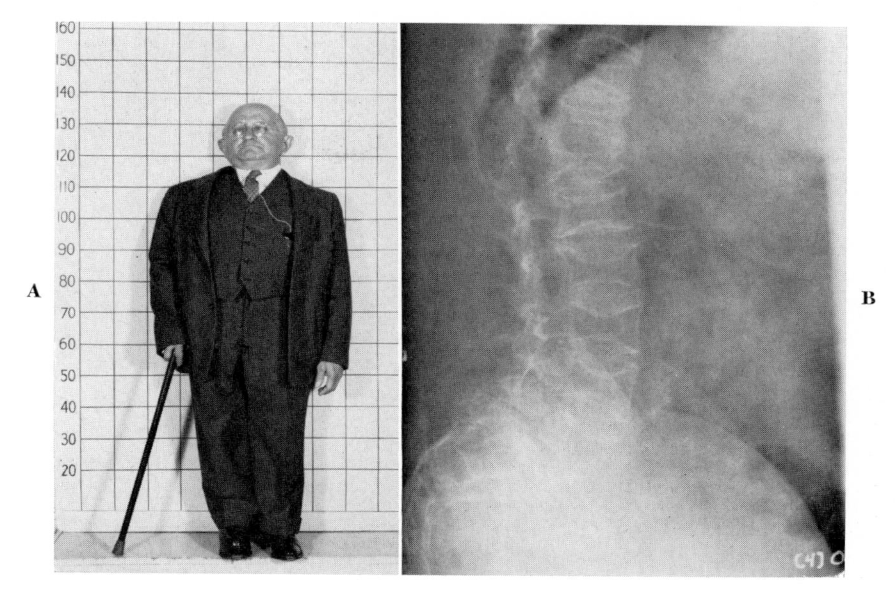

Fig. 6-14. I. L. (455357), white male born in 1902, was apparently a sporadic case of osteogenesis imperfecta. He was first seen at the Johns Hopkins Hospital for a fracture at age 8 years. He had numerous fractures, necessitating admission thereafter. The diagnosis of OI was first made at the age of 21 years (1923). The last fracture occurred in 1932 (age 30 years). At the age of 45 years a bout of acute cholecystitis requiring cholecystectomy was withstood in a normal manner. Hypertension was first discovered then. Hearing defect was first noted in 1951 and a hearing aid was applied. The patient died of coronary occlusion at the age of 60 years. Examination in 1961 showed blue sclerae, deafness, characteristically shaped skull with overhang above the ears, and short stature, **A.** Profound osteoporosis of the spine was demonstrated, **B.**

Prevalence and inheritance

Among the seven disorders under principal discussion in this book, osteogenesis imperfecta vies with the Marfan syndrome for first place as to incidence. It was relatively easy to accumulate more than a hundred apparently unrelated propositi for purposes of this study.* Between 1920 and 1940 forty cases of OI were seen at the Mayo Clinic.[41] Of these, eleven had a story of the disease in other members of the family. Almost half of those with positive family histories had otosclerosis, whereas deafness occurred in only about one sixth of those without a positive family history.

There is no peculiar racial distribution of OI, cases having been described in Jews[160] and American Negroes,[104,160,248] and in natives of Japan,[139,175] China,[53] India,[112] Egypt,[10,11] and Russia,[247] as well as all the western European countries.

The evidence is overwhelming that OI is usually inherited as an autosomal dominant. Bell[22] found such to be the case for blue sclerotics in seventy-three kinships with a total of 463 affected persons. In an analysis of eighty-nine families with 1,000 individuals, of whom 515 were affected, Fuss[92] demonstrated autosomal dominance for the syndrome of bone fragility and blue sclerotics. One of the best-

*Patients from Baltimore or Maryland and patients who have been seen at some time at Johns Hopkins Hospital have been reported in several previous publications.[79,80,81,120,196,216]

studied pedigrees is that of a family of the eastern shore of Maryland, reported by Hills and McLanahan.[120] Twenty-seven of fifty-one members of five generations were affected. A number of other pedigrees with affected persons in five successive generations have been published. Scores of "dominant" pedigrees are on record.[58,116,135,143,188,189]

Seedorff,[210] after studying fifty-five kinships with 180 affected individuals, constructed a complicated schema based on the theories that each component of the syndrome is the result of a separate gene and that three separate genes control the bone fragility, with mutation in one, two, or three being responsible, respectively, for OIT levis, OIT gravis, and OIC. This complex schema is untenable because of the arguments against a multiple-gene basis of hereditary syndromes (Chapter 1) and because of the probability, on clinical and histopathologic grounds, that the three arbitrarily designated states are in fact different grades of severity of the same disorder of connective tissue.

Freda and co-workers[84] estimated the frequency of OIC to be about 1 in 40,000 births and quoted others as estimating the frequency as less than 1 in 60,000 births.

Frequently the statement appears[102,120] that the so-called congenital form of the disease probably is not inherited, in many instances, or is inherited in a different manner (e.g. as a recessive) than the other forms.* Many of such instances—severely affected stillborn children of normal parents—may be *de novo* mutations. The rarity of families in which two infants with OIC are born from indubitably normal parents speaks against recessive inheritance in the majority of cases. Obviously, identical twins with OIC[78,204,254] (Fig. 6-5*A*) are not a contradiction to this statement. Occurrence of the disorder in identical twins is evidence of the genetic basis of the "congenital" form of OI. Furthermore, the rarity of parental consanguinity is against the view that OIC is recessive. Even if the parents had to be considered normal by every gauge, suspicion of subtle abnormality would remain. When a severely affected offspring from very mildly affected parents is encountered, there is the possibility that both parents are heterozygous and the child homozygous.[149]

Seedorff[210] thought, from the cases in the literature and from his own cases, that OIC occurred much more frequently in females. Among his seven cases of OIC, only one was male. This might be construed as evidence that OIC is a distinct entity. In our own experience, however, defining as OIC any case in which abnormality referrable to the skeleton was described at birth, the sex ratio does not deviate significantly from one. The question of recessive inheritance of some cases of OIC is discussed further below.

There have been advocates for the view that there is an entity called osteopsathyrosis idiopathica of Lobstein and distinct from the triad of blue sclerotics, deafness, and fragilitas ossium.[121,153] Some permit deafness in patients of the presumably distinct osteopsathyrosis group but insist that a main differentiating feature is the absence of blue sclerotics. Holcomb[121] wrote as follows: "In the Davis family, whose history I have investigated, the tendency to break bones

---

*A comparable question exists in connection with congenital cystic disease of the kidneys, a disorder in which two forms may truly exist: a congenital form, which proves fatal very early in life, and a late form, with average age of death at about 50 years.[66]

with abnormal frequency, especially in childhood, occurred in a number of persons in five generations of the family, but in no case was there the slighest indication of the blue sclera or progressive deafness."* This type of evidence does not necessarily indicate that a separate entity is involved, since it is clear that in a given family the individual components of a syndrome may display considerable independence in penetrance and expressivity. An alternative possibility is the existence of multiple alleles.

In surveying the genetics of OI, Herndon[117] writes as follows: "In my opinion we do not have sufficient critical information to permit us to distinguish between the possibilities of (1) a minority of cases representing the homozygous state of a different or possibly the same gene; (2) a mutation rate for a dominant gene that is quite high in relation to the number of clinically recognized cases, but not necessarily high in terms of mutant genes per generation; (3) a considerable reduction in penetrance of a dominant gene, with the rate of penetrance probably being different in different family groups, modified either by unrecognized environmental factors or possibly by modifying genes; (4) any possible combination of the first three factors."† These are some of the same factors as are discussed in connection with the "cause" of "sporadic" cases of hereditary disease, pp. 11 and 12.

Twins, both of whom were affected by OIC, were described by Schultze.[204] The report is of further note because the father had blue sclerae and deafness but no apparent fragility of the bones; support for the identity of OIC and OIT is, therefore, provided. Others[142,195] have reported families in which one or more members were affected by the congenital form of OI and other members by the late form. Bierring[29] described OIC in mother and daughter.

Bell[22] found, in tabulating reported cases of bone fragility with blue sclerae on the one hand, and cases of bone fragility alone, on the other, a seemingly highly significant difference in sex incidence and mode of inheritance (whether through mother or father) in the two groups. The explanation for a bias, if such existed, is not apparent. Also, the use of published data rather than those accumulated in a uniform manner by the researcher himself is beset with such pitfalls that it is doubtful that one is justified in concluding—and Bell does not so conclude—that a fundamental difference is involved. On the basis of other experience, it is entirely likely that blue sclerotics and fragilitas ossium of otherwise indistinguishable character can occur as isolated, heritable anomalies genetically distinct from osteogenesis imperfecta. It is, of course, well known that otosclerosis clinically identical with that of osteogenesis imperfecta occurs even more commonly as an isolated anomaly than as part of this syndrome. (In the family reported by Macgregor and Harrison,[158] otosclerosis and recessively inherited total color blindness occurred, by chance, together in some members.) This is a situation somewhat comparable to that involved in the ectopia lentis of the Marfan syndrome: the manifestations may occur alone or as part of a complex syndrome.

Consanguinity is not impressively frequent in the pedigrees of OI. Liber[153] reported on the offspring of a marriage of first-cousin children of first-cousin parents. The proband had bone disease and deafness. The mother "was short and squat, had a large skull, and was and apparently always had been almost totally

---

*From Holcomb, D. Y.: J. Hered. **22**:105, 1931.

†From Herndon, C. N.: Clin. Orthop. **8**:132, 1956.

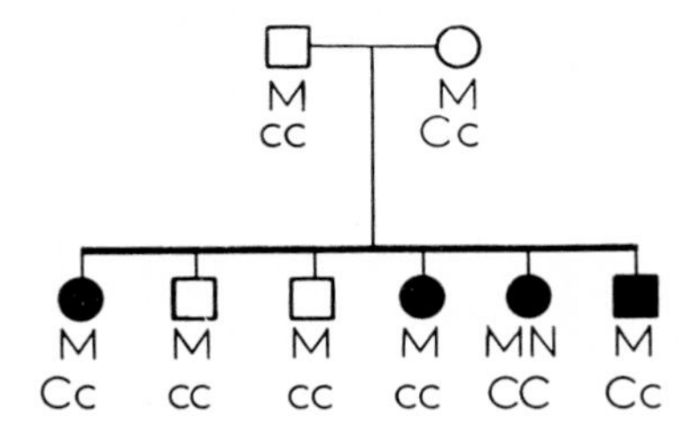

Fig. 6-15. Pedigree of family in which four sibs had osteogenesis imperfecta and both parents were seemingly unaffected. The blood group data indicate that the fifth child is not the progeny of the stated father. It is possible that the mother has the gene for OI, which is only very mildly expressed in her. (Redrawn from Smårs, G., Beckman, L., and Böök, J. A.: Acta Genet. **11**:133, 1961.)

deaf." A child of the proband had multiple fractures. Thus the consanguinity probably played no role. On the other hand, Komai and associates[149] made reference to the consanguineous mating of two individuals with only blue sclerotics, resulting in a child with the full-blown syndrome.

"Skipped generations" have been described[58,121,266] in well-studied families. Because of the exceedingly wide range of expressivity it is not surprising if manifestations in fundamentally affected persons are at times too mild to be recognized clinically. Smårs and associates[219,220] described an interesting family (Fig. 6-15) in which four of six children were affected but both parents could pass as unaffected. One of the affected children was proved by blood group data to be illegitimate, making recessive inheritance unlikely and also suggesting that the mother was heterozygous. In fact, the mother had had one fracture from falling from a bicycle and was slightly deaf in one ear.

Even with the excellent system for indexing hereditary diseases in Denmark, Seedorff[210] concluded that one is not justified in attempting to calculate the mutation rate for this anomaly. Furthermore, Seedorff could find no conclusive evidence that the parents of patients with osteogenesis imperfecta tend to be older, as seems to be the case in chondrodystrophic dwarfism.[169] In his group of cases of OIT, Seedorff[210] concluded that these individuals are 1.4 times more productive of children than their normal siblings. So far as perpetuating the disease is concerned, each affected individual produced, on the average, 0.75 affected children. If it were not for constantly occurring new cases on the basis of mutation, the disease would in time disappear. Seedorff estimated that in Denmark one infant with OIC is born each year.

Komai and associates[149] attempted a crude estimate of the mutation rate in OI, assuming that all cases of OIC represent new dominant mutation, that the female preponderance in OIC is genuine, that four out of five affected male fetuses die before birth whereas none of the affected female fetuses die in utero, and finally that the frequency of OIC is about 2 per 100,000 births. OIC cases represent by this estimate a mutation rate of 1.67×10^{-5} per gene per generation. Also, there is no reproduction in the severe form of OI tarda, which, according to Seedorff, is 2.14 times as frequent as OIC. In addition, the reduced effective fertility of late cases would bring the total estimate of mutation rate to about 4×10^{-5} per gene per generation.

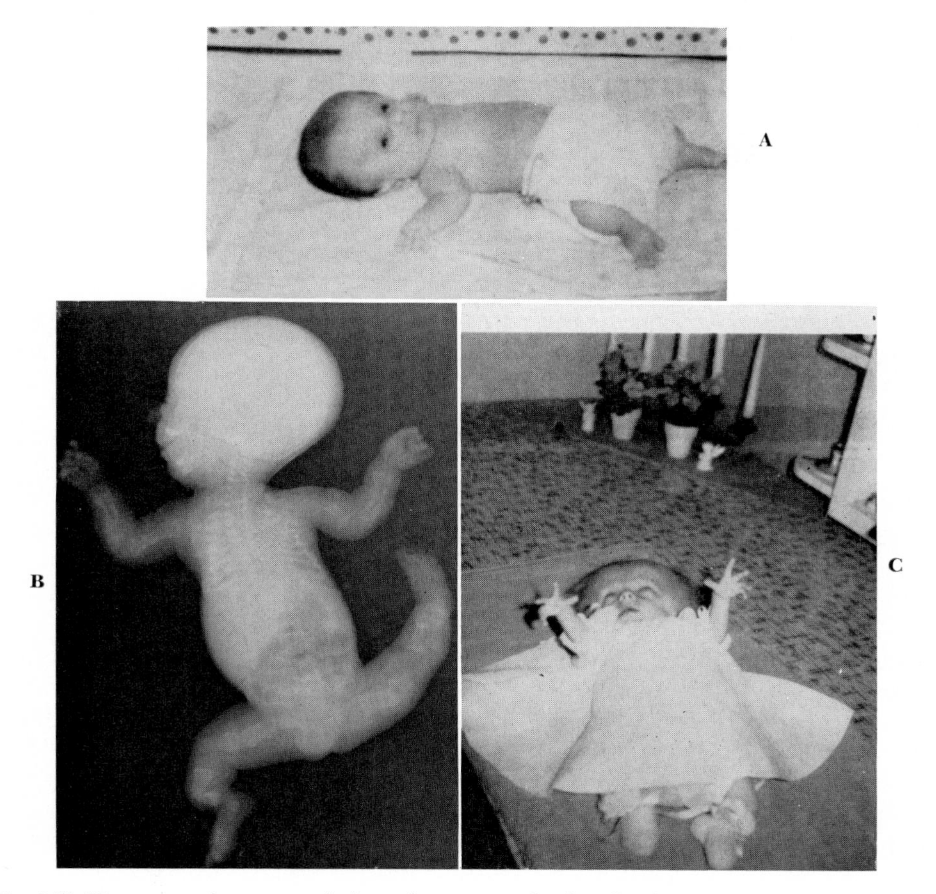

Fig. 6-16. Two cases of osteogenesis imperfecta congenita in offspring of ostensibly normal parents. **A** and **B,** Typical clinical and radiologic appearance in newborn infant. **C,** View at 10 months with development of hydrocephalus. A male sib with identical changes confirmed by x-ray examination died at the age of 2 days. Another sib is normal. The parents are not related. (From McKusick, V. A.: Medical genetics 1958-1960, St. Louis, 1961, The C. V. Mosby Co.)

Accumulating experience suggests that in some cases osteogenesis imperfecta congenita may be an autosomal recessive disorder separate from the autosomal dominant one. Goldfarb and Ford[105] described OIC in two consecutive female sibs with normal parents. Chawla[50] observed OIC in four sibs with normal parents. A comparable experience is illustrated in Fig. 6-16. Awwaad and Reda[12] described two cases of OIC in one sibship, offspring of consanguineous but unaffected parents. Hein[115] observed OIC in the offspring of a first-cousin marriage. Hanhart[111] described a recessive form of "osteopsathyrosis congenita." Meyer[166] described "atypical osteogenesis imperfecta" in three of the eleven offspring of incestuous mating between a mentally defective woman and her father. Manifestations were spontaneous fractures, generalized osteoporosis, and Wormian bones in the region of the lamboidal sutures. Blue sclerae were absent. Mental retardation requiring institutionalization and microphthalmos were also present but appeared to be segregating independently in this sibship.

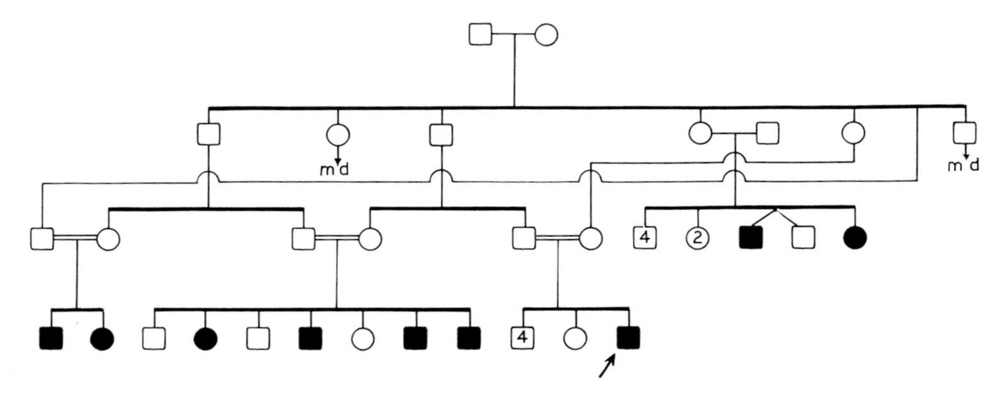

Fig. 6-17. Osteogenesis imperfecta congenita in kindred reported by Kaplan and Baldino.[138] **md,** Many descendants.

Studying the same family, Berry[25] demonstrated cystinuria in the three sibs with atypical OI. Since arginine, ornithine, and lysine were also present and since other amino acids, glucose, and protein were not present in the urine in excess, the biochemical disorder seemed to be classic recessive cystinuria and not the Fanconi syndrome. Thus, these same three patients with atypical OI had cystinuria. Five of the eleven children mentioned above survived; the two without osteogenesis imperfecta and cystinuria are also mentally retarded.

The condition called "periosteal dysplasia of Porak and Durante" by French authors is probably the same as osteogenesis imperfecta, and several examples of recessive inheritance have been reported. Kaplan and Baldino[138] dscribed a case in an inbred, Arabic-speaking, polygamous sect called the Mozabites living in southern Algeria. Nine cases had occurred among the descendants of one marital couple, in a pattern supporting autosomal recessive inheritance (Fig. 6-17). The proband had bulging head and eyes, bent limbs (as in Fig. 6-2), slate-blue sclerae, mosaic skull bones, scoliosis, multiple fractures of ribs and bones of the extremities, and hernia. Reference was made to several other reported instances of apparent recessive inheritance, e.g. that by Glanzmann,[103] of an affected 9-year-old girl and her affected 4-month-old brother. Also identity to Vrolik's type of osteogenesis imperfecta (i.e. the congenital form) was suggested.

Confusion with hypophosphatasia (p. 443) must be avoided in any consideration of a recessive form of congenital OI.

If there is indeed a recessive form of OIC, an enzyme defect is likely to be found, rather than a structural change in a connective tissue protein, which on theoretical grounds (p. 16) is more likely in the dominantly inherited, usual form of OI.

In summary, an autosomal recessive disorder with all the features of OIC probably exists. However, this disorder probably accounts for only a small proportion of OIC cases. Therefore, the following statement relevant to genetic counselling is valid: "In the case of normal parents (i.e. without brittle bones and blue sclerae) who have one infant affected with OIC, the possibility of giving birth to a second affected child is almost negligible."*

---

*From Freda, V. J., Vosburgh, G. J., and Di Liberti, C.: Osteogenesis imperfecta congenita: a presentation of 16 cases and review of the literature, Obstet. Gynec. **18:**535, 1961.

Pathology[132,250,258]

Histologically, the cortical layer of the bones and the trabeculae of the spongiosa are thin. The periosteum may appear normal, but some have reported reduction in the number of subperiosteal osteoblasts. A peculiar, basophilic, periodic acid and Schiff–positive material has been found in place of osteoid. In other tissue, only argyrophilic reticulin fibers and no mature collagen are demonstrated. Histochemically, phosphatase activity is not demonstrably disturbed, epiphyseal cartilage appears to be completely normal,[79] and invasion of the regularly arranged cartilage cell columns by capillaries is normal. The metaphysis shows calcified cartilage but no true bone or osteoid. This calcified cartilage tends to fracture and fragment. Organic bone matrix fails to be deposited, and in its stead a peculiar basophilic material makes its appearance. As stated above, the material stains with periodic acid and leucofuchsin and, furthermore, is argyrophilic. Follis[81] suggests that it may represent immature bone matrix in the manner that reticulin, which it resembles in its staining properties, may represent immature collagen.

Swedish workers using recently developed biophysical techniques demonstrated disorganization of the collagen matrix.[24,75] The specific techniques that they employed were microradiography, polarized light microscopy, and x-ray diffraction. Their findings are by no means inconsistent with those of Follis: ". . . in osteogenesis imperfecta the compact bone has a quite abnormal distribution of mineral salts and arrangement of organic fibers. . . . The immature fibrillar bone normally seen in the foetus and newborn infant resembles in several ways the tissue found in osteogenesis imperfecta. Normally this primary bone tissue is rapidly replaced by secondary bone after birth, but in osteogenesis imperfecta this secondary bone tissue is not found."*

Osteoblasts and osteoclasts are usually present in normal numbers. Chemically, calcium and phosphorus are present in the bones in a normal ratio; the total content of bone salts is reduced, however.

In the skin, Follis[80] found absence of normal adult collagen fibers and substitution by argyrophilic fibers with other properties of reticulin. However, the shrinkage temperature of the skin was normal.

In the eye, decreased thickness of the sclera was described as early as 1841 by von Ammon[244] and more recently by Buchanan,[42] Casanovas,[48] and Follis,[79] but normal thickness was found by Bronson[40] and Voigt.[243] Ruedemann[196] has found histologic changes in cornea and sclera fundamentally identical to those described by Follis[79] in the corium. Clearly, the blue coloration is the result of the brown-pigmented choroid showing through the thin sclera.[252]

In sections of the teeth, "clodlike" calcification of quite abnormal type is seen. Rushton[197] showed that peripheral pulp cells produce "precollagenous" argyrophilic fibers but that these are not converted into collagen except in the immediate vicinity of blood vessels. These observations are in complete agreement with those of Follis, in bone, skin, and sclera.

Histologically the changes in the ear in osteogenesis imperfecta are quite distinct from those of otosclerosis, despite the close clinical similarities, according to the studies made by Ruttin,[200] Gimplinger,[98] and others. Still others[173] maintain that, although the changes in the bone of the labyrinthine capsules are ad-

---

*From Engfeldt, B., Engstrom, A., and Zetterstrom, R.: J. Bone Joint Surg. **36-B**:654, 1954.

mittedly distinctive, deafness does not develop unless histologically typical otosclerosis is present. It is my impression that the precise pathogenetic relationship of deafness to the rest of this syndrome is in the main unknown.

The fundamental defect

A generalized mesenchymal defect has been assumed for several decades. The histologic investigations of Follis (described above) appear to indicate that the fundamental difficulty may be in the maturation of collagen beyond the reticulin fiber stage. (This assumes that one can subscribe without reservation to the view that reticulin fibers are immature collagen fibers.[159] Even if this is not the case, it can be stated that the collagen fibers in OI are abnormal and resemble reticulin fibers in many respects.) So far as the bones are concerned, the disease must be considered a disorder of osteoblastic activity. Normal chondroblastic activity is suggested by the fact that growth and development of cartilage are normal.

It has been claimed by Seedorff[210] that a condition in cattle called anosteoplasia congenita[128] is an identical disorder. In 1958 Coop[60] wrote as follows: "Osteogenesis imperfecta is a condition recognized with increased frequency in cats during the last eight years, especially in the Siamese and Burmese breeds."* It was thought that study of such animals could be very useful to the understanding of the disease in man. That the disease seemed to behave as an autosomal recessive in cats[123,124,218] might be an indication (p. 16) that its basic nature was different from that of the disease in man. Hereditary spherocytosis in mice is recessive and in man is dominant.[170] However, studying a kindred of Burmese cats, Scott and co-workers[208] showed that fractures did not develop after the diet was changed from horse meat and ground beef heart to fish catfood, skim milk, and table scraps and that under these dietary circumstances even the offspring of two "homozygotes" had no skeletal abnormality. Riser[190] similarly concluded that "osteogenesis imperfecta" in cats is the result of calcium deficiency.

Calkins and associates[45] observed a disorder resembling osteogenesis imperfecta in the standard French poodle and in the Norwegian elkhound. The frequency of fractures diminished at puberty. Clinical differences from the disease in man were attributed to early weight bearing and rapid leg growth in dogs. A reduction in the net rate of collagen formation seemed to be present. Holmes and associates[122] described "osteogenesis imperfecta" in lambs.

Giordano[100] in Milan, Italy, has been studying histochemical enzymatic reactions in OI. Caniggia and associates[46] claimed that the collagen in OI has an abnormally high proline content.

Summer[233] studied serum levels of proline after oral administration of proline in six children with OIT and in one with OIC. Peak levels in the first hour were less high in the OI cases than in normal subjects.

Chowers and colleagues[52] demonstrated aminoaciduria in six members of two families and postulated a renal tubular defect in OI. The affected persons had radiologic features consistent with osteogenesis imperfecta but not eye or ear abnormality, and inheritance was rather clearly autosomal recessive. It is likely that they were dealing with an entity related to the Fanconi syndrome and not

*From Coop, M. C.: J. Amer. Vet. Med. Ass. **132**:299, 1958.

with true OI. Brigham and Tourtellotte[37] reported in brief an increased urinary excretion of glycine, serine, threonine, ethanolamine, and valine, with a reduced level of these substances in the plasma, and suggested a renal tubular defect in OI. A detailed report has not yet appeared.

Although such a suggestion must remain speculative at this stage, one wonders if there may not be synthesized, in osteogenesis imperfecta and possibly in some others of the hereditary disorders of connective tissue, an atypical species of fibrous connective tissue protein. Do the amino acid sequences of collagen, in OI, differ from those in the "normal" by a single amino acid substitution, comparable to the recently demonstrated differences in several of the hemoglobin variants?

Miscellaneous considerations

In general, a decrease in the incidence of fractures is observed after puberty[41] with, possibly, an increase in this incidence after the menopause. The father of one of my patients (C. B., 351637) had numerous fractures up to the age of 16 years but thereafter was well enough that he served in the Navy for several years! Both sexes show the improvement at puberty. Both clinical experience in man[4] and experimental evidence from animals[93] indicate an important role of sex hormones in the normal formation of bone matrix. This hormonal influence may explain in large part the observations cited above; increased vigilance on the part of the patient may be in part responsible for the improvement after puberty.

Estrogens and testosterone are worthy of more extensive trial in these patients.[194] Certainly it is important to avoid the superimposition of postmenopausal osteoporosis on the osteoporosis of this heritable disease.[168] Nonmasculinizing forms of androgens[106] might be a boon. Sex hormones are said[60] to be beneficial in osteogenesis imperfecta of cats. Serum albumin, which seems to be a precursor for bone matrix, is beneficial when administered to patients with certain acquired varieties of osteoporosis.[3] It apparently has not been used in osteogenesis imperfecta. Strontium has also not been tested,[212] with the exception of one study[35] in which the author thought the results were favorable and rendered further study worth while. As one might expect, many kinds of medication have been employed for this distressing and long-standing disorder—for example, thymus extract.[209] Furthermore, because of difficulties in evaluating results, the variable course of the disease, and wishful thinking on the part of physicians and patients, overly enthusiastic reports have at times been forthcoming.

Unless quite by accident some efficacious therapeutic measure is discovered, no definitive progress in the therapy of OI can be anticipated until the precise reason for the failure of normal development and/or maturation of collagen is understood. Only then can measures directed at correcting the specific deficit be devised. There is every reason to anticipate that the biochemical defect in hereditary disorders such as this will be precisely defined in the future. Optimism in regard to possibilities of correcting or modifying the basic defect is justified.

Osteogenesis imperfecta and the Marfan syndrome were thought to be present in the same patient, by at least two authors. Although arachnodactyly may have been present, it is not certain that the specific entity of the Marfan syndrome was also present. Fromm and colleagues[89] and Weil[251] described precocious menarche, blue sclerae, multiple fractures, and irregular cutaneous pigmentation—many of the features of Albright's polyostotic fibrous dysplasia. Although Fromm referred to it as osteogenesis impretecta, it seems doubtful that this was fundamentally the same disease as that to which we have applied the designation OI in a rather specific manner in this discussion.

As in acquired forms of osteoporosis, it is highly important to avoid immobilization of the patient because of the further depletion of bone matrix occasioned thereby. It is doubtful that a high intake of calcium, phosphorus, and vitamin D is helpful, and the combination of these with immobilization may have dire effects: C. B. (J.H.H. 242806) developed large bladder stones and a *Proteus* infection of the urinary tract after immobilization for eleven weeks in a cast and a "bone-building diet" that included several quarts of milk a day and added calcium and vitamin D. The pinning and plating of fractures have much to recommend them because they reduce the necessity for immobilization.

Osteotomies and related procedures of orthopedic surgery are employed to correct deformities. Fixation by an intramedullary rod has also been recommended.[7,161,165,233]

In severely affected women, pregnancy is not to be encouraged, not only because of the 50% chance of the child's being affected but also because of adverse effects of the pregnant and the parturient[177] state on the skeleton. Deafness from otosclerosis often begins or is aggravated during pregnancy. (Some, like Nager,[174] doubt a relationship, however.) Because of the pelvic deformities of the disease, delivery may be mechanically very difficult.[66] One patient[160] has fractured her coccyx with each of the deliveries. There is a strikingly high incidence of breech presentation in cases of infants with OIC born of normal mothers.

Because of inactivity it is easy for victims of this disease to become obese. Obviously, this is to be avoided. In young patients, Fröhlich's syndrome is sometimes suspected without basis.

Idiopathic osteoporosis of childhood or adolescence without blue sclerae and other stigmata of osteogenesis imperfecta is occasionally observed.[9,130] Sometimes more than one sib is affected but usually not.[69] This appears to represent an entity distinct from osteogenesis imperfecta; whether it is genetic is unclear. Possibly this is the condition that Chowers and colleagues[52] were dealing with in the six cases, five of them familial, with radiologic features of osteogenesis imperfecta but no blue sclerae or deafness. Aminoaciduria and low serum uric acid levels were demonstrated by these patients. Because of these findings and rather clear autosomal recessive inheritance, the cases may be more accurately classified as a form of renal tubular defect related to the Fanconi syndrome.

Lifelong osteoporosis with codfish vertebrae and susceptibility to fracture occurs also in homocystinuria (Chapter 4) and might be confused with osteogenesis imperfecta.

As mentioned earlier (p. 256), hypophosphatasia (p. 443) must not be confused with osteogenesis imperfecta congenita.

Among the genetically determined skeletal disorders having osseous fragility as a feature is a newly recognized disorder, pycnodysostosis. The features are autosomal recessive inheritance, bone sclerosis with proneness to fracture, persistently wide cranial fontanelles, micrognathism with virtual absence of the ramus of the mandible, hypoplasia of the clavicles, and osteolysis in the terminal phalanges of the fingers. Some of the features resemble those of cleidocranial dysostosis, with which pycnodysostosis has sometimes been confused but which shows dominant inheritance. Lamy and Maroteaux[163] first described and named pycnodysostosis. Seedorff[210] suggested that Henri de Toulouse-Lautrec (1864-1901), French painter, suffered from osteogenesis imperfecta. His appearance as displayed in photographs (Fig. 10-28) is certainly consistent. Particularly suggestive of OI are Lautrec's short legs; Jose Ferrer, when playing Lautrec in the motion picture *Moulin Rouge,* walked about on his knees. Review of available information has led Maroteaux and Lamy[164] to believe that Lautrec in fact suffered from pycnodysostosis. His parents were first cousins. The failure to grow dated from an early age. He was apparently already infirm, for he was using a stick when his first recognized fracture (of the left femur) occurred at age 14 from a fall as he tried to get out of a chair. The following year fracture of the right femur occurred when he slipped into a shallow ditch while on a walk. Photographs[171] do not suggest blue sclerae, and those in swimming garb show no bowing deformity of the legs. Maroteaux and Lamy[164] conclude that photographs suggest micrognathia and they suggest further that Lautrec's perpetual wearing of a hat was prompted by an open anterior fontanelle!

Achondroplasia is a frequent misdiagnosis in these patients. Confusion may occur at birth (see Fig. 6-2) or in later life. The patient described by Ruth[198] was diagnosed as having achondroplasia because of the big head and short limbs. At the age of about 50 years he was selling papers from a wheelchair. In discussion of a patient 53 years old (I. L., Sinai 70327), the following conclusion was stated: "In regard to the developmental anomaly of this patient: I believe he is an achondroplastic dwarf with typically well-built torso and relatively short spindly legs."

OI, a hereditary form of osteoporosis, is accompanied by blue sclerae. In other forms of osteoporosis, such as Cushing's syndrome, prolonged administration of adrenal steroids, and senile (or postmenopausal) osteoporosis, it is likely that the connective tissue defect is more extensive than merely involving the organic matrix of bone. I have in isolated instances (e.g. M. H., 738167) been impressed with the occurrence of blue sclerae in senile osteoporosis.

Vaughn[242] noted an increase in the blueness of the sclerae in a case of OI, with episodes of stress such as fractures. This observation, as well as the declining frequency of fractures at puberty (and possible increase after the menopause) may represent an interaction of hormonal effects with the hereditary disorder of connective tissue.

Blue sclerotics cannot, of course, as a rule be used as the only criterion for the diagnosis of OI. Evaluation is especially difficult in children, who normally have bluish sclerae.

It is of interest that an Osteogenesis Imperfecta Foundation has been established under the laws of the state of Texas, with headquarters in Fort Worth.*

SUMMARY AND CONCLUSIONS

Osteogenesis imperfecta is a generalized disorder of connective tissue involving, in addition to bone, the skin, ligaments, tendons, fascia, sclera, and inner ear. Although the most frequent functionally important manifestations are

---

*Address: Box 892, Fort Worth, Texas.

brittle bones and deafness, blue sclerae are a dramatic feature, and thin skin, loose-jointedness, and hernia occur as manifestations of a single basic defect.

An exceptionally wide range of expressivity has resulted in the description of several different syndromes, all of which may be but different expressions of a single type of connective tissue disorder, inherited as a Mendelian autosomal dominant. The existence of an autosomal recessive form presenting usually as osteogenesis imperfecta congenita is likely, however.

Studies to date are most consistent with the view that the basic defect is one which involves either the maturation of the collagen fiber beyond the stage of the argyrophilic, reticulin fiber or the synthesis of a different species of collagen with tinctorial resemblance to reticulin.

REFERENCES

1. Adair-Dighton, C. A.: Four generations of blue sclerotics, Ophthalmoscope **10**:188, 1912.
2. Adatia, M. D.: J. Indian Med. Prof. **4**:1810, 1957.
3. Albright, F., Bartter, F. C., Dempsey, E. F., Forbes, A. P., Henneman, P. H., and Reifenstein, E. C., Jr.: Serum albumin and bone matrix, Macy Conferences, Metabolic interrelations with special referene to calcium, New York, 1953.
4. Albright, F., and Reifenstein, E. C., Jr.: The parathyroid glands and metabolic bone disease, selected studies, Baltimore, 1948, The Williams & Wilkins Co., p. 150.
5. Alexander, J. B.: Fragilitas ossium associated with blue sclerotics in four generations, Brit. Med. J. **1**:677, 1922.
6. Altmann, F.: The temporal bone in osteogenesis imperfecta congenita, Arch. Otolaryng. **75**:486, 1962.
7. Anon.: Fragilitas ossium, J.A.M.A. **161**:773, 1956.
8. Apert, E.: Les hommes de verre, Presse Méd. **36**:805, 1928.
9. Archibald, R. M., New York City: Personal communication.
10. Attiah, M. A. H.: Blue sclerotics, Bull. Ophthal. Soc. Egypt **26**:96, 1933.
11. Attiah, M. A. H., and Sobhy Bey, M.: Blue sclerotics, Bull Ophthal. Soc. Egypt **24**:67, 1931.
12. Awwaad, S., and Reda, M.: Osteogenesis imperfecta. Review of literature and report on three cases, Arch. Pediat. **77**:280, 1960.
13. Axmann, E.: Merkwürdige Fragilität der Knochen ohne dyskrasische Ursache als krankhafte Eigenthümlichkeit dreier Geschwister, Ann. Ges. Heilk. (Karlsruhe) **4**:58, 1831.
14. Baker, S. L.: Hyperplastic callus simulating sarcoma in two cases of fragilitas ossium, J. Path. Bact. **58**:609, 1946.
15. Bantz, W.: Ueber einen Fall von Osteogenesis imperfecta tarda mit gleichzeitger habitueller Schultergelenksluxation beiderseits, Zbl. Chir. **68**:1726, 1941.
16. Bartter, F. C., and Bauer, W.: Fragilitas ossium. In Cecil, R. L., and Loeb, R. F.: Textbook of medicine, ed. 9, Philadelphia, 1955, W. B. Saunders Co., p. 1447.
17. Bauer, K. H.: Ueber Osteogenesis imperfecta, Deutsch. Zschr. Chir. **154**:166, 1920.
18. Bauer, K. H.: Ueber Identität und Wesen der sogenannten Osteopsathyrosis idiopathica und Osteogenesis imperfecta, Deutsch. Zschr. Chir. **160**:289, 1920.
19. Bauer, K. H.: Erbkonstitutionelle "Systemerkrankungen" und Mesenchym, Klin. Wschr. **2**:624, 1923.
20. Becks, H.: Histologic study of tooth structure in osteogenesis imperfecta, Dent. Cosmos **73**:737, 1931.
21. Behr, C.: Keratokonus, blaue Sklera, habituelle Luxationen, Monatsbl. f. Augenh. **1**:281, 1913.
22. Bell, J.: Blue sclerotics and fragility of bone. Treasury of human inheritance., vol. 2, part III, Cambridge and London, 1928, University of London, Cambridge University Press.
23. Bergman, G.: The incremental pattern of the dentine in a case of osteogenesis imperfecta, Oral Surg. **13**:70, 1960.
24. Bergman, G., and Engfeldt, B.: Studies on mineralized dental tissues. IV. Biophysical studies in osteogenesis imperfecta, Acta Path. Microbiol. Scand. **35**:537, 1954.

25. Berry, H. K.: Cystinuria in mentally retarded siblings with atypical osteogenesis imperfecta, Amer. J. Dis. Child. **97**:196, 1959.
26. Bert, J. M.: Les formes de transition entre les syndromes familiaux de fragilité osseuse (type Lobstein) et de grande hyperlaxité-ligamentaire (type Morquio), Presse Med. **50**:290, 1942.
27. Biebl, E., and Streitmann, B.: Elastosis perforans bei einem Fall von Osteogenesis imperfecta, Z. Haut. Geschlechtskr. **35**:333, 1963.
28. Biering, A., and Iversen, T.: Osteogenesis imperfecta associated with Ehlers-Danlos syndrome, Acta Paediat. **44**:279, 1955.
29. Bierring, K.: Contribution to the perception of osteogenesis imperfecta congenita and osteopsathyrosis idiopathica as identical disorders, Acta Chir. Scand. **70**:481, 1933.
30. Bigler, M.: Ueber das gleichzeitige Vorkommen von Osteopsathyrose und blauer Verfärbung der Skleren bei Otosklerose, Arch. Ohr. Nas Kehlkopfheilk. **5**:233, 1923.
31. Blattner, R. J., Heyes, F., and Robinson, H. B. G.: Osteogenesis imperfecta and odontogenesis imperfecta (hereditary opalescent dentin), J. Dent. Res. **21**:325, 1942.
32. Blegvard, O., and Haxthausen, H.: Blue sclerotics and brittle bones, with macular atrophy of the skin and zonular cataract, Brit. Med. J. **2**:1071, 1921.
33. Blencke, A.: Ueber das gemeinsame Vorkommen von Knochembrüchigkeit mit blauen Skleren und Schwerhörigkeit, Zschr. Orthop. Chir. **45**:406, 1924.
34. Bonnet, P., and Wertheimer, C.: Un cas d'osteopsathyrose, Bull. Soc. Ophtal. Franc., p. 119, 1935.
35. Breuer, J.: Zur Therapie der Osteopsathyrosis mit blauen Skleren, Deutsch. Med. Wschr. **56**:1735, 1930.
36. Brickley, D. W.: Otosclerosis and blue scleras, Arch. Otolaryng. **46**:230, 1947.
37. Brigham, M. P., and Tourtellotte, C. D.: Amino acid changes in blood and urine in osteogenesis imperfecta (abstract), Fed. Proc. **21**:167, 1962.
38. Broca, A., and Herbinet: De l'osteopsathyrosis ou fragilité osseuse dite essentielle, Rev. Chir. **77**:284, 1905.
39. Bromer, R. S.: Rickets and infantile scurvy occurring in case of osteogenesis imperfecta, Amer. J. Roentgen. **55**:30, 1946.
40. Bronson, E.: On fragilitas ossium and its association with blue sclerotics and otosclerosis, Edinburgh Med. J. **18**:240, 1917.
41. Bryan, R. S., Cain, J. C., and Lipscomb, P. R.: Hereditary osteogenesis imperfecta. A mother and son with their family tree, Mayo Clin. Proc. **31**:475, 1956.
42. Buchanan, L.: Case of congenital maldevelopment of the cornea and sclerotic, Trans. Ophthal. Soc. U.K. **23**:267, 1903.
43. Bull, J.: Paget's disease of the skull with platybasia, Proc. Roy. Soc. Med. **40**:85, 1946.
44. Caffey, J.: Pediatric x-ray diagnosis, ed. 2, Chicago, 1950, Year Book Medical Publishers, Inc., p. 41.
45. Calkins, E., Kahn, D., and Diner, W. A.: Idiopathic familial osteoporosis in dogs; "osteogenesis imperfecta," Ann. N.Y. Acad. Sci. **64**:410, 1956.
46. Caniggia, A., Ravenni, G., and Del Giovane, L.: On the pathogenesis of fragilitas ossium hereditaria, Panminerva Med. **3**:67, 1961.
47. Caniggia, A., Stuart, C., and Guideri, R.: Fragilitas ossium hereditaria tarda (Eckman-Lobstein disease), Acta Med. Scand., supp. 340:1, 1958.
48. Casanovas, J.: Blue scleras and fragilitas ossium, Arch. Ophth. Hispano-Amer. **34**:133, 1934.
49. Chamberlain, W. E.: Basilar impression (platybasia). A bizarre developmental anomaly of the occipital bone and upper cervical spine with striking and misleading neurologic manifestations, Yale J. Biol. Med. **11**:487, 1939.
50. Chawla, S.: Intrauterine osteogenesis imperfecta in four siblings, Brit. Med. J. **1**:99, 1964.
51. Chont, L. K.: Osteogenesis imperfecta; report of 12 cases, Amer. J. Roentgen. **45**:850, 1941.
52. Chowers, I., Czaczkes, J. W., Ehrenfeld, E. N., and Landau, S.: Familial aminoaciduria in osteogenesis imperfecta, J.A.M.A. **181**:771, 1962.
53. Chu, H. I., Liu, S. H., Chen, K. C., Yü, T. F., Su, C. C., Wang, C. W., and Cheng, T. Y.: Osteogenesis imperfecta. II. Observations on the effect of vitamins C and D, and thyroid and pituitary preparations on the calcium, phosphorus and nitrogen metabolism with a report of bone analysis, Chin. Med. J. (supp.) **3**:539, 1940.

54. Cleminson, F. J.: Otosclerosis associated with blue sclerotics and osteogenesis imperfecta, Proc. Roy. Soc. Med. **20**:471, 1927.
55. Cocchi, U.: Hereditary diseases with bone changes. In Schinz, H. R.: Roentgen-diagnostics, New York, 1951, Grune & Stratton, Inc.
56. Colden, C.: Blaue Skleren mit eigenartigem ophthalmoskopischen Befund, Klin. Mbl. Augenheilk. **74**:360, 1925.
57. Committee on Otosclerosis, American Otological Society: Otosclerosis; a résumé of the literature to July, 1928, New York, 1929, Paul B. Hoeber, Inc., Medical Book Department of Harper & Row, Publishers.
58. Conlon, F. A.: Five generations of blue sclerotics and associated osteoporosis, Boston Med. Surg. **169**:16, 1913.
59. Conlon, F. A.: Blue sclerotics; a note upon associated otosclerosis, Amer. J. Ophthal. 1 (series 3):726, 1918.
60. Coop, M. C.: A treatment for osteogenesis imperfecta in kittens, J. Amer. Vet. Med. Ass. **132**:299, 1958.
61. Cornil, L., Berthier, J., and Sild, A.: Sur l'adjonction à osteopsathyrose hereditaire de deux nouveaux signes: tympans bleus et amyotrophie diffuse, Rev. Neurol. **67**:89, 1937.
62. Criscitiello, M. G., Ronan, J. A., Jr., Besterman, E. M. M., and Schoenwetter, W.: Cardiovascular abnormalities in osteogenesis imperfecta, Circulation **31**:255, 1965.
63. Cronental, R.: Ueber die Osteopsathyrosis hereditaria, Deutsch. Arch. Klin. Med. **174**:228, 1932.
64. Crooks, J.: Two unusual examples of osteogenesis imperfecta, Brit. Med. J. **1**:705, 1932.
65. Crowe, F. W., Schull, W. J., and Neel, J. V.: A clinical pathological and genetic study of multiple neurofibromatosis, Springfield, Ill., 1956, Charles C Thomas, Publisher, p. 36.
66. Dalgaard, O.: Bilateral polycystic disease of the kidneys, Copenhagen, 1957, Ejnar Munksgaard Forlag.
67. Danelius, G.: Osteogenesis imperfecta intrauterin diagnostiziert, Arch. Gynaek. **154**:160, 1933.
68. Daubenspeck, K.: Pseudoarthrosenbehandlung bei Osteopsathyrosis, Zbl. Chir. **67**:370, 1940.
69. Dent, C. E., and Friedman, M.: Idiopathic juvenile osteoporosis, Quart. J. Med. **34**:177, 1964.
70. Dessof, J.: Blue sclerotics, fragile bones and deafness, Arch. Ophthal. **12**:60, 1934.
71. Eddowes, A.: Dark sclerotics and fragilitas ossium, Brit. Med. J. **2**:222, 1900.
72. Ekman, O. J.: Dissertatio medica descriptionem et casus aliquot osteomalaciae sistens, Upsala, 1788.
73. Elefant, E., and Tošovsky, V.: Osteogenesis imperfecta congenita, Ann. Paediat. **202**:285, 1964.
74. Ellis, R. W. B.: Four cases of fragilitas ossium and blue sclerotics, Proc. Roy. Soc. Med. (Sect. Dis. Child.) **24**:1054, 1931.
75. Engfeldt, B., Engstrom, A., and Zetterstrom, R.: Biophysical studies of the bone tissue in osteogenesis imperfecta, J. Bone Joint Surg. **36-B**:654, 1954.
76. Fairbank, H. A. T., and Baker, S. L.: Hyperplastic callus formation with or without evidence of fracture in osteogenesis imperfecta with account of the histology, Brit. J. Surg. **36**:1, 1948.
77. Fairbank, Sir Thomas: An atlas of general affections of the skeleton, Baltimore, 1951, The Williams & Wilkins Co.
78. Faxén, N.: Case of twins with osteogenesis imperfecta, Acta Paediat. **14**:251, 1932.
79. Follis, R. H., Jr.: Osteogenesis imperfecta congenita; a connective tissue diathesis, J. Pediat. **41**:713, 1952.
80. Follis, R. H., Jr.: Maldevelopment of the corium in the osteogenesis imperfecta syndrome, Bull. Hopkins Hosp. **93**:225, 1953.
81. Follis, R. H., Jr.: Histochemical studies on cartilage and bone. III. Osteogenesis imperfecta, Bull. Hopkins Hosp. **93**:386, 1953.
82. Fraser, I.: Fragilitas ossium tarda, Brit. J. Surg. **22**:231, 1934.
83. Fraser, J. S.: Otosclerosis associated with fragilitas ossium and blue sclerotics; clinical report of 3 cases, Proc. Roy. Soc. Med. **12**:126, 1918.
84. Freda, V. J., Vosburgh, G. J., and Di Liberti, C.: Osteogenesis imperfecta congenita: a presentation of 16 cases and review of the literature, Obstet. Gynec. **18**:535, 1961.

85. Frerking, H. W., and Zink, O. C.: A case of osteogenesis imperfecta diagnosed in utero, Amer. J. Roentgen. **67**:103, 1952.
86. Freytag, G. T.: Ueber blaue Sklera und Knochenbrüchigkeit, Klin. Mbl. Augenheilk. **66**:507, 1921.
87. Friedberg, C. K.: Zur Kenntnis des vererbbaren Syndroms: Abnorme Knochenbrüchigkeit, blaue Skleren und Schwerhörigkeit, Klin. Wschr. **10**:830, 1931.
88. Friedenwald, J. S., and others: Ophthalmic pathology: an atlas and textbook, Philadelphia, 1952, W. B. Saunders Co.
89. Fromm, G. A., Parisier, H., Roca, J., and Defilippi Novoa, C. A.: Osteogenesis imperfecta associated with cutaneous pigmentation and other congenital malformations, Amer. J. Dis. Child. **96**:344, 1958.
90. Fulconis, H.: La fragilité osseuse congénitale (maladie de Durante), Paris, 1939, Masson et Cie.
91. Funk, P.: Beitrag zur Kenntnis der Osteopsathyrose (Typus Lobstein), Schweiz. Med. Wschr. **70**:473, 1940.
92. Fuss, H.: Die erbliche Osteopsathyrosis, Deutsch Z. Chir. **245**:279, 1935.
93. Gardner, W. V., and Pfeiffer, C. A.: Influence of estrogen and androgens on the skeletal system, Physiol. Rev. **23**:139, 1954.
94. Gautier, P., and Guinard-Daniol, J.: Un cas de maladie de Lobstein associée à une thrombasthenie héréditaire et familial de Glanzmann, Bull. Soc. Méd. Hôp. Paris **68**:577, 1952.
95. Gebala, A.: Acid hyperphosphatasia in three families with osteogenesis imperfecta, Lancet **2**:1084, 1956.
96. Geipert, G.: Beitrag zur Erblichkeit der sog. Osteopsathyrosis, Z. Menschl. Vererb. Konstitutionsl. **19**:691, 1936.
97. Gillanders, L. A.: Osteogenesis imperfecta diagnosed in utero, Brit. J. Radiol. **30**:500, 1957.
98. Gimpliner, E.: Blaue Verfärbung der Skleren und Herderkrankung der Labyrinthkapsel, Arch. Ohr. Nas. Kehlkopfheilk. **13**:345, 1925.
99. Ginsberg, D. M.: Normal serum acid phosphatase levels in ostetogenesis imperfecta, Ann. Intern. Med. **56**:141, 1962.
100. Giordano, A.: Hereditary diseases of the osteo-cartilaginous system. Comparative morphological basis, Acta Genet. **7**:155, 1957.
101. Glanzmann, E.: Hereditäre hämorrhagische Thrombasthenie (ein Beitrag zur Pathologie des Blutplättchen), Jahrb. Kinderheilk. **88**:113, 1918.
102. Glanzmann, E.: Osteogenesis imperfecta (Typus Vrolik) und Osteopsathyrosis idiopathica (Typus Lobstein), Schweiz. Med. Wschr. **66**:1122, 1936.
103. Glanzmann, E.: Familiäre Osteogenesis imperfecta (Typus Vrolik) und ihre Behandlung mit Vitamin D-Stoss, Bull. Schweiz. Akad. Med. Wiss. **1**:180, 1945.
104. Gleich, M.: Osteogenesis imperfecta tarda; report of 4 cases in one family, New York J. Med. **30**:850, 1930.
105. Goldfarb, A. A., and Ford, D.: Osteogenesis imperfecta in consecutive siblings, J. Pediat. **44**:264, 1954.
106. Gordan, G. S., Eisenberg, E., Moon, H. D., and Sakamoto, W.: Methylandrostenediol, a protein anabolic steroid with little androgenic activity, J. Clin. Endocr. **11**:209, 1951.
107. Greenberg, E. I., and Faegenburg, D.: The antepartum diagnosis of osteogenesis imperfecta congenita: a report of two cases recognized in utero, J. Mount Sinai Hosp. N.Y. **31**:90, 1964.
108. Gurlt, E.: Handbuch der Lehre von den Knochenbruchen, Berlin, 1862-1865, vol. 1, pp. 147-154.
109. Gutzeit, R.: Ueber blaue Sklera und Knochenbrüchigkeit, Klin. Mbl. Augenheilk. **68**:771, 1922.
110. Hanhart, E.: Ergebnisse der Erforschung von Erbkrankheiten und Missbildungen in der Schweiz, Arch. Klaus Stift. Vererbungsforsch. **18**:632, 1943.
111. Hanhart, E.: Ueber eine neue Form von Osteopsathyrosis congenita mit einfachrezessivem Erbgang, sowie vier neue Sippen mit dominantem Erbgang und die Frage der Vererbung der sog. Osteogenesis imperfecta, Arch. Klaus Stift. Vererbungsforsch. **26**:426, 1951.
112. Harnett, W. L.: Two cases of osteogenesis imperfecta with blue sclerotics in natives of India, Brit. J. Surg. **22**:269, 1934.
113. Hass, J.: Zur Kenntnis der Osteopsathyrosis idiopathica, Med. Klin. **15**:1112, 1919.

114. Hatteland, K.: T. Norske Laegeforg. **77**:75, 1957. Quoted in Brit. Med. J. **1**:1172, 1957.
115. Hein, B. J.: Osteogenesis imperfecta with multiple fractures at birth: an investigation with special reference to heredity and blue sclera, J. Bone Joint Surg. **10**:243, 1928.
116. Henley, F. A.: A case of congenital osteopsathyrosis with genealogical tree of the family, Brit. Med. J. **1**:326, 1942.
117. Herndon, C. N.: Osteogenesis imperfecta; some clinical and genetic considerations, Clin. Orthop. **8**:132, 1956.
118. Heys, F. M., Blattner, F. J., and Robinson, H. B. G.: Osteogenesis imperfecta and odontogenesis imperfecta: clinical and genetic aspects in eighteen families, J. Pediat. **56**:234, 1960.
119. Hilgenfeldt, O.: Beitrag zum Krankheitsbilde der idiopathischen abnormen Knochenbrüchigkeit, Deutsch. Z. Chir. **238**:433, 1933.
120. Hills, R. G., and McLanahan, S.: Brittle bones and blue scleras in five generations, Arch. Intern. Med. **59**:41, 1937.
121. Holcomb, D. Y.: A fragile-boned family; hereditary fragilitas ossium, J. Hered. **22**:105, 1931.
122. Holmes, J. R., Baker, J. R., and Davies, E. T.: Osteogenesis imperfecta in lambs, Vet. Rec. **76**:980, 1964.
123. Holzworth, J.: Osteogenesis imperfecta, Vet. Bull. (Lederle) **15**:18, 1956.
124. Holzworth, J.: Disease conditions prominent in cats, Univ. Pennsylvania Bull. School Vet. Med., Veterinary Extension Quart. **58**:101, 1958.
125. Hunter, D.: A case of osteogenesis imperfecta, Lancet **1**:9, 1927.
126. Hursey, R. J., Witkop, C. J., Jr., Miklashek, D., and Sackett, L. M.: Dentinogenesis imperfecta in a racial isolate with multiple hereditary defects, Oral Surg. **9**:641, 1956.
127. Hurwitz, L. J., and McSwiney, R. R.: Basilar impression and osteogenesis imperfecta in a family, Brain **83**:138, 1960.
128. Inderbitzin, A.: Ueber Anosteoplasia congenita beim Kalbe, Virchow Arch. Path. Anat. **269**:665, 1928.
129. Ivancie, G. P.: Dentinogenesis imperfecta, Oral. Surg. **7**:984, 1954.
130. Jackson, W. P. U.: Osteoporosis of unknown cause in younger people. Idiopathic osteoporosis, J. Bone Joint Surg. **40-B**:420, 1958.
131. Jacobsen, J. G., Matienzo, J. A., Forbes, A. P., and Rourke, G. M.: Serum acid phosphatase in osteogenesis imperfecta, Metabolism **10**:483, 1961.
132. Jeckeln, E.: Systemgebundene mesenchymale Erschöpfung. Eine neue Bergriffsfassung der Osteogenesis imperfecta, Virchow Arch. Path. Anat. **280**:351, 1931.
133. Jelnes, K. T.: Osteogenesis imperfecta and otosclerosis, Ugeskr. Laeg. **111**:1262, 1949.
134. Jewell, F. C., and Lofstrom, L. E.: Osteogenic sarcoma occurring in fragilitas ossium, Radiology **34**:741, 1940.
135. Joachim, H., and Wasch, M. G.: Fragilitas ossium in five generations, Ann. Intern. Med. **7**:853, 1934.
136. Johansson, S.: Ein Fall von Osteogenesis imperfecta mit verbreiteten Gefassverkalkungen, Acta Radiol. **1**:17, 1921.
137. Johnson, W. A., and Karrer, M. C.: Osteogenesis imperfecta in pregnancy, report of a case, Obstet. Gynec. **10**:642, 1957.
138. Kaplan, M., and Baldino, C.: Dysplasie periostale paraissant familiale et transmise suivant le mode mendélien recessif, Arch. Franc. Pediat. **10**:943, 1953.
139. Katsu, Y.: An instance of osteogenesis imperfecta congenita, Jap. J. Obstet. **16**:171, 1933.
140. Kaul, B.: Ein Abortivfall von Osteogenesis imperfecta congenita kombiniert mit Missbildungen der Blutgefasse (Osteoangiogenesis imperfecta), Frankfurt. Z. Path. **53**:289, 1939.
141. Keats, T. E.: Diffuse thickening of the calvarium in osteogenesis imperfecta, Radiology **69**:408, 1957.
142. Keats, T. E., and Anast, G. S.: Circumscribed skeletal rarefactions in osteogenesis imperfecta, Amer. J. Roentgen. **84**:492, 1960.
143. Kellogg, C. S.: Osteogenesis imperfecta; study of five generations, Arch. Intern. Med. **80**:358, 1947.
144. Kersley, G. D.: Fragilitas ossium and allied conditions, St. Barthodomew's Hosp. Rep. **68**:159, 1935.
145. Key, J. A.: Brittle bones and blue sclerae (hereditary hypoplasia of the mesenchyme), Arch. Surg. **13**:523, 1926.

146. Khoo, F. Y.: Congenital pseudarthrosis of the tibia and its relation to fragilitas ossium. Amer. J. Dis. child. **77**:201, 1949.
147. Kidd, F.: Case for diagnosis: imperfecta osteogenesis? Proc. Roy. Soc. Med 4 (Clin. Sect.): 106, 1911.
148. Knaggs, L.: Osteogenesis imperfecta, Brit. J. Surg. **11**:737, 1924.
149. Komai, T., Kunai, H., and Ozaki, Y.: A note on the genetics of van der Hoeve's syndrome, with special reference to a large Japanese kindred, Amer. J. Hum. Genet. **8**:110, 1956.
150. Krabbe, K. H.: La maladie de Henri de Toulouse-Lautrec, Acta. Psychiat. Neurol. Scand., supp. 108:211, 1956.
151. Lamy, M.: L'infirmité de Toulouse-Lautrec, Presse Méd. **64**:249, 1956.
152. Leicher, H., and Hass, E.: Labyrinthausfall bei Osteopsathyrosis, Z. Laryng. **36**:190, 1957.
153. Liber, B.: Fragilitas ossium, J.A.M.A. **162**:700, 1956.
154. Lobeck, H.: Ein Beitrag zur Osteogenesis imperfecta, Franfurt, 1938, A. M. Dissertation, p. 32. Cited by Seedorff.[210]
155. Lobstein, J.G.C.F.M.: Lehrbuch der pathologischen Anatomie, Stuttgart, 1835, vol. 2, p. 179.
156. Looser, E.: Zur Kenntnis der Osteogenesis imperfecta congenita et tarda, Mitt. Grenzgeb. Med. Chir. **15**:161, 1906.
157. Lovett, R. W., and Nichols, H.: Osteogenesis imperfecta. With the report of a case with autopsy and histological examination, Brit. Med. J. **2**:915, 1906.
158. Macgregor, A. G., and Harrison, R.: Congenital total color blindness associated with otosclerosis, Ann. Eugen. **15**:219, 1950.
159. McKinney, R.: Studies on fibers in tissue cultures. III. The development of reticulum into collagenous fibers in cultures of adult rabbit lymph nodes, Arch. Exp. Zellforsch. **9**:14, 1929.
160. McKusick, V. A.: Unpublished observations.
161. McKusick, V. A., and colleagues: Medical genetics 1963, J. Chronic Dis. **17**:1077, 1964.
162. McKusick, V. A.: Hereditary disorders of connective tissue, Bull. N.Y. Acad. Med. **35**:143, 1959.
163. Maroteaux, P., and Lamy, M.: La pycnodysostose, Presse Méd. **70**:999, 1962.
164. Maroteaux, P., and Lamy, M.: The malady of Toulouse-Lautrec, J.A.M.A. **191**:715, 1965.
165. Messinger, A. L., and Teal F.: Intramedullary nailing for correction of deformity in osteogenesis imperfecta, Clin. Orthop. **1**:221, 1955.
166. Meyer, H.: Atypical osteogenesis imperfecta; Lobstein's disease, Arch. Pediat. **72**:182, 1955.
167. Milne, M. D., Stanbury, S. W., and Thomson, A. E.: Observations on Fanconi syndrome and renal hyperchloraemic acidosis in adults, Quart. J. Med. **21**:61, 1952.
168. Moldawer, M.: Senile osteoporosis. The physiological basis of treatment, Arch. Intern. Med. **96**:202, 1955.
169. Mørsch, E. T.: Chondrodystrophic dwarfs in Denmark. In Opera ex domo biologiae hereditarie humanae Universitatis Hafniensis, vol. 3, Copenhagen, 1941, Ejnar Munksgaard.
170. Motulsky, A., Heustis, R., and Anderson, R.: Hereditary spherocytosis in mouse and man, Acta Genet. (Basel) **6**:240, 1956.
171. Murray, D., and Young, B. H.: Osteogenesis imperfecta treated by fixation with intramedullary rod, Southern Med. J. **53**:1142, 1960.
172. Mussio, T. J.: Osteogenesis imperfecta congenita: report of a case discovered in utero, Obstet. Gynec. **15**:361, 1960.
173. Nager, F. R.: Otosklerose bei infantiler Osteopsathyrosis und Blaufärbung der Skleren, Schweiz. Med. Wschr. **51**:660, 1921.
174. Nager, F. R.: Pathology of the labyrinthine capsule, and its clinical significance. In Nelson loose-leaf medicine of the ear, New York, 1939, Thomas Nelson & Sons, p. 237.
175. Naita, S.: Klinische und histologische Untersuchungen des Zahngewebes bei Osteogenesis imperfecta, etc., Mitt. Med. Fakült. Kais. Univ. Kyushu, Fukuoka. **9**:97, 1924. Ref. Zbl. Kinderheilk. **18**:822, 1925.
176. Nielsen, H. E.: Familial occurrence of osseus fragility, blue sclera and deafness, Nord. Med. **15**:2203, 1942.
177. Nordin, B. E., and Roper, A.: Post-pregnancy osteoporosis; a syndrome? Lancet **1**:431, 1955.

178. Noyes, F. B.: Hereditary anomaly in structure of dentin (abstract), J. Dent. Res. **15**:154, 1935.
179. O'Connell, J. E. A., and Turner, J. W. A.: Basilar impression of the skull, Brain **73**:405, 1950.
180. Ormerod, E. L.: An account of a case of mollities ossium, Brit. Med. J. **2**:735, 1859.
181. Pelner, L., and Cohen, J. N.: Osteogenesis imperfecta tarda, Amer. J. Roentgen. **61**:690, 1949.
182. Perruchot, H.: Toulouse-Lautrec (translated by Humphrey Hare), Cleveland and New York, 1960, The World Publishing Co.
183. Peters, A.: Blaue Sklera und Knochenbrüchigkeit, Klin. Mbl. Augenheilk. **51**:594, 1913.
184. Posner, A. C., and Goldman, J. A.: A case of osteogenesis imperfecta congenita diagnosed in utero, Amer. J. Obstet. Gynec. **73**:1143, 1957.
185. Puppel, E.: Osteogenesis imperfecta, Mschr. Geburtsh. Gyn. **82**:269, 1929.
186. Reed, W. B., and Pidgeon, J. W.: Elastosis perforans serpiginosa with osteogenesis imperfecta, Arch. Derm. (Chicago) **89**:342, 1964.
187. Rennert, H., and Popella, E.: Abortive Fälle von Osteopsathyrose mit Marfan-Symptomatik, Med. Mschr. **9**:106, 1955.
188. Riddell, W. J. B.: A pedigree of blue sclerotics, brittle bones and deafness, with colour blindness, Ann. Eugen. **10**:1, 1955.
189. Rieseman, F. R., and Yater, W. M.: Osteogenesis imperfecta. Its incidence and manifestations in seven families, Arch. Intern. Med. **67**:950, 1941.
190. Riser, W. H.: Juvenile osteoporosis (osteogenesis imperfecta)—a calcium deficiency, J. Amer. Vet. Med. Ass. **139**:117, 1961.
191. Roberts, E., and Schour, I.: Hereditary opalescent dentine—dentinogenesis imperfecta, Amer. J. Orthodont. **25**:267, 1939.
192. Rogers, T. R.: Otosclerosis associated with blue sclerotics and fragilitas ossium, Proc. Roy. Soc. Med. **29**:1107, 1936.
193. Rolleston, J. D.: Inherited syphilis and blue sclerotics, Ophthalmoscope **9**:321, 1911.
194. Ropes, M. W., Rossmeisl, E. C., and Bauer, W.: The effect of estrin medication in osteogenesis imperfecta, Conference on Metabolic Aspects of Convalescence, New York, 1946, Trans. 14th meeting, Josiah Macy Jr. Foundation, p. 87.
195. Rosenbaum, S.: Osteogenesis imperfecta and osteopsathyrosis, a contribution to the study of their identity and their pathogenesis, J. Pediat. **25**:161, 1944.
196. Ruedemann, A. D., Jr.: Osteogenesis imperfecta congenita and blue sclerotics: a clinicopathologic study. Arch. Ophthal. **49**:6, 1953.
197. Rushton, M. A.: The structure of the teeth in a late case of osteogenesis imperfecta, J. Path. Bact. **48**:591, 1939.
198. Ruth, E. B.: Osteogenesis imperfecta. Anatomic study of a case, Arch. Path. **36**:211, 1943.
199. Ruttin, E.: Ohrbefund bei Osteopsathyrose, Mschr. Ohrenheilk. **53**:305, 1919.
200. Ruttin, E.: Osteopsathyrose und Otosklerose, Arch. Ohr. Nas. Kehlkopfheilk. **3**:263, 1922.
201. Sarma, V.: A case of intrauterine osteogenesis imperfecta, Brit. Med. J. **2**:1856, 1960.
202. Scherr, D. D.: A severely deformed patient with osteogenesis imperfecta at the age of fifty-four, J. Bone Joint Surg. **46-A**:159, 1964.
203. Schmidt, M. B.: Die allgemeinen Entwicklüngshemmungen der Knochen, Ergebn. Allg. Path. **4**:612, 1897.
204. Schultze, F.: Beitrag zur idiopathischen Osteopsathyrose, Arch. Klin. Chir. **47**:327, 1894.
205. Schulze, C.: Erbbedingte Strukturanomalien menschlicher Zähne, Munich and Berlin, 1956, Urban u. Schwarzenberg.
206. Schwarz, E.: Hypercallosis in osteogenesis imperfecta, Amer. J. Roentgen. **85**:645, 1961.
207. Scott, D., and Stiris, G.: Osteogenesis imperfecta tarda. A study of three families with special reference to scar formation, Acta Med. Scand. **145**:237, 1953.
208. Scott, P. P., McKusick, V. A., and McKusick, A. B.: The nature of "osteogenesis imperfecta" in cats. Evidence that the disorder is primarily nutritional, not genetic, and therefore not analogous to the disease in man, J. Bone Joint Surg. **45-A**:125, 1963.
209. Second, E. W., Wilder, R. M., and Henderson, M. S.: Osteogenesis imperfecta tarda (osteopsathyrosis) treated with thymus extract (Hanson), Proc. Mayo Clin. **11**:1, 1936.
210. Seedorff, K. S.: Osteogenesis imperfecta. A study of clinical features and heredity based

on 55 Danish families comprising 180 affected persons, Copenhagen, 1949, Ejnar Munksgaard.

211. Shambaugh, G. E., Jr.: Fenestration operation for otosclerosis; experimental investigations and clinical observations in 2,100 operations over period of 10 years, Acta Otolaryng., supp. 79: pp. 1-101, 1949.
212. Shorr, E., and Carter, A. C.: The usefulness of strontium as an adjuvant to calcium in the remineralization of the skeleton in man, Bull. Hosp. Joint Dis. **13**:59, 1952.
213. Shugrue, J. J., Rockwood, R., and Anderson, E. W.: Fragilitas ossium and deafness, Arch. Intern. Med. **39**:98, 1927.
214. Siegel, B. M., Friedman, I. A., and Schwartz, S. O.: Hemorrhagic disease in osteogenesis imperfecta. Study of platelet functional defect, Amer. J. Med. **22**:315, 1957.
215. Simmons, C. C.: Osteogenesis imperfecta and idiopathic fragilitas ossium, Am. Surg. **46**:179, 1907.
216. Simsky: Blue sclerotics, fragility of the bones and deafness, Amer. J. Ophthal. **9**:844, 1926.
217. Sisk, J. N.: Fragilitas ossium in twins, Wisconsin Med. J. **30**:273, 1931.
218. Skaggs, J. W., and Theobald, J. A.: Osteogenesis imperfecta in a kitten, J. Amer. Vet. Med. Ass. **130**:450, 1957.
219. Smårs, G.: Osteogenesis imperfecta in Sweden: clinical, genetic, epidemiological and sociomedical aspects, Stockholm, 1961, Svenska Bokförlaget.
220. Smårs, G., Beckman, L., and Böök, J. A.: Osteogenesis imperfecta and blood groups, Acta Genet. **11**:133, 1961.
221. Smith, O. N., and Mitchell, J. M.: The serum phosphatase in osteogenesis imperfecta, Amer. J. Med. Sci. **190**:765, 1935.
222. Snapper, I.: Medical clinics on bone diseases, ed. 2, New York, 1949, Interscience Publishers.
223. Spurway, J.: Hereditary tendency to fracture, Brit. Med. J. **2**:844, 1896.
224. Stapes, P. P., Jr., and Riva, H. L.: Maternal osteogenesis imperfecta; report of two cases in sisters, Obstet. Gynec. **4**:557, 1954.
225. Stein, F. H.: Nogen tilfaelder av osteopsathyrosis idiopathica med nedarvning i 4 led, T. Norske Laegeforen. **47**:557, 1927. Cited by Seedorff.[210]
226. Stenvers, H. W.: Röntgenologische Bemerkungen zur vorhergehenden Arbeit von J. van der Hoeve und A. de Kleyn, Arch. Ophthal. **95**:94, 1918.
227. Stephenson, S.: Blue sclerotics, Trans. Ophthal. Soc. U.K. **35**:274, 1915.
228. Stilling, H.: Osteogenesis imperfecta, Virchow Arch. **115**:357, 1889.
229. Stobie, W.: The association of blue sclerotics with brittle bones and progressive deafness, Quart. J. Med. **17**:274, 1924.
230. Stool, N., and Sullivan, C. R.: Osteogenesis imperfecta in a 95-year-old woman, Proc. Mayo Clin. **34**:523, 1959.
231. Strack, E.: Beobachtung von Fragilität der Knochen in der Jugend, ein Beitrag zu der Lehre von den Knochenkrankheiten, J. Pract. Arzneyk. Wundarzneyk. **25**:163, 1807.
232. Strach, E. H.: Hyperplastic callus formation in osteogenesis imperfecta; report of a case and review of the literature, J. Bone Joint Surg. **35-B**:417, 1953.
233. Summer, G. K.: Oral proline tolerance in osteogenesis imperfecta, Science **134**:1527, 1961.
234. Sundberg, C. G.: Discussion of paper by G. Zander, Nord. Med. **1**:802, 1939. Quoted by Seedorff.[210]
235. Taylor, A. R., and Chakravorty, B. C.: Clinical syndromes associated with basilar impression, Arch. Neurol. **10**:475, 1964.
236. Terrien, F., Sainton, P., and Veil, P.: Deux cas de syndrome de van der Hoeve (oeil bleu; fragilité osseuse; surdité), Arch. Ophthal. **44**:293, 1927.
237. Terry, W. I.: Hereditary osteopsathyrosis, Trans. Am. S. A. **36**:317, 1918.
238. Toto, P. D.: Osteogenesis imperfecta tarda with dentinogenesis imperfecta, Oral Surg. **6**:772, 1953.
239. Vallery-Radot, P., and Aris, P.: Osteopsathyrosis hereditaire, Bull. Soc. Pédiat. Paris **22**:291, 1924.
240. Van der Hoeve, J., and de Kleyn, A.: Blaue Sclerae, Knochenbrüchigkeit und Schwerhörigkeit, Arch. Ophthal. **95**:81, 1918.
241. Vander Veer, E. A., and Dickinson, A. M.: Fragilitas ossium, Ann. Surg. **74**:629, 1921.
242. Vaughan, J. H. (Richmond): Personal communication, 1956.

243. Voigt, O.: Ein Fall von Osteogenesis imperfecta, Freiburg, 1926, Dissertation. Cited by Seedorff.[210]
244. Von Ammon, F. A.: Klinische Darstellungen der angeborenen Krankheiten und Bildungsfehler des menschlichen Auges, Berlin, 1841, G. Reimer, p. 73.
245. Voorhoeve, N.: Blue sclerotics, in connection with other hereditary or congenital abnormalities, Lancet **2**:740, 1918.
246. Vrolik, W.: Tabulae ad illustrandam embryogenesim hominis et mammalium, tam naturalem quam abnormem, Amstelodami, 1849.
247. Vyropaer, D.: Cited by Seedorff.[210]
248. Wagoner, G. W.: Idiopathic osteopsathyrosis, Ann. Surg. **80**:115, 1924.
249. Watkyn-Thomas, F. W.: Diseases of the throat, nose and ear, Springfield, Ill., 1953, Charles C Thomas, Publisher, p. 612.
250. Weber, M.: Osteogenesis imperfecta congenita, a study of its histopathogenesis, Arch. Path. **9**:984, 1930.
251. Weil: Pubertas praecox und Knochenbrüchigkeit (abstract), Klin. Wschr. **2**:2114, 1922.
252. Weinmann, J. P., and Sicher, H.: Bone and bones, ed. 2, St. Louis, 1955, The C. V. Mosby Co.
253. Weinmann, J. P., Svoboda, J. F., and Woods, R. W.: Hereditary disturbances of enamel formation and calcification, J. Amer. Dent. Ass. **32**:397, 1945.
254. Welz, W. E., and Lieberman, B. L.: Report of a case of osteogenesis imperfecta in twins, Amer. J. Obstet. Gynec. **14**:49, 1927.
255. Werner, R.: Mehrfaches Vorkommen einer Neigung zu Knochenbrüchen und Sarkomentwicklung in einer Familie, Z. Krebsforsch. **32**:40, 1940.
256. Wiechmann, E., and Paal, H.: Zur Klinik der sogenannten blauen Skleren, München. Med. Wschr. **72**:213, 1925.
257. Wilson, G. W., and Steinbecker, M.: Hereditary hypoplasia of dentine, J. Amer. Dent. Ass. **16**:866, 1929.
258. Wilton, A.: Die Skelettveränderungen bei einem Spätfalle von Osteogenesis imperfecta nebst Erörterung der Entstehungsweise unter Berücksicktigung anderer Skelettkrankheiten, Virchow Arch. Path. **283**:778, 1932.
259. Winter, G. R., and Maiocco, P. D.: Osteogenesis imperfecta and odontogenesis imperfecta, Oral Surg. **2**:782, 1949.
260. Wirth, M.: Blaue Skleren und Knochenbrüchigkeit, Klin. Mbl. Augenheilk. **74**:505, 1925.
261. Witkop, C. (Bethesda, Md.): Personal communication.
262. Wyatt, T. C., and McEachern, T. H.: Congenital bone dysplasia (osteogenesis imperfecta) associated with lesions of parathyroid glands, Amer. J. Dis. Child. **43**:403, 1932.
263. Wyllie, W. G., and Schlesinger, B.: Osteogenesis imperfecta presenting with delay in walking, two cases, Proc. Roy. Soc. Med. **42**:80, 1949.
264. Yeoman, P. M.: Multiple osteotomies and intramedullary fixation of the long bones in osteogenesis imperfecta, Proc. Roy. Soc. Med. **53**:946, 1960.
265. Zander, G. S. F.: Case of osteogenesis imperfecta tarda with platyspondylisis, Acta Radiol. **21**:53, 1940.
266. Zurhelle, E.: Osteogenesis imperfecta bei Mutter und Kind, Z. Geburtsh. Gyn. **74**:942, 1913.

7

Alkaptonuria

Historical note

Garrod[30] gave the following early history of alkaptonuria:

> Until the early years of the nineteenth century no distinction was drawn in medical writings between urines which were black when passed and such as darkened on exposure to air, but it is difficult to suggest any other diagnosis than that of alkaptonuria for some cases referred to in works of the sixteenth and seventeenth centuries, such as that mentioned by G. A. Scribonius (in 1584) of a schoolboy who, although he enjoyed good health, continuously excreted black urine, and that cited by Schenck (in 1609) of a monk who exhibited a similar peculiarity and stated that he had done so all his life. The most interesting record of this kind is to be found in the work of Zacutus Lusitanus, published in 1649. The patient was a boy who passed black urine and who, at the age of fourteen years, was submitted to a drastic course of treatment which had for its aim the subduing of the fiery heat of his viscera which was supposed to bring about the condition in question by charring and blackening his bile. Among the measures prescribed were bleedings, purgation, baths, a cold and watery diet, and drugs galore. None of these had any obvious effect, and eventually the patient, who tired of the futile and superfluous therapy, resolved to let things take their natural course. None of the predicted evils ensued, he married, begat a large family, and lived a long and healthy life, always passing urine black as ink.*

In 1859 Boedeker[15] recognized that the reducing properties of the urine from a patient with alkaptonuria differed from those of urine containing glucose. Bismuth hydroxide was, for example, not reduced. Because of the avid uptake of oxygen in alkaline solutions he gave the name alkaptonuria to the condition: ". . . in alkalischer Lösung bei gewöhnlicher Temperatur den Sauerstoff begierig zu verschlucken und nannte ihn danach Alcapton (freilich recht barbarisch zusammengesetzt aus dem arabischen *al kali* und dem griechischen καπτειν, begierig verschlucken)."† In 1861, Boedeker[16] spelled the name *alkaptonurie,*

---

*Knox[42] called attention to this interesting historical note.

†From Boedeker, C.: Z. Rat. Med. 7:130, 1859. Translation: ". . . in alkaline solution at ordinary temperature avidly to absorb the oxygen and named it accordingly alcapton (admittedly somewhat barbarously compounded from the Arabic *al kali* and the Greek καπτειν, to suck up greedily)."

a practice which has been followed in the German literature. The French spell it *alcaptonurie,* and English writers use "c" and "k" interchangeably.

The morbid anatomy of ochronosis was described by Virchow in 1866[85] on the basis of findings in a 67-year-old man. Although the gross coloration was gray to blue-black, an ochre color was observed microscopically, hence Virchow's designation *ochronosis.* Not until the early part of this century was the connection between ochronosis and alkaptonuria recognized—by Albrecht in 1902[3] and by Osler in 1904.[64] Boedeker's patient[15,16] had severe pain in the lumbar spine "so severe that he lay mostly in bed and could take only a few steps." The development of severe arthritis in the course of alkaptonuria with ochronosis was emphasized by Gross and Allard[33] in 1907. The characteristic roentgenographic appearance of the spine in ochronosis was described by Söderbergh[79] in 1913.

The chemical structure of "alkapton" was established in 1891 by Wolkow and Baumann,[88] who identified it as 2, 5-dihydroxyphenylacetic acid and named it homogentisic acid because of its close structural similarity to gentisic acid (2, 5-dihydroxybenzoic acid).

Alkaptonuria is *par excellence* Garrod's disease.[31,42] Archibald Garrod (see frontispiece) greatly extended knowledge of the nature of the disorder and on the basis of these studies conceived the principle underlying most inborn errors of metabolism, the last being his terminology. As Beadle[9] pointed out in his Nobel lecture, the concept of one-gene—one-enzyme was essentially Garrod's. As Garrod[30] stated in 1908: "Of inborn errors of metabolism, alkaptonuria is that of which we know most, and from the study of which most has been learnt." In most research, following the lead of Wolkow and Baumann,[88] alkaptonuria had been viewed as a specific form of infection of the alimentary tract—a concept that was undoubtedly influenced by the thinking of the Bacteriology Era in which he worked—but Garrod[29] thought of alkaptonuria as an enzyme defect:

> We may further conceive that the splitting of the benzene ring in normal metabolism is the work of a special enzyme, [and] that in congenital alcaptonuria this enzyme is wanting. . . . The experiments of G. Embden and others upon perfusion of the liver suggest that organ as the most probable seat of the change.*

Garrod's contemporaries such as Osler[64] considered alkaptonuria to be a "freak" of metabolism, comparable to morphologic freaks, and to be of no pathologic importance. Indeed, it is likely that many of Garrod's contemporaries viewed his work in alkaptonuria as a harmless but practically noncontributory pastime. There is the tone of the *apologia* in Garrod's writings on the value of studying rare diseases (see quotation in the Preface). Clearly, Garrod was ahead of his time.

The juxtaposition of Garrod and Bateson and the rediscovery of Mendel's work were important factors in the development of the concept of inborn errors of metabolism. Bateson's *Mendel's Principles of Heredity* did much to acquaint the English-speaking world with "genetics," the term he applied to this field.[7] Because of the occurence of affected sibs with normal parents and the high proportion of parents who are consanguineous, he suggested to Garrod that alkaptonuria is a recessively inherited disorder. In 1932 Hogben and colleagues[38]

---

*From Garrod, A. E.: Lancet **2**:1484, 1901.

analyzed statistically the family data on alkaptonuria and supported the recessive hypothesis. There were, however, anomalous pedigrees in which alkaptonuria was transmitted through many successive generations, suggesting dominant inheritance, e.g. that of Pieter,[66] reported from Santo Domingo. The interpretation of these as quasidominance due to marriage, in successive generations, of affected homozygous persons with carrier heterozygous persons, in an inbred population, was demonstrated by restudy in the Dominican Republic by Milch.[53]

The question as to whether homogentisic acid is a normal metabolite, which in alkaptonuria accumulates in unusual concentration behind an enzyme block (the view of Garrod), or whether it is an abnormal compound formed by an abnormal series of reactions was resolved by 1928 in favor of the former view, by Neubauer[62] and by others.

In 1958 La Du and associates[45] succeeded in demonstrating deficiency of homogentisate oxidase in liver, as predicted by Garrod. The importance of ochronotic connective tissue changes in producing arthritis and cardiovascular pathology has become generally recognized only in the last few decades, although some contemporaries of Garrod[36,83] emphasized it. The pathogenesis of connective tissue alterations in alkaptonuria is the most recent chapter in the history of the disease.

Clinical manifestations

The phenotypic features of alkaptonuria are blackness of urine, pigmentation of cartilaginous and collagenous structures (ochronosis), and degenerative joint and vascular changes.

The urine turns dark on sitting. Darkening is hastened by alkalinization of the urine. Black diapers are sometimes the first clue to the presence of the disease. Washing with soap exaggerates the pigmentation of the diaper rather than removing it. Some patients never note black urine, the conditions for darkening apparently never being present. One patient first noted dark urine at age 93.[28] Garrod[29] observed that in the first hours after birth alkaptonuria may not be demonstrable although it appears in the second day of life and continues without interruption thereafter. It is probable that immaturity of the enzyme systems involved in tyrosine oxidation accounts for the failure of expression from the very beginning. As a reducing substance homogentisic acid produces a positive reaction in some urinary tests for glycosuria, such as that using Benedict's solution, but of course not with enzyme tests specifically for glucose. The proper interpretation of an atypical test for reducing substance in the urine is the most frequent means of diagnosing alkaptonuria. A specific enzymatic method for quantitative determination of homogentisic acid in blood and urine is available.[72]

Pigmented prostatic calculi were described by Young[89] and by others and probably occur in all alkaptonuric men over age 50. These calculi are usually calcified, as well, and evident by x-ray study. Enlargement of the stone-filled prostate may require prostatectomy.[14,43] Death in uremia from prostatic obstruction has been observed.[8,65] Apparently the alkalinity of the prostatic secretions promotes polymerization of homogentisic acid and this pigment then affords a nidus for stone formation.

Renal stones also occur in ochronosis.[25,35,37,43,47,48,49,65] Deposition of pigment in the renal parenchyma occurs but *per se* does not interfere with renal func-

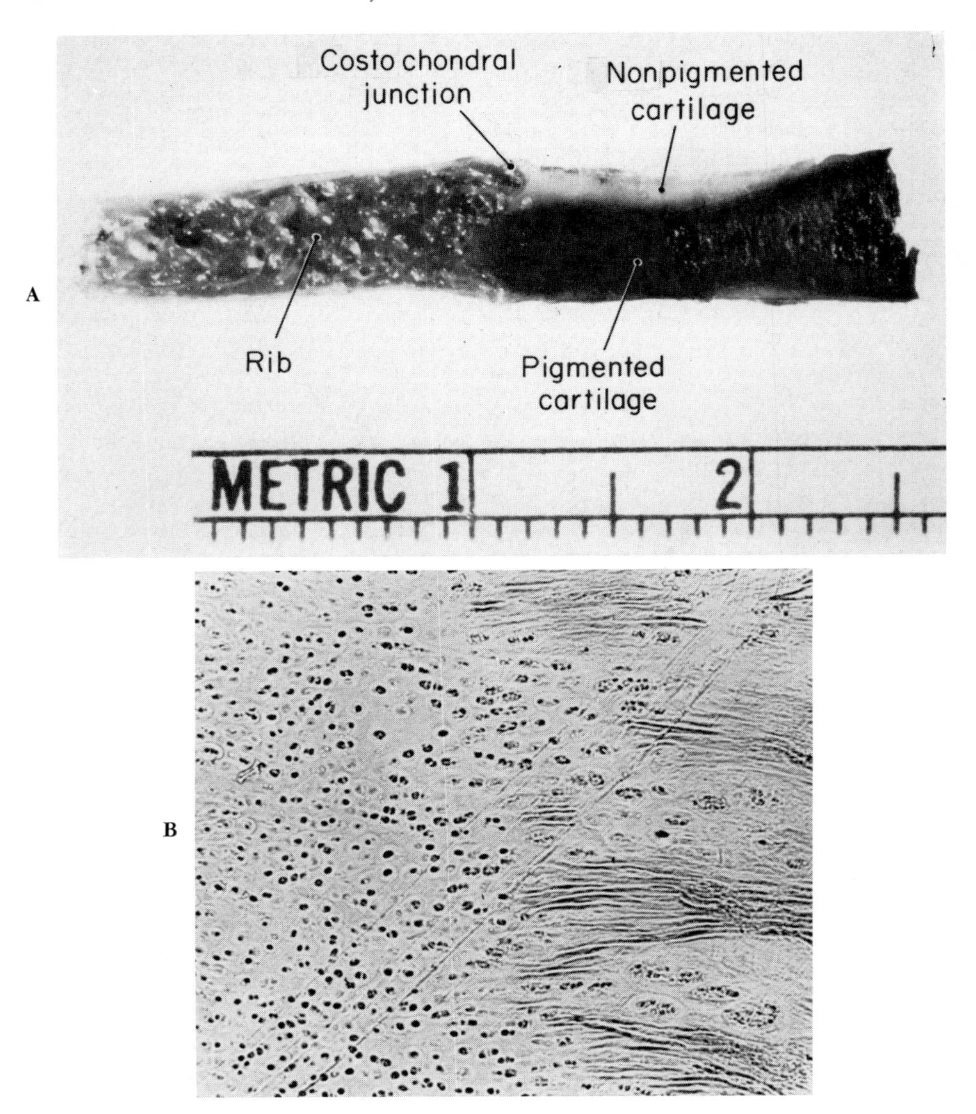

Fig. 7-1. A, Deeply pigmented costal cartilage in patient with alkaptonuria. Note that the periphery of the cartilage is not pigmented. **B,** Histologic appearance of cartilage from specimen shown in **A.** The pigmented area is on the right half. Sparsity of cells and artifactual streaks produced in sectioning, because of stiffness of the specimen, are evident. (Courtesy Dr. Robert A. Milch.)

tion. Patients with alkaptonuria who have renal failure due to an unrelated renal abnormality show greatly aggravated ochronosis, e.g. the 11-year-old boy with polycystic kidneys reported by Arcangeli and co-workers.[5]

Ochronotic pigmentation of blue-black hue is most evident in the sclera and in ear cartilages, but pigmentation of many cartilaginous and collagenous structures is found at surgical operation or autopsy—for example, costal cartilages (Fig. 7-1) and heart valves. Pigmentation does not become evident, as a rule, until the twenties or thirties. The scleral pigmentation is usually concentrated about midway between the corneal limbus and the inner and outer canthi, at the sites of insertion of the rectus muscles. Pigmentation of the cornea, concentrated peripherally at the three and nine o'clock positions, has been observed,[78] as well as pigmentation of the tarsal plates and eyelids. In one case[76] the pigmentation was mistaken for melanosarcoma and the eye was removed. Pigmentation of the nasal cartilages is sometimes evident at the tip of the nose. Pigmentation of the pinnae is best demonstrated by transillumination. The ear becomes stiff, also, so that it cannot be folded with the normal ease. Calcification and even ossification are radiographically demonstrable. The cerumen is jet black and the eardrum often shows steel blue pigmentation. It is said[44] that pigmentation of tendons in the hand may be evident through the skin in some cases. The pigment is excreted in the sweat. Clothing in contact with the axilla may be stained, and the skin of the axillary and inguinal area, as well as the malar area of the face, may show brownish coloration. In one exceptional case a bluish gray discoloration of the fingernails was described.[27]

Ochronotic arthropathy was succinctly and graphically described by the late Joseph J. Bunim and his colleagues[63] in the following manner:

> The anatomic distribution and sequence of spinal and peripheral joint involvement in ochronosis are characteristic. The course is chronic and progressive, beginning early in the fourth decade with back pain and stiffness. During the ensuing ten years the knees become involved and later the shoulders and hips are affected. The patient becomes increasingly crippled and by sixty years of age may be totally disabled.
>
> Two acute manifestations may develop during the chronic course: herniation of the intervertebral discs and synovial effusion following negligible trauma. Acute rupture of a nucleus pulposus may be the first manifestation of ochronotic spondylosis. It occurs principally in males in early adult life. Articular structures in ochronosis seem to be vulnerable; pain and effusion may follow minor injuries. The friable articular cartilages are readily fragmented and embedded in the synovial lining with consequent effusion and pain.
>
> In males, joint involvement occurs more frequently, develops at an earlier age, and is of greater severity than in females. Ruptured discs are especially more common in males.*

These authors also provided a useful table, comparing the joint changes in males and females (Table 7).

Low back pain, limitation of motion in the lumbar spine, and symptoms of root pressure by extruded intervertebral disc[23] are matched by the x-ray finding of narrowing of the intervertebral space and collapse and calcification of the intervertebral discs of the lumbar spine (Fig. 7-2). Some degree of fusion of the vertebral bodies occurs. Unlike rheumatoid spondylitis, little calcification of spinal ligaments occurs. The radiographic findings are sufficiently typical that studies of Egyptian mummies[73,87] have led to the conclusion that certain of them are the bodies of persons with alkaptonuria.

Large joints such as the hips and knees usually show degenerative changes by x-ray, with calcium deposits around the joint or present as loose bodies in the joint.[82] Frequently, ochronotic arthritis is of such severity as to keep the patient bedridden for many years. Severe pain over the symphysis pubis occurs rather

*From O'Brien, W. M., La Du, B. N., and Bunim, J. J.: Amer. J. Med. 34:813, 1963.

Table 7. Comparison of arthropathy in males and females*

Data	*Males*	*Females*
Number	116 cases	47 cases
Severity	Often severe	Usually mild
Spine	Onset in late thirties with loss of range of motion in lumbar and thoracic spine, loss in height	Onset in mid-forties, usually milder and more insidious course than in men
Disc rupture	Onset in late twenties, occurs in about 20%	Rare (4% or less)
Knee	Onset in early forties, often severe and disabling early in course with contracture and joint bodies	Onset in early fifties, usually milder than in men
Shoulder	Onset in early fifties, usually only loss in range of motion	Same as in men
Hip	Onset in early fifties with gradual progression—only occasionally severe	Onset in early fifties with gradual progression, frequently severe

*From O'Brien, W. M., La Du, B. N., and Bunim, J. J.: Amer. J. Med. **34**:813, 1963.

frequently.[35,50,58,82] By x-ray film the pubic synchondrosis in such cases may present irregular sclerosis, narrowing, and destructive changes.[67,68] Rupture of the Achilles tendon, which was found to be deeply pigmented, has been reported in at least two instances.[1,22]

A review[77] of case reports of alkaptonuria indicates a high frequency of cardiovascular abnormality. Generalized arteriosclerosis[20,28] and abnormalities of the heart valves, particularly calcific aortic stenosis, are frequent. Myocardial infarction is a frequent cause of death.[86]

Auditory impairment occurs in some cases. (See review by O'Brien and coworkers.[63]) Long-standing severe hoarseness,[32] fixed vocal cords, and pigmentation of the larynx observed by direct laryngoscopy[39] have been described.

The oldest individual with alkaptonuria was probably the one reported by Galdston and associates,[28] who died at age 99.

Pathology

Coal black pigmentary changes in the costal, laryngeal, and tracheal cartilages, as well as others, are striking in elderly alkaptonuric patients. Fibrous tissues such as tendons, ligaments, endocardium, and heart valves are likewise pigmented. Microscopically the pigment is found deposited both intracellularly and extracellularly and may be either granular or homogeneous. Ochronotic pigment can be distinguished histologically from melanin only with difficulty if at all.[21] Probably no patient with alkaptonuria escapes ochronosis, if survival to at least early adulthood occurs. Histopathologic changes in the eye were described by Rones[70] and by Allen and co-workers[4] and changes in the ear, by Brunner.[18]

Cardiovascular abnormalities have been observed in a high proportion of autopsied cases. In 1910 Beddard[10] found that of eleven persons with ochronosis eight had chronic mitral and aortic "valvulitis," one had aortic aneurysm, and one had aneurysm of the left ventricle. Generalized arteriosclerosis,[28] calcification of the heart valves, particularly calcific aortic stenosis, and calcified annulus

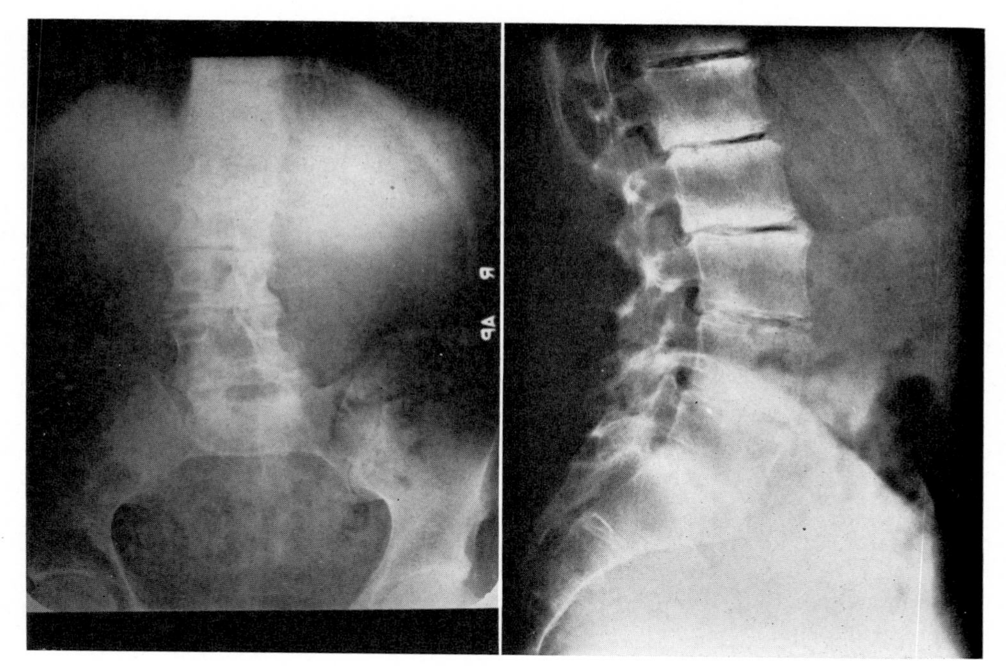

Fig. 7-2. Characteristic spinal changes of ochronotic arthropathy in 34-year-old man (R. S., 761270).

fibrosus mitralis[47] have been noted. Many have suggested that ochronotic patients suffer accelerated arteriosclerosis. However, O'Brien and associates,[63] from a review of reported cases, challenged this suggestion. The matter cannot be considered settled.

In one case[21] severe renal disease referred to as "ochronotic nephrosis" was observed, but this may have been coincidence of an unrelated nephritis, since no other similar case has been reported.

Basic defect and pathogenesis

Patients with alkaptonuria have been demonstrated to have a deficiency of homogentisic acid oxidase in liver[45] and in kidney.[92] (Normally the enzyme is present only in these tissues.) Because of the enzyme deficiency and the lack of an alternative pathway for the degradation of homogentisic acid, this substance, a normal intermediary in tyrosine metabolism (Fig. 7-3), is excreted in the urine. Whether enzyme protein lacking normal activity is present or no protein whatever is formed is not known. The level of homogentisic acid oxidase has not been measured in heterozygotes.

The alkaptonuric adult usually excretes from 4 to 8 gm. of homogentisic acid a day.

Zannoni and co-workers[91] presented reasons for believing that benzoquinone-acetic acid, the quinone of homogentisic acid, is mainly responsible for the ochronotic pigmentation of connective tissue in alkaptonuria.

Milch[52,54] found that, although homogentisic acid does not bind to collagen, polymerized auto-oxidized homogentisic acid (HGA-OP) is bound to hide pow-

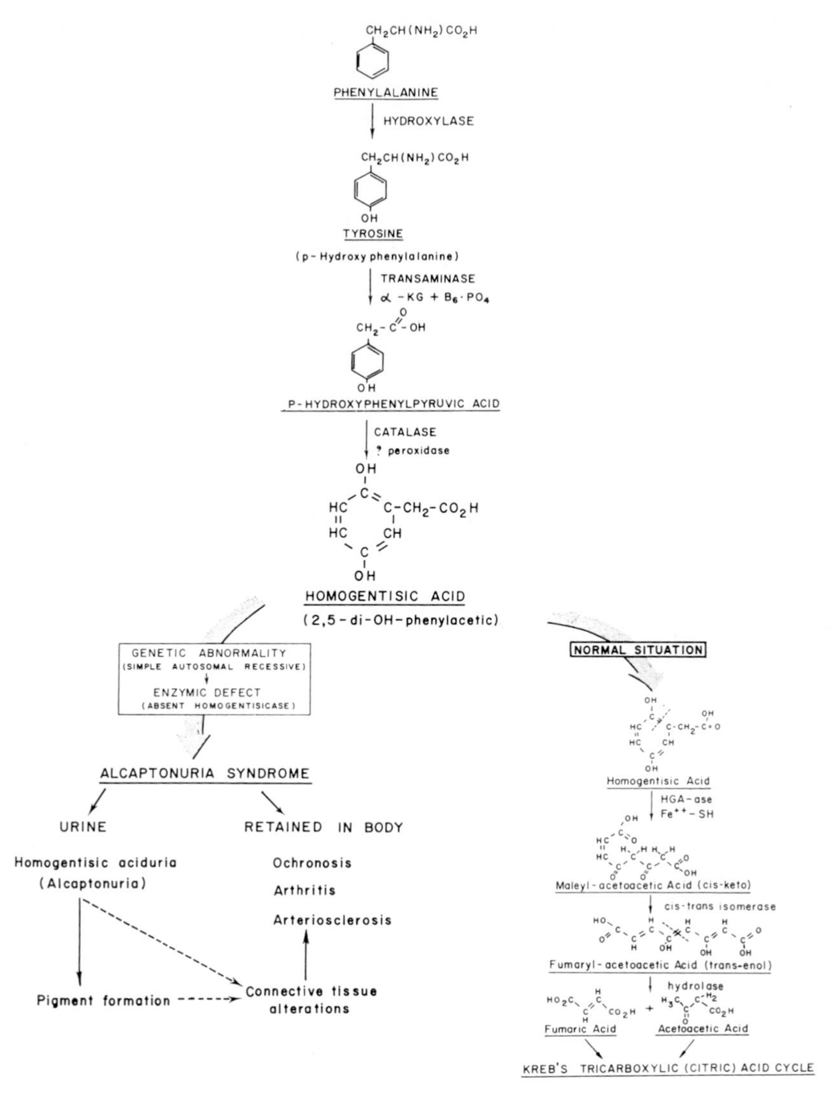

Fig. 7-3. The normal pathway for metabolism of tyrosine, and the defect in alkaptonuria. (Courtesy Dr. Robert A. Milch.)

der in solution. Furthermore, degradation of collagen by collagenase is interfered with appreciably when the collagen is treated with HGA-OP. Milch concluded: "Coupled with previous observations it is suggested that HGA-OP can act as a potent tanning agent for collagen. It is further suggested that ochronosis and degenerative joint disease observed in patients with alkaptonuria may possibly be explained by the *in vivo* occurrence of such a phenomenon."* (See Figs. 7-4 and 7-5.)

*From Milch, R. A.: Proc. Soc. Exp. Biol. Med. **107**:183, 1961.

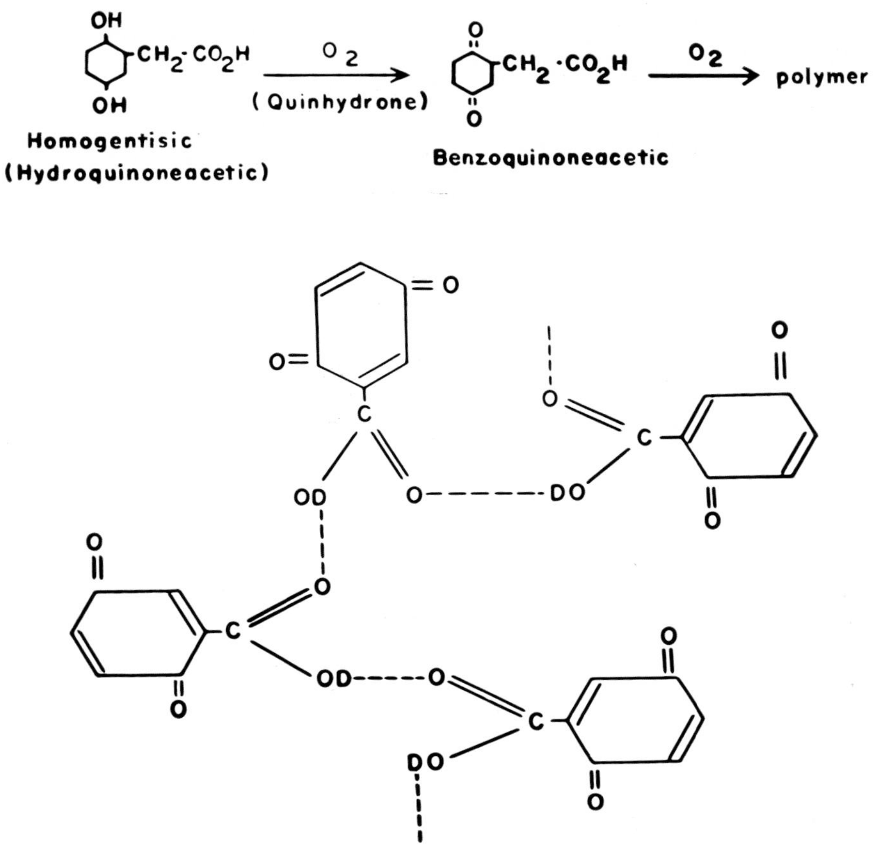

Fig. 7-4. Proposed conversion of homogentisic acid to a polymer by auto-oxidation (top). Proposed structure of the deuterium-labelled polymer, based on infrared spectrography (below). (Courtesy Dr. Robert A. Milch.)

Moran and Ynis[59] produced clinical arthritis and typical joint changes of ochronosis by injecting homogentisic acid into the joints of rabbits.

Prevalence and inheritance

As shown in Table 8, autosomal recessive inheritance of alkaptonuria was demonstrated by the analysis of Hogben and associates,[38] who used alkaptonuria to test the so-called Lenz-Hogben, or *a priori,* method of segregation analysis. This method of testing the recessive hypothesis assumes complete, or truncate, ascertainment. The close agreement with the predictions of the recessive hypothesis supports the correctness of the assumption of complete ascertainment. Apparently the probability of ascertainment of a given family was not dependent on the number of sibs affected. The usual unaffected state of parents of affected sibships likewise supports the recessive hypothesis.

In northern Ireland in 1957 Stevenson[81] found two families with alkaptonuria: a father and daughter and a brother and sister. The population numbered about 1,400,000 at that time. Dent is quoted[63] as estimating the phenotype

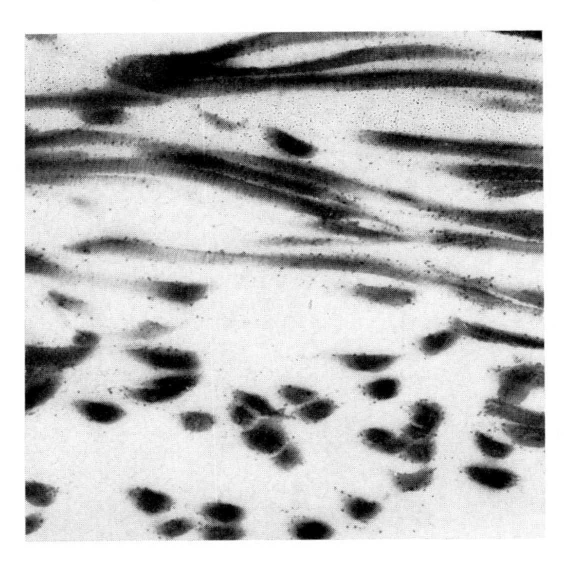

Fig. 7-5. Electron micrograph of collagen fibers from patient with ochronosis. The electron-dense ochronotic polymer is demonstrated as granules closely associated with, and presumably bound to, the collagen fibers. (Courtesy Dr. Robert A. Milch.)

Table 8. Segregation analysis of alkaptonuria*

Sibship size	*Number of sibships*	*Alkaptonuric members* *Observed*	*Expected*	*Variance*
1	5	5	5	0
2	8	10	9.14	0.97960
3	5	8	6.48	1.31485
4	2	4	2.93	0.84010
5	3	4	4.92	1.77534
6	3	8	5.47	2.32785
7	2	5	4.04	1.94048
8	3	5	6.67	3.51720
9	1	4	2.43	1.38020
10	1	2	2.65	1.59170
11	3	7	8.61	5.41590
14	1	4	3.56	2.44640
Total	37	66	61.90	23.52962

*From Hogben, L., Worrall, R. L., and Zieve, I.: Proc. Roy. Soc. Edinburgh **52:**264, 1932.

frequency as 1 in 100,000. Like other recessive disorders, e.g. acatalasia, Tay-Sachs disease, familial Mediterranean fever, etc., the frequency is not uniform; unusually high frequencies have been found in the Dominican Republic[35] and in the region around Piestany, Czechoslovakia.[19,75] (See Figs. 7-6 and 7-7.) In these areas of high gene frequency and high inbreeding, transmission of alkaptonuria through several generations creates a pedigree pattern simulating dominance.[41,51] This quasidominance is clearly the result of repeated marriage of homozygous affected with heterozygous carrier persons. No evidence for the existence of a

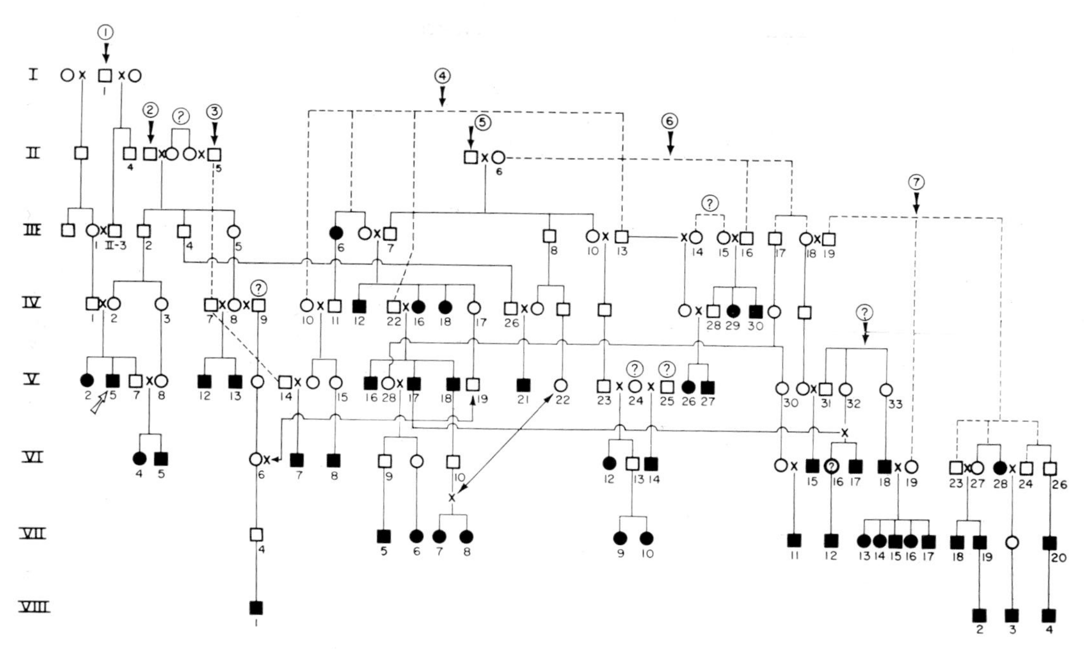

Fig. 7-6. Pedigree of inbred group in Dominican Republic with many cases of alkaptonuria, some in successive generations. (Courtesy Dr. Robert A. Milch.)

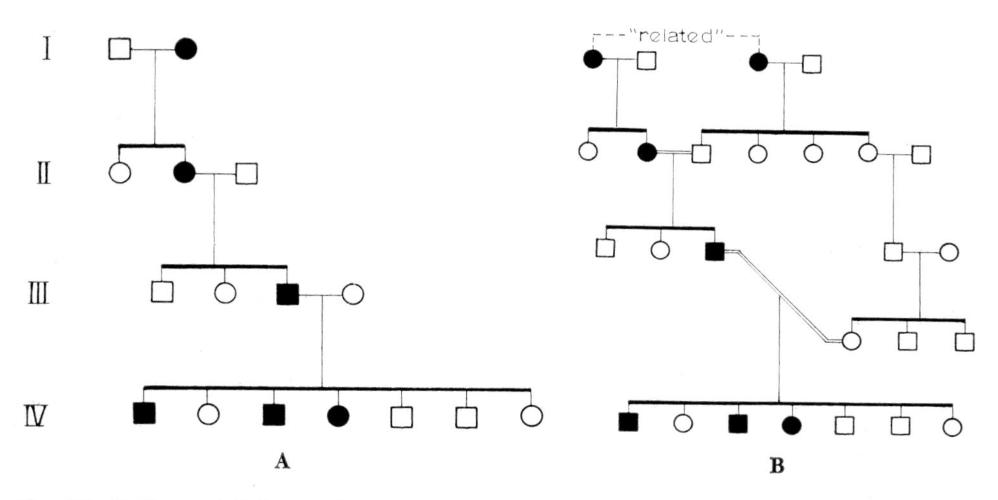

Fig. 7-7. Pedigree of Lebanese family with alkaptonuria. **A,** The pedigree suggests autosomal dominant inheritance. **B,** Consanguinity is indicated by the more complete pedigree. The spouses of the affected persons in the first, second, and third generations are presumably heterozygotes. (Based on data from Khachadurian, A., and Abu Feisal, K. A.: J. Chronic Dis. 7:455, 1958.)

dominant form of alkaptonuria (or of more than one basically distinct recessive form) has been discovered.

The wide distribution of alkaptonuria is indicated by its description in Japanese,[1] Asiatic Indians,[61,71,74,84] American Negroes,[2] and the Bantu.[6] Furthermore, its antiquity is supported by the finding of typical ochronotic spondylosis in Egyptian mummies.[73,87]

In the study of Hogben and associates[38] it was noted that the reported cases included 100 males and 46 females. Since the proband was much more often a male, they concluded that the more frequent urine examination of males in connection with insurance, military service, and employment accounted for the distorted sex ratio. The explanation was supported by the finding that among infants slightly more females than males were detected. A higher frequency of arthritis in male alkaptonurics may contribute to the higher number of ascertained males. In the review of reported cases by O'Brien and co-workers[63] 60% of 520 patients were male.

Simple methods for recognizing heterozygotes—for use in genetic counselling, for example—are not available. Oral homogentisic acid loading tests show no difference between the relatives of alkaptonurics and normal controls.[44,63]

Other considerations

Treatment with vitamins, brewer's yeast, tyrosinase, insulin, adrenocortical extract,[28] vitamin C,[60] vitamin B_{12},[26] cortisone,[13,90] and phenylbutazone[12] has no effect on alkaptonuria. Whether cortisone or vitamin C has any beneficial effects with regard to the ochronotic changes in connective tissue is not known.

An excellent example of a phenocopy (a nongenetically produced phenotype resembling a gene-determined one) is provided by the ochronosis that develops after the prolonged use of carbolic acid dressings for chronic cutaneous ulcers.[10,11,17,24,36]

Presumed spontaneous alkaptonuria in a rabbit[46] and ochronosis in cattle, dogs, and horses[49,69] have not been investigated biochemically and genetically for possible homology to the disease in man. La Du and co-workers[45] found that a generalized pigmentation of connective tissues in the silky bantam fowl is not due to alkaptonuria.

Several authors have pointed out that understanding the pathogenesis of joint changes in ochronosis may provide important clues for research in primary osteoarthritis and perhaps other types of arthritis. Evidence is now available indicating a significant genetic contribution to the pathogenesis of osteoarthritis in men[40] and in mice.[80] It is not unreasonable to suspect that a biochemical defect may be present in osteoarthritis.

As has been reviewed above, in alkaptonuria, excessive metabolites resulting from the failure of degradation of homogentisic acid appear to act as a cross-linking agent on mature collagen. A comparable role may be played by low molecular weight aliphatic aldehydes in producing many of the changes in connective tissue, such as aorta, with aging in nonalkaptonuric persons.[56,57]

SUMMARY

Like homocystinuria, alkaptonuria is an inborn error of metabolism, inherited as an autosomal recessive, in which important connective tissue changes occur. The clinical manifestations are dark urine, urinary and prostatic calculi, pigmentation of connective tissues (especially cartilage), progressive arthropathy of characteristic type, and probably cardiovascular lesions including valvular sclerosis and accelerated arteriosclerosis. The biochemical defect is a deficiency of homogentisic acid oxidase, an enzyme normally present in liver and kidney.

REFERENCES

1. Abe, Y., Oshima, N., Hatanaka, R., Amako, T., and Hirohata, R.: Thirteen cases of alkaptonuria from one family tree with special reference to osteo-arthrosis alkaptonurica, J. Bone Joint Surg. **42-A**:817, 1960.
2. Abbott, L. D., Jr., Mandeville, F. B., and Rein, W. J.: Complete roentgen and ophthalmologic examination for ochronosis in two alcaptonuric children, Virginia Med. Monthly **70**:615, 1943.
3. Albrecht, H.: Ueber Ochronose, Z. Heilk. **23**:366, 1902.
4. Allen, R. A., O'Malley, C., and Straatsma, B. R.: Ocular findings in hereditary ochronosis, Arch. Ophthal. **65**:657, 1961.
5. Arcangeli, A., Colloridi, V., and Chiarini, M.: Una eccezionale associazione morbosa congenita: rene policistico ed alcaptonuria con ochronose, Arch. Ital. Pediat. **20**:66, 1959.
6. Baldachin, B. J., and Rothman, W. T.: Alkaptonuric arthritis; report of a case in a Bantu, Cent. Afr. J .Med. **5**:287, 1959.
7. Bateson, W.: Mendel's principles of heredity, London, 1902, Cambridge University Press.
8. Bauer, O.: Ueber Steinbildungen in den Harnwegen bei Ochronose (Lithiasis ochronotica), Mitt. Grenzgeb. Med. Chir. **41**:451, 1929.
9. Beadle, G. W.: Genes and chemical reactions in neurospora, Science **129**:1715, 1959.
10. Beddard, A. P.: Ochronosis associated with carboluria, Quart. J. Med. **3**:329, 1910.
11. Beddard, A. P., and Plumtre, C. M.: A further note on ochronosis associated with carboluria, Quart. J. Med. **5**:505, 1912.
12. Biggs, T. G., Jr., and Cannon, E., Jr.: Ochronosis: report of a case, J. Louisiana Med. Soc. **105**:395, 1953.
13. Black, R. L.: Use of cortisone in alkaptonuria, J.A.M.A. **155**:968, 1954.
14. Bluefarb, S. M.: Alkaptonuria and ochronosis, Quart. Bull. Northwest. Univ. Med. School **32**:101, 1958.
15. Boedeker, C.: Ueber das Alcapton; ein neuer Beitrag zur Frage: welche Stoffe des Harns können Kupferreduction bewirken? Z. Rat. Med. **7**:130, 1859.
16. Boedeker, C.: Das Alkapton; ein Beitrag zur Frage: welche Stoffe des Harns können aus einer alkalischen Kupferoxydlösung Kupferoxydul reduciren? Ann. Chem. Pharm. **117**:98, 1861.
17. Brogren, N.: Case of exogenetic ochronosis from carbolic acid compresses, Acta Dermatovener. **32**:258, 1952.
18. Brunner, H.: Ueber die Verändergungen des Schläfenbeines bei der Ochronose, Mchr. Ohrenheilk. **63**:997, 1929.
19. Červeňanský, J., Sitaj, Š., and Urbánek, T.: Alkaptonuria and ochronosis, J. Bone Joint Surg. **41-A**:1169, 1959.
20. Coodley, E. L., and Greco, A. J.: Clinical aspects of ochronosis, with report of a case, Amer. J. Med. **8**:816, 1950.
21. Cooper, J. A., and Moran, T. J.: Studies on ochronosis, Arch. Path. **64**:46, 1957.
22. DiFiore, J. A.: Ochronosis, Arthritis Rheum. **3**:359, 1960.
23. Eisenberg, H.: Alkaptonuria, ochronosis, arthritis and ruptured intervertebral disk, Arch. Intern. Med. **86**:79, 1950.
24. Fishberg, E. H.: Ueber die Carbolochronose, Virchow Arch. Path. Anat. **251**:376, 1924.
25. Fisher, R. G., and Williams, J.: Ochronosis associated with degeneration of an intervertebral disc, J. Neurosurg. **12**:403, 1955.
26. Flaschenräger, B., Halawani, A., and Nabeh, I.: Alkaptonurie und Vitamin B_{12}, Klin. Wschr. **32**:131, 1954.
27. Friderich, H., and Nikolowski, W.: Endogene Ochronose, Arch. Dermat. u. Syph. **192**:273, 1951.
28. Galdston, M., Steele, J. M., and Dobriner, K.: Alcaptonuria and ochronosis with a report of three patients and metabolic studies in two, Amer. J. Med. **13**:432, 1952.

29. Garrod, A. E.: About alkaptonuria, Lancet **2**:1484, 1901.
30. Garrod, A. E.: The Croonian lectures on inborn errors of metabolism. Lecture II. Alkaptonuria, Lancet **2**:73, 1908.
31. Garrod, A. E.: Inborn errors of metabolism, London, 1909, Frowde, Hodder & Stoughton.
32. Gonnermann, R.: Kasuistischer Beitrag zur Ochronose, Beitr. Path. Anat. **100**:598, 1938.
33. Gross, O., and Allard, E.: Untersuchungen über Alkaptonuria, Z. Klin. Med. **64**:359, 1907.
34. Hammond, G., and Powers, H. W.: Alkaptonuric arthritis: report of a case, Lahey Clin. Bull. **11**:18, 1958.
35. Harrold, A. J.: Alkaptonuric arthritis, J. Bone Joint Surg. **38-B**:532, 1956.
36. Heile: Ueber die Ochronose und die durch Formol verursachte pseudo-ochronotische Färbung der Knorpel, Virchow Arch. **160**:148, 1900.
37. Hendel, H., and Ben-Assa, B. J.: Report about a Bedouin family affected by alkaptonuria (comprising two cases of uro-lithiasis), Ann. Paediat. **195**:77, 1960.
38. Hogben, L., Worrall, R. L., and Zieve, I.: The genetic basis of alkaptonuria, Proc. Roy. Soc. Edinburgh **52**:264, 1932.
39. Janecek, M.: Osteoarthrosis ochronotica (alcaptonurica), Lek. Listy **2**:536, 1947.
40. Kellgren, J. H.: Osteoarthrosis in patients and populations, Brit. Med. J. **2**:1, 1961.
41. Khachadurian, A., and Abu Feisal, K.: Alkaptonuria. Report of a family with seven cases appearing in four successive generations with metabolic studies in one patient, J. Chronic Dis. **7**:455, 1958.
42. Knox, W. E.: Sir Archibald Garrod's "Inborn errors of metabolism," II. Alkaptonuria, Amer. J. Hum. Genet. **10**:95, 1958.
43. Koonce, D. M.: Ochronosis: report of three cases in siblings, J. Tennessee Med. Ass. **51**:85, 1958.
44. La Du, B. N.: Alcaptonuria. In Stanbury, J. B. Wyngaarden, J. B., and Fredrickson, D. S., editors: The metabolic basis of inherited disease, New York, 1960, Blakiston Division, McGraw-Hill Book Co., Inc., pp. 394-427.
45. La Du, B. N., Zannoni, V. G., Laster, L., and Seegmiller, J. E.: The nature of the defect in tyrosine metabolism in alcaptonuria, J. Biol. Chem. **230**:251, 1958.
46. Lewis, J. H.: Alcaptonuria in a rabbit, J. Biol. Chem. **70**:659, 1926.
47. Lichtenstein, L., and Kaplan, L.: Hereditary ochronosis. Pathological changes observed in two necropsied cases, Amer. J. Path. **30**:99, 1954.
48. Manson-Bahr, P., and Ransford, O. N.: Some pigmentations of the skin occurring in patients from the tropics: carotinaemia, haemochromatosis and alkaptonuria, Trans. Roy. Soc. Trop. Med. Hyg. **32**:395, 1938.
49. Martin, W. J., Underdahl, L. O., and Mathieson, D. R.: Alkaptonuria: report of 3 cases, Proc. Mayo Clin. **27**:193, 1952.
50. McKenzie, A. W., Owen, J. A., and Ramsay, J. H. R.: Two cases of alcaptonuria, Brit. Med. J. **2**:794, 1957.
51. Milch, R. A.: Direct inheritance of alcaptonuria, Metabolism **4**:513, 1955.
52. Milch, R. A.: Studies of alcaptonuria: binding of homogentisic acid solutions to hide powder collagen, Proc. Soc. Exp. Biol. Med. **106**:68, 1961.
53. Milch, R. A.: Studies of alcaptonuria: inheritance of 47 cases in eight highly inter-related Dominican kindreds, Amer. J. Hum. Genet. **12**:76, 1960.
54. Milch, R. A.: Studies of alcaptonuria: collagenase degradation of homogentisic-tanned hide powder collagen, Proc. Soc. Exp. Biol. Med. **107**:183, 1961.
55. Milch, R. A., and Robinson, R. A.: Studies of alcaptonuria: content and density of the water and solid phases of ochronotic cartilage, J. Chronic Dis. **12**:409, 1960.
56. Milch, R. A.: Hydrothermal shrinkage of metabolite-treated aortae, J. Atheroscler. Res. **5**:215, 1965.
57. Milch, R. A.: Reaction of collagen-cross-linking aldehydes with phenylenediamines, Nature **205**:1108, 1965.
58. Minno, A. M., and Rogers, J. A.: Ochronosis: report of a case, Ann. Intern. Med. **56**:179, 1957.
59. Moran, T. J., and Ynis, E. J.: Studies on ochronosis. II. Effects of injection of homogentisic acid and ochronotic pigment in experimental animals, Amer. J. Path. **40**:359, 1962.
60. Mosonyi, L.: A propos de l'alcaptonurie et de son traitement, Presse Méd. **47**:708, 1939.
61. Natarajan, M.: Ochronotic arthritis (a report of three cases), Indian J. Surg. **22**:222, 1960.

62. Neubauer, O.: Intermediärer Eiweisstoffwechsel, Handb. Norm. Path. Physiol. **5**:671, 1928.
63. O'Brien, W. M., La Du, B. N., and Bunim, J. J.: Biochemical, pathologic and clinical aspects of alcaptonuria, ochronosis and ochronotic arthropathy. Review of world literature (1584-1962), Amer. J. Med. **34**:813, 1963.
64. Osler, W.: Ochronosis: the pigmentation of cartilages, sclerotics and skin in alkaptonuria, Lancet **1**:10, 1904.
65. Pagan-Carlo, J., and Payzant, A. R.: Roentgenographic manifestations in a severe case of alcaptonuric osteoarthritis, Amer. J. Roentgen. **80**:635, 1958.
66. Pieter, H.: Une famille d'alcaptonuriques, Presse Méd. **33**:1310, 1925.
67. Pomeranz, M. M., Friedman, L. J., and Tunick, I. S.: Roentgen findings in alcaptonuric ochronosis, Radiology **37**:295, 1941.
68. Poschl, M.: Röntgenbild und Röntgenbestrahlung bei der Arthrosis alkaptonurica, Fortschr. Roentgenst. **76**:97, 1952.
69. Poulsen, V.: Ueber Ochronose bei Menschen und Tieren, Beitr. Path. Anat. **48**:346, 1910.
70. Rones, B.: Ochronosis oculi in alkaptonuria, Amer. J. Ophthal. **49**:440, 1960.
71. Sarin, L. R., and Bhargava, R. K.: Alkaptonuria with ochronosis, J. Indian Med. Ass. **28**:481, 1957.
72. Seegmiller, J. E., Zannoni, V. G., Laster, L., and La Du, B. N.: An enzymatic spectrophotometric method for the determination of homogentisic acid in plasma and urine, J. Biol. Chem. **236**:774, 1961.
73. Simon, G., and Zorab, P. A.: The radiographic changes in alkaptonuric arthritis, Brit. J. Radiol. **34**:384, 1961.
74. Sinha, H. K.: A case of alkaptonuria, Indian Med. Gaz. **65**:153, 1930.
75. Šitaj, S., and Urbánek, T.: Alkaptonuria, Rev. Czech. Med. **2**:288, 1956.
76. Skinsnes, O. K.: Generalized ochronosis. Report of an instance in which it was misdiagnosed as melanosarcoma, with resultant enucleation of an eye, Arch. Path. **45**:552, 1948.
77. Smith, H. P., and Smith, H. P., Jr.: Ochronosis: report of two cases, Ann. Intern. Med. **42**:171, 1955.
78. Smith, J. W.: Ochronosis of the sclera and cornea complicating alkaptonuria; review of the literature and report of four cases, J.A.M.A. **120**:1282, 1942.
79. Söderbergh, G.: Ueber Ostitis deformans ochronotica, Neur. Zbl. **32**:1362, 1913.
80. Sokoloff, L., Crittenden, L. B., Yamamoto, R. S., and Jay, G. E., Jr.: The genetics of degenerative joint disease in mice, Arthritis Rheum. **5**:531, 1962.
81. Stevenson, A. C. (Oxford): Personal communication.
82. Sutro, C. J., and Anderson, M. E.: Alkaptonuric arthritis: cause for free intraarticular bodies, Surgery **22**:120, 1947.
83. Umber, G., and Burger, M.: Zur Klinik intermediarer Stoffwechselstörungen (Alkaptonurie mit Ochronose und Osteo-Arthritis deformans; Zystinurie), Deutsch. Med. Wschr. **39**:2337, 1913.
84. Vaishnava, S., and Pulimood, B. M.: Alkaptonuria, Indian J. Pediat. **25**:518, 1958.
85. Virchow, R.: Ein Fall von allgemeiner Ochronose der Knorpel und knorpelähnlichen Theile, Arch. Path. Anat. **37**:212, 1866.
86. Wagner, L. R., Knott, J. L., Machaffie, R. A., and Walsh, J. R.: Clinical and pathological findings in ochronosis, J. Clin. Path. **13**:22, 1960.
87. Wells, C., and Maxwell, B. M.: Alkaptonuria in an Egyptian mummy, Brit. J. Radiol. **35**:679, 1962.
88. Wolkow, M., and Baumann, E.: Ueber das Wesen der Alkaptonurie, Z. Physiol. Chem. **15**:228, 1891.
89. Young, H. H.: Calculi of the prostate associated with ochronosis and alkaptonuria, J. Urol. **51**:48, 1944.
90. Yules, J. H.: Ochronotic arthritis. Report of a case, Bull. New Eng. Med. Center **16**:168, 1954.
91. Zannoni, V. G., Malawista, S. E., and La Du, B. N.: Studies on Ochronosis. II. Studies on benzoquinoneacetic acid, a probable intermediate in the connective tissue pigmentation of alcaptonuria, Arthritis Rheum. **5**:547, 1962.
92. Zannoni, V. G., Seegmiller, J. E., and La Du, B. N.: Nature of the defect in alcaptonuria, Nature, London **193**:952, 1962.

8

Pseudoxanthoma elasticum

Historical note

The first description of the skin changes is that by Rigal[98] in 1881, and the first autopsy report was provided by Balzer[6] in 1884. Because of the yellow and elevated appearance of the skin lesions, the disorder was grouped with the xanthomatoses by Rigal and Balzer and by Chauffard.[18] The disease was identified as a separate and nonxanthomatous entity by Darier[24] in 1896.

In 1889 Chauffard,* at a meeting of the Société Médicale des Hôpitaux in Paris described a patient destined to occupy a prominent role in the histoy of this disease. His case was separately reported, during the next fifteen years, by Besnier and Doyon[12]; by Darier,[24] who established the histopathology and offered the name *pseudoxanthoma elasticum* with the alternative *elastorrhexis;* and by Hallopeau and Laffitte,[49] who described dramatic changes in the fundus oculi. The patient's well-documented story is of further interest because it demonstrates the typical feaures of the syndrome from which he suffered: changes in the skin, repeated massive gastrointestinal hemorrhages, weak peripheral pulses, and failing vision. Chauffard's description[18] follows†:

> This is a man of 35 years. . . . At 24 years of age, while doing his military service in New Caledonia, he suffered a large hematemesis. This accident repeated itself several times (at ages 26, 31, and 33). This summer he was admitted to the Hôtel Dieu for a hematemesis.
>
> In 1880 L. was discharged and returned to France; and it was shortly afterward, he states, when he noted the beginning of his skin affection. . . . The xanthomatous eruption is composed of a series of evolving groups, perfectly symmetrical and confined exclusively to the several flexural folds—the base of the neck, the two axillary creases, the folds of the elbows, the anterior abdominal wall, especially just below the umbilicus, the two inguinal triangles, the inferior aspect of the penis, around the anus, the two popliteal fossae. . . . The center of the group is formed by an almost confluent agglomeration of intradermal plaques, soft to the touch, projecting to some extent like papules, separated by small folds of skin. Their coloration is rather pale, resembling that of fresh butter or yellow chamois; the size of

*Anatole Chauffard (1855-1932), an internist, is better known for his discovery (with Minkowski) of congenital hemolytic icterus (1900), now more generally called hereditary spherocytosis, and of the increased osmotic fragility of the erythrocytes in this condition (1907).[3]
†Translation mine.

> the largest plaque is scarcely greater than that of a pea. . . . If one retracts both lips, one sees that the mucosa of the inner aspect is involved. It demonstrates a cluster of small, yellowish intramucosal nodules, resting on a richly vascular background traversed by numerous dilated and tortuous capillaries. . . . In February there developed an unusual phenomenon, of which there is today scarcely any trace remaining. The peripheral zone of the eruptive groups in the skin was traversed by rather large, violaceous rose networks that were not elevated and formed a congestive halo around the yellow plaques. . . . Today traces of this perinodular hyperemia remain only in the pectoral regions, on the anterior extension of the axillary groups. . . .
>
> The pulse is feeble and compressible and gives with the sphygmometer of Verdin a tension of 650, rather than of 750, the average normal figure.

In August, 1896, at the Third International Dermatologic Congress in London, Darier[24] reported histologic studies on the skin of Chauffard's patient. By 1903, this patient had developed amblyopia; and Hallopeau and Laffitte[49] reported that there was "chorioretinitis of the central region, involving the macula, with secondary atrophy of the optic disc."

Although Hallopeau and Laffitte in 1903 speculated that there might be some connection between the changes in the skin and those in the fundus oculi of Chauffard's patient, it was not until 1929 that the relationship of angioid streaks and pseudoxanthoma elasticum was established by Ester Grönblad,[44] an ophthalmologist, and James Strandberg,[118] a dermatologist, both of Stockholm. Angioid streaks had been described by Doyne[27] in 1889, and the name was assigned by Knapp[65] in 1892. Knapp thought angioid streaks have a vascular basis. Their origin as a result of crazing of Bruch's membrane was first suggested by Kofler[66] in 1917.

Involvement of the peripheral arteries in this syndrome and the physiologic consequences thereof have been studied in the last twenty-five years by Carlborg,[16] Van Embden Andres,[132] Scheie and Freeman,[105] Urbach and Wolfram,[131] Prick,[59,95] Guenther,[45] Wolff and associates,[140] and Goodman and colleagues,[43] among others. Gastrointestinal hemorrhage was emphasized by several of these authors and particularly by Revell and Carey[97] in 1948. During the early 1950's the suggestion that this disease is an abnormality of collagen fibers rather than elastic fibers was advanced by Hannay,[50] who used standard histologic techniques, and by Tunbridge and collaborators,[130] who used electron microscopy. Return to the view that the elastic fiber is primarily involved came from the work of Rodnan and associates,[100] Fisher and co-workers,[33] Goodman and colleagues,[43] and others.

Pseudoxanthoma elasticum is the name usually given this syndrome. With the renewed evidence that the elastic fiber is the main site of abnormality, "elasticum" seems accurate and the skin and arterial changes certainly justify the designation "pseudoxanthoma." The only eponym that has been applied to this syndrome at all frequently, Grönblad-Strandberg, is not easily remembered or spoken and has not attained wide use. The abbreviation PXE is the term that will be used frequently in this presentation to refer to the entire syndrome.

Clinical manifestations

Clinical expression of PXE is found mainly in three areas: the skin, the eye, and the cardiovascular system. Because of the widespread involvement of the muscular arteries, hemorrhagic symptoms referable to virtually every organ system may occur. The following descriptions are based in part on more than twenty-five cases observed at the Johns Hopkins Hospital.

Skin and mucosa. The changes in the skin (Figs. 8-1*A* and 8-2) are often not recognizable clinically before the second decade of life or later. The face, neck, axillary folds, cubital areas, inguinal folds, and periumbilical area are particularly prone to involvement. The skin in the perioral area, including the creases of the skin, another zone of particular wear and tear, is likely to show changes. (It is of note that senile "elastotic degeneration" [see below] occurs frequently

A

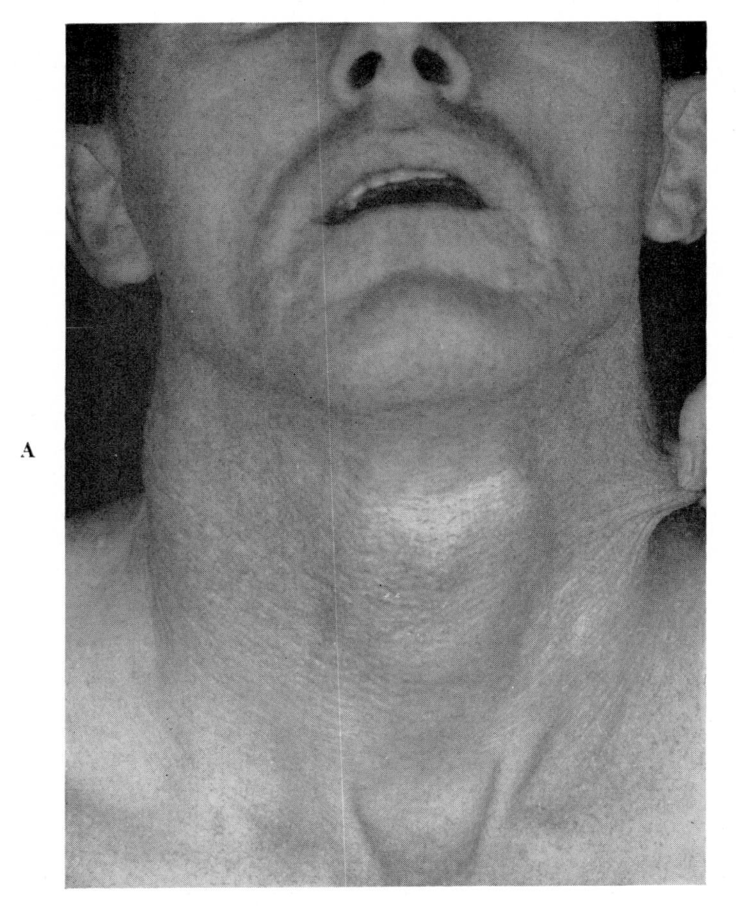

Fig. 8-1. C. T. (582989), a 32-year-old man. **A** and **B,** The skin is lax, rigid, and grooved, with a yellowish tint. **C,** Angioid streaks and proliferative changes in fundus oculi. **D,** Calcification of deep femoral artery (photograph retouched). **E,** Calcification of posterior tibial artery (photograph retouched). **F,** Histologic changes in the skin. Elastic tissue stain. (×50.) **G,** Same as in **F.** (×125.) The skin of the neck, axillae, and groin is involved. Both second toes have a congenital flexion deformity ("hammertoe"). Beginning at the age of 30 years, the patient has had a total of about ten massive gastrointestinal hemorrhages necessitating hospitalization and transfusion. No bleeding site has ever been identified. X-ray film of the lungs reveals peculiar nodular densities diffusely distributed throughout both lung fields. (**B** from McKusick, V. A.: Bull. N. Y. Acad. Med. **35:**143, 1959.)

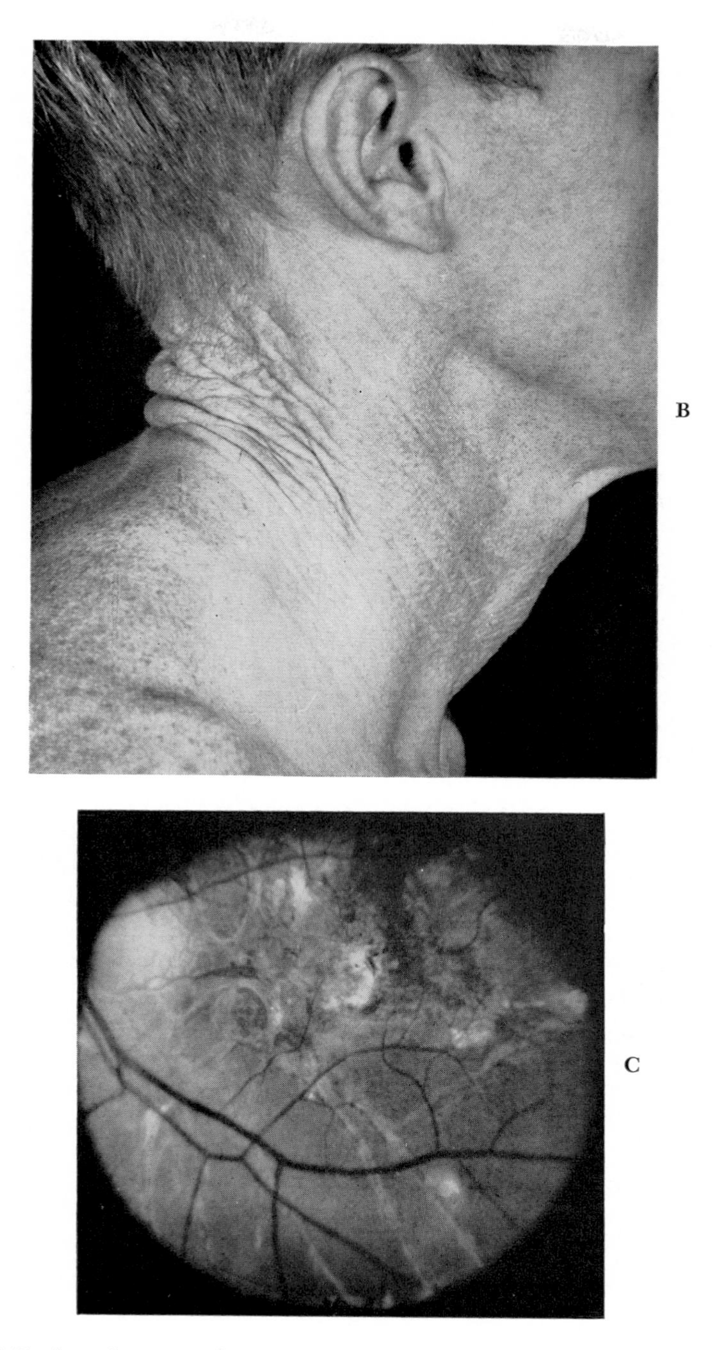

Fig. 8-1, cont'd. For legend see opposite page.

Continued.

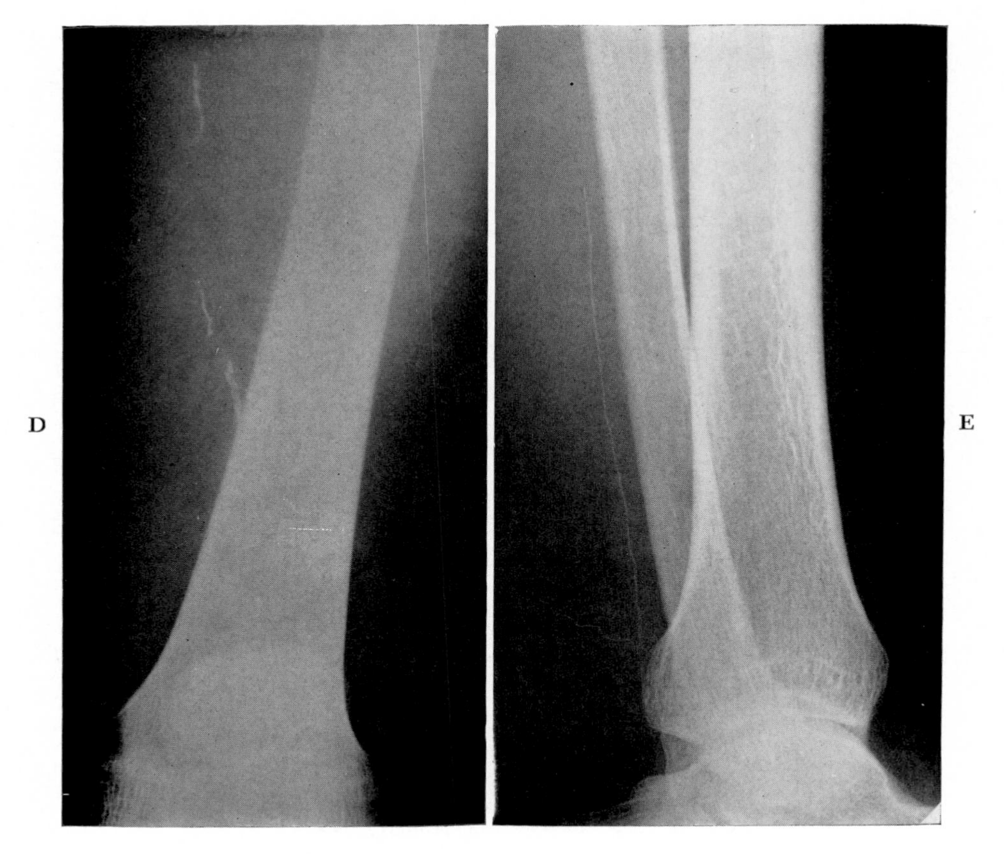

Fig. 8-1, cont'd. For legend see p. 288.

in the same area, as indicated by the frequency with which this histologic change is seen in specimens of lip carcinoma. Surgical pathologists and skin pathologists become very familiar with senile elastosis because of its frequency in specimens with neoplasms of the skin in older individuals.) The skin becomes thickened and grooved like coarse-grained Moroccan leather. The areas between the grooves, diamond-shaped, rectangular, and polygonal, are elevated and yellowish. *Cutis rhomboidalis nuchae* and *la peau citréïne,* although terms more often used for conditions distinct from PXE, would be appropriate for the changes seen in some of these patients.[123] "Crepelike" in another suggested description.[85] The skin in the involved areas becomes lax, redundant, and relatively inelastic. In girls (and the female is more often affected by this disorder) the cosmetically undesirable changes in the skin, especially that of the neck, are often occasion for consulting a physician. Exaggeration of the nasolabial folds and chin creases is often striking (Fig. 8-3) and may create a "hound-dog" appearance of the face. Profound laxity of skin in the neck, axillary folds, and abdominal wall is observed in some. Striking lesions in the inguinal triangles and on the penis occur in some patients (Fig. 8-4).

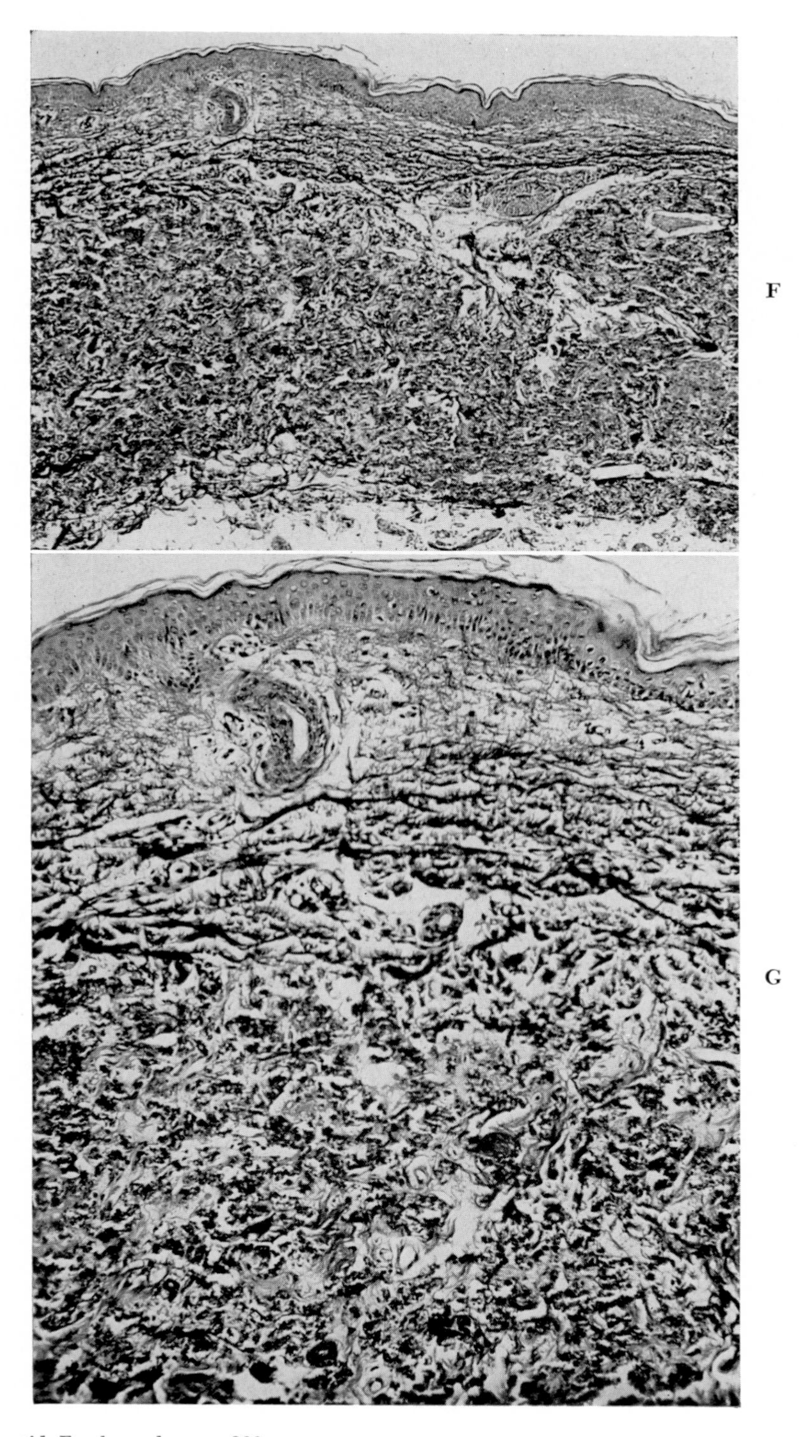

Fig. 8-1, cont'd. For legend see p. 288.

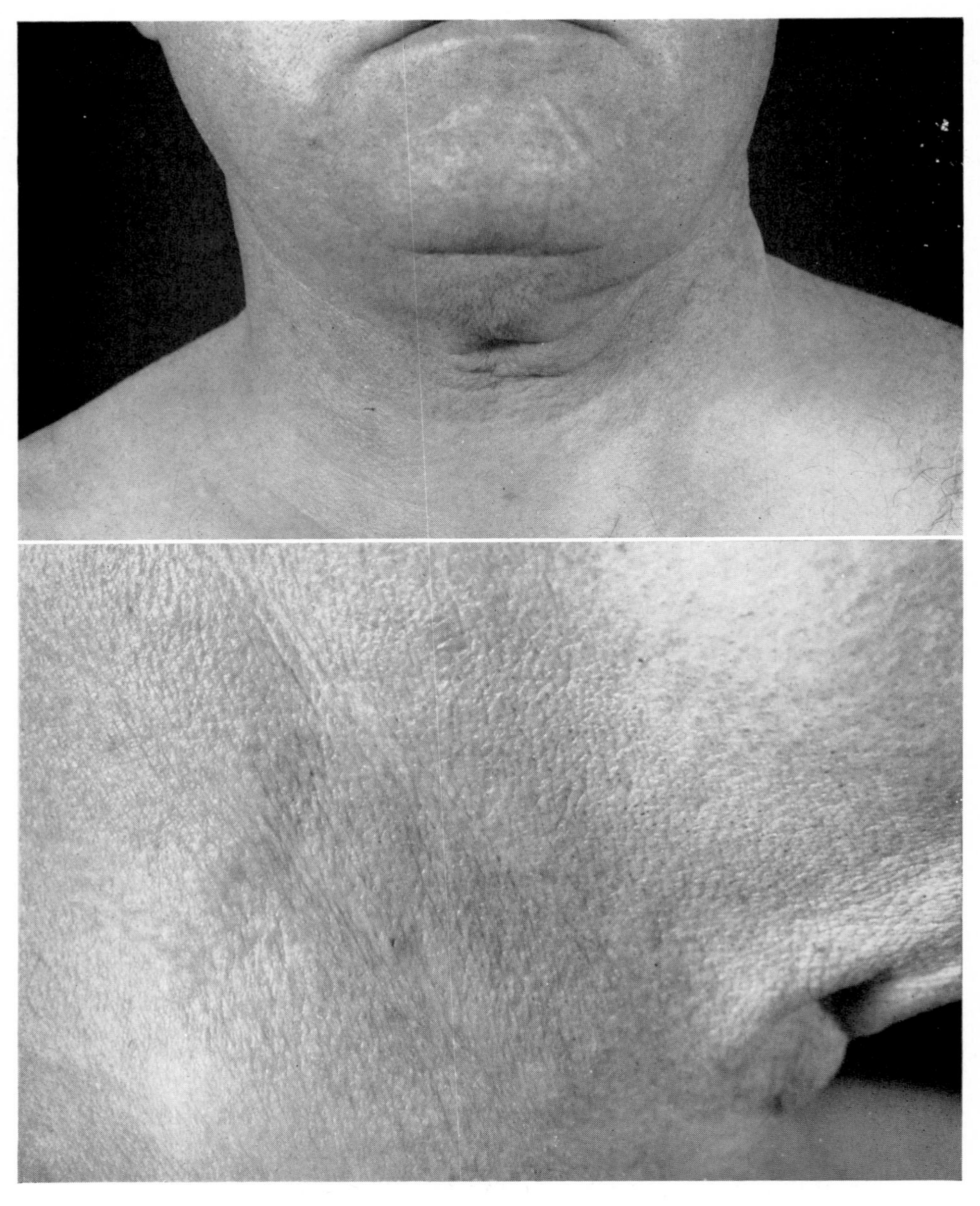

Fig. 8-2. P. J. G. (J.H.H. 721600), 45 years old, had a severe gastrointestinal hemorrhage at the age of 34 years. No basis was discovered and there was no recurrence. He was told at that time that he had hemorrhage in the right eye. For several years, especially in winter, he noted cramping and fatigability of the legs. At the age of 44 years there was onset of progressive failure of vision. There are no similar abnormalities in the family. Examination revealed only minimal changes in the skin of the neck. The skin would have been passed as normal were it not for the rest of the clinical picture. The skin elsewhere was normal except possibly for slightly increased looseness in flexure areas. Both fundi showed large areas of old hemorrhage and fibrosis in the macular area, typical angioid streaks, and hyaline bodies near the optic discs. No pulses were palpable in the legs below the femorals. Blood pressure and electrocardiogram were normal. The aorta was moderately tortuous, and serum cholesterol was 355 mg.%. (Patient seen through courtesy of Dr. J. R. Krevans.)

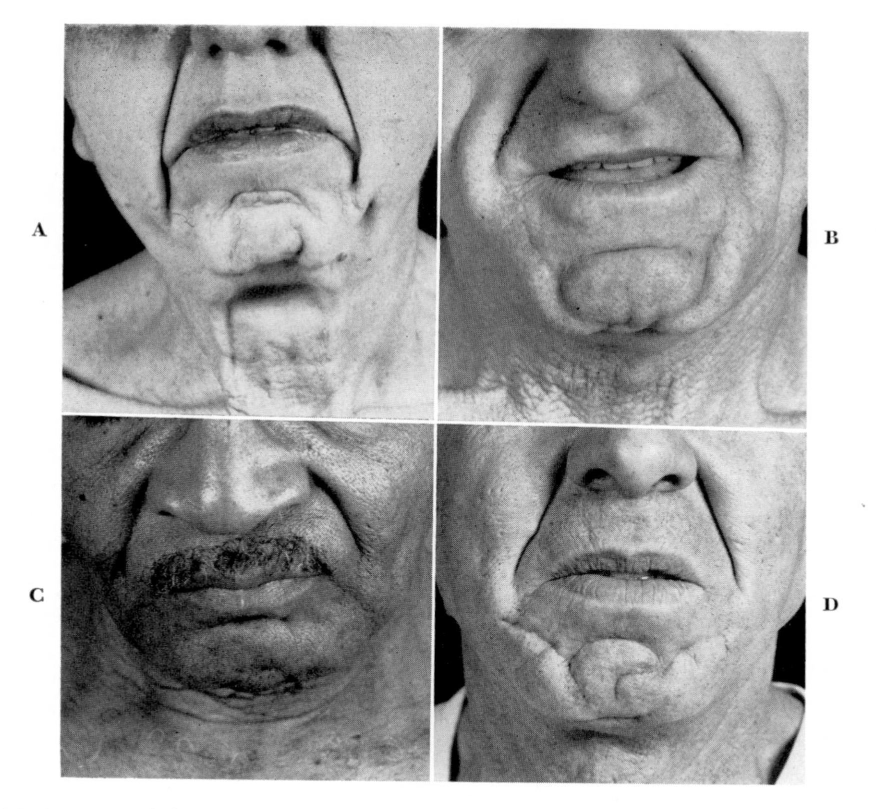

Fig. 8-3. Accentuated facial folds and creases in four patients with PXE. Those shown in **A, B,** and **D** are sibs. (From Goodman, R. M., Smith, E. W., Paton, D., Bergman, R. A., Siegel, C. L., Ottesen, O. E., Shelley, W. M., Pusch, A. L., and McKusick, V. A.: Medicine **42:**297, 1963.)

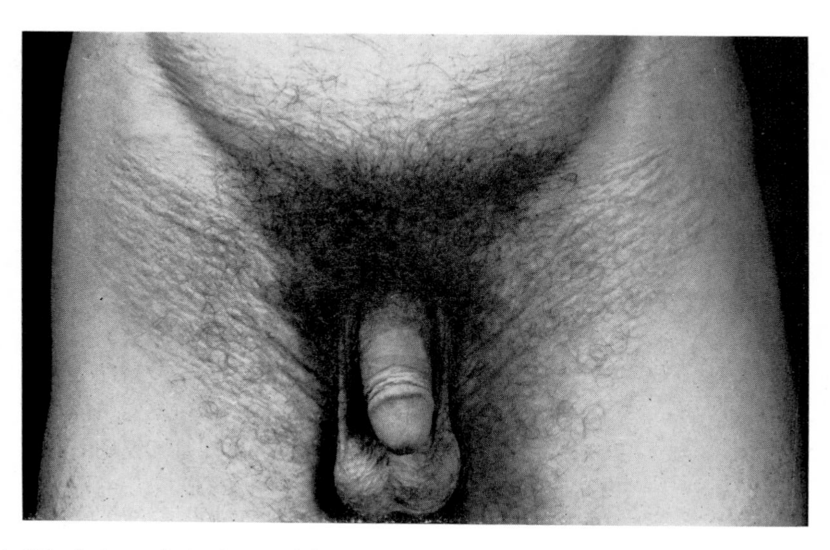

Fig. 8-4. Skin lesions of the lower abdomen, femoral triangles, and penis in a 33-year-old man (C. G., 456025). (From Goodman, R. M., Smith, E. W., Paton, D., Bergman, R. A., Siegel, C. L., Ottesen, O. E., Shelley, W. M., Pusch, A. L., and McKusick, V. A.: Medicine **42:**297, 1963.)

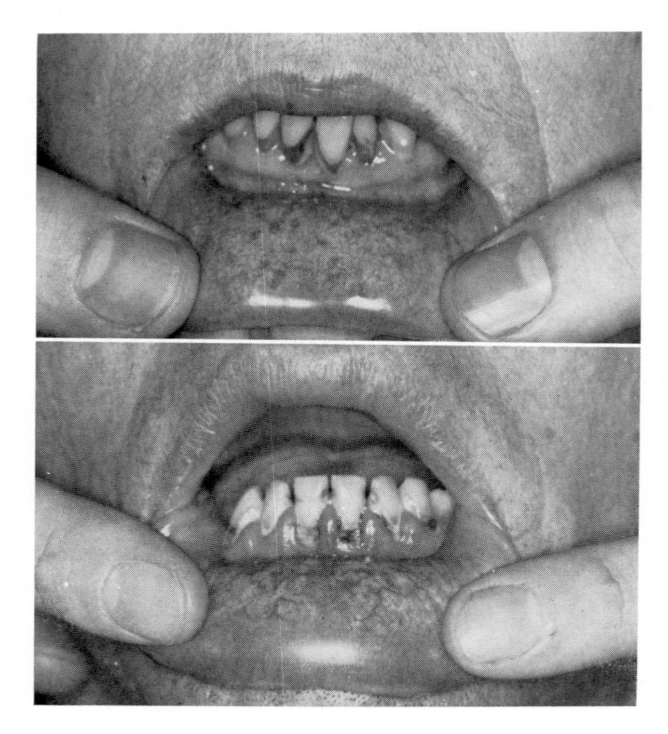

Fig. 8-5. Lesions of the labial mucosa.

The soft palate often shows changes grossly and histologically identical to those in the skin[39]; the inner aspect of the lips and the buccal mucosa are commonly affected areas[85] (Fig 8-5). At times the mucosa of the rectum and vagina is affected.[16] In some patients the cutaneous changes are exceedingly mild despite advanced ocular and arterial changes (Fig. 8-2). Van Embden Andres[132] described four patients with only minimal clinical but typical histologic changes in the skin. In two other cases of his, there were no clinically detectable changes in the skin, yet there were positive findings on biopsy. Goodman and colleagues[43] described similar experiences; see Fig. 8-3. Rubbing or stretching of the skin may make the lesions more evident.[85] Sometimes the patients report expressing "matter" from the nodular lesions of the neck and about the chin. In Gold's case[42] ulceration and drainage of the skin lesions occurred.

In addition to the classic features, some patients have localized skin changes of a different type on the neck, axilla, or anterior abdominal wall. These consist of large (3 by 4 cm.) circinate plaques of closely grouped, hyperkeratotic papules, 1 to 2 mm. in size. A hyperkeratotic cap can be dislodged to leave a small bloody depression. This lesion[111] is termed reactive perforating elastoma (elastoma perforans serpiginosa, Miescher's elastoma, etc.).

The skin changes about the neck were noted by the mother at birth of one patient. In others they have been noted in early childhood. In some patients no remarkable peculiarity is evident to the patient until the changes are pointed out by the physician consulted because of failing vision or gastrointestinal hemorrhage.

Calcification in the middle and deeper layers of the dermis is identifiable by radiographic techniques (Fig. 8-6). In three of ten patients who were appropriately studied Goodman and colleagues[43] found calcinosis cutis.

The eye. The characteristic changes in the eye are demonstrated by funduscopic examination and consist of angioid streaking of the fundus (Fig. 8-1*C*). These streaks are red, brownish, or gray and are four or five times wider than veins but resemble vessels in the manner in which they course over the fundus.[138] That the streaks lack pigmentation can be demonstrated by applying sufficient pressure to the eye to occlude the retinal artery. Pallor of the avascular retina produced by this maneuver decreases visible contrasts and in many patients leads to virtual disappearance of the streaks. That the streaks are cracks in a membrane beneath the retina is clinically substantiated by observation of their tapering and their complementary zigzag borders. They always underlie the retinal vessels. In later stages the streaks are bordered by proliferating scar tissue and retinal pigment epithelium producing cuffing of the type shown. (Figs. 8-7 to 8-9.) Electroretinography usually shows no abnormality until late stages.

The angioid streaks are probably not present at birth but, like the skin changes, they usually develop in the second decade or later. They may be the only ocular sign of PXE for many years. The development of hemorrhage and the appearance of chorioretinal scarring are ominous signs. Although complete blindness does not occur, macular involvement frequently results in diminution of visual acuity to 20/200, 20/400, or the ability to see fingers at a few feet. When chorioretinal scarring and accompanying retinal pigment proliferation are ex-

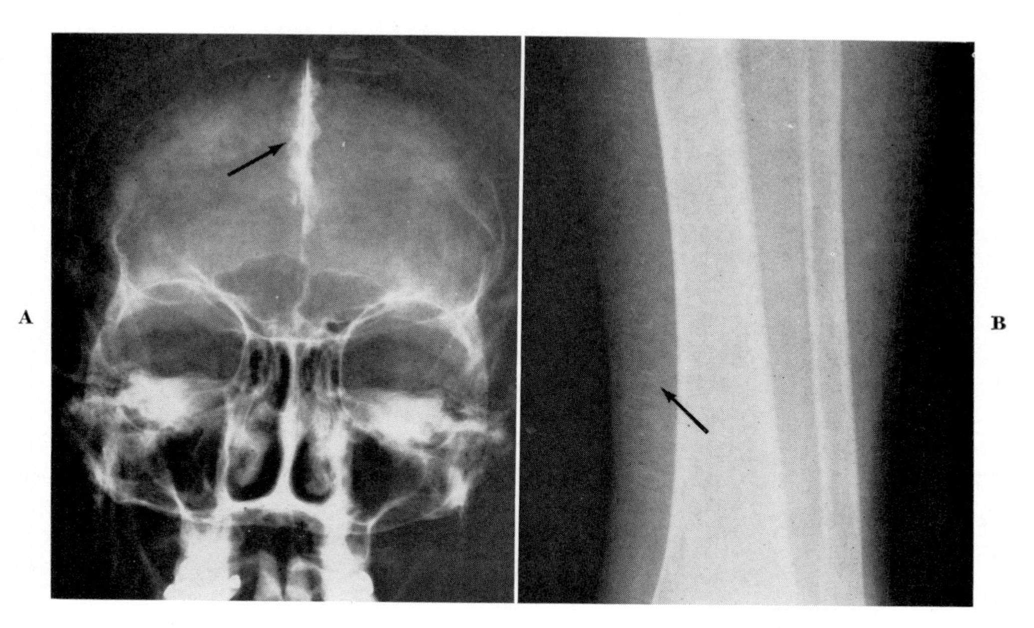

Fig. 8-6. Calcification of the falx cerebri, **A**, and of the skin, **B**, in D. G. (757257), 54-year-old white female (shown also in Fig. 8-14). (From Goodman, R. M., Smith, E. W., Paton, D., Bergman, R. A., Siegel, C. L., Ottesen, O. E., Shelley, W. M., Pusch, A. L., and McKusick, V. A.: Medicine **42**:297, 1963.)

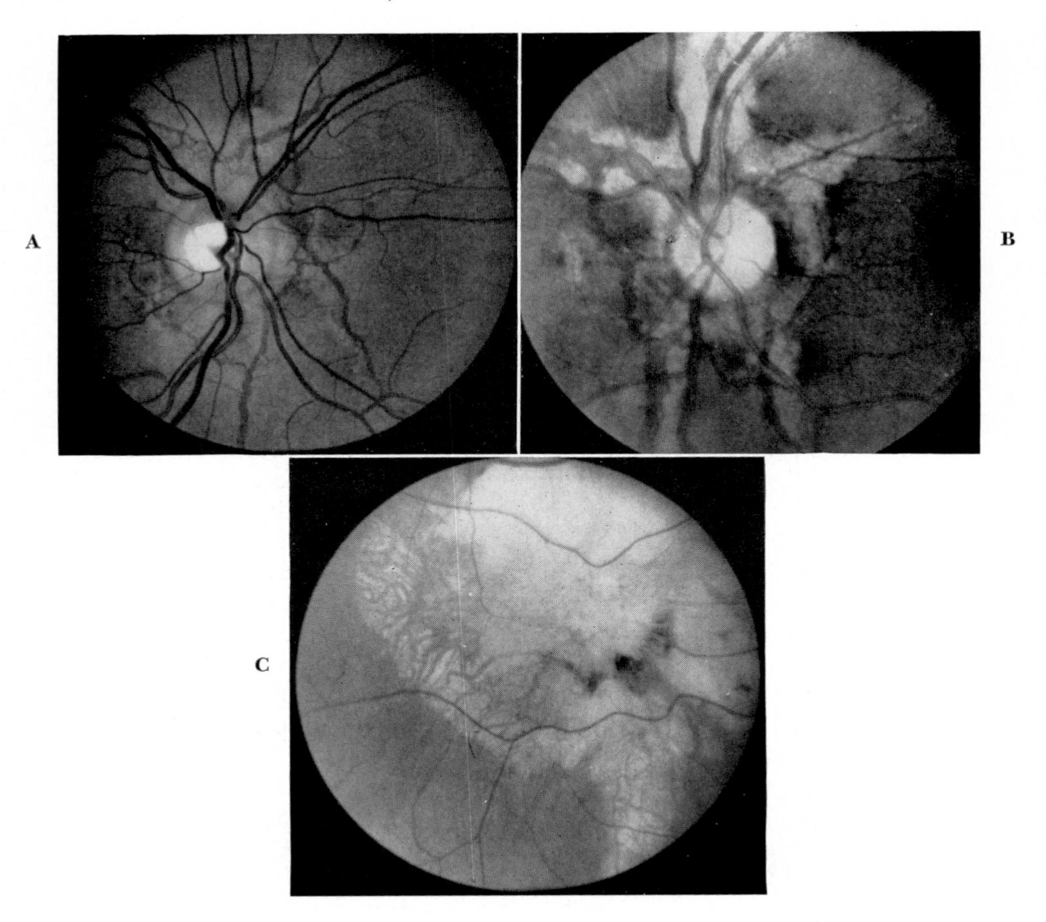

Fig. 8-7. Fundus photographs in PXE. **A,** Angioid streaks in typical configuration. Note that the streaks underlie retinal vessels. Choroidal vessels are not seen. **B,** Extensive fibrous cuffing accompanies the angioid streaks. **C,** Late stage, showing absence of angioid streaks in the area photographed and increased visibility of choroidal vessels inferior to the heavily scarred macular region. (From Goodman, R. M., Smith, E. W., Paton, D., Bergman, R. A., Siegel, C. L., Ottesen, O. E., Shelley, W. M., Pusch, A. L., and McKusick, V. A.: Medicine **42**:297, 1963.)

tensive, angioid streaks may be obscured, although indistinct remnants of streaks usually persist at the periphery of such scars.

In some cases the occurrence of retinal hemorrhage can be related to trauma such as, for example, that sustained in one patient by high diving. White or yellowish dots referred to as colloid bodies, or *Drüsen,* are described[140] and were present in the vicinity of the discs in the patient whose skin changes are demonstrated in Fig. 8-2.

Some patients show only pigmentary mottling of the fundus.[43,109] This change is interpreted as the earliest manifestation of alteration in Bruch's membrane.

Although angioid streaks are the ocular hallmark of PXE, not infrequently only a less specific central chorioretinitis is present.[10,132] This may have been the case with Chauffard's famous patient.[49] Like the hemorrhages, the central chorioretinitis is a grave threat to vision because of involvement of the macular areas.

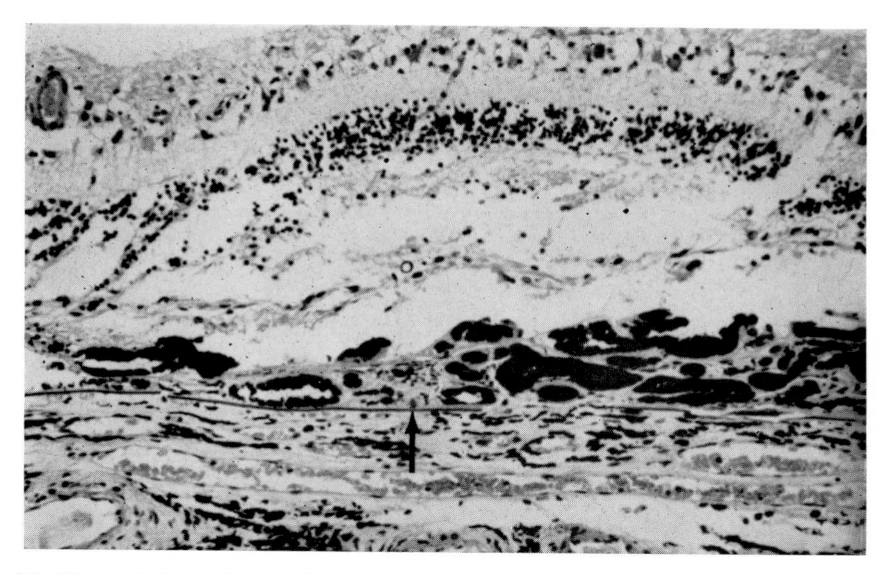

Fig. 8-8. Histopathology of angioid streaks. Bruch's membrane is indicated by the arrow. Breaks are shown in the right of the picture. (Courtesy Dr. David Paton.)

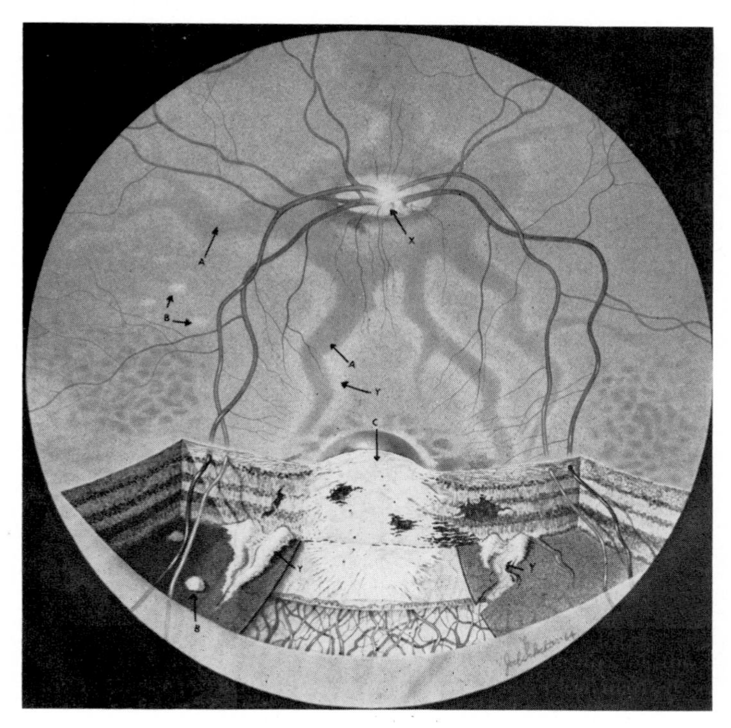

Fig. 8-9. Diagram correlating the funduscopic and histologic features of the eye in PXE. **A,** Angioid streaks; **B,** drusen of Bruch's membrane; **C,** mound of vascularized scar tissue at the macula; **X,** hyaline body of the optic disc; **Y,** fibrous tissue cuffing an angioid streak. In the lower part of the diagram the retina is shown in cross section and between two angioid streaks. Bruch's membrane and the choriocapillaris have been cut away, showing the pattern of underlying choroidal vessels. (Courtesy Dr. David Paton.)

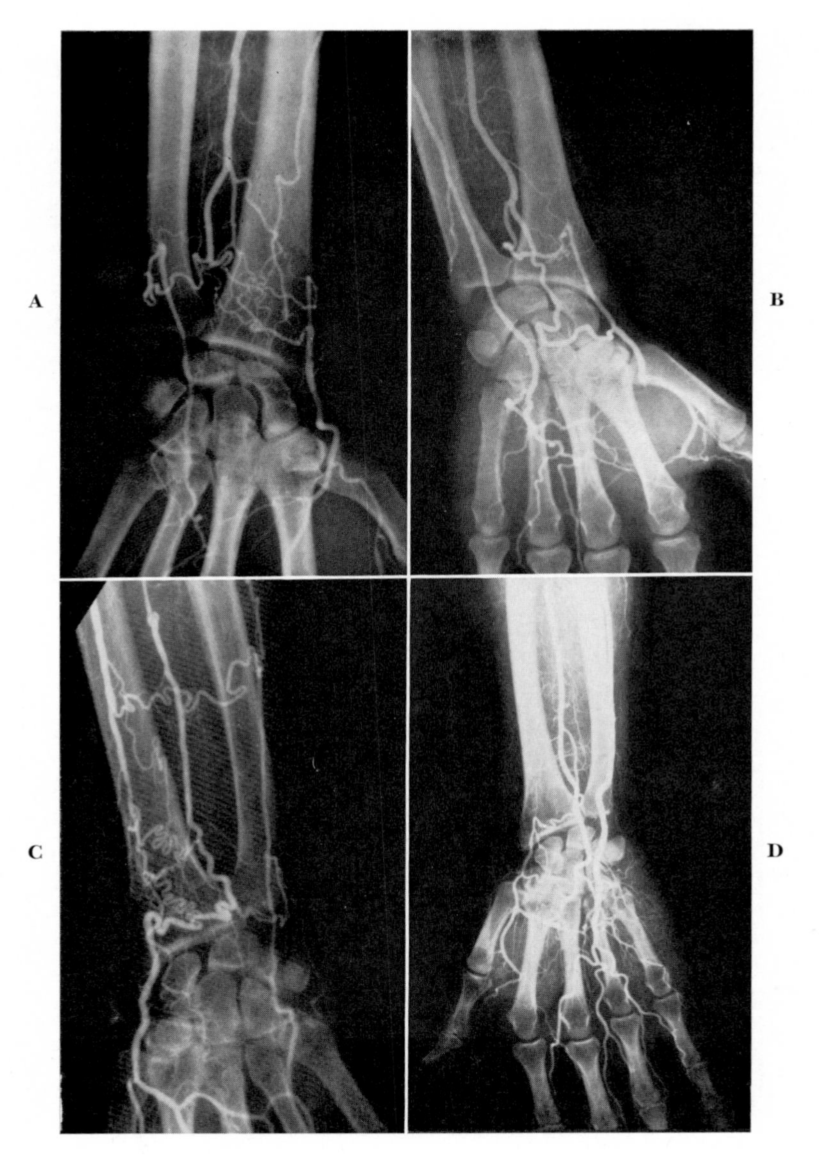

Fig. 8-10. Findings of brachial arteriography in PXE. **A,** Obstruction of both the radial and the ulnar artery, with refilling from a dilated interosseous artery, in J. C. (279288), 65-year-old Negro male. **B,** Obstruction of the radial artery, with refilling from the interosseous, in C. G. (456025), 33-year-old white male. **C,** Occlusion, narrowing, and irregularity of the main arteries in the forearm, with marked collateral formation, in R. T. (1022161), 54-year-old white female. **D,** Occlusion of the radial artery in D. W. (1023639), 50-year-old white female.

Anderson[2] described a family in which PXE of the skin was associated with choroidal sclerosis in four males. The choroidal sclerosis alone was present in a fifth male. Short angioid streaks seem evident in certain of the illustrations, however. Funduscopic findings in heterozygotes are discussed on p. 312.

The cardiovascular system. Clinically the arterial involvement is expressed by pulse changes and symptoms of arterial insufficiency in the extremities, by x-ray evidence of premature medial calcification of peripheral arteries, by symptoms of coronary insufficiency, by hemorrhage in one or more of many different areas, and by hypertension.

Weakness or absence of pulses in the extremities is a frequent finding. Fatigability or frank intermittent claudication may occur in the legs. The development of these manifestations by the third decade or earlier and the involvement of the arms as well as the legs aid in the differentiation of these changes from those of ordinary arteriosclerosis. Fig. 8-1*D* and *E* give examples of arterial calcification that began to develop at least as early as the latter part of the third decade of life. Calcification as early as the age of 9 years has been described[140]; in this child, intermittent claudication, loss of pulsations in the distal arteries of the limbs, calcification of the arteries, and repeated attacks of melena (see below) were present. A brother, 25 years of age, had similar symptoms.

The radial and/or ulnar pulses are sometimes absent in PXE. Substituting for these pulses may be an arterial pulsation in an anomalous position near the middle of the volar surface of the wrist. Ischemic symptoms almost never occur in the upper extremity. Bäfverstedt and Lund[5] found no abnormality of the brachial arteriogram in a 9-year-old child with PXE. Carlborg and co-workers[17] found narrowing of arteries in the forearm in one of four cases studied. Goodman and colleagues[43] found drastic changes in the brachial arteriograms of six pa-

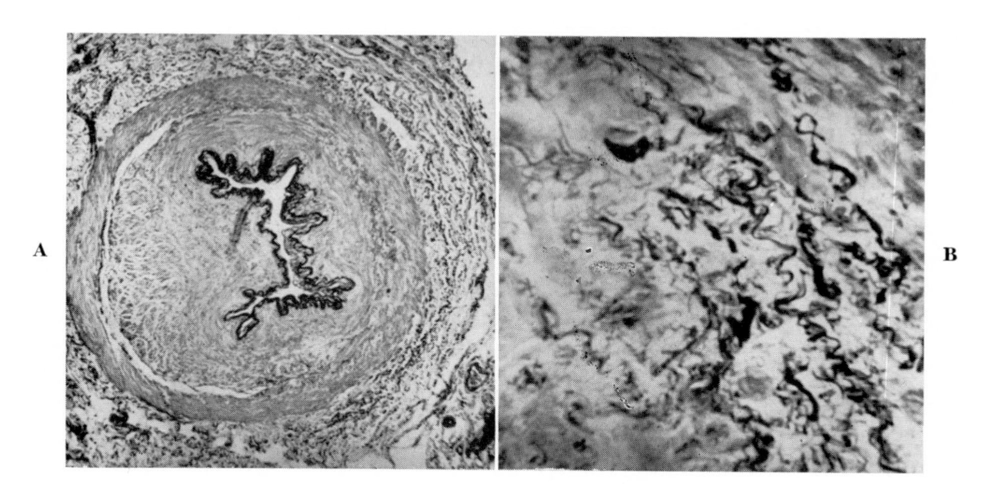

Fig. 8-11. Biopsy of radial artery in R. T. (1022161), 54-year-old white female with PXE. The lumen is almost completely occluded due to marked fibrous proliferation in the media. The intima is delicate and the internal elastic membrane appears normal. Elastic fibers in the region of the external elastic membrane are ruptured and irregular. The cleft shown laterally is an artifact of sectioning; it probably occurred in a weakened part of the wall. **A,** Verhoeff stain. (× 100.) **B,** Region of external elastic membrane, Verhoeff stain. (×600.)

tients, of whom the youngest was 33 years old at the time of study. In all, the radial and/or ulnar arteries were occluded or markedly narrowed. The interosseous arteries were little, if any, affected and had undergone dilatation. In cases of occluded radial and ulnar arteries, terminal collaterals from the interosseous arteries provided apparently adequate filling of the arterial system in the hand. These changes are illustrated in Figs. 8-10 and 8-11.

Reduced pulse wave velocity in the arteries of the extremities was found in most cases of PXE.[16,132] The pulse wave was, furthermore, of reduced amplitude and plateau configuration. The dicrotic notch may be lost. The peak is attained more slowly than normal.[5,108] The fact that the 9-year-old child studied by Bäfverstedt and Lund[5] showed these changes in the pulse curves, despite normal arteriograms, suggests that occlusive changes are not essential to the alterations in the pulse curves.

Angina pectoris, electrocardiographic changes compatible with myocardial ischemia, radiographic evidence of coronary artery calcification,[85] and myocardial infarction[85] are observed in patients with PXE and leave little doubt that the coronary arteries are involved in this disorder. In one patient (N. G., 1136343) with substernal pain and nonspecific electrocardiographic changes, an electrocardiographic-exercise test was negative, and coronary arteriograms showed no definite abnormality.

Hemorrhages constitute the major medical problem in most cases of PXE that come to the attention of the internist. Gastrointestinal hemorrhage is common[58] and may be fatal.[47,127] It may occur from a lesion such as peptic ulcer or hiatal hernia, which per se can produce hemorrhage, but in most cases of PXE the source of bleeding is not evident on clinical study. In cases of peptic ulcer, the arterial disease plays a strong contributory role to hemorrhages, similar to that of arteriosclerosis and primary amyloid disease. Superficial ulceration has been discovered by gastroscopy[75] or on gastrectomy.[58] Hemorrhage from the jejunum has been described.[103] In my own experience, gastrointestinal bleeding in PXE has occurred as early as 6½ years of age (Fig. 8-12). In cases of gastrointestinal hemorrhage, the physician should almost automatically look for the skin changes of this syndrome just as one should look for Kayser-Fleischer rings in patients with liver disease, and for cutaneous telangiectasia in these same patients with gastrointestinal hemorrhage. Some patients visit many different clinics, seeking the cause of bleeding. Some have repeated abdominal explorations and repair of some lesion, such as hiatal hernia, which may or may not be incidental. The reports of massive gastrointestinal hemorrhage during pregnancy in three women with PXE[77,141] suggest that pregnancy has an aggravating influence. Nellen and Jacobson[85] noted flushing of the skin lesions with each episode of hematemesis. (See p. 287 for a description of perinodular hyperemia in Chauffard's patient.)

In addition to gastrointestinal bleeding, the types of hemorrhage by location include subarachnoid, retinal, renal, uterine,[132] bladder, and nasal. Spontaneous hemarthroses occur.[132] Excessive bleeding from cuts of the skin does not seem to be a problem, although hemorrhages in the skin lesions have been described[36,81]; Foerster's patient[34] sought medical advice because of purpura on the legs and, later, on the left forearm. At the age of 16 years, one of the patients in my series (R. E. H., J.H.H. 193470) had a severe illness diagnosed as "black (hemorrhagic) measles." It is possible that the connective tissue disease was responsible for the hemorrhagic manifestations of the measles. Subarachnoid hemorrhage is commonly a cause of death.

Hypertension is frequent in PXE and in some cases has been convincingly shown to be the result of vascular disease, of the PXE type, in the renal vessels. The occurrence of hypertension is unfortunate because of its aggravating influence on the tendency to hemorrhage. In one patient,[26] 29 years old, intra-

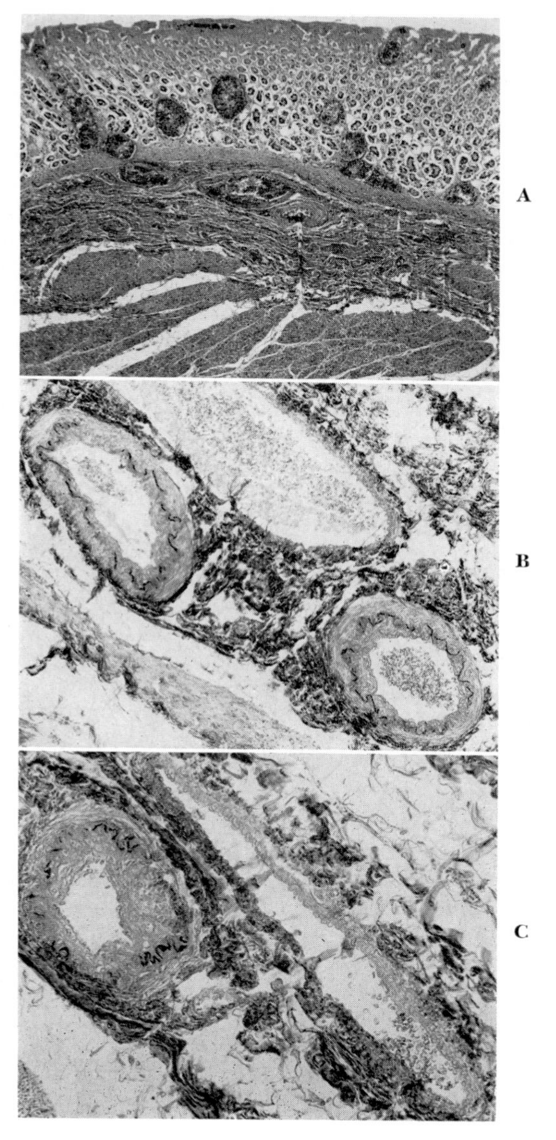

Fig. 8-12. Vessels of gastrointestinal tract in N. C. (p. 319). **A,** Dilated gastric mucosal vessels, some of which are probably ruptured. **B** and **C,** Submucosal vessels showing rupture of elastic membranes and surrounding reaction.

cranial "berry" aneurysm occurred in association with skin changes and angioid streaks. Scheie and Hogan[106] had a similar case. Another patient (E. W., J.H.H. 69818), seen in the past in Johns Hopkins Hospital and twice reported,[55,97] died of cerebral hemorrhage at the age of 43 years. Severe hypertension and pronounced albuminuria were persistently present in the last few years of life. Rosenheim[101] tells me of a case of PXE in a teen-ager, with severe hypertension and with calcification of both renal arteries. Parker and colleagues[89] reported two sisters with PXE in whom the presenting manifestation was hypertension, at age 10 in one and at 6 in the other.

Calcification in peripheral arteries (both arms and legs) has been determined radiologically by a number of observers, including Sanbacka-Holström,[104] Zentmayer,[145] Silvers,[109] Silvers and Wolfe,[110] Carlborg,[16] Scheie,[105] Wolff,[140] and Goodman and associates.[43] Both medial and intimal calcification can be demonstrated. (Fig. 8-13.) Calcification, probably also of vascular location, is sometimes

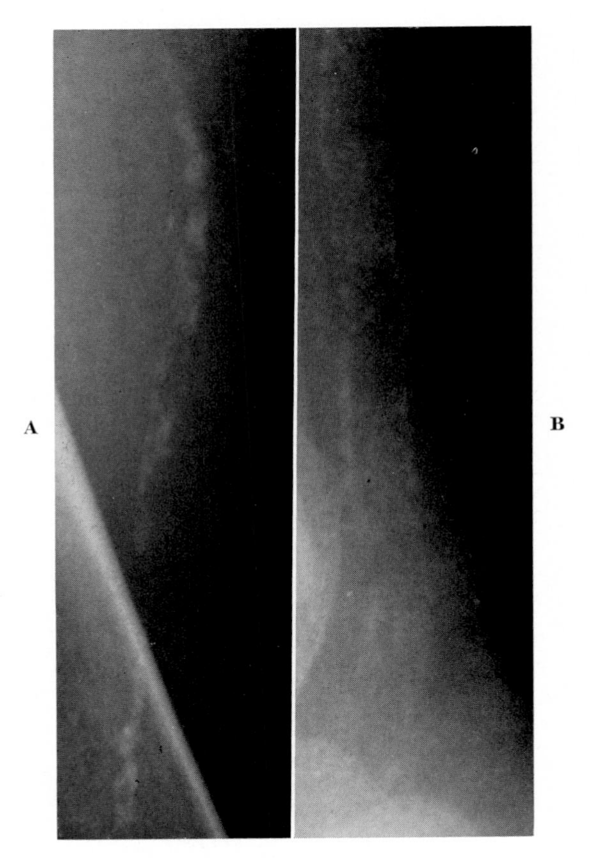

Fig. 8-13. Arterial calcification. **A,** The femoral artery of C. T. (1022514), 52-year-old man, shows intimal (dense patches) and medial (fine mottling) calcification. **B,** The radial artery of D. C. (863132), 58-year-old man, shows medial calcification. (From Goodman, R. M., Smith, E. W., Paton, D., Bergman, R. A., Siegel, C. L., Ottesen, O. E., Shelley, W. M., Pusch, A. L., and McKusick, V. A.: Medicine **42**:297, 1963.)

demonstrated in the choroid plexus[106,132] on skull x-ray film. It was demonstrated in the siphon of the internal carotid artery in a 30-year-old patient of this series and in reported cases.[106,145] In a 31-year-old European woman living in South Africa, Nellen and Jacobson[85] demonstrated calcification of the coronary arteries radiographically. Calcification of the falx cerebri and of the pineal was also present. (See Fig. 8-6 for another example of calcification of the falx cerebri.) A 34-year-old brother with skin lesions had coronary thrombosis. Scheie and Hogan[106] described a case of PXE with "bilateral calcified carotid artery aneurysms." Hypercholesterolemia is not a necessary factor in the premature vascular change, although its presence probably exaggerates pathologic alterations. We have one patient (J. C., 279228) with typical cutaneous and fundal changes of PXE and equally typical Leriche syndrome (thrombotic obliteration of the bifurcation of the aorta) for which successful homografting was performed. In another patient, a 48-year-old woman (Fig. 8-14), there is extensive calcification in the abdominal aorta. Both manifestations may bear no relation to the PXE.

Dilatation of the aorta has been remarked on in several of the cases. This was the case, for instance, in Joffe's 30-year-old patient[56] and in the 35-year-old normotensive patient of Marchionini and Turgut.[82] Whether this finding bears a direct relationship to the fundamental defect is unclear. Case 9 of Carlborg[16] demonstrated marked dilatation (phlebectasia) of the jugular veins.

Other features. Psychiatric disorders seem to occur with abnormally high frequency in these patients. Whether these can be explained on the basis of cerebral vascular changes is difficult to state. Certainly the high incidence of neurologic abnormalities is attributable to the vascular disease and hypertension. The nature of the neurologic abnormalities will not be discussed in detail because they are highly variable, yet per se are not unlike what one customarily encounters with advanced arteriosclerosis and/or hypertension. The unusual feature is the relatively early age at which the neurologic accidents and deterioration occur.

Pathology

In the skin, the characteristic changes occur in the deeper and middle zones of the corium (Fig. 8-1*F*). Large aggregations of material with the staining property of elastic fibers dominate the field. This material is granular for the most part, but in places rodlike structures are seen. Tuberculoid areas with giant cells[126,136] occur in the area of degeneration. (See Fig. 2-C in reference 14.) Calcification of the degenerated material occurs to a pronounced degree. This was established by Finnerud and Nomland,[32] using the von Kossa stain, and by Lobitz and Osterberg,[74] using microincineration. Actual bone formation is claimed.[8] Goodman and colleagues[43] have presented evidence that calcium deposition in elastic fibers is the earliest demonstrable histopathologic change in PXE. Elastic fibers surrounding sweat glands may, for example, show early changes. Later the elastic fibers become fragmented. (See Figs. 8-11 and 8-15.) Exposure of the tissue section to collagenase does not alter the appearance of the foci of calcified elastic fibers. Elastase, however, removes many of the elastic fiber ends that project from the edge of large concretions. Densely calcified fibers are usually not affected by elastase treatment.

Most histologic studies of the eye[13,37,47,64,133] have shown basophilia and tears

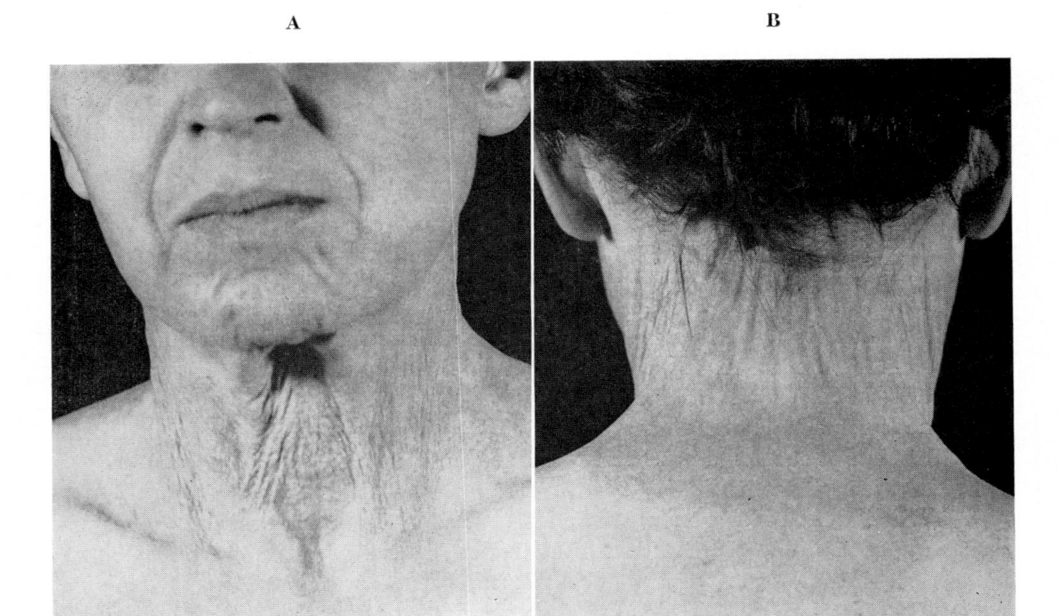

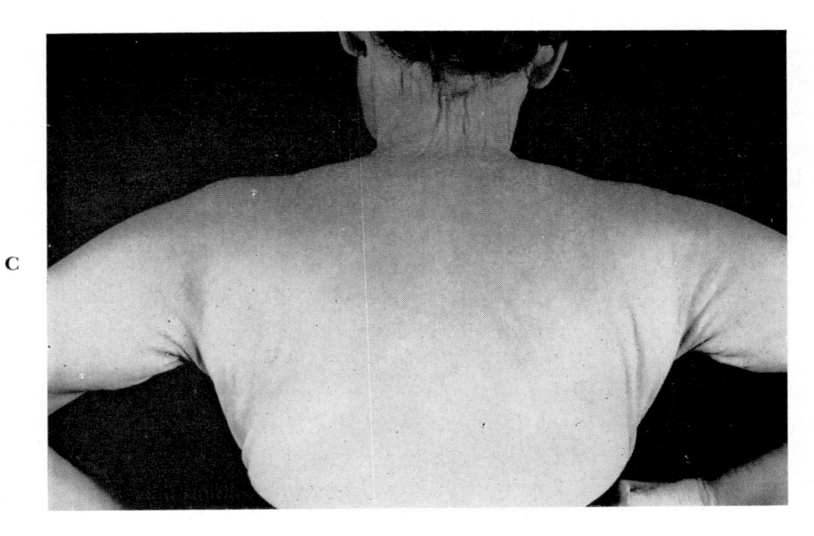

Fig. 8-14. D. G. (757275), 48 years of age at the time of study, has extensive cutaneous and mucosal changes and fundus changes. In her early twenties several massive hematemeses occurred, for which gastric resection was performed. It may be significant that the skin changes first appeared after measles at the age of 3 years. No pulses were palpable in the feet. X-ray films showed extensive calcification in the abdominal aorta. In this patient the diagnosis might be suspected from the chest x-ray film, which showed folds of redundant skin in both axillary areas. This patient had congenital short thumbs (short terminal phalanx), probably as an independent hereditary anomaly. Stecher[114] suggested that the abnormality is inherited as a recessive, although numerous other studies have proposed dominant inheritance. **A** and **B,** Changes in the skin of the neck. **C,** The neck and axillae. **D,** The anterior abdominal wall. **E** and **F,** The neck before and after plastic surgical repair.

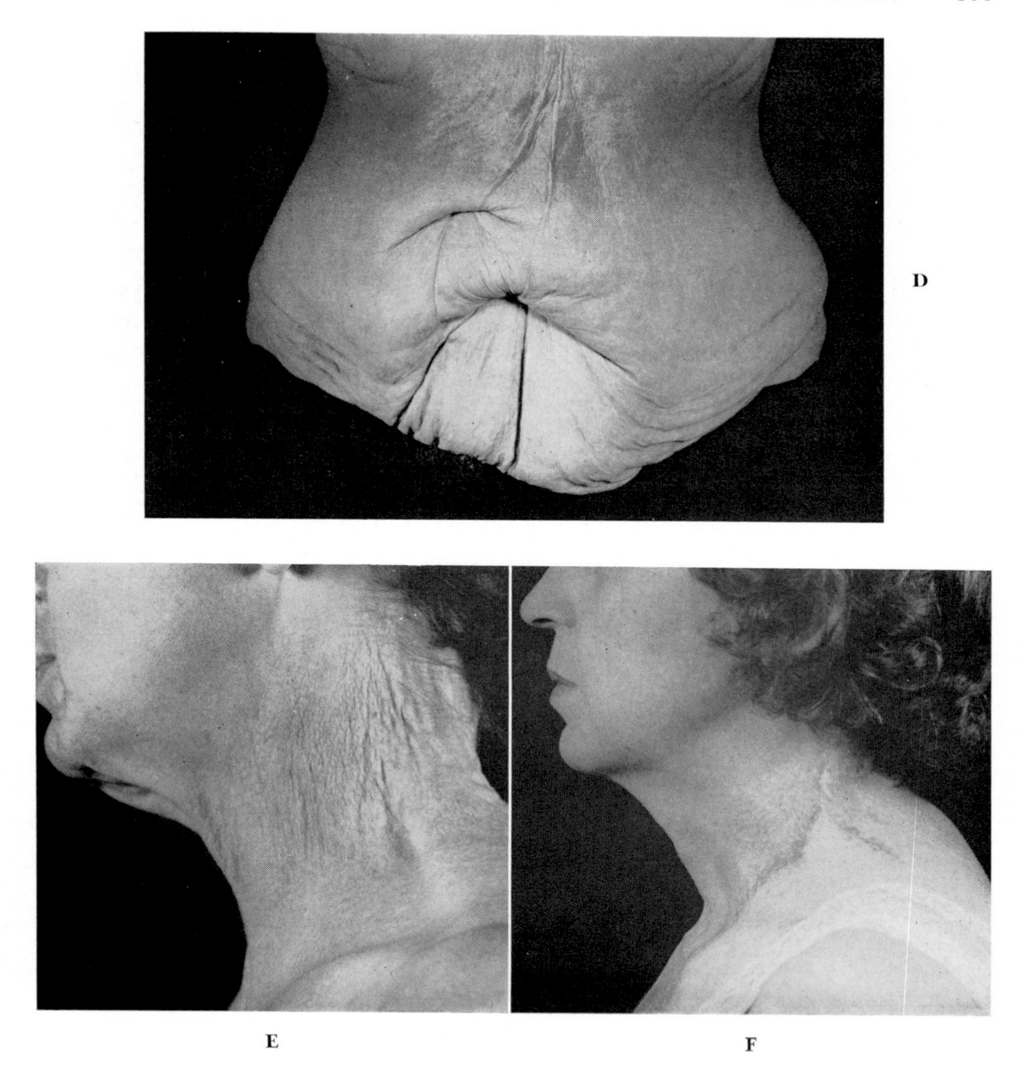

Fig. 8-14, cont'd. For legend see opposite page.

in the lamina elastica of Bruch's membrane; Benedict[9] and Law[69] failed to find these, however. Most observers, furthermore, have found advanced sclerotic changes in the choroidal vessels. When tears are present in Bruch's membrane, scar tissue tends to occupy the breaks or extend through beneath the pigment epithelium.[37] The breaks correspond to the streaks seen on funduscopic examination. Basophilia of the lamina elastica is encountered not infrequently in the eyes of older individuals; it occurs more regularly and at a younger age in PXE. Descemet's membrane of the cornea has chemical, physical, and tinctorial resemblances to the lamina elastica of Bruch's membrane. However, clinical or histologic evidence of involvement of the cornea has apparently not been observed in PXE.

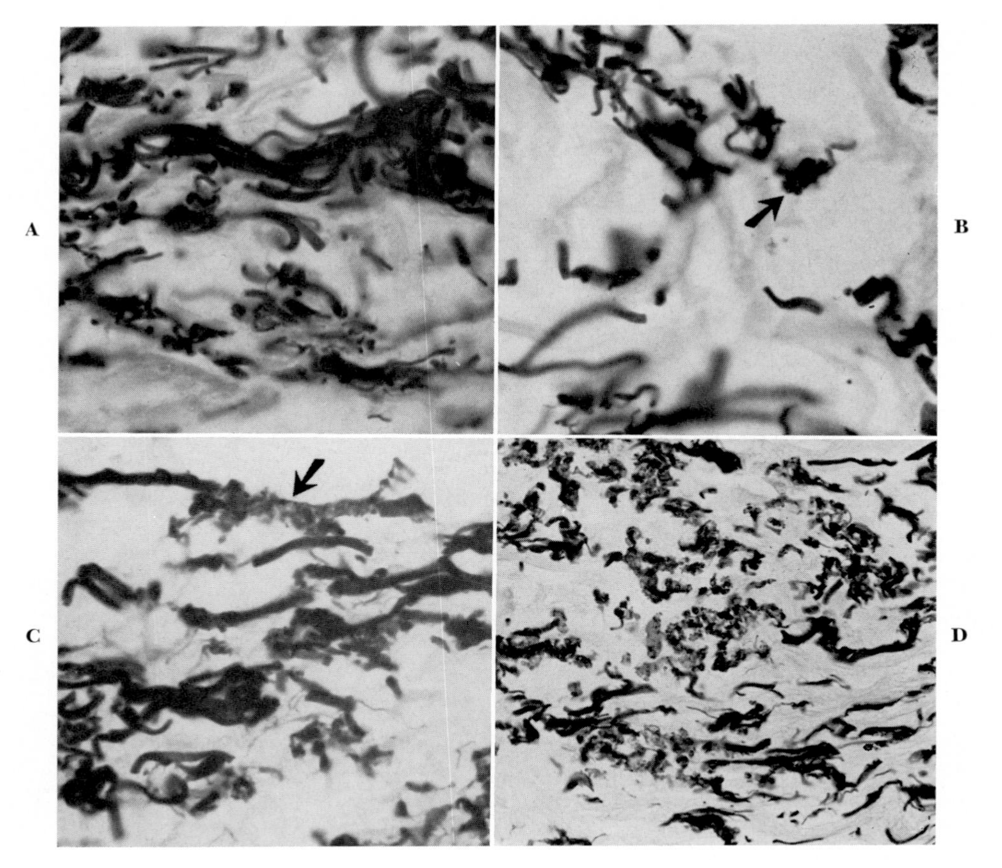

Fig. 8-15. Elastic fibers in skin. **A,** Normal. **B,** The arrow indicates a focus of altered elastic tissue in the skin of a patient with PXE. **C,** More extensive granular degenerative change in PXE. **D,** Advanced elastic tissue change in PXE.

Gross and histologic studies of the cardiovascular system are few. In the original case of Balzer[6] whitish thickening of the endocardium of the right atrium was described, as well as plaques of the same description on the pericardium and on the ventricular endocardium. Histologically, degeneration, thought to involve elastic elements, was demonstrated at these sites and in the walls of the pulmonary alveoli. (I have observed identical findings in two of three autopsied cases described in detail below, as did also Carlborg and colleagues.[17]) In Prick's case[59,95] the patient had hypertension and died at the age of 45 years of a cerebrovascular accident. Histologic changes interpreted as degeneration of elastic fibers were described in the coronary, renal, pancreatic, uterine, cutaneous, and mesenteric arteries, as well as the splenic trabeculae, hepatic veins, and Bruch's membrane of the eye. In the patient of Urbach and Wolfram,[131] a 49-year-old man who died with a Korsakoff-type psychosis and who had widening of the aorta, as seen by x-ray examination, identical histologic changes were found in the brachial, cutaneous, and cerebral arteries and in Bruch's membrane. They also described and illustrated histologic changes in the aorta, which are, in my opinion, probably merely those seen in the senile aorta, sometimes even at the age of 49 years. Coffman and Sommers[21] thought there were specific aortic changes in their patient. Furthermore, these authors attributed valvular disease to PXE; mitral stenosis in one individual was thought to have this basis.

Carlborg[16] recorded autopsy observations made by another physician without particular knowledge of, or attention to, this syndrome. Klein[64] also reported an autopsied case. Three other autopsied cases are described below.

In the original case, Balzer[6] described degenerative changes involving presumably the elastic fibers in the walls of the pulmonary alveoli. However, the patient was a 49-year-old stonemason, who died of extensive pulmonary tuberculosis. This may have been responsible for any changes observed in the lungs. Furthermore, in the autopsied cases of Prick[95] and Urbach,[131] no abnormality of pulmonary elastic tissue was found. One can only speculate about the possible basis of a miliary mottling of one lung field described in x-ray examination of one patient[140] and observed in both lung fields of one of my patients (C. T., J.H.H. 582989). It is possible that repeated small interstitial hemorrhages with resultant hemosiderosis are responsible. Calcification in small vessels is another possible explanation. In this same patient, there are no evidences of pulmonary hypertension, and studies of pulmonary function show no definite abnormality. In patients studied by Van Embden Andres,[132] no abnormality of residual air volume, maximum breathing capacity, and vital capacity was discovered.

In the thyroid arteries removed during thyroidectomy there were described[59] abnormalities of the type seen in small coronary arteries in the first autopsied case below. Scheie and Freeman[105] biopsied the ulnar artery in one case and described "elastic tissue degeneration" with compensatory muscular hypertrophy. Identical findings were reported by Goodman and colleagues,[43] as shown in Fig. 8-13. The intima was found to be delicate. The lumen was almost completely obliterated as a result of the medial process. Without illustration, Kaplan and Hartman[58] described degeneration of elastic elements, especially internal elastic lamella, in the vessels of the stomach removed in a 23-year-old white woman because of gastrointestinal bleeding. Beadlike microaneurysms were also present. Woo and Chandler[141] report similar findings. In one case of Revell and Carey[97] there were changes demonstrated in the peritonsillar tissues.

Many of the patients have advanced and premature arterial changes indistinguishable from ordinary atherosclerosis and arteriosclerosis. By changes in the media PXE probably sets the stage for the development of intimal changes, unusually early in life and in unusually severe degree.

The basic defect

Whether PXE is a dystrophy of elastic fibers or of collagen fibers has been much debated. Certainly the degenerate material that develops in the skin has certain tinctorial characteristics of elastic fibers.

The evidence that PXE is an abiotrophy of collagenous rather than elastic fibers is as follows[50,132]: (1) Normally the skin contains relatively few elastic fibers. Elastin makes up only about 2% of the dry weight of skin.[31] Collagen, on the other hand, constitutes about 72%. The few elastic fibers present are concentrated immediately beneath the epidermis and serve, according to one view,[31] a principal function of attaching the epidermis to the corium. (A defect in these fibers[124] may be responsible for the lesions of epidermolysis bullosa. This point is moot, however.) The lesions of PXE are located in the deeper layers of the corium and are more extensive than can be accounted for on the basis of the normal amount of elastic fibers in the skin. The skin of the soles and palms is more liberally supplied with elastic fibers, but PXE lesions do not occur there ordinarily. (2) The arteries predominantly involved are the so-called muscular arteries, the media of which contains collagenous fibers but little elastic tissue. (3) The tunica elastica interna of these vessels (except in one report[58]) remains intact. (4) Except for their orceinophilia, most of the abnormal fibers resemble collagen fibers more than elastic fibers, because of their width. (5) Electron microscopic studies[130] reveal that the dystrophic fibers, although abnormal in other respects, have the characteristic 640 Å. periodicity of collagen. It appears, then, that in PXE the collagen may undergo dystrophic chemical or physico-chemical changes, with resulting acquisition of the tinctorial characteristics of elastic fibers. (6) There has been no acceptable clinical or pathologic evidence of abnormality arising from a defect of elastic tissue in the lungs or aorta.

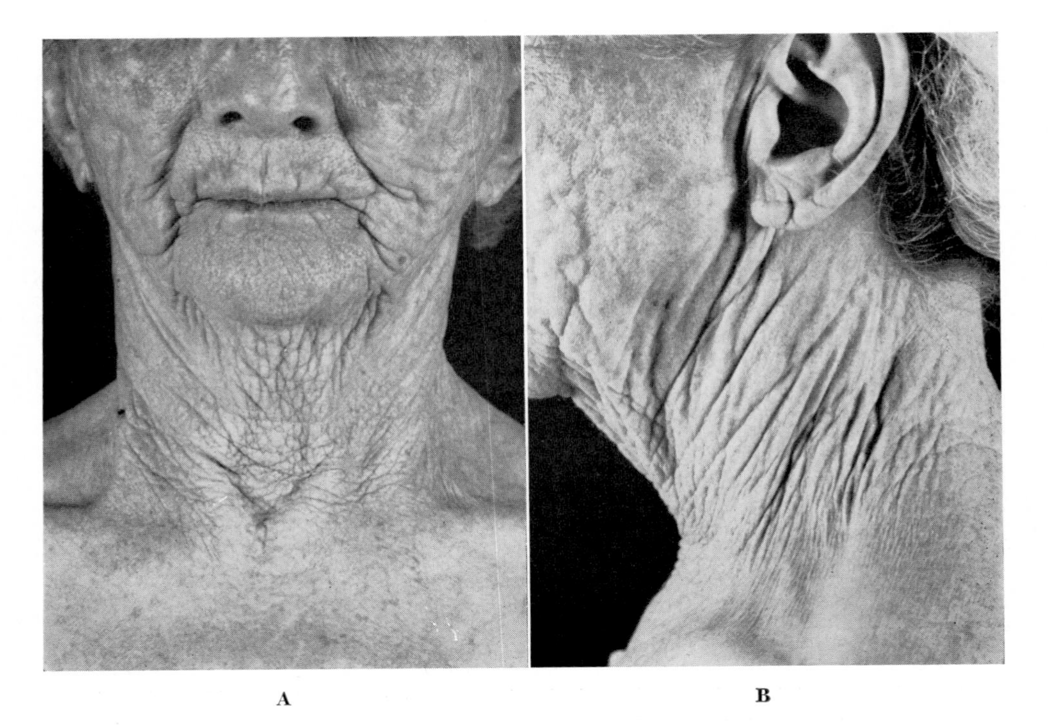

A B

Fig. 8-16. Senile elastosis. A. H. (775457), 73-year-old female, was admitted because of bleeding from the lower bowel. The changes in the skin, **A** and **B,** resemble those of PXE but differ in the relative absence of changes in the axillae, **D.** The changes on the hands, **C,** are more striking than those usually seen in PXE. There were no angioid streaks in the fundi, and the peripheral arteries showed very little calcification. The histologic appearance, **E** and **F,** probably is distinct from that in PXE. Note that there is very little granular material. In **E** is presented the results of hematoxylin and eosin stain of the skin biopsy. Note the broad ribbons of connective tissue fibers, suggesting fragmented collagen. In **F** is presented the orcein stain of the same tissue. Both are at $\times 100$ magnification. The cause of the lower bowel bleeding has not been identified.

Gillman and co-workers[40] make important observations on what appears to be a rather widely occurring phenomenon. This they term "elastotic degeneration of collagen fibers." Irradiation, trauma, and aging (Fig. 8-16) appear to be responsible. In addition to degeneration of existing collagen fibers, the authors admit the possibility that there may be a disturbance of formation of new collagen fibers, resulting in simulation of elastic fibers. By means of a battery of many staining procedures they showed that there are distinct differences between "normal" elastic fibers of skin and arteries and "elastotically degenerated" colla-

C D

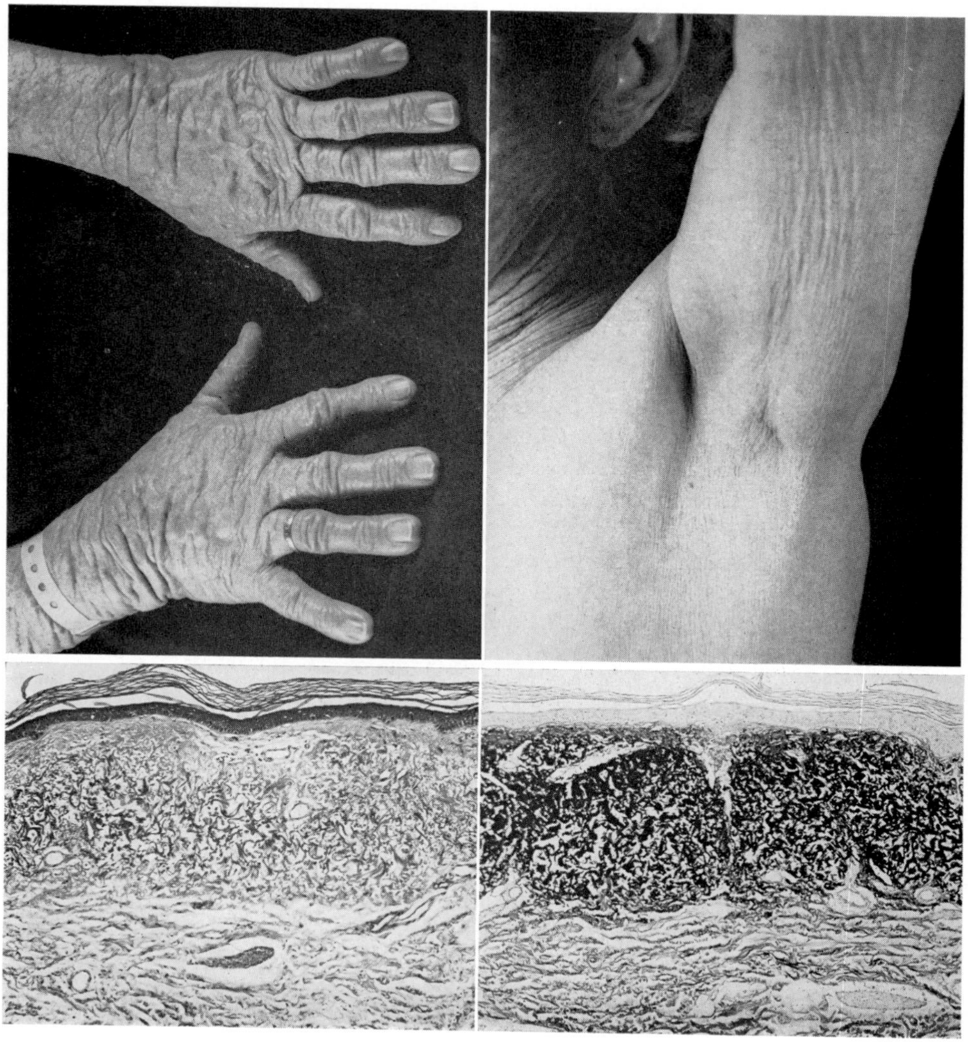

E F

Fig. 8-16, cont'd. For legend see opposite page.

gen fibers at the same site. Although no studies of PXE were made, the important observations of the South African group are probably pertinent in connection with this hereditary syndrome: "elastotic degeneration" of collagen can occur on either an acquired or a hereditary basis. In both, fragmentation and calcification occur. Gillman and colleagues[40] maintain that Mallory's phosphotungstic acid–hematoxylin stain differentiates the presumed degenerated collagen of PXE from normal elastic fibers.

Tunbridge and co-workers[130] noted that enzymatic digestion of skin increases "elastic staining" and results in an increase in amorphous material. Keech and Reed,[60] working in the same group, using electron microscopy, conclude that by a variety of means, physical, chemical, and enzymatic, one can produce so-called "moth-eaten" fibers (MEF) from either collagenous or elastic fibers, that MEF represent an intermediate form, and finally that "collagen and elastin are not two separate and distinct entities but are probably intimately associated *in vivo*." (See also references 15 and 61.)

The view that collagen is the source of the degenerated material has been challenged and the earlier "elastic theory" defended by Rodnan and associates[100] and by Moran and Lansing,[83] who in histochemical studies, studies by elastase digestion and microincineration, and examinations by fluorescence and electron microscopy concluded that there is a striking resemblance to elastic tissue in the following respects: brilliant autofluorescence, lack of periodicity in ultrastructure, liability to elastase, inhibition of affinity for elastic tissue dyes following methylation, and strong proclivity to calcium incrustation.

Calcification of the elastic fibers has been viewed as a secondary phenomenon comparable to the calcification of degenerated tissues as in chronic inflammation, atherosclerosis, hematomas, etc. Goodman and colleagues,[43] after finding that calcium accretion on elastic fibers is the earliest demonstrable histologic change, proposed that deposition of calcium may lead to brittleness and subsequent fracture of elastic fibers. A similar sequence of events has been proposed in the case of Bruch's membrane and the development of angioid streaks. If this view of the pathogenesis is accurate, the question of the nature of the basic defect resolves itself into the question of what causes the increased affinity of the elastic fibers for calcium.

Findlay[31] reported that the enzyme elastase removes the degenerate material from sections of skin from PXE patients. An earlier objection was that elastase is not entirely specific; for example, it is said[48] to dissolve mucoproteins, behaving, therefore, fundamentally as a mucase. Furthermore, other studies[7] with elastase indicate some effects on normal collagen. More recently, elastase has been purified, and it has been demonstrated[73,102] that elastase digestion is relatively specific for elastic tissue.

The argument that elastic fiber normally present is insufficient to account for the relatively large amount of degenerate material is disputed by Moran and Lansing,[83] who feel that there are sufficient elastic fibers in the deeper layers of the corium and further suggest that proliferation of elastic fibers may occur in this disease. They point to the occurrence of macrophages and giant cells[87,126] as a characteristic more of degenerate elastic fiber than of collagen. A similar reaction in the lung, presumbably to degenerated elastic tissue, described by Walford and Kaplan,[134] was referred to by Moran and Lansing, who state also that there is "a definite increase in collagenous tissue in the involved areas." They suggest that it would be easy, under these circumstances, to conclude that all fibers had the electron microscopic characteristics of collagen, simply through inaccurate selection of the fields of study.

Potentially very important observations have been made by Weidman and associates,[135] Pautrier,[92] and Lever[71]: young asymptomatic individuals may show in the skin abundant, irregularly branching, thick, nonfragmented fibers with the tinctorial characteristics of elastic fibers. The implication has been that these are individuals who would subsequently develop typical PXE and/or are members of kinships containing other definite cases. However, to my knowledge, this implication has not been established except possibly in one patient of Van Embden Andres,[132] who had central chorioretinitis of the type seen in PXE and, by skin biopsy, "hyperplasia of elastic fibers without elastorrhexis." If it is further confirmed that these individuals with what Weidman calls "juvenile elastoma" do indeed represent instances of predegeneration PXE, it would mean that a quite unique type of connective tissue fiber is produced in these persons and undergoes degeneration with physiologic stresses. It would mean, furthermore, that the efforts to relate the basic defect to collagen or to elastica are pointless. I find it difficult to believe that these cases of Weidman and others are related to PXE, mainly because there should be identifiable, in one and the same individual, areas of as yet nondegenerate "elastoma" and other areas of typical PXE.

The pathogenesis of the angioid streaks has been considered to be unsettled.[23] The theory propounded by Kofler[66] in 1917 is that breaks in Bruch's membrane explain this finding. After reviewing the matter, Cowper[23] concluded that the original view (that the primary difficulty is a degeneration and sclerosis of the choroidal arteries with secondary changes in the retina and in Bruch's membrane) seems more consistent with the known facts. When the other conditions in which angioid streaks occur (p. 313) are considered, as well as the histologic findings of breaks in Bruch's membrane, Kofler's theory seems almost certainly the correct one. Adelung[1] demonstrated that the lines of force within the eye, resulting from pull of the intrinsic and extrinsic ocular muscles on the relatively fixed site of the optic nerve, have the same configuration as the peripapillary interlacement and radial extensions of angioid streaks. Such forces acting upon a weakened Bruch's membrane undoubtedly account for the distribution of angioid streaks.

As mentioned on p. 17, recessive inheritance suggests an enzyme defect. Possibly some as yet unidentified metabolic defect in some way damages the elastic fibers so that degeneration occurs, or some enzyme important to the integrity of the elastic fiber protein or a substance closely associated with it may be deficient.

Whatever the nature of the basic defect, the clinical behavior of PXE is that of an abiotrophy. The predominant involvement of areas of the skin exposed to maximum wear and tear, such as flexion folds, belt line,[10] pressure points, etc., is striking. Szymanski and Caro[120] describe a lesion at a site of trauma. No clinical or pathologic changes in the joints have been encountered. (Gold[42] described Still's disease in a child with PXE, but the association may have been a coincidence.)

Prevalence and inheritance

PXE probably occurs quite generally without particular racial distribution. The two autopsied patients at Johns Hopkins Hospital (see below) were both

Negroes and several other Negro patients with PXE have been seen here (e.g. J. C., 279288). In addition to being described in natives of many European countries, including Turkey,[82] it has been observed in Japanese.[86]

Some indication of the frequency of PXE is provided by the fact that 125 cases of associated skin and fundus changes and sixty-eight cases of skin changes alone had been described prior to 1940.[123] Several hundred cases have by now been reported. Berlyne and colleagues[11] estimated the frequency to be between 1 in 160,000 and 1 in one million persons. It is my impression that it occurs more frequently than 1 in 160,000.

Tabulations of cases of PXE in the literature show a preponderance of females.[20,28,128] Since women are more prone to seek medical advice, especially regarding a cosmetic problem created by the skin involvement, the female preponderance may be factitious. A review of 106 cases from the Mayo Clinic showed a 1 to 1.2 ratio of males to females.[22] Within this group there were thirty-two cases with only angioid streaks; the ratio in this group was 2.2 to 1, males to females.

Increased frequency of parental consanguinity,[51,125,132] the occurrence of multiple affected sibs, both males and females, and the rarity of the disorder in successive generations[21,54,82,115] suggest autosomal recessive inheritance. The occasional observation of affected parent and child may be explained by marriage of the affected homozygous parent with a heterozygote or by occasional manifestation in a heterozygous person.

Berlyne and colleagues[11] thought that in given sibships affected persons are usually either all males or all females. On this basis they proposed that the mode of inheritance is that of partial sex linkage, as would be observed if the responsible gene were located on a homologous segment of the X and Y chromosomes. Cytologic and genetic evidence would suggest, however, that this mechanism of inheritance does not exist in man.[79] Furthermore, in our personal experience, several sibships have had affected members of both sexes.

The occasional instance of affected parent and child (e.g. reference 88) may have resulted because the unaffected parent was heterozygous.

Berlyne and colleagues[11] reported that persons presumed to be heterozygous for the PXE gene had an abnormally prominent choroidal vascular pattern and suggested that this resulted from atrophy of the choriocapillaris. In family members studied by Goodman and colleagues[43] and in those patients with early ocular involvement the choroidal vessels were not unusually prominent, although they were in some patients with advanced changes (Fig. 8-7). Since the choriocapillaris lies below Bruch's membrane, any increased density in the latter structure in early stages of PXE os as a possible heterozygous manifestation should render the choroidal vascular layer *less* visible. The increased visibility of these vessels in later stages of PXE is readily accounted for by damage to, and atrophy of, the pigment epithelium of the retina.

Miscellaneous considerations

There is no definitive treatment for this disorder. Tocopherol (vitamin E) was said[117] to effect dramatic improvement in the skin and eyes of one patient. Others[4] also claim improvement. No beneficial effect was observed in one patient studied. Adrenocortical steroids have been used in several patients. In one patient

(N. G., 1136343) the treatment was continued for over a year. Although the results are difficult to evaluate, no clear benefit has been noted. Although the reactive process in the skin, eye, and arteries might be reduced by such treatment, the chronic, indeed lifelong, nature of the disease process makes steroid therapy impractical. Good cosmetic effects have been reported by plastic surgeons,[19,94] who have removed the loose, excess skin around the neck, which may be distressingly unsightly, especially in women. Fig. 8-14 demonstrates a patient in whom plastic surgery was performed.

It seems conceivable that a funduscopic picture indistinguishable from that of the angioid streaks seen with PXE may occur on other bases than this particular genetic one. For example, angioid streaks are encountered in association with Paget's disease.[84] However, PXE is the most common basis for the finding. Scholz[107] stated that, previous to 1941, 59% of 139 cases of streaks had the skin condition. On the other hand, in a series collected from the literature, Goedbloed[41] found fifty-seven cases with skin involvement among sixty-seven with streaks, and Sanbacka-Holström[104] found eighty-seven out of one hundred cases. Not only may angioid streaks occur with either PXE or Paget's disease, but also there are a few adequately documented instances of the occurrence of changes in the skin, fundus oculi, and bones of the same individual. Woodcock[142] described a 54-year-old white man with bilateral angioid streaks, skin changes of PXE in the axillae, and Paget's disease as manifested by cephalic enlargement, bowing of the legs, spontaneous fractures, renal calculi, and characteristic radiologic changes. Sanbacka-Holström[104] refers in passing to such a patient, and there are loose references to the coincidence of the three manifestations in textbooks and reviews. Shaffer and colleagues[108] have described a 58-year-old woman with angioid streaks and evidences of Paget's disease from the age of 40 years. The only skin lesion was an "elliptical lemon-yellow plaque 1.0 cm. long on the left posterior axillary fold." The histology was typical of PXE. One sister had mild Paget's disease. Larmande and Margaillan[68] had a case of combined disease. Dr. David Paton[91] tells me of two patients he has studied, in whom there is association of PXE skin changes, angioid streaks, calcification in peripheral vessels, and Paget's disease of bone.

There may be reason (Chapter 10) to think that there is no fundamental relationship between PXE and at least one common variety of Paget's disease. One reason is that Paget's disease usually behaves like an autosomal dominant. Furthermore, it is more frequent in men. In Paget's disease, as in PXE, calcification occurs in the media of arteries. Calcium deposition in Bruch's membrane is probably responsible for the development of angioid streaks in this condition.

Angioid streaks have been observed in one patient with familial hyperphosphatemia and metastatic calcification,[80] in a patient with idiopathic thrombocytopenic purpura,[144] and in several instances of lead poisoning.[25] Depositions in Bruch's membrane may account for the development of cracks in these disorders also.

At least ten cases of sickle cell disease with angioid streaks have been described.[38,43,90] Skin changes of PXE were present in at least three cases.[38,43,119] In those cases with only angioid streaks with sickle cell anemia it is likely that deposition of iron renders Bruch's membrane brittle.

Clinically, the skin changes in "senile elastosis" (Fig. 8-16) are somewhat similar to those of PXE. *Actinic elastosis* is the term recommended by the American Dermatological Association, inasmuch as age and senility probably are not primary factors. Clinical differences from PXE include involvement of the hands in actinic elastosis and sparing of the axillae and other unexposed areas commonly affected in PXE. The histologic appearance in actinic elastosis is different, being characterized by diffuse involvement in the superficial parts of the corium, less intense basophilia of the connective tissue fibers, and usually absence of fragmentation of the involved fibers into granular material. Percival and associates[93] concluded that this condition is a dystrophy of collagen. However, Smith and associates[112] concluded that the electron microscopic features, enzyme susceptibilities, and amino acid composition indicate an increase in elastic fibers. There is, however, a decrease in collagen, mainly in the insoluble fraction.

Case reports, with autopsy observations

Case 1. R. K. (J.H.H. 156572), a Negro man born in 1891, died in 1954 from accidental mercury poisoning.

The family history was largely unknown. He had no children.

About 1932 the patient was found to have a positive serologic test for syphilis, and treatment with arsenicals, mercury, and bismuth was given at another hospital where he had gone because of failing vision. He was first seen at this hospital in 1938 because of continuing dimming of vision. He had worn spectacles for about six years with no apparent staying of the visual failure in spite of several changes. Bilaterally the entire macular area was the site of atrophy and scarring. The vessels were normal. Running out from each disc in all directions were wide, branching, brownish streaks. About the neck he was noted to have many linear 4 or 5 mm. yellowish papules about 1 mm. thick. These were arranged parallel to the clavicle and coalesced in many areas to form short streaks several centimeters in length. The diagnosis of PXE with angioid streaks was made and confirmed by skin biopsy (Skin Path. No. 9606). On general examination the patient was noted to have an arcus senilis bilaterally. The blood pressure was 170/90 mm. Hg. No pulse change or circulatory abnormality in the legs or elsewhere was detected by history or examination.

The patient was visited in his home several times late in 1953 but refused to come to the hospital for investigation of the connective tissue disorder. He was now almost completely blind. For many years he had been suffering from intermittent swelling and pain of the proximal interphalangeal joints. He had also had much pain in the tibial and calf areas, as well as the knees. He had developed ulcerations of the pretibial area and made a practice of soaking these with bichloride of mercury solution. He took Dolcin, a proprietary analgesic, for his aches and pains. Several years previously he had been told that he had diabetes mellitus.

About 6 A.M. on Jan. 11, 1954, the patient intended to take Dolcin tablets for relief of pains in both shins and, because of his faulty vision, took three tablets of bichloride of mercury instead. He first noted burning of his mouth and thereafter pain in the mid-epigastrium, accompanied by the vomiting first of a large amount of clear yellow fluid and later of bright red blood of unknown quantity. Severe persistent bloody diarrhea followed. He was seen by his family physician, who could record no blood pressure and sent him to the hospital, where he arrived about eight hours after the accidental ingestion of mercury.

The patient had been noted to be easily confused in recent years, and therefore the exact details of the history of the final days of life are not entirely certain.

Physical examination revealed the skin of the neck, axillae, inguinal areas, and anterior abdominal wall to be nodular and leathery. It was strikingly inelastic, but this may have been in part the result of dehydration. All interphalangeal joints showed fusiform enlargement, and nodules were located around the knuckles. The heart showed a loud blowing apical systolic murmur and rather numerous extrasystoles. Femoral pulses were present, but none could be felt in the popliteal fossae or feet. There were two large depigmented scars with some unhealed and scabbed areas on both pretibial prominences.

The patient was virtually anuric throughout his hospital stay and died on the sixth hospital day. The diagnosis of mercury poisoning was corroborated by the finding of 6 mg. Hg^{++} per

20 ml. of stomach fluid taken at admission. Death occurred despite the use of BAL and supportive measures.

Autopsy (No. 24837) was performed ten hours after death by Dr. H. M. Hill. (In spite of the delay, fibroblasts grew out in tissue culture from explants of skin and of aortic adventitia.) The body weighed 50 kilograms and measured 168 cm. in length. The changes in the skin and joints and the juxta-articular nodules were observed as during the clinical examination.

The heart weighed 325 grams and did not appear to be enlarged. A most impressive finding was thickening of the endocardium of the right atrium. This was somewhat yellowish, and over the trabecular ridges there were peculiar nodular thickenings. The posterior leaflet of the tricuspid valve had a smooth, thickened, firm, rolled edge without excrescenses. The aortic leaflet of the mitral valve was similarly thickened at the edge, and there was marked calcific change at its attachment. The coronary ostia were normal, but everywhere the coronary arteries were exceedingly sclerotic and calcified, with reduction of their caliber to little more than a pin point.

The aorta was of normal caliber, with only minimal atherosclerosis in the abdominal portion and normal elasticity by gross test. There were marked calcification and narrowing of the femoral, popliteal, and posterior tibial arteries. These changes were particularly striking at areas of bending, such as in the popliteal fossae. The posterior tibial arteries were exceedingly beaded. The vessels at the base of the brain were sclerotic. Grossly and histologically there were characteristic changes of mercury poisoning in the kidney and gastrointestinal tract.

Histologically, the corium, the sclera, and the subendocardial area of the right atrium showed the same changes which have been frequently described previously in the skin of patients with PXE. Faintly basophilic (by hematoxylin and eosin stain), fragmented material was concentrated most heavily in the mid-dermis. Present in great abundance in the clinically involved areas and present sparsely elsewhere, it had the tinctorial characteristics of elastic tissue. The popliteal and coronary arteries showed marked medial and intimal sclerosis and calcification. As demonstrated in Fig. 8-17*C*, branches of the coronary sinus near the right atrium showed changes in the media comparable to those in the atrial endocardium and corium. Small arteries showed similar changes.

Comment. Of particular interest are the histologic changes in the endocardium of the right atrium and in the sclera. Neither site normally demonstrates more than a very sparse distribution of elastic fibers. The deforming arthropathy is likewise of special note. The manifestation has not been commented on previously in cases of PXE, except for the patient with Still's disease reported by Gold.[42] Unfortunately, no histologic studies of either joint structures or juxta-articular nodules were performed.

Case 2. C. J. (J.H.H. 292168), a Negro woman born in 1896, was seen here on several occasions in 1943 and died at the hospital on Jan. 1, 1944.

Her mother died of a stroke at the age of 48 years. The patient had four brothers: two died in childhood and one shortly after discharge from the Army in World War I; the other was living and well. The patient had sixteen children, of whom seven were living in 1943. No other instance of PXE is known to have occurred in the family. However, the family has not been traced and studied with this point specifically in mind.

The patient's eyesight had always been poor but had become worse in the last year of life. She noted tarry stools on several occasions and complained at times of epigastric burning. Early in 1943 she developed anginal symptoms for the first time.

Examinations revealed a blood pressure of 190/110 mm. Hg. There was evidence of marked weight loss (about 50 pounds in one year). The skin everywhere was very loose, due in part to PXE. The neck veins were full and dilated but not the arm veins. The heart was enlarged to the left anterior axillary line. The patient was so debilitated that carcinoma was suspected. Directly above the umbilicus there was a plaque of smooth skin containing small, hard, elevated nodular areas. Histologically (Skin Path. No. 5157) there were changes typical of PXE. The fundi showed no angioid streaking, but there were fairly marked hypertensive and sclerotic changes in the arteries, many hemorrhages, and in the macula area many yellow shiny plaques.

Total serum protein was 8.3 gm.%, of which 5.5 gm.% was globulin. Hemoglobin was 10.5 gm.%. Electrocardiogram revealed left axis deviation, left ventricular strain pattern, and prolonged A-V conduction. On chest x-ray examination, calcification in superficial vessels in the left axilla was demonstrated. The aorta was dilated and tortuous. On barium swallow the esophagus was relaxed and tortuous. Gastric analysis revealed normal acidity.

After four months away from the hospital, during which time she had become steadily

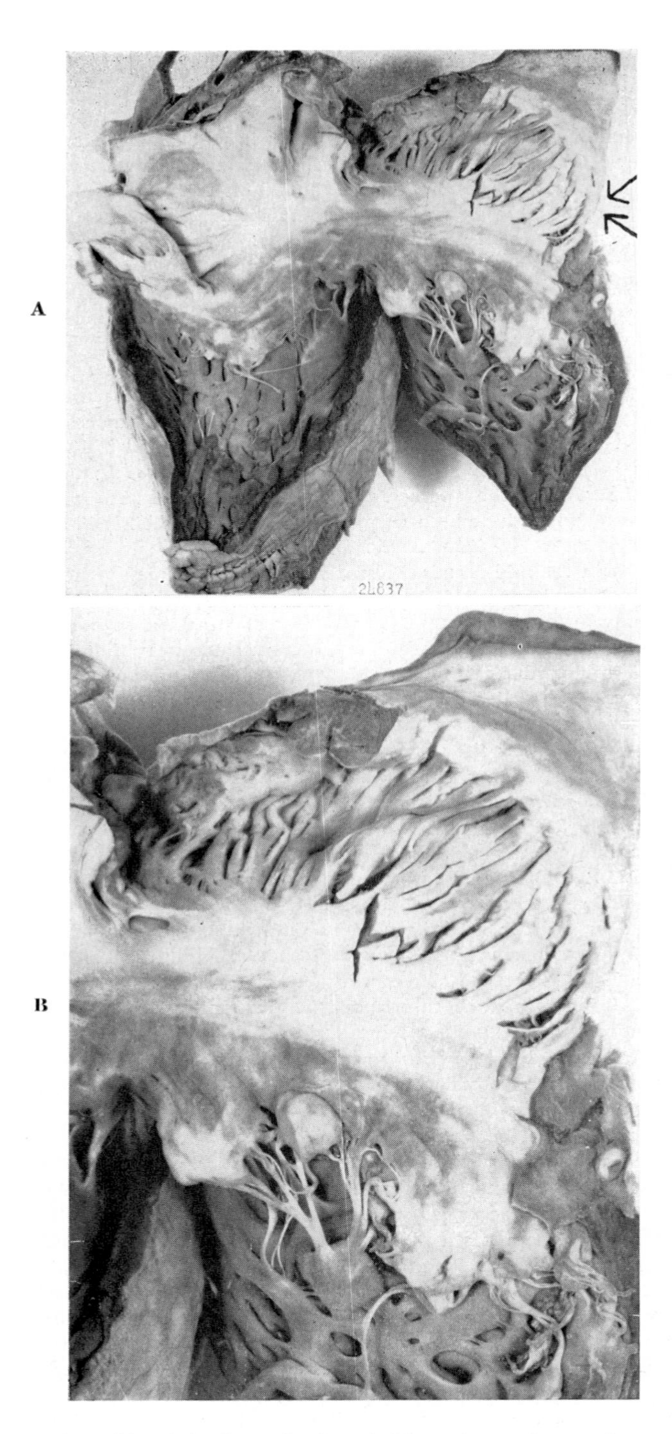

Fig. 8-17. A, The right side of the heart in Case 1. There is an abnormal, pearly thickening of the endocardium, with yellowish, irregularly nodular lesions in the area indicated by the arrows. The latter lesions look not unlike those in the skin. **B,** Enlarged view of part of heart shown in **A.**

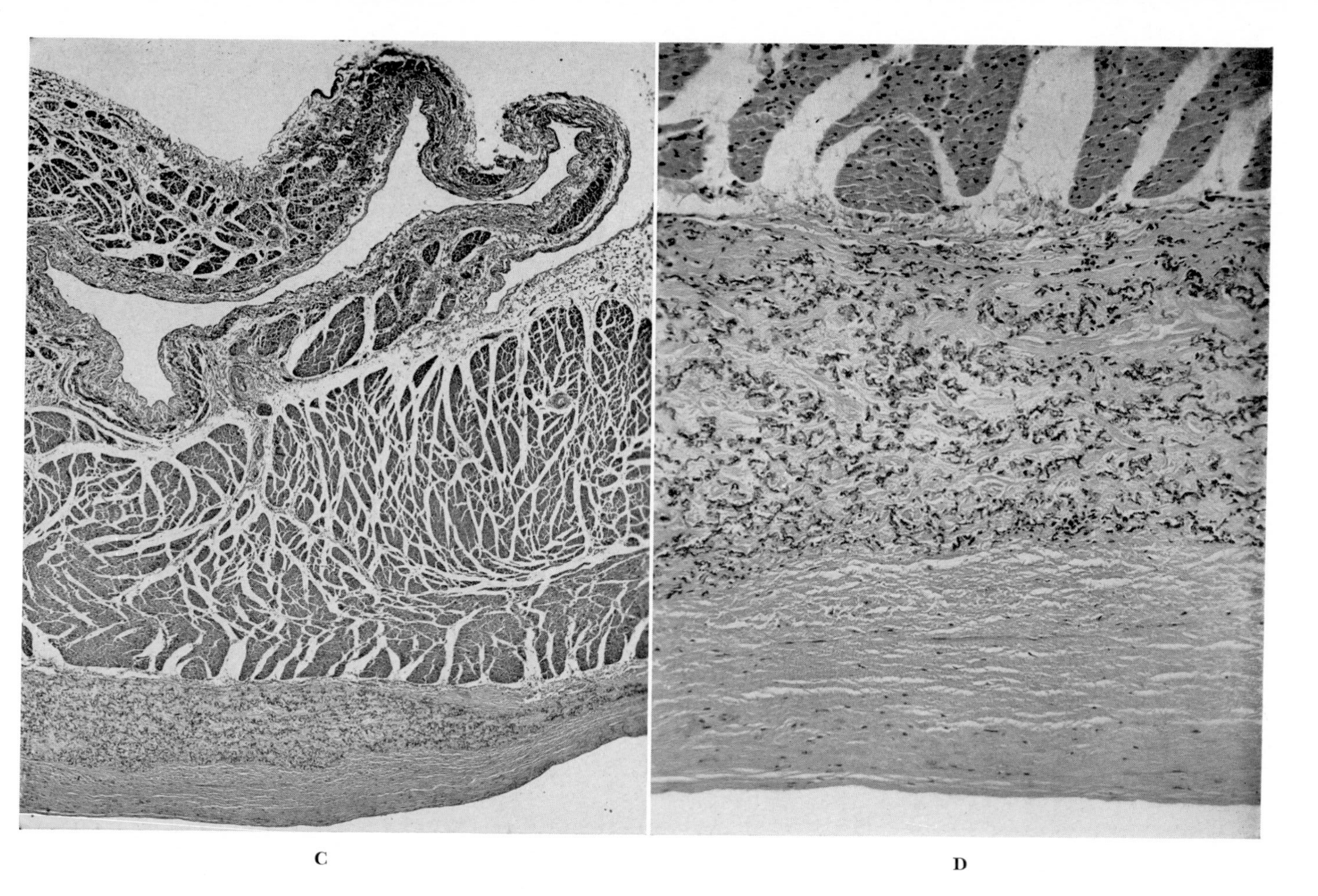

Fig. 8-17, cont'd. Wall of right atrium. (Hematoxylin and eosin stain; ×25.) On the endocardial surface (below) one of the opaque, elevated plaques is seen in section. On the epicardial surface a branch of a cardiac vein is seen. **D,** Enlarged view of one part of the field in **C**. (Hematoxylin and eosin stain; ×100.) Striking similarity to the changes in the skin is evident (see Fig. 8-1*F* and *G*.)

Continued.

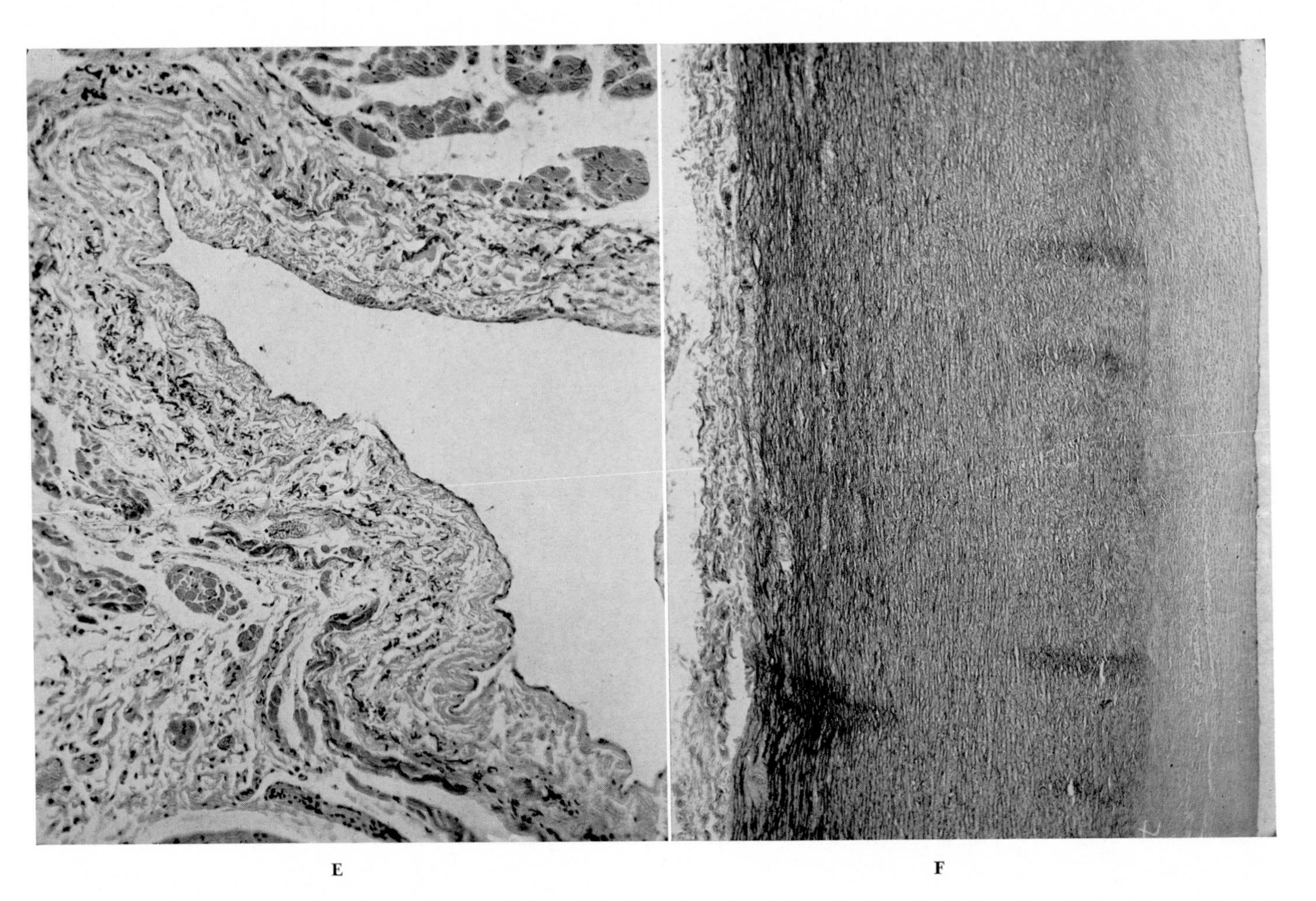

Fig. 8-17, cont'd. E, Enlarged view of another part of the field in **C** to show the changes in the wall of the vein, which again are identical to those in the skin and endocardium. (Hematoxylin and eosin stain; ×100.) **F,** Elastic fiber stain of aorta. The intima (on right) is thickened, but the media shows no striking disorganization. (×50.)

weaker, the patient was brought back to the hospital with massive leg edema and ascites and with Cheyne-Stokes breathing. She died two hours later.

Autopsy (No. 18717) revealed marked generalized arteriosclerosis, arteriosclerotic and arteriolosclerotic nephritis with Kimmelstiel-Wilson type lesions of glomeruli, and coronary sclerosis with myocardial scarring. In addition, there were tuberculous peritonitis and caseous obstruction of the thoracic duct with chylous ascites. The aorta was atheromatous, with a few ulcerations.

Comment. Hyperglobulinemia was probably due to tuberculosis. It is of interest that Kimmelstiel-Wilson lesions occurred in this nondiabetic individual. In general, premature and severe arteriosclerosis dominated the clinical picture and the findings at autopsy. What relation there may have been between the skin changes and the vascular disease is unclear. In general, however, this patient demonstrates the early and rapidly progressive dissolution of the vascular system characteristic of patients with PXE.

Case 3. N. C. was 13 years old at the time of death from gastrointestinal hemorrhage Hematemeses and/or melena had occurred repeatedly during the previous 6½ years, necessitating nine hospital admissions. Death occurred in 1945. The diagnosis was always in doubt clinically. At autopsy, too, the precise diagnosis was not made. PXE was first diagnosed in the brother, R. C., then (1957) age 35 years, on the basis of typical skin and eye changes and a history of gastrointestinal hemorrhage at the age of 15 years. On review of the medical records of the proband (N. C.), it was found that on a hospital admission four years before death it was noted that "over the cervical region is a raised pebbly eruption." Later it was recorded that "over the neck, chest, abdomen, and flexor surfaces of the arm there were elevated, small white papules, some discrete, others confluent, which appear like scar tissue." On one occasion the diagnosis of PXE, along with other possibilities, was suggested by a dermatologist, but the total picture was not put together. An ophthalmologist commented as follows: "The eyegrounds are essentially negative. Over a broad area temporally from the fovea in both eyes, there is a peculiar light brown mottling. The patient's brother is said to have this too and also the same sort of bleeding."

Histologic studies showed striking focal or segmental vascular changes, especially in the stomach and small intestine, but also to some extent in many other organs, including the heart, pancreas, kidney, and the brain. In some vessels there was fragmentation of the elastica, with deposition of collagenous material between it and the lumen, as well as loss of muscle (Fig. 8-12*A*). In the walls of some vessels, there was material which in part stained brilliantly red with picro-Mallory dye, like "fibrinoid." Mucosal vessels in the stomach and intestine were widely dilated and exceedingly thin walled (Fig. 8-12*B*). The wall of the atrium showed dense elastosis of the endocardium (Fig. 8-17*C* and *D*) of the type seen in Case 1 and reported in several instances in the literature.[6,17,79]

SUMMARY AND CONCLUSIONS

The clinical manifestations of pseudoxanthoma elasticum include (1) characteristic skin changes, occurring especially in areas of wear and tear; (2) angioid streaks of the fundus oculi; and (3) hemorrhage, symptoms of ischemia, and hypertension, resulting from arterial degeneration. Gastrointestinal hemorrhage is the complication of most importance to the internist.

Evidence on the nature of the basic defect is reviewed, and it is concluded that the elastic fiber is primarily involved in this abnormality, which behaves as an abiotrophy.

Descriptions of three autopsied cases are added to the meager information available on the state of tissues other than the skin and eye. In two cases, changes unique to PXE were demonstrated in the endocardium of the right atrium and in the coronary vessels.

Pseudoxanthoma elasticum is inherited as an autosomal recessive.

REFERENCES

1. Adelung, J. C.: Zur Genese der Angioid Streakes (Knapp), Klin. Mbl. Augenheilk. **119:**241, 1951.

2. Anderson, B.: Familial central and peripapillary choroidal sclerosis associated with familial pseudoxanthoma elasticum, Trans. Amer. Ophthal. Soc. **46:**326, 1948.
3. Anon.: Obituary of A. Chauffard, Bull. Soc. Franc. Hist. Méd. **26:**402, 1932.
4. Ayres, S., Jr., Discussion of paper of Shaffer et al.,[108] Arch. Derm. Syph. **76:**632, 1957.
5. Bäfverstedt, B., and Lund, F.: Pseudoxanthoma elasticum and vascular disturbances with special reference to a case in a nine-year-old child, Acta dermatovener. **35:**438, 1955.
6. Balzer, F.: Récherches sur les charactères anatomiques du xanthélasma, Arch. Physiol. **4** (series 3):65, 1884.
7. Banga, I.: Thermal contraction of collagen and its dissolution with elastase, Nature **172:**1099, 1953.
8. Beeson, B. B.: Pseudoxanthoma elasticum (Darier) associated with formation of bone, Arch. Derm. Syph. **34:**729, 1936.
9. Benedict, W. L.: The pathology of angioid streaks in the fundus oculi, J.A.M.A. **109:**475, 1937.
10. Benedict, W. L., and Montgomery, H.: Pseudoxanthoma elasticum and angioid streaks, Amer. J. Ophthal. **18:**205, 1935.
11. Berlyne, G. M., Bulmer, H. G., and Platt, R.: The genetics of pseudoxanthoma elasticum, Quart. J. Med. **30:**201, 1961.
12. Besnier, E., and Doyon, P. A. A.: Annotations et appendices en traité des maladies de la Peau, de Kaposi, ed. 2, 1891, p. 336. Cited by Darier.[24]
13. Böck, J.: Zur Klinik und Anatomie der gefässähnlichen Streifen im Augenhintergrund, Z. Augenheilk. **95:**1, 1938.
14. Bronner, A.: Considérations sur la syndrome de Groenblad et Strandberg, Bull. Soc. Franc. Derm. Syph. **61:**78, 1954.
15. Burton, D., Hall, D. A., Keech, M. K., Reed, R., Sax, H., Tunbridge, R. E., and Wood, M. J.: Apparent transformation of collagen fibrils into elastin, Nature **176:**966, 1955.
16. Carlborg, U.: Study of circulatory disturbances, pulse wave velocity and pressure pulses in larger arteries in cases of pseudoxanthoma elasticum and angioid streaks. A contribution to the knowledge of the function of the elastic tissue and the smooth muscles in larger arteries, Acta. Med. Scand., supp. 151:1-209, 1944.
17. Carlborg, U., Ejrup, B., Grönblad, E., and Lund, F.: Vascular studies in pseudoxanthoma elasticum and angioid streaks, Acta Med. Scand. **350:**1, 1959.
18. Chauffard, A.: Xanthélasma disséminé et symétrique sans insuffisance hépatique, Bull. Soc. Méd. Hôp. Paris **6** (series 3):412, 1889.
19. Chikelair, G. F.: Pseudoxanthoma elasticum treated surgically, Plast. & Reconstr. Surg. **12:**152, 1953.
20. Cockayne, E. A.: Inherited abnormalities of the skin and its appendages, London, 1933, Oxford University Press and Humphrey Milford, pp. 319-321.
21. Coffman, J. D., and Sommers, S. C.: Familial pseudoxanthoma elasticum and valvular heart disease, Circulation **19:**242, 1959.
22. Connor, P. J., Juergens, J. L., Perry, H. O., Hollenhorst, R. W. and Edwards, J. E.: Pseudoxanthoma elasticum and angioid streaks, a review of 106 cases, Amer. J. Med. **30:**537, 1961.
23. Cowper, A. R.: Angioid streaks; tears in Bruch's membrane or pigmented choroidal vessels? Arch. Ophthal. **51:**762, 1954.
24. Darier, J.: Pseudoxanthoma elasticum, Mschr. Prakt. Derm. **23:**609, 1896.
25. DeSimone, S., and DeConcilliis, U.: Strie angioidi della retina (considerazioni cliniche e patogenetiche), Arch. Ottal. **62:**161, 1958.
26. Dixon, J. M.: Angioid streaks and pseudoxanthoma elasticum with aneurysm of the internal carotid artery, Amer. J. Ophthal. **34:**1322, 1951.
27. Doyne, R. W.: Choroidal and retinal changes; the result of blows on the eyes, Trans. Ophthal. Soc. U.K. **9:**129, 1889.
28. Eddy, D. D., and Farber, E. M.: Pseudoxanthoma elasticum. Internal manifestations: a report of cases and a statistical review of the literature, Arch. Derm. **86:**729, 1962.
29. Edwards, H.: Haematemesis due to pseudoxanthoma elasticum, Gastroenterologia **89:**345, 1958.
30. Felsher, Z.: Collagen, reticulin, and elastin. In Rothman, S.: Physiology and biochemistry of the skin, Chicago, 1954, University of Chicago Press, p. 391 ff.

31. Findlay, G. H.: On elastosis and the elastic dystrophies of the skin, Brit. J. Derm. Syph. **66:**16, 1954.
32. Finnerud, C. W., and Nomland, R.: Pseudoxanthoma elasticum; proof of calcification of elastic tissue; occurrence with and without angioid streaks of the retina, Arch. Derm. Syph. **35:**653, 1937.
33. Fisher, E. R., Rodnan, G. P., and Lansing, A. I.: Identification of the anatomic defect in pseudoxanthoma elasticum, Amer. J. Path. **34:**977, 1958.
34. Foerster, O. H.: Transactions of the Dermatological Conference of the Mississippi Valley, Arch. Derm. Syph. **30:**280, 1934.
35. Fontan, P., Mérand, A., and Pfister, R.: Syndrome de Groenblad-Strandberg, Bull. Soc. Franc. Derm. Syph. **62:**101, 1955.
36. Franceschetti, A., and Roulet, E. L.: Le syndrome de Groenblad et Strandberg (striés angioïdes de la rétine et pseudoxanthome élastique) et ses rapport avec les affections du mésenchyme, Arch. Ophtal (Paris) **53:**401, 1936.
37. Friedenwald, J. S., and others: Ophthalmic pathology; an atlas and textbook, Philadelphia, 1952, W. B. Saunders Co.
38. Geereats, W. J., and Guerry, D.: Angioid streaks and sickle cell disease, Amer. J. Ophthal. **50:**213, 1960.
39. Giesen, H.: Beitrag zur Kasuistik des Pseudoxanthoma elasticum, Inaugural dissertation, Erlangen, 1936.
40. Gillman, T., Penn., J., Bronks, D., and Roux, M.: Abnormal elastic fibers; appearance in cutaneous carcinoma, irradiation injuries, and arterial and other degenerative connective tissue lesions in man, Arch. Path. **59:**733, 1955.
41. Goedbloed, J.: Syndrome of Groenblad and Strandberg; angioid streaks in the fundus oculi, associated with pseudoxanthoma elasticum, Arch. Ophthal. **19:**1, 1938.
42. Gold, S. C.: Still's disease with pseudoxanthoma elasticum, Proc. Roy. Soc. Med. **50:**473, 1957.
43. Goodman, R. M., Smith, E. W., Paton, D., Bergman, R. A., Siegel, C. L., Ottesen, O. E., Shelley, W. M., Pusch, A. L., and McKusick, V. A.: Pseudoxanthoma elasticum, a clinical and histopathological study, Medicine **42:**297, 1963.
44. Grönblad, E.: Angioid Streakes—Pseudoxanthoma elasticum: vorläufige Mitteilung, Acta Ophthal. **7:**329, 1929.
45. Guenther, E.: Untersuchungen über den Pulsverlauf in den grösseren distalen Arterien der Extremitäten in einigen Fällen von Pseudoxanthoma elasticum cum angioid streakes (Grönblad-Strandbergs Syndrom), Acta Med. Scand. **123:**482, 1946.
46. Haber, H.: Histological report on a case shown by Dr. Fenner at the Royal Society of Medicine, Proc. Roy. Soc. Med. (Sect. Derm.) **42:**136, 1949.
47. Hagedoorn, A.: Angioid streaks, Arch. Ophthal. **21:**746, 935, 1939.
48. Hall, D. A., Reed, R., and Tunbridge, R. E.: Structure of elastic tissue, Nature **170:**264, 1952.
49. Hallopeau and Laffitte: Nouvelle note sur un cas de pseudo-xanthome élastique, Ann. Derm. Syph., Paris **4:**595, 1903.
50. Hannay, P. W.: Some clinical and histopathological notes on pseudoxanthoma elasticum, Brit. J. Derm. **63:**92, 1951.
51. Hartung, H.: Ueber familiäre angioide Pigmentstreifenbildung des Augenhintergrundes, Klin. Mbl. Augenheilk. **88:**43, 1932.
52. Hermann, H.: Das Grönblad-Strandberg-Syndrom in erbbiologischer Betrachtung, Z. Haut. Geschlechtskr. **20:**314, 1956.
53. Hoffmann, D.: Kardiovaskuläre Erkrankunkgen beim Strandberg-Grönblad-Syndrom, Z. Menschl. Vererb. Konstitutionsl. **33:**389, 1956.
54. Hubler, W. R.: Two cases of pseudoxanthoma elasticum, Arch. Derm. Syph. **50:**51, 1944.
55. Jacoby, M. W.: Pseudoxanthoma elasticum and angioid streaks; report of a case, Arch. Ophthal. **11:**828, 1934.
56. Joffe, E., and Joffe, M.: Zur Aetiologie des Pseudoxanthoma elasticum (Darier), Arch. Derm. u. Syph. **165:**713, 1932.
57. Jones, J. W., Alden, H. S., and Bishop, E. L.: Pseudoxanthoma elasticum. Report of five cases illustrating its association with angioid streaks of the retina, Arch. Derm. Syph. **27:**423, 1933.

58. Kaplan, L., and Hartman, S. W.: Elastica disease; case of Grönblad-Strandberg syndrome with gastrointestinal hemorrhage, Arch. Intern. Med. **94**:489, 1954.
59. Kat, W., and Prick, J. J. G.: A case of pseudoxanthoma elasticum with anatomico-pathological irregularities of the thyroid arteries, Psychiat. Neurol. (Basel) **44**:417, 1940.
60. Keech, M. K., and Reed, R.: Enzymatic elucidation of the relationship between collagen and elastin; an electron-microscopic study, Ann. Rheum. Dis. **16**:35, 1957.
61. Keech, M. K., Reed, R., and Wood, M. J.: Further observations on the transformation of collagen fibrils into "elastin" and electron-microscopic studies, J. Path. Bact. **71**:477, 1956.
62. Kennedy, C. B.: Discussion of paper of Shaffer et al.,[108] Arch. Derm. Syph. **76**:631, 1957.
63. Kissmeyer, A., and With, C.: Clinical and histological studies on the pathological changes in the elastic tissue of the skin, Brit. J. Derm. **34**:175, 1922.
64. Klein, B. A.: Angioid streaks; a clinical and histopathologic study, Amer. J. Ophthal. **30**:955, 1947.
65. Knapp, H.: On the formation of dark angioid streaks as an unusual metamorphosis of retinal hemorrhage, Arch. Ophthal. **21**:289, 1892.
66. Kofler, A.: Beitrag zur Kenntnis der Angioid Streakes (Knapp), Arch. Augenheilk. **82**:134, 1917.
67. Kupfer, C.: Personal communication.
68. Larmande, A., and Margaillan, A.: Maladie de Paget et syndrome de Groenblad-Strandberg, Bull. Soc. Franc. Ophtal. **70**:206, 1957.
69. Law, F. W.: A contribution to the pathology of angioid streaks, Trans. Ophthal. Soc. U.K. **58**:191, 1938.
70. Lee, M. M. C.: Physical and structural age changes in human skin, Anat. Rec. **129**:473, 1957.
71. Lever, W. F.: Histopathology of the skin, ed. 2, Philadelphia, 1949, J. B. Lippincott Co., p. 56.
72. Levy, G., and Brewer, R. L.: Pseudoxanthoma elasticum. Report of a case, Amer. J. Med. **26**:157, 1959.
73. Lewis, U. J., Williams, D. E., and Brink, N. G.: Pancreatic elastase; purification, properties and function, J. Biol. Chem. **222**:705, 1956.
74. Lobitz, W., and Osterberg, A. E.: Pseudoxanthoma elasticum; microincineration, J. Invest. Derm. **15**:297, 1950.
75. Loria, P. R., Kennedy, C. B., Freeman, J. A., and Henington, V. M.: Pseudoxanthoma elasticum (Groenblad-Strandberg syndrome). A clinical, light- and electron-microscope study, Arch. Derm. Syph. **76**:609, 1957.
76. Lynch, F. W.: Elastic tissue in fetal skin, Arch. Derm. Syph. **29**:57, 1934.
77. McCaughey, R. S., Alexander, L. C., and Morrish, J. A.: The Grönblad-Strandberg syndrome. A report of three cases presenting with massive gastrointestinal hemorrhage during pregnancy, Gastroenterology **31**:156, 1956.
78. McKusick, V. A.: Hereditary disorders of connective tissue, Bull. N. Y. Acad. Med. **35**:143, 1959.
79. McKusick, V. A.: On the X chromosome of man, Quart. Rev. Biol. **37**:69, 1962. Also AIBS monograph, Washington, D. C., 1964.
80. McPhaul, J. J., Jr., and Engel, F. L.: Heterotopic calcification, hyperphosphatemia and angioid streaks of the retina, Amer. J. Med. **31**:488, 1961.
81. Marchesani, O.: and Wirz, F.: Die Pigment-streifenerkrankung der Netzhaut—das Pseudoxanthoma elasticum der Haut—eine Systemerkrankung, Arch. Augenheilk. **104**:522, 1931.
82. Marchionini, A., and Turgut, K.: Ueber Pseudoxanthoma elasticum hereditarium, Derm. Wschr. **114**:145, 1942.
83. Moran, T. J., and Lansing, A. I.: Studies on the nature of the abnormal fibers in pseudoxanthoma elasticum, Arch. Path. **65**:688, 1958.
84. Morrison, W. H.: Osteitis deformans with angioid streaks, Arch. Ophthal. **26**:79, 1941.
85. Nellen, M., and Jacobson, M.: Pseudoxanthoma elasticum (Grönblad-Strandberg disease) with coronary artery calcification, S. Afr. Med. J. **32**:649, 1958.
86. Ohno, T.: Ueber Pseudoxanthoma elasticum und dessen Histologie, Arch. Derm. u. Syph. **149**:420, 1925.
87. Ormsby, O. S., and Montgomery, H.: Diseases of the skin, ed. 8, Philadelphia, 1954, Lea & Febiger, p. 747.

88. Osbourn, R. A., and Olivo, M. A.: Pseudoxanthoma elasticum in mother and daughter, Arch. Derm. Syph. **63**:661, 1951.
89. Parker, J. C., Friedman, A. E., Kien, S., Levin, S., and Bartter, F. C.: Pseudoxanthoma elasticum and hypertension, New Eng. J. Med. **271**:1204, 1964.
90. Paton, D.: Angioid streaks and sickle cell anemia, Arch. Ophthal. **62**:852, 1959.
91. Paton, D.: Personal communication.
92. Pautrier, L. M.: À propos de deux affections d'élastine du revêtement cutané, témoins d'affections généralisées de l'élastine de tout l'organisme, Arch. Belg. Derm. Syph. **4**:259, 1948.
93. Percival, G. H., Hannay, P. W., and Duthie, D. A.: Fibrous changes in the dermis, with special reference to senile elastosis, Brit. J. Derm. **61**:269, 1949.
94. Pickrell, K. L., Kelley, J. W., and Marzoni, F. A.: The plastic surgical treatment of pseudoxanthoma elasticum, Plast. Reconstr. Surg. **3**:700, 1948.
95. Prick, J. J. G.: Pontine pseudobulbar-paralyse bei Pseudoxanthoma elasticum. Eine klinische anatomische Studie, Doctoral thesis, Maastricht, 1938.
96. Reinertson, R. P., and Farber, E. M.: Pseudoxanthoma elasticum with gastrointestinal bleeding, Calif. Med. **83**:94, 1955.
97. Revell, S. T. R., Jr., and Carey, T. N.: Pseudoxanthoma elasticum as a disseminated disease, Southern Med. J. **41**:782, 1948.
98. Rigal, D.: Observation pour servir à l'histoire de la chéloide diffuse xanthélasmique, Ann. Derm. Syph. **2**:491, 1881.
99. Rizzuli, A. B.; Angioid streaks with PXE; a case followed with fundus photography over a period of 27 years, Amer. J. Ophthal. **40**:387, 1955.
100. Rodnan, G. P., Fisher, E. R., and Warren, J. E.: Pseudoxanthoma elasticum: clinical findings and identification of the anatomic defect (abstract), Clin. Res. **6**:236, 1958.
101. Rosenheim, M. (London): Personal communication.
102. Rosenthal, T. B., and Lansing, A. I.: Isolation and assay of elastase from pancreatin (abstract), Anat. Rec. **124**:356, 1956.
103. Sames, C. P.: Pseudoxanthoma elasticum: severe melaena from the jejunum treated by resection, Proc. Roy. Soc. Med. **54**:519, 1961.
104. Sanbacka-Holström, I.: Das Grönblad-Strandbergische Syndrome. Pseudoxanthoma elasticum—angioid streaks—Gefässveränderungen, Acta Dermatovener. **20**:684, 1939.
105. Scheie, H. G., and Freeman, N. E.: Vascular disease associated with angioid streaks of the retina and pseudoxanthoma elasticum, Arch. Ophthal. **35**:3, 1946.
106. Scheie, H. G., and Hogan, T. F., Jr.: Angioid streaks and generalized arterial disease, Arch. Ophthal. **57**:855, 1957.
107. Scholz, R. O.: Angioid streaks, Arch. Ophthal. **26**:677, 1941.
108. Shaffer, B., Copelan, H. W., and Beerman, H.: Pseudoxanthoma elasticum. A cutaneous manifestation of a systemic disease. Report of a case of Paget's disease and a case of calcinosis with arteriosclerosis as manifestations of this syndrome, Arch. Derm. Syph. **76**:622, 1957.
109. Silvers, S.: Pseudoxanthoma elasticum with angioid streaks of retina, Arch. Derm. Syph. **42**:155, 1940.
110. Silvers, S. H., and Wolfe, H. E.: Pseudoxanthoma elasticum with angioid streaks. The syndrome of Groenblad and Strandberg, Arch. Derm. Syph. **45**:1142, 1942.
111. Smith, E. W., Malak, J., Goodman, R. M., and McKusick, V. A.: Reactive perforating elastoma: a feature of certain genetic disorders, Bull. Hopkins Hosp. **11**:235, 1962.
112. Smith, J. G., Jr., Davidson, E. A., and Clark, R. D.: Dermal elastin in actinic elastosis and pseudoxanthoma elasticum, Nature **195**:716, 1962.
113. Smith, J. G., Jr., Sams, W. M., Jr., Davidson, E. A., and Clark, R. D.: Pseudoxanthoma elasticum. Histochemical and biochemical alterations, Arch. Derm. **86**:741, 1962.
114. Stecher, R. M.: The physical characteristics and heredity of short thumbs, Acta Genet. (Basel) **7**:217, 1957.
115. Stegmaier, O. C.: Pseudoxanthoma elasticum associated with angioid streaks of the retina, Arch. Derm. Syph. **70**:530, 1954.
116. Storsteen, K. A., and Janes, J. M.: Arteriography and vascular studies in Paget's disease of the bone, J.A.M.A. **154**:472, 1954.
117. Stout, O. M.: Pseudoxanthoma elasticum with retinal angioid streaking, decidedly improved on tocopherol therapy, Arch. Derm. Syph. **63**:510, 1951.

118. Strandberg, J.: Pseudoxanthoma elasticum, Z. Haut Geschlechtskr. **31**:689, 1929.
119. Suerig, K. C., and Siefert, F. E.: Pseudoxanthoma elasticum and sickle cell anemia, Arch. Intern. Med. **113**:135, 1964.
120. Szymanski, F. J., and Caro, M. R.: Pseudoxanthoma elasticum. Review of its relationship to internal diseases and report of an unusual case, Arch. Derm. **71**:184, 1955.
121. Tannenhein, V.: Zur Kenntnis des Pseudoxanthoma elasticum (Darier), Wein. Klin. Wschr. **14**:1038, 1901.
122. Teller, H., and Vester, G.: Elektronenmikroskopiche Untersuchungsergebnisse an der kollagenen Interzellularsubstanz des Koriums beim Pseudoxanthoma elasticum, Derm. Wschr. **136**:1373, 1957.
123. Témine, P.: Contribution à l'étude de l'élastorrhexie systématisée, Paris thesis, Paris, 1940, Jouve & Cie.
124. Terry, T. S.: Angioid streaks and osteitis deformans, Trans. Amer. Ophthal. Soc. **32**:555, 1934.
125. Throne, B., and Goodman, H.: Pseudoxanthoma elasticum, Arch. Derm. Syph. **6**:419, 1921.
126. Tominaga, B., Harada, S., and Hashimoto, T.: A case of pseudoxanthoma elasticum with tuberculoid granulation tissue, Arch. Derm. Syph. **30**:864, 1934.
127. Touraine, A.: L'elastorrhexie systématisée, Bull. Soc. Franc. Derm. Syph. **47**:255, 1940.
128. Touraine, A.: L'élastorrhexie systématisée, Presse Méd. **49**:361, 1941.
129. Touraine, A., and James: Pseudoxanthome élastique (élastorrhexis), Bull. Soc. Franc. Derm. Syph. **47**:217, 1940.
130. Tunbridge, R. E., Tattersall, R. N., Hall, D. A., Astbury, W. T., and Reed, R.: The fibrous structure of normal and abnormal skin, Clin. Sci. **11**:315, 1952.
131. Urbach, E., and Wolfram, S.: Ueber Veränderungen des elastischen Gewebes bei einem autoptisch untersuchten Fälle von Groenblad-Strandbergschem Syndrom, Arch. Derm. u. Syph. **176**:167, 1938.
132. Van Embden Andres, G. H.: Afwijkingen, aan de inwendige organen bij Pseudoxanthoma Elasticum en Angioide Stregpen, Groningen, 1952.
133. Verhoeff, F. H.: Histological findings in a case of angioid streaks, Brit. J. Ophthal. **32**:531, 1948.
134. Walford, R. L., and Kaplan, L.: Pulmonary fibrosis and giant-cell reaction with altered elastic tissue; endogenous "pneumoconiosis," Arch. Path. **63**:75, 1957.
135. Weidman, F. D., Anderson, N. P., and Ayres, S.: Juvenile elastoma, Arch. Derm. Syph. **28**:183, 1933.
136. Welti, M. H.: Pseudoxanthoma elasticum (Darier) in Verbindung mit einer tuberculoiden Granulationsbildung, Arch. Derm. u. Syph. **163**:427, 1931.
137. Whitecomb, F. F., Jr., and Brown, C. H.: Pseudoxanthoma elasticum. Report of twelve cases: massive gastrointestinal hemorrhage in one patient, Ann. Intern. Med. **56**:834, 1962.
138. Wilmer, W. H.: Atlas fundus oculi, New York, 1934, The Macmillan Co., plate 92.
139. Winer, L. H.: Elastic fibers in unusual dermatoses, Arch. Derm. Syph. **71**:338, 1955.
140. Wolff, H. H., Stokes, J., and Schlesinger, B.: Vascular abnormalities associated with pseudoxanthoma elasticum, Arch. Dis. Child. **27**:82, 1952.
141. Woo, J. C., Jr., and Chandler, F. W.: Pseudoxanthoma elasticum with gastric hemorrhage. Report of a case, Ann. Intern. Med. **49**:215, 1958.
142. Woodcock, C. W.: Transactions of the Cleveland Dermatological Society, Arch. Derm. Syph. **65**:623, 1952.
143. Woringer, F.: Sur deux aspects histologiques différents de pseudoxanthome élastique, Bull. Soc. Franc. Derm. Syph. **61**:80, 1954.
144. Yatzkan, D. N.: Angioid streaks of the fundus, Amer. J. Ophthal. **43**:219, 1957.
145. Zentmayer, W.: Angioid streaks of the fundus oculi observed over a period of thirty-six years; report of a case, Arch. Ophthal. **35**:541, 1946.

9

The mucopolysaccharidoses

Historical note

The disorder (or group of disorders) now called, among other names, the Hurler syndrome is said by Henderson[109] to have been recognized in three siblings by John Thompson of Edinburgh between about 1900 and 1913. Berkhan's case,[18] reported in 1907, may have been the Hurler syndrome. The first definitive description was that of Charles H. Hunter* whose report appeared in the *Proceedings of the Royal Society of Medicine* in 1917, while he was serving in England as a major in the Canadian Army Medical Corps. This beautifully detailed and descriptive report concerned two brothers, 10 and 8 years of age, respectively, who were admitted to the Winnipeg General Hospital in 1915. The habitus was typically dwarfed. There were deafness, widely spaced teeth, short neck, protuberant abdomen with hepatosplenomegaly, inguinal hernias, short, broad, thick, stiff hands, semiflexed knees, and noisy respiration. The elder boy had cardiomegaly and "a distinct diastolic murmur audible in the third and fourth left interspaces close to the sternum . . .; at the apex, a systolic murmur was conducted towards the axilla." Twelve illustrations, including many x-ray films demonstrating typical changes (such as "shoe-shaped" sella), were presented by Hunter. The boys appeared to be normally intelligent; clouding of the cornea was not observed; the spine was straight with loss of the normal contour, but there was no gibbus. We have been able to obtain follow-up information (Fig. 9-1). Hunter's patients probably suffered from the X-linked form of this disease, called MPS II below.

In 1919 Gertrud Hurler of Munich[121] published cases at the suggestion of Professor Meinhard von Pfaundler,[223] who was chief of the University Clinic of Pediatrics and who had presented two patients with this syndrome to the Munich Society for Pediatrics on June 27 of the same year. The patients of Hurler and Pfaundler were infants; gibbus was present, as were corneal clouding and retardation of intellect. They probably suffered from the autosomal recessive form of the disease referred to below as MPS I.

---

*Hunter was later Professor of Medicine in the University of Manitoba, Winnipeg. He died March 18, 1955, at the age of 82 years (Canad. Med. Ass. J. **72**:712, 1955).

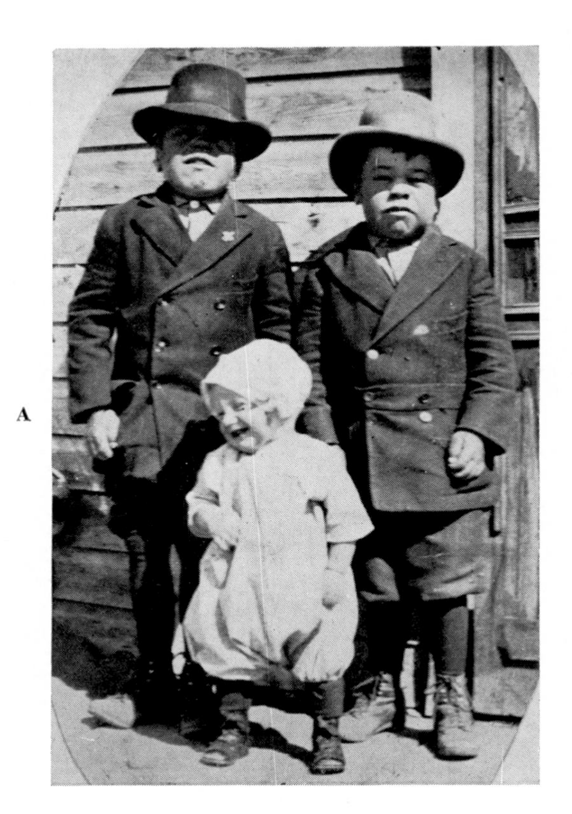

A

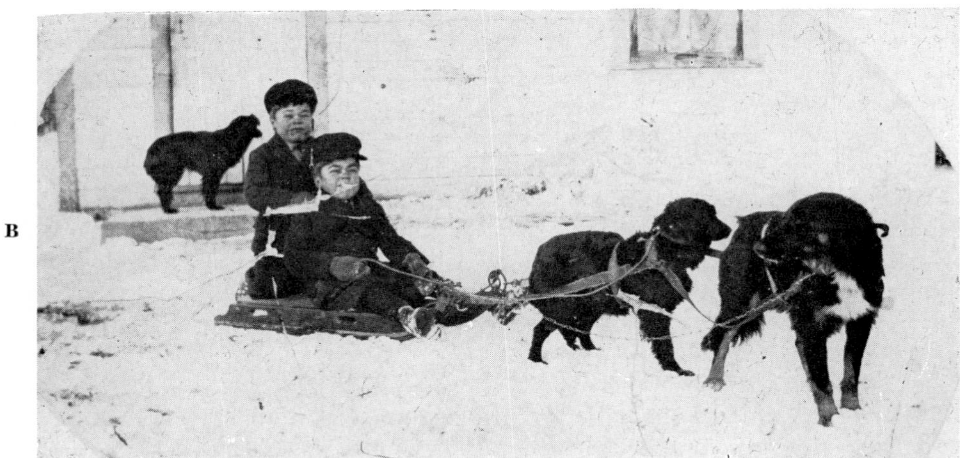

B

Fig. 9-1. Previously unpublished photographs of the patients Hunter described in 1917.[120] The younger brother (G. B. C., born in 1907) died in 1918 of pneumonia, and the elder one (R. W. C., born in 1904) died in 1920 of "dropsy." The youngest sibling in **A** was apparently unaffected. The characteristic facies and clawhands are evident. These brothers are thought to have had the sex-linked recessive form of mucopolysaccharidosis (MPS II). (Photographs and follow-up information courtesy Dr. Nancy Gemmell and Dr. L. G. Bell, University of Manitoba, Winnipeg.)

It is surprising that Hunter's beautiful publication received, compared to Hurler's, relatively little attention. Subsequently, even in the English-speaking medical world, it was principally Hurler's paper that was referred to and the names of Hurler and Pfaundler that became most firmly associated with the syndrome. (A similar situation exists in connection with the Morquio syndrome, which was described in England by Brailsford slightly earlier than by Morquio of Montevideo.)

The first case from the United States was that reported by Putnam and Pelkan[226] in 1925 under the title "Scaphocephaly with malformations of the skeleton and other tissues." The nosography of the Hurler syndrome has now advanced to the point where the limits of the syndrome and its several clinical and pathologic features are reasonably well described, although mildly affected persons are still difficult to identify with certainty except by chemical test (p. 376). A tabular survey of the cases reported up to 1950 was presented by Jervis.[133] Emanuel[75] estimated that over 200 cases had been reported, by 1954. In 1952, Brante[28] classified the Hurler syndrome as a mucopolysaccharidosis. Discovery of mucopolysacchariduria by Dorfman and Lorincz[67] and by Meyer and colleagues[196] firmly established the nature of the disease.

On clinical and genetic grounds an X-linked form was distinguished by several observers, beginning with Njå[214] in 1946. Chemical methods for characterizing the mucopolysacchariduria, combined with clinical characterization, resulted in delineation of four other mucopolysaccharidoses—referred to below as MPS III (Sanfilippo syndrome), MPS IV (Morquio syndrome), MPS V (Scheie syndrome), and MPS VI (Maroteaux-Lamy syndrome). Nosography of the Morquio syndrome, which in its earlier stages closely simulates the Hurler syndrome, has an interesting and somewhat complex history, which will be detailed later.

Many different names have been suggested for this group of disorders. Most are now of historic interest, only. Husler[122] suggested "dysostosis multiplex." Ellis and co-workers,[73] Cockayne,[46] and other English authors used the term "gargoylism."* Washington[298] suggested "lipochondrodystrophy," believing this to be a disorder of lipid metabolism. This is the term used by the *Cumulated index medicus.* However, it is a misnomer, as indicated by present evidence bearing on the basic defect of the disease. This is another instance demonstrating the desirability of using noncommittal terms in connection with syndromes in which the basic defect is as yet unknown.

The six distinct mucopolysaccharidoses that have been differentiated by combined clinical, genetic, and biochemical study are more or less arbitrarily designated MPS I through VI. Since the numerical designations are not easily remembered, eponyms are proposed as alternatives. MPS I (Hurler snydrome) is the prototype mucopolysaccharidosis. MPS II (Hunter syndrome) is the X-linked form of the disease. MPS III (Sanfilippo syndrome) and MPS V (Scheie syndrome) were previously considered "Hurler variants." MPS IV (Morquio syndrome) is now known to have a characteristic mucopolysacchariduria and dis-

*This seems an unnecessarily cruel term in view of the fact that the intellect may be little impaired and survival to adulthood is not infrequent. It is scarcely a diagnosis that can be cited to a parent, for example. Families sometimes raise legitimate objections to such statements (all too frequent in the literature) as these: "He is a typical gargoyle" or "there are three gargoyles in this family."

tinctive skeletal and extraskeletal features. The newest addition to the group, MPS VI, was first clearly delineated as an entity separate from the others by Maroteaux and Lamy and their colleagues.[185a,186]

MUCOPOLYSACCHARIDOSIS I (MPS I, Hurler syndrome)

As the prototype mucopolysaccharidosis, MPS I will be described in especially full detail.

Clinical manifestations

This form of the disease becomes clinically evident in infancy or early childhood. Of the six mucopolysaccharidoses it produces death at the earliest age, on the average. The infant usually develops normally for a few months and then progressively deteriorates mentally and physically. Lumbar gibbus, stiff joints, chest deformity, or rhinitis may first prompt the parents to seek medical advice. Dwarfing is accompanied by radiologic changes in the skeleton that are more or less typical of this specific entity (Figs. 9-2*C* and 9-4). Progressive clouding of the

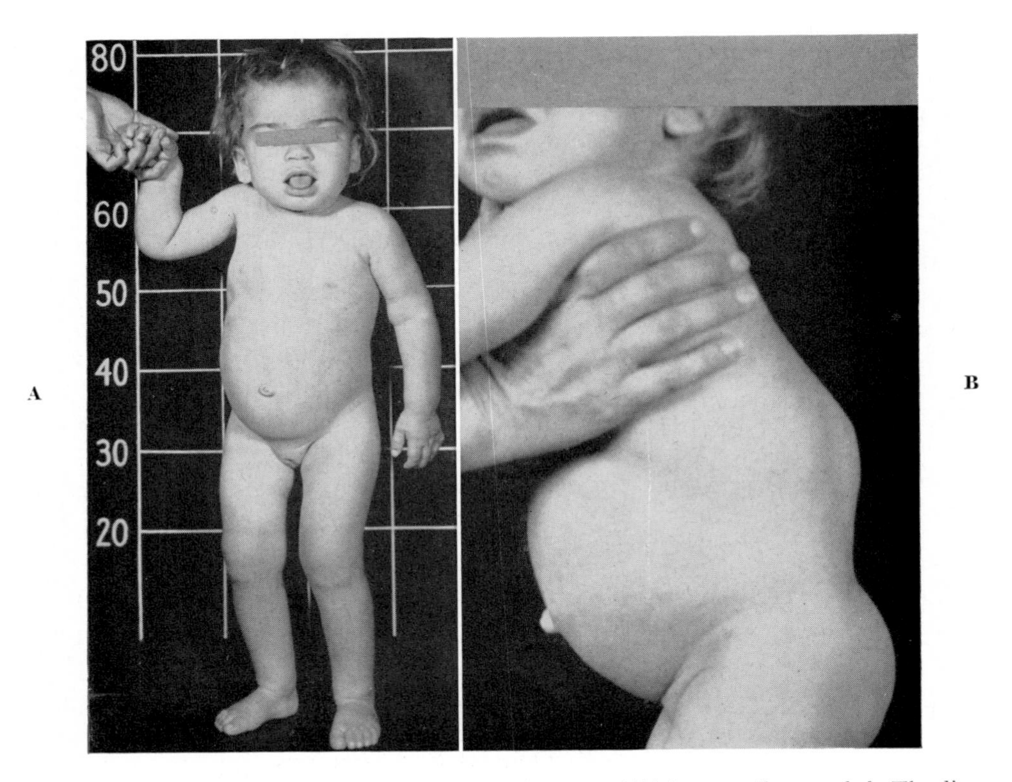

Fig. 9-2. Thirty-four-month-old child (S. S., B3747). The child is mentally retarded. The liver and spleen are enlarged, the corneas cloudy, and the teeth short, abnormally formed, and late in appearing. The fingers show flexion contractures as do other joints to a slight extent. There is constant nasal congestion so that the patient is a mouth-breather. Most of these features are evident in **A.** In **B** the lower dorsal, upper lumbar gibbus is evident. The skeletal basis for this appearance is shown by the x-ray film of the spine in **C.** Note the lumbar kyphos, beaking of the lumbar vertebrae, the sabre-shaped ribs, and hepatosplenomegaly.

cornea occurs in all cases and may conceal retinal degeneration that is occurring concurrently. The liver and spleen are enlarged as a result of mucopolysaccharide deposits. The usual causes of death, which in most cases occurs before 10 years of age, are respiratory infection and cardiac failure. The anatomic basis for the cardiac features is the deposition of mucopolysaccharide in the intima of the coronary arteries (Fig. 9-6*B* to *D*) and in the heart valves.

Mental development, which appears to be normal for the first year or so of life, shows regression thereafter. Hydrocephalus may be obvious, and even in those cases in which it develops more slowly so that the skull sutures close, internal hydrocephalus (Fig. 9-6*A*), probably the result of meningeal deposits, is a frequent finding at autopsy.

The line along which development occurs in these patients is so similar from patient to patient that—as in the Marfan syndrome, myotonic dystrophy, mongolism, and some other conditions—the patients, even though unrelated, tend to resemble each other more than their unaffected siblings.

The head is large and bulging, often with prominent scalp veins in the case of

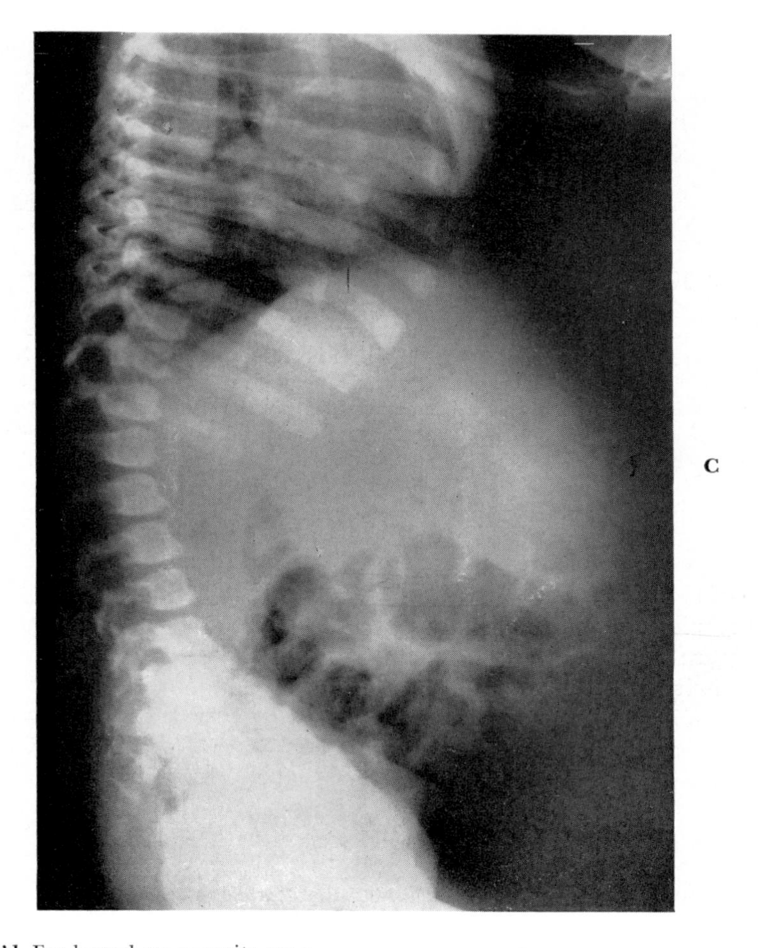

C

Fig. 9-2, cont'd. For legend see opposite page.

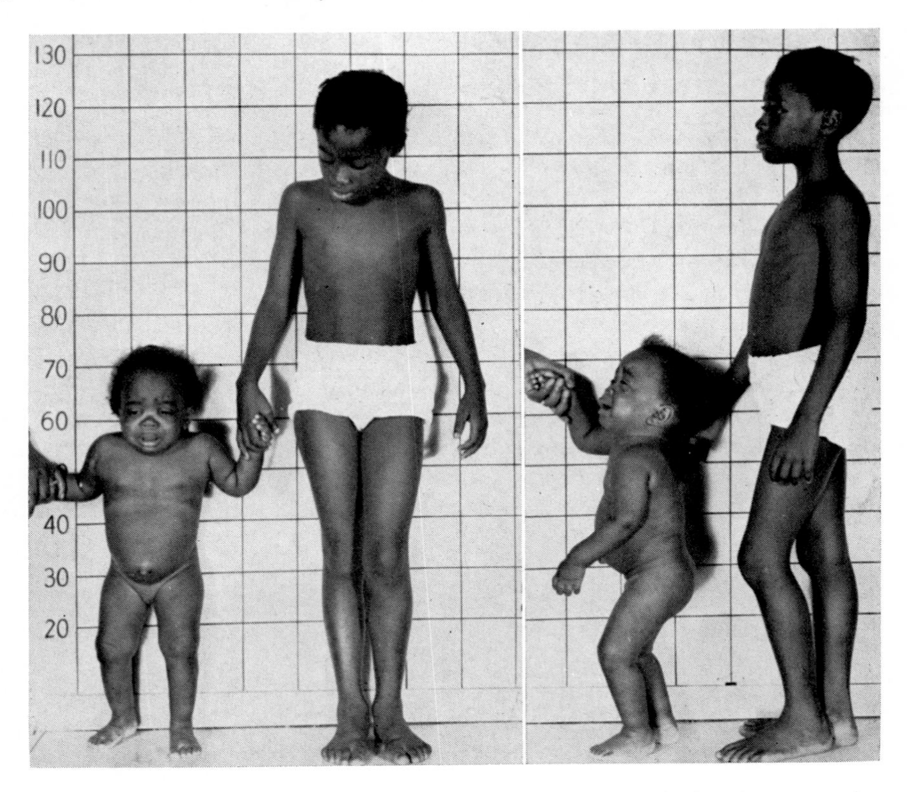

Fig. 9-3. The Hurler syndrome. On the left of each view: C. D. (B41371), 2½ years of age, is a member of the only Negro family with the Hurler syndrome I have seen. The head is large and the facies characteristic of the Hurler syndrome. The elbows, shoulders, knees, and other joints show reduced mobility, preventing full extension. The hands are short, and the terminal phalanges cannot be fully extended. Both the liver and the spleen are enlarged. Nasal breathing is obstructed by a continuous mucopurulent discharge. Both corneas are clouded. Of six children, three—two boys and this girl—have been affected with the autosomal recessive form of the Hurler syndrome. A normal 8-year-old sister is also shown here. The two other affected children died at the ages of 3 and 4 years. (From McKusick, V. A.: Bull. N. Y. Acad. Med. **35:**143, 1959.)

small children. The bridge of the nose is flattened, creating a saddle appearance. The tip of the nose is broad with wide nostrils. Hypertelorism is usual. The skull is often scaphocephalic,* i.e. shaped like the keel of a boat, seemingly as a result of premature closure of the sagittal and metopic sutures with hyperostosis in those areas. This hyperostosis often creates a longitudinal (sagittal) ridge, which may cross the forehead. Radiologic changes in the sella turcica, in the form of unusual length and shallowness and an anterior "pocketing" (Figs. 9-4*C* and 9-7*C*) are striking. This type of sella is called "shoe-shaped" by Ullrich,[284] who found in other cases a shallow "shell-shaped" or a deeper "bowl-shaped" fossa.

The lips are large and patulous. These, with the apathetic facies, the open

*There is usually no difficulty in distinguishing the Hurler syndrome from the specific conditions given the generic names *acrocephaly* and *scaphocephaly*,[220] although in the earlier days of the nosography of Hurler's syndrome such confusion did occur.[134]

mouth, and frequently enlarged tongue, may lead to a false diagnosis of cretinism. In general, the facial features are coarse and ugly. The teeth are usually small, stubby, widely spaced, and malformed. In many of the cases there is hypertrophy both of the bony alveolar ridges and of the overlying gums.[51] An actual bone cyst of the alveolar ridge was present in one of Caffey's cases.[35] Chronic "rhinitis" with noisy mouth breathing is virtually universal in this group of patients. X-ray films of the facial bones usually show marked deformities, which are probably responsible for the nasal manifestations. On lateral view of the skull, it can often be seen that a mass of adenoid tissue in the nasopharynx is narrowing or obliterating the normal air shadow.

The neck is exceedingly short, and the thorax, on which the head appears to rest directly, is deformed. There is usually a flaring of the lower rib cage, probably due in part to the hepatosplenomegaly. Kyphosis with gibbus in the lower thoracic and upper lumbar area is likely to be present. Myelograms in one case revealed partial obstruction of the spinal canal at the level of the gibbus. Radiologic examination usually shows wedge-shaped deformity of the body of the vertebrae, with anterior hooklike projection, so-called beaking of the vertebrae. In some instances there appears to be anterior herniation of the nucleus pulposus with pressure atrophy of the upper anterior margin of the subjacent vertebral body (usually the second lumbar). This atrophy may be the mechanism of the anterior hook in some cases. (See Fig. 9-2*C* and reference 35.) The gibbus is often the first observed abnormality. When the infant begins to sit, he is likely to assume a posture like a cat's in sitting (Fig. 9-2*B*), the "cat-back deformity."

The hands are usually broad, with stubby fingers.[261] The fifth fingers are often bent radially, and, in general, there is likely to be at least partial flexion contracture of the fingers as well as of the larger joints. The terminal phalangeal bones are often hypoplastic by x-ray examination and this is evident clinically. Clawhand is present in most patients more than a few years old. (See Figs 9-1, 9-7, and 9-10.) This deformity results from stiffening of the phalangeal joints, with inability of full extension.

Limitation in extensibility of joints is usually striking.[121] This feature may be due in part to deformity of the joint surfaces but more likely to changes in the tendons and ligaments surrounding the joints. As a result, the patients often find it necessary to walk on their toes, especially if they have been in bed a good deal. A deformity of the wrist may superficially suggest rickets. However, the stiff joints (along with many other features) help distinguish the Hurler syndrome[117]; the joints in rickets are more limber than normal. The limitation of motion of joints seems to extend to the thorax, which often is relatively fixed in position.[75]

In addition to the radiologic changes already described in the skull and in the vertebral column, the bones of the extremities are abnormal in appearance. Caffey[35] pointed out that metaphyseal changes are minimal and that the predominant change involves the diaphysis. The tubular bones show a swelling of the shaft due to expansion of the medullary cavity. The cortex may be thinned. Changes tend to be more striking in the bones of the arms than in those of the legs. A curious narrowing of the proximal third of the femora to a caliber less than half the normal has been noted.[35] The phalangeal bones, for example, are short and misshapen (Fig. 9-4*C*). The ribs are characteristically broad, sabre-shaped, or spatulate (Figs. 9-4*A* and 9-5). The vertebral ends of the ribs are

A

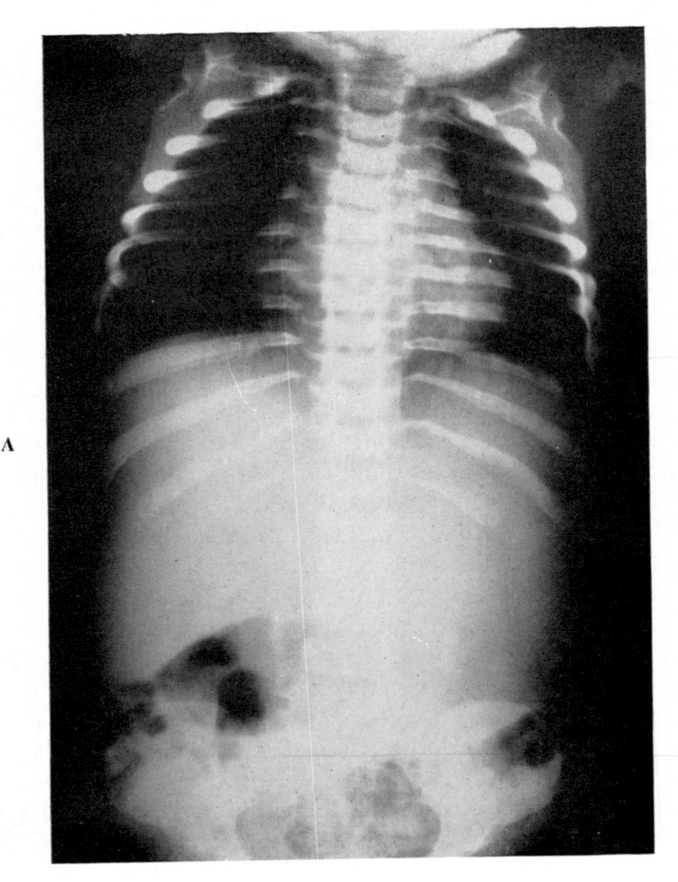

Fig. 9-4. Skeletal changes in the Hurler syndrome. **A,** The lower ribs are unusually broad and spatulous. Note the evidence of hepatosplenomegaly.

unusually narrow, particularly by comparison with the rest of the rib. Horrigan and Baker[115] found that the superior surface of the condyle of the mandible has a concave contour.

Genu valgum, coxa valga, pes planus, talipes equinovarus, and other deformities occur frequently. Deformity of the sternum has been said[123] not to be a feature; however, congenital deformity of one type or another has been seen (Fig. 9-7).[140] "Funnel chest" was present in one of Hurler's cases[133] and in one of mine.

The abdomen is protuberant, due in part to hepatosplenomegaly, in part to the defect of the supporting tissues. Both liver and spleen may be so large that their lower borders dip into the pelvis. One patient developed pancytopenia and epistaxes, possibly on the basis of hypersplenism.[261] Lindsay[158] described an abnormal hippuric acid test in one patient and, in another, prolonged elevation of galactose in the blood after intravenous injection. The number of patients tested was not stated. Although no systematic study has been made, the impression is given that surprisingly little functional impairment results from the marked gross and histologic involvement of the liver.

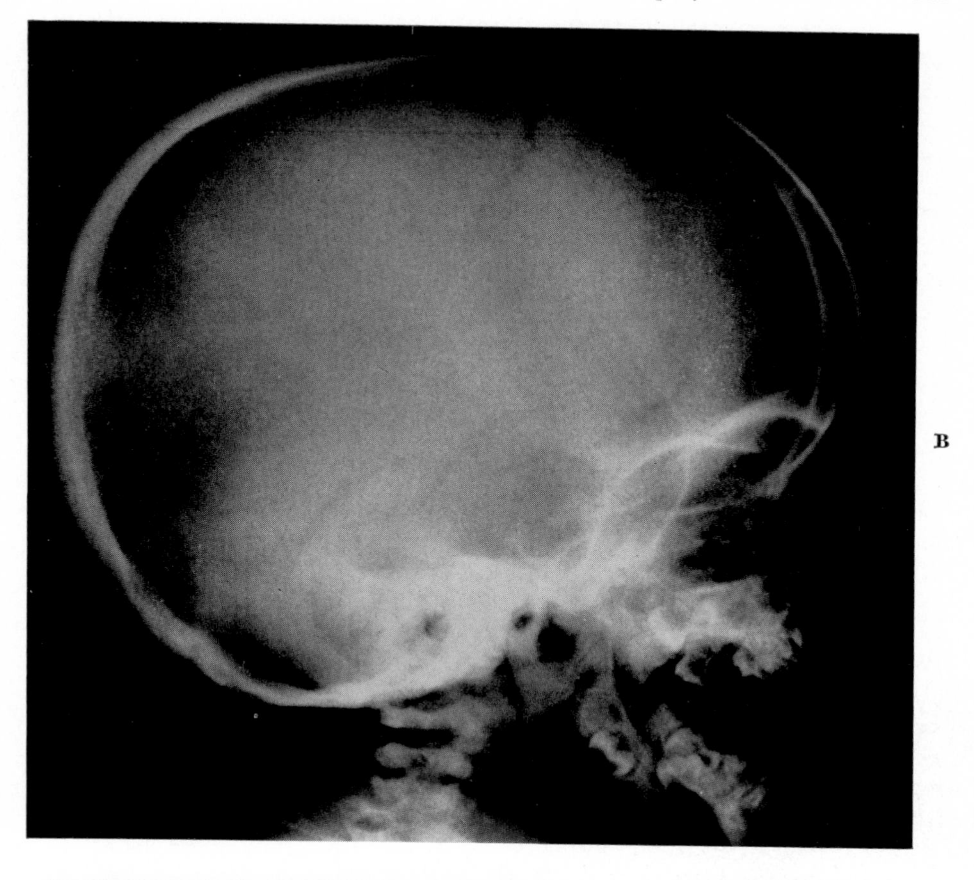

B

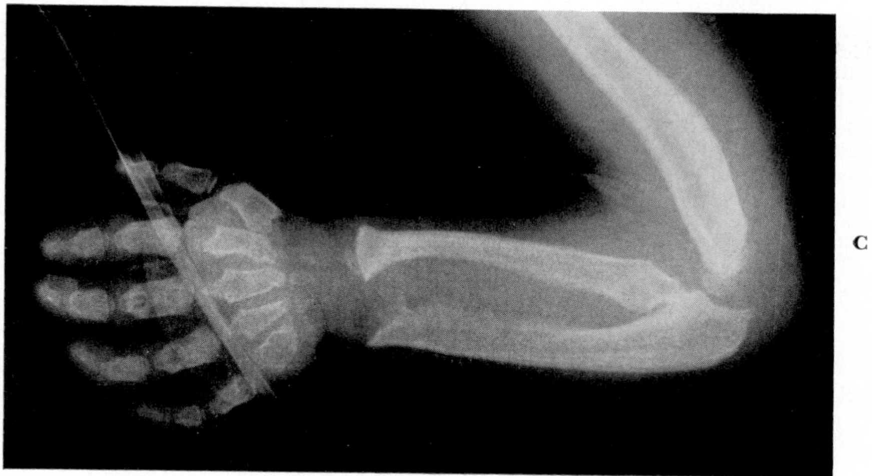

C

Fig. 9-4, cont'd. B, The anterior pocketing of the sella, "shoe-shaped" sella, is highly characteristic. Furthermore, pronounced abnormality in the region of the paranasal sinuses is evident. **C,** The long bones of the arm are abnormally short and broad. The bones of the hand are strikingly abnormal in configuration. Again their shape is virtually pathognomonic of the Hurler syndrome.

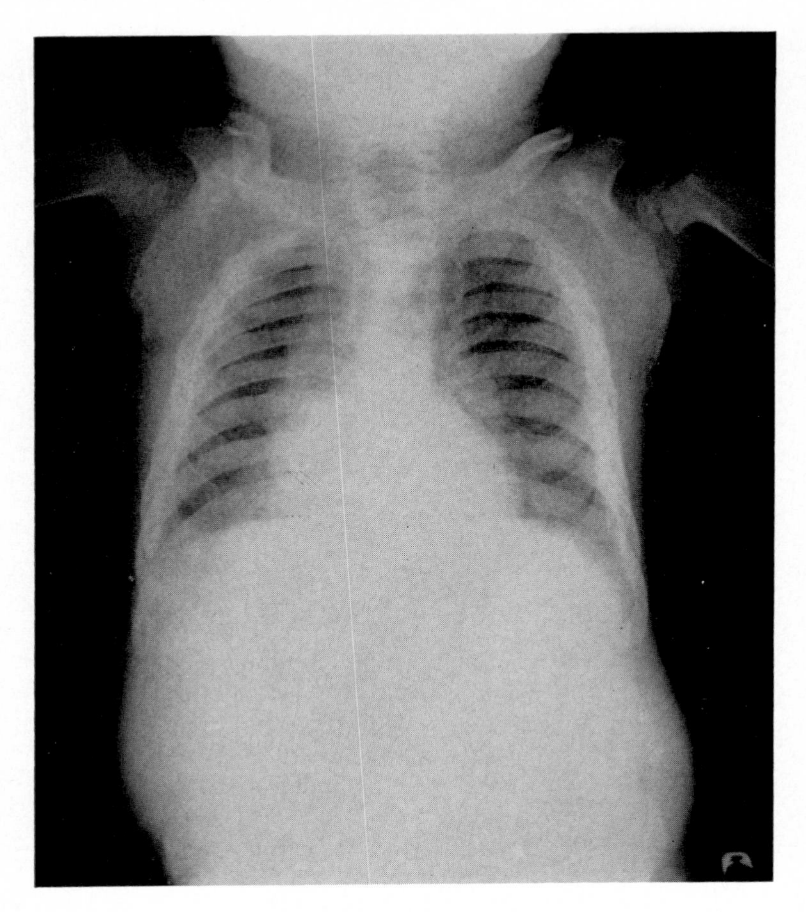

Fig. 9-5. Chest x-ray film of G. V. D., Jr. (B2188), 4½ years of age. This patient has the Hurler syndrome in entirely typical form. He reached a peak of intellectual development at about 2 years and has deteriorated since then. Gibbus was noted at 1 year. Thick skin, lanugo, "shoe-shaped" sella, and ground-glass corneas are present. Hydrocele and right inguinal hernia were treated surgically at the age of 1½ years. The central infiltration of the lung fields was present in an unchanged form for at least six months. Tuberculin skin tests are negative. The changes are believed to be the result of chronic bronchitis. However, interstitial pulmonary infiltration as part of the disease and analogous to the infiltrations elsewhere cannot be excluded. The opacification of the upper abdomen by hepatosplenomegaly, the broad ribs, and the abnormality of the proximal ends of the humeri are evident.

McCormick[171] reported fatal rupture of the stomach in a 6-year-old boy who had suffered from repeated episodes of gastric dilatation. Diastasis recti and umbilical hernia are almost invariable, and inguinal hernia is frequent. Engel[77] described scrotal hernias the size of a child's head. Bilateral hydrocele is also seen.[107]

In most of the cases the entire surface of the body, both trunk and extremities, is covered by fine, lanugo-like fuzz. In older patients, too, hairiness is quite striking, especially over the arms and hands (Fig. 9-7*B* and *C*), this being a feature of all the mucopolysaccharidoses. Nodular thickening of the skin, of the type described later under MPS II, may be unusual in MPS I.

No consistent endocrine abnormality is clinically detectable, in spite of the histologic evidence of cellular deposits in most glands of internal secretion. Thyroid enlargement without dysfunction has been described and is probably related to the histologic infiltration referred to. Hypoglycemia from hepatic involvement is thought to be a risk but has not actually been demonstrated, to my knowledge. The deformity of the sella turcica is part of the disorder of bone and not a result of enlargement of the pituitary.

Clouding of the cornea probably develops in all cases of MPS I. The cornea usually has merely a steamy appearance in earlier stages. On inspection this feature is most apparent if light is shined on the cornea from the side. Slit-lamp examination confirms the finding. The opacities are located in the medial and deeper layers of the cornea. The epithelium and endothelium are spared. Other ocular abnormalities such as buphthalmos[58] and megalocornea[19,73,133,202] have been described. There may be a retinal element in visual impairment, since histopathologic changes in the retina have been described,[159] and the electroretinogram is diminished or "extinguished" in many cases.[93]

Mental retardation is a conspicuous feature of all cases of MPS I. Hydrocephalus may occur in severely affected infants.[9,158] Some cases may show simple dilatation of the ventricles, secondary to cortical atrophy.[284] There is true internal hydrocephalus in some cases; the ventricular dilatation is too marked to be accounted for on the basis of cortical atrophy alone (Fig. 9-6*A*). The mental deterioration is likely to be progressive, resembling juvenile amaurotic idiocy in this respect.[133] There may be accompanying neurologic signs such as motor paralysis, increase in muscular tone, and the Babinski sign.

One would presume that the deafness is, in the main, secondary to the bone disease, as in osteogenesis imperfecta. In a 16-month-old child and a 2-year-old child studied by Dr. William G. Hardy of the Johns Hopkins Hearing and Speech Clinic, the deafness was of the conductive type, and in a 3-year-old patient hearing was unimpaired. Because of the deformity of the nasopharynx, these patients probably have more than the average susceptibility to middle ear infection. Furthermore, the ossicles have shown deformity with limitation of joint motion as in other joints and bones.[304] Therefore, a conductive element in the deafness of some patients is to be expected.

Nasal congestion, noisy mouth breathing, and frequent upper respiratory infections occur in essentially all patients with the Hurler syndrome. The malformation of the facial and nasal bones is probably in large part responsible. Ellis and associates[73] commented on this feature. Most other writers have also emphasized it and considered malformation of the nasopharynx to be its basis.

Murmurs also were described by Meyer and Okner[202] Engel[77] and others. Ashby and co-workers[9] described "congenital heart disease" as the cause of death at 9 years of age in one child and in a 19-year-old patient who died suddenly. Mouth breathing and dyspnea from thoracic deformity and restriction of expansion[75] (which may be very striking), abnormality of the bronchial cartilages, and, finally, frequent attacks of bronchitis make it difficult to dissect out that part of the dyspnea which is on a cardiac basis. The best specific descriptions of the cardiovascular aspects of the Hurler syndrome are those of Lindsay[158] and Emanuel.[75] Emanuel described in two brothers cardiac signs he interpreted as being those of pulmonary hypertension. In one, cardiac catheterization was performed with demonstration of a much elevated pulmonary artery pressure (88/50

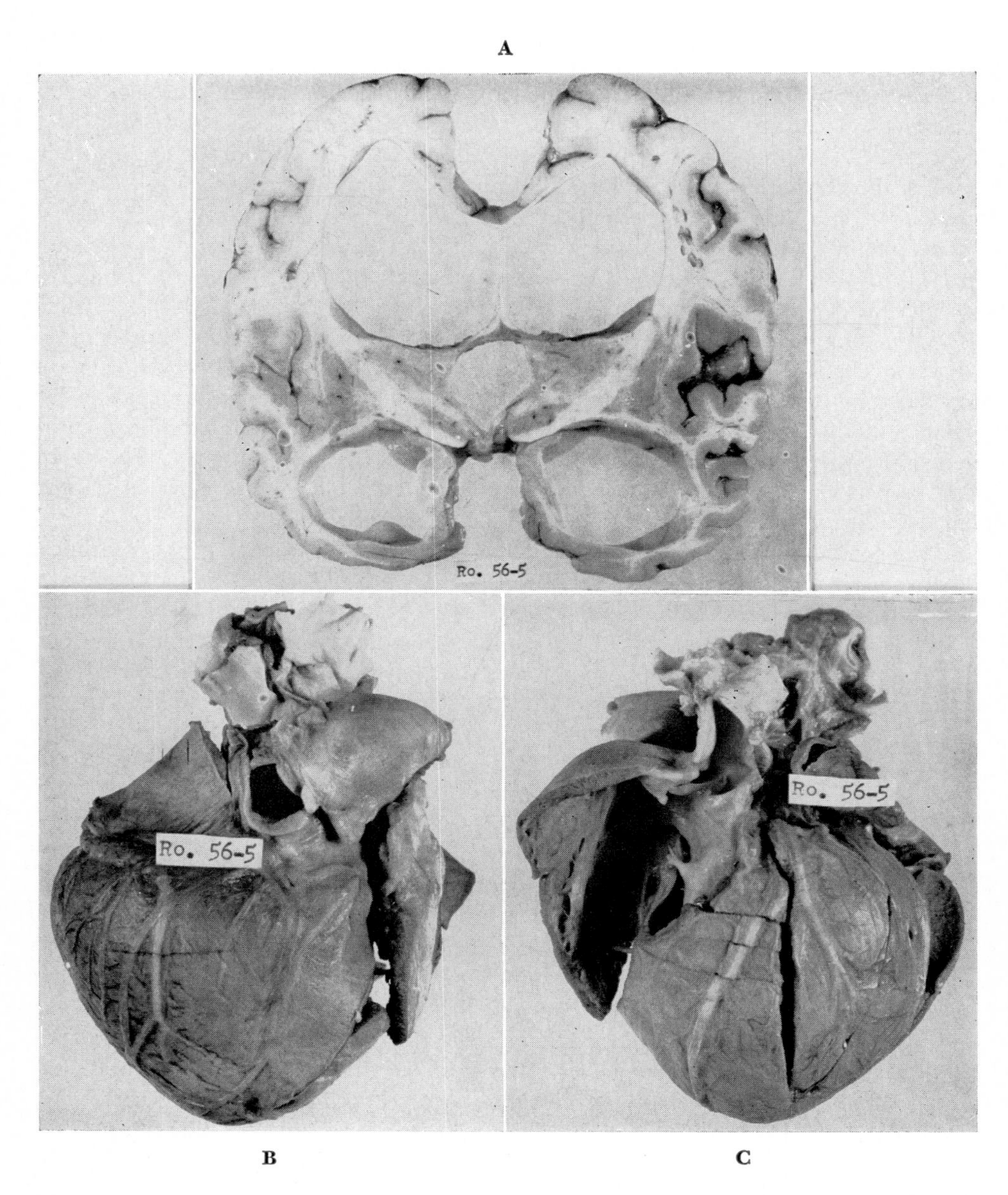

Fig. 9-6. Case of the Hurler syndrome in 10-year-old male. **A,** Pronounced hydrocephalus. Possible involvement of the meninges is responsible. **B** and **C,** Two views of the heart. The coronaries are obviously thickened.

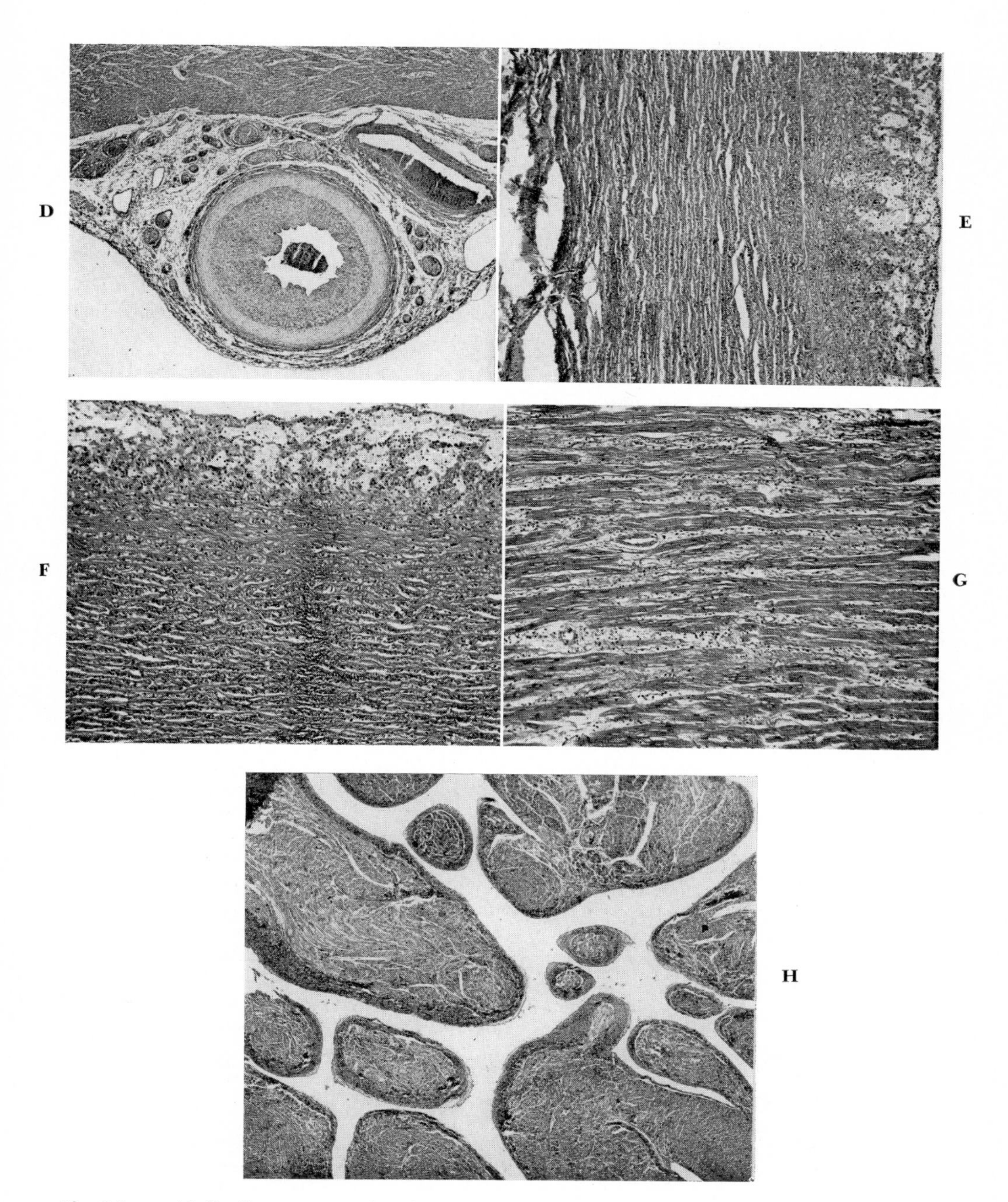

Fig. 9-6, cont'd. D, Coronary arteries showing pronounced thickening of intima. (×30; reduced ⅝.) **E,** Section of pulmonary artery showing enormous thickening of intima. (×67; reduced ⅝.) **F,** Section of aorta showing, in addition to intimal deposit, inclusion-laden connective tissue cells between the elastic lamellae. **G,** Section of myocardium showing infiltration of connective tissue cells laden with inclusion material. (× 100; reduced ⅝.) **H,** Endocardial thickening surrounding the carneous trabeculae of the ventricle is evident. (×30; reduced ⅓.)

mm. Hg). The peripheral arteries of the arms were described as thickened in a 6½-year-old child[159] and there was hypertension (132/100 mm. Hg). Some of the above cases were probably instances of MPS II (p. 346). Catheterization and angiocardiographic studies were reported by Krovetz and associates.[145]

What was interpreted as angina pectoris occurred[51] as early as 4¾ years of age in a child who died at the age of 7 years. The extensive occlusive disease of the coronary arteries discovered at autopsy in this child would suggest that this is the basis of sudden death in many of these patients (Fig. 9-6).

Lindsay[158] stated that systolic murmurs along the left sternal border were so striking in these patients that four of sixteen were suspected of having an interventricular septal defect. There was a similar clinical experience in the group of cases at the Johns Hopkins Hospital. The experience with other heritable disorders of connective tissue, specifically the Marfan and Ehlers-Danlos syndromes, in which cardiac malformations of the conventional types occur with predictably increased frequency, suggests that the same might occur in the Hurler syndrome. Pathologic studies have not corroborated this suspicion (see below). Although some cardiovascular abnormality was present in the great majority of patients who have died, all the changes have been of a specific type, as described later.

The clinical diagnosis is confirmed biochemically by identifying excessive mucopolysaccharide in the urine and by finding metachromatic granules in the circulating lymphocytes or bone marrow cells. Methods for these tests are detailed later (p. 377).

The following narrative by an intelligent and observing father outlines the evolution of the Hurler syndrome up to the age of about 4 years:

> My impression is that her most difficult period was roughly that of her first to second year. Deafness appeared, so far as we could tell, shortly after her first birthday, becoming complete by about 16 to 18 months of age. Around this time the more pronounced abdominal swelling also began to show, and she was sick much of the time. Nights were very difficult for her and everyone during this time, and until a bit beyond 2 years of age, she would cry for hours, perhaps in pain. On the other hand, she has seemed to be a bit less sensitive to outside pain than the other children. After the crying spells began to diminish, her personality became more buoyant. During the last year or more, *angelic* would scarcely be too strong a word. She radiates love and affection and thoughtfulness, coupled with a good sense of humor. Her motor skills have kept up remarkably well; she ate with a spoon before 1 year and has kept it up with normal increase in proficiency; she was diaper-trained by about 2½ years and bed-trained by about 3¼ years, with no unusual effort; although the gait is a bit awkward because of underdevelopment of leg muscles and a very large abdomen, she loves to run and dance and slide and swing. Picture books are great favorites; animals are adored, as are dolls and cuddly toys, toward which she is quite maternal. Vision seems still acute, although cloudiness is apparent in the cornea. She dresses and undresses herself as far as her build permits and is almost fastidious about putting away clothes, hanging things up, removing dishes to the sink after eating, etc. (this behavior pronounced since 3 years of age). Simple cutout jigsaw puzzles she handles well. She understands gestures and expressions perfectly and uses them herself for very efficient communication. During April and May of this year (at the age of 3¾ years) she was a day pupil at a nursery school for the deaf. Since September she has been a Monday to Friday boarding pupil at a state institution for deaf children. Here a very capable teacher seems to be making progress with lip reading and vocalization instruction. Other than the direct Hurler's symptoms, her general health has been reasonably

good: chickenpox; several periods of respiratory infection each year; and occasional (every six weeks or so?) flash fevers to about 103°F., which are over in a few hours, leaving her worn out for a day. Her teeth have never developed fully, even now being little more than widely separated stumps; however, she can handle, and seems to enjoy, practically any kind of food.

My wife and I feel that, at least until quite recently, her intelligence has been essentially normal. She usually learns new patterns of action, or placement of objects, or play, after only one or two repetitions—unless something arouses the stubbornness, of which she has a powerful streak. She watches the other children playing, with close comprehension of their actions and antics, often either joining or copying, nearly always enjoying. She knows all the clothing in the house, often bringing the appropriate items, in proper order, to those of us getting dressed. In driving, she will often back-seat drive, telling me which turns to take, by murmurs and gestures, even when we are several miles from home but headed for it. She sets great store on the proper way of doing things! Her sleep is now peaceful, 11 hours a night and usually an hour's nap; even when she is tired her personality holds up cheerfully. When hurt in any way she usually cries but little; however, the offended member *must* be kissed to make the hurt go away.

It is possible that her rate of development is slowing down; she is learning, or at least responding, among the slowest members of her eighteen-pupil nursery class. Also, recently there has been pronounced increase in the swelling. Our local pediatrician believes that the liver is almost entirely responsible for the more than double normal girth, and that x-ray treatment might offer her a palliative. Should the swelling become much greater, walking will become extremely difficult. Difficulties with respiratory disease might have been too much for her system already, before modern drugs; except for a couple of summer months, there is a constant nasal discharge of varying rate of flow. Her circulation seems to have its troubles, in that lips and fingernails are often very blue.

As further illustration, the following two patients, brothers, are described in detail:

Case 1. P. H. (J.H.H. 818143), the product of a normal pregnancy, is the elder son of unrelated, healthy parents. He was considered a healthy baby, and initial development was uneventful, but a gibbus of the thoracolumbar spine and pectus excavatum were noted at 3 months of age. No specific diagnosis was made until the age of 13 months, when the patient already exhibited many of the classic features of the autosomal recessive Hurler syndrome. He stood at 9 months but walking was poor, partly, the parents feel, because corneal clouding was already dimming vision. Other Hurler features at the age of 13 months included the "gargoyle facies" and broad, short, stubby fingers with clawhands. Most of the other joints also showed early limitation of movement, with flexion contractures in some. The abdomen was prominent, though without hernias, and the lower thoracic cage was flared; the neck was short and thick, and there was a pronounced sagittal ridge. The teeth were widely spaced and poorly formed, and respirations were noisy. Deafness was marked, although there was no evidence of past otitis media.

By 21 months, progression of the disease was obvious, with marked impairment of intellect and enlargement of the head, and the child had ceased to walk. Attempts at toilet training had been unsuccessful. Gross motor and sensory nervous functions were normal and there were no heart murmurs. While showing severe deafness to pure tones of 2,000 and 4,000 cycles per second at 80 to 90 decibels, the child babbled in a relatively normal fashion, indicating that at one time hearing must have been nearly normal.

Laboratory studies at 21 months yielded normal results and included routine hematology, urinalysis, fasting blood sugar, total cholesterol, calcium, phosphorus, albumin and globulin, and alkaline phosphatase. Reilly bodies were not found in the peripheral leukocytes. An electrocardiogram and lumbar puncture were normal, but an electrocencephalogram showed mild diffuse abnormalities. An intravenous infusion of glucose showed a diabetic pattern, but there were no other diabetic stigmata. Glucagon stimulation and an insulin tolerance test were normal.

X-ray films at this time showed slight cardiac enlargement. The long bones showed shortening and widening of the shafts with lack of tubulation. The distal ends of the radii and humeri showed abnormalities in angulation and configuration. The skull was enlarged, with prominence of the frontal and parietal bones, and in the lateral view the sella turcica showed the typical slipper shape. The spinal x-ray films revealed angulation between L1 and L2, with beaking along the arterior surfaces of these vertebrae. The pelvis was wide, with large, shallow, angulated acetabular shelves; coxa vara was present. The metacarpals and phalanges showed shortening and broadening, with the proximal ends pointed, while the ribs were broad and spatulate.

Urinary studies of mucopolysaccharide excretion were performed at the ages of 5 and 7 years. On both occasions considerable amounts of both chondroitin sulfate B and heparitin sulfate were found.

The patient, now 7 years of age, is completely bedfast, exhibiting huge hydrocephalus, with an open anterior fontanelle. Undoubtedly this is playing a large part in the general picture, particularly as a cause of the extreme apathy. The facial features have become progressively more gross, and the corneas are opaque to the extent that the pupils cannot be visualized. Estimates of the hepatomegaly, over the years, have varied from 3 to 8 cm. and of the splenomegaly, from 0 to 2 cm. below the costal margin. At no time has there been evidence of valvular heart damage.

Case 2. M. H. (J.H.H. 1038296), the younger and only sib of Case 1, was noted at birth to have a curved back and a depression of the front of the chest. Despite this he was considered to be a normal baby until, between the ages of 6 and 12 months, his facial features were noted to be taking on appearances similar to those of his brother. He walked at 2 years and learned to utter a few syllables; true speech, however, was never attained. From an early age respirations were noisy, and bilateral inguinal hernias were repaired at 6 weeks and 7 months, respectively.

By the age of 4 years mental retardation was severe, and examination revealed most of the signs of Hurler syndrome. These are tabulated and compared to those of his brother in Table 9. X-ray films at this time were also classic. The spine showed vertebral changes, af-

Table 9. Two brothers with Hurler syndrome (MPS I)

Case 1 *P. H. (J.H.H. 818143)* *5 years*	*Case 2* *M. H. (J.H.H. 1038296)* *4 years*
Weight, 40 pounds	Weight, 42 pounds
Length, 36½ inches; chest, 23 inches	Length, 39 inches; chest, 24 inches
Head circumference, 27 inches (hydrocephalic)	Head circumference, 21½ inches
Severe mental retardation	Mental retardation
Unable to sit or talk; deaf	Able to walk but not talk; deaf
Typical Hurler facies	Same
Edema of eyelids	Same
Wide-spaced teeth	Same
Corneal opacity	Same
Low-set ears	Same
Lanugo	Same
Hands and feet wide, with clawhand	Same
Cool lower extremities	Warm
Slight lumbar gibbus	Large lumbar gibbus
Stiff joints	Moderately stiff joints
Pectus excavatum	More severe pectus excavatum
Ronchi	Same
Liver edge 3 cm. below costal margin	Same
No palpable spleen	Spleen tip 2 cm. below costal margin
No hernia	Surgical repair of inguinal hernias
Decreased femoral pulses	Pulses normal
Uncircumcized	Circumcized

fecting D12, L1, and L2 in particular, and there was anterior "beaking." The bones of the upper extremity were thickened and short, particularly the metacarpals, which showed "pointing" at both proximal and distal ends. The skull was somewhat enlarged, with hyperostosis of the sagittal suture, and the sella turcica was elongated. The pelvis showed shallow acetabula and there was coxa vara. The ribs were typically broad and spatulate with coarse trabeculations.

Urinary studies at the age of 4 years revealed increased excretion of mucopolysaccharide, composed of a large fraction of chondroitin sulfate B and a smaller heparitin sulfate fraction. Routine study of a peripheral blood film revealed no abnormality.

At the age of 5, the boy described as Case 2 has deteriorated further and has ceased to walk, preferring to crawl. His eyesight is poor due to corneal opacities, and his mental function approaches the imbecile level.

Peripheral blood smears were taken from both boys and stained with toluidine blue. Definite metachromatic granules were seen in the cytoplasm of 18% of the lymphocytes of Case 1 and in 10% of those of Case 2.

Pathology

At least forty autopsies have been reported: many individual case reports,[9,15,61,75,97,110,136,143,146,181,203,250,261,270,271,282,284,287,298] two by Jervis,[133] eight by Lindsay and co-workers,[159] and so on. Jackson[123] and others have reported on biopsies of the liver.

Abnormalities have been identified in, among other sites, cartilage, fasciae, tendons, periosteum, blood vessels, heart valves, meninges, and cornea. All of these may contain cells that are thought to be of the fibroblast line and distended with large amounts of deposited material. These are appropriately called "clear cells" by Millman and Whittick,[203] but perhaps it would be preferable to use the more specific designation "gargoyle cells."[277] In addition, collagen in many of these areas has been said to look abnormal in a poorly defined way. Collagen fibers are described by some (e.g. reference 158) as swollen, homogeneous, and lacking in their normal fibrillary characteristics. Material presumably identical to that in the fibroblasts balloons the nerve cells of both the central nervous system and the peripheral ganglia, the nerve cells in the nuclear layer of the retina,[159] the Kupffer cells of the liver, the parenchymal cells of the liver, the reticulum cells of the spleen and lymph nodes, and the epithelial cells of several endocrine organs such as the pituitary[146] and testis. Mental retardation and hepatosplenomegaly are explained by these deposits.

Enlargement and vacuolization of the chondrocytes and osteocytes, as well as of the periosteal cells, are described[24,159] and probably are intimately related to the skeletal malformation.

In the heart, in persons dying after a few years of life, the aortic and mitral valves almost invariably have shown some degree of nodular thickening,[75,159] as well as changes in the chordae tendineae.[24] Functionally both stenosis and regurgitation can result. In the case of Smith and co-workers[261] the histologic picture in the heart valves was dominated by the presence of "gargoyle cells." These have also been seen in the coronary arteries.[49,159,181] Grossly[75] even in young individuals the coronary arteries may "stand out like white cords." Virtually complete occlusion may result from the extensive intimal deposits.[51,59] The aorta[181] and pulmonary artery[75] may also show intimal deposits, presumably of the same material as forms the vacuoles of the cells of various organs. The myocardial cells may show marked ballooning by vacuoles (see photomicrograph, reference 22). Patchy thickening of the endocardium and epicardium is described.[75,159,271]

Of the peripheral arteries, changes have been described in those of the brain, spleen, pancreas, and kidney, as well as in the mesenteric, carotid, radial, and anterior tibial arteries.

Emanuel[75] was able to find thirty-two autopsy reports, with specific description of the heart provided in twenty-six. (Some were undoubtedly instances of MPS II.) Of these, twenty-two had cardiovascular abnormalities (85%). In fifteen patients the mitral valve was deformed, in nine the aortic, in seven the tricuspid, and in two the pulmonary. In three (including Emanuel's case) all four valves, the epicardium, the endocardium, the coronary arteries, and the aorta and pulmonary artery were involved.[159,271]

It is of note that the order of incidence of involvement of the heart valves—mitral, aortic, tricuspid, pulmonary—is precisely as in rheumatic fever. In both situations there are probably operating at least two prominent factors: the metabolic aberration (in one case acquired, in the other inherited) and the hemodynamic stresses. The peak pressures* sustained by the four valves in the position of closure are in the same sequence as the incidence of valve involvement: mitral, 120 mm. Hg; aortic, 80 mm. Hg; tricuspid, 25 mm. Hg; pulmonary, 12 mm. Hg.

Vanace and co-workers[290] described advanced mitral stenosis in a boy who died at the age of 5½ years. No clouding of the cornea was noted, but slit-lamp examination was not done. Lagunoff and associates[147] studied the mitral valve in one case and concluded that two types of cells are present, one containing glycolipid and one containing acid mucopolysaccharide.

A conventional type of congenital malformation of the heart has been thought clinically to be present in three of the patients seen at this hospital. Seemingly, however, no such malformation has been revealed by any of the pathologic studies.

Abnormality of the tracheobronchial cartilages together with that of the upper airways may be responsible for the susceptibility to respiratory infection in these patients. Bronchopneumonia is a frequent cause of death.[133]

Kobayashi[144] demonstrated granules of acid mucopolysaccharide in the epithelial cells of the glomeruli of three patients. He discussed the relationship to the mucopolysacchariduria and the Reilly granules. Cole and associates[47] illustrate a histologic section of skin that was interpreted as showing "marked fragmentation of collagen fibers and mucinous degeneration."

Vacuolated cells have been described in Bowman's membrane by Berliner[19] and by others. Lindsay and co-workers[159] described highly metachromatic granules in the cornea. The literature on the corneal histopathology was reviewed by Scheie and co-workers[248] with addition of information from several cases. The basal layer of the epithelium shows edema, cytoplasmic vacuolization, and metachromatic cytoplasmic granules. Bowman's membrane is replaced in part by large cells with vacuolated cytoplasm and metachromatic cytoplasmic granules. Corneal corpuscles in the stroma likewise contain metachromatic granules. Conjunctival biopsy may be positive in all cases with corneal clouding and has been recommended[248] as a simple diagnostic procedure. The connective tissue of the conjunctiva shows monocytes with toluidine blue–positive granules in the cytoplasm.

---

*All values here are approximations.

These corneal and conjunctival findings are also present in MPS V and probably in MPS IV.

The skin of the fingers was shown by Hambrick and Scheie[103] to be useful for biopsy in MPS I (as well as in MPS V):

> The characteristic cellular lesion of Hurler's was present within the skin from all sites, clinically normal or abnormal. This consisted of a peculiar, granular vacuolization of the cytoplasm of epithelial cells and fibrocytes of the dermis. The degree of involvement of the epidermis may be quite extensive, particularly in the skin of the involved fingers.*

The granules have metachromatic tinctorial properties and are positive for stains relatively specific for mucopolysaccharides.

Extensive changes in the leptomeninges were described by Magee.[181] The coincidence of subdural hematoma in his case makes these changes difficult to interpret. However, others report extensive changes in the meninges.[59,97,243] Millman and Whittick[203] found thickening of the leptomeninges over the cerebral hemispheres and "clear cells" histologically. In Njå's[214] Case 2, an instance of MPS II, there was hydrocephalus with "thickened and milky leptomeninges." The hydrocephalus[243] may be the result of interference with drainage, produced by the deposits characteristic of the disease.[98] The frequency of hydrocephalus (Fig. 9-6*A*) has been underestimated. It is probably an important factor in the cerebral impairment in these patients.

Greenfield and associates[98] describe the central nervous system changes as being predominantly distention of the nerve cells of the cerebral cortex with little or no defect of myelination. A peculiar feature of the Hurler syndrome is "the presence in the centrum semi-oval and medullary cores of the gyri of greatly enlarged perivascular spaces."

Formalin or alcohol dissolves the vacuolar material.[24] Some reported failures[59,159,270] to stain the material in postmortem tissues may have their bases in this fact. Dioxane-dinitrophenol fixative has been useful[159] in preserving the deposited material. To study mucopolysaccharides in the tissues of cases of mucopolysaccharidosis, the best method, in the opinion of Haust and Landing[106] is to cut frozen sections of unstained tissue and then fix in a 1:1 mixture of tetrahydrofuran and acetone. In their view, lead acetate is a poor fixative because it preserves mucopolysaccharide poorly and interferes with metachromatic staining. Scheie and associates[248] found that absolute alcohol, Carnoy's solution, trichloracetic acid, acridine, and lead acetate, in descending order, gave the best preservation of mucopolysaccharides in skin biopsies.

Some have reported that the intracellular deposits take conventional fat stains.[22,105,282] Most, however, have found that the vacuoles do not stain as fat, or stain atypically.[261] Analyses of hepatic and splenic tissue for fat reveal no increase.[110,270,277] The material may stain with periodic acid—Schiff's reagent (PAS) or with Best's carmine. It displays striking metachromasia.[287] Bishton and colleagues[24] suggest that even if precautions are taken to prevent solution of the material deposited in the liver, one cannot expect satisfactory staining of "heparin-type" polysaccharides by the periodic acid–Schiff technique. They recommend use of toluidine blue as a stain in these cases.

---

*From Hambrick, G. W., and Scheie, H. G.: Arch. Derm. **85**:455, 1962.

Histochemical studies led Lindsay and collaborators[159] to suspect that the storage material is glycoprotein. Brante[28] isolated a material, polysaccharide in nature, having 0.9% sulfur, 27% hexosamine, and 26% glucuronic acid, containing no fatty acids by hydrolysis, and representing 10% of the dry weight of the liver. Uzman[287] described two storage materials isolated from the liver and spleen of these patients: (1) a complex polysaccharide containing glucose, galactose, hexosamines, and sulfate, soluble in water and formaldehyde but insoluble in other organic solvents, and staining metachromatically with toluidine blue; (2) a glycolipid, soluble in water and ethanol but not in other organic solvents, and containing fatty acids, sphingosine, neuraminic acid, hexuronic acid, hexosamines, glucose, and galactose. These Uzman refers to as fractions P and S, respectively. Stacey and Baker[265] reported the presence of sulfated polysaccharide fractions as well as of nonsulfated fractions, the latter somewhat related to blood group-specific substances. Brown[30] has proposed a possible molecular structure of the material he isolated in large amounts from the liver of patients with the Hurler syndrome and has referred to it as an oligosaccharide. By his evidence the material is composed exclusively of D-glucosamine and D-glucuronic acid units combined in glycosidic linkage. The material in point may be identical to the type of mucopolysaccharide called heparitin sulfate by Meyer.[193] Meyer and colleagues[196] found large amounts of heparitin sulfate in the liver of one patient.

Dawson[59] thought that the deposits in the brain consisted of phospholipid, although those elsewhere seemed to be mucopolysaccharide. Uzman[287] did not study brain. Meyer[194] found that mucopolysaccharide (both chondroitin sulfate B and heparitin sulfate) was deposited in the brain in appreciable amounts.

The fundamental defect

Straus and associates[270] thought that the Hurler syndrome might be a dystrophy of collagen, and Cole and co-workers[47] also subscribed to this view. These authors based their opinions mainly on the lack of good evidence of this being a lipid storage disease and the fact that contractures of joints and hernia occur, as well as skin changes that Cole interpreted as involving primarily collagen.

On the other hand, Ellis and colleagues[73] considered gargoylism (as they called it) a disorder of lipid metabolism. Washington[298] in his term "lipochondrodystrophy" implied the same theory.

De Lange and co-workers[62] and Strauss[271] thought the storage material might be a glycogen. Lindsay and co-workers[159] suggested that the stored material might be a polysaccharide (such as glycogen) or glycoprotein. Brante[28] studied three cases clinically and histologically and came to the conclusion that the Hurler syndrome is a "congenital enzyme disturbance as regards the metabolism of the mucopolysaccharide or of some of its components, or as regards the binding of the mucopolysaccharide to protein, etc." The qualitatively and/or quantitatively abnormal mucopolysaccharide accumulates at various sites, according to the last view.

Uzman[287] took a slightly different view. He held that the genetic defect is one concerning the metabolism (i.e. synthesis) of "structural polysaccharides," which are normally important building blocks of connective tissue elements.[94]

Dorfman and Lorincz[67] and Meyer and associates[196] found considerable amounts of chondroitin sulfate B and heparitin sulfate in the urine and tissues of patients with the Hurler syndrome—a nice corroboration of the view that this disease is a mucopolysaccharidosis. These polysaccharides have been identified in the brain also.[100] Meyer and collaborators[196] found large amounts of heparitin sulfate in the liver of a patient, and Stacey and Baker[265] found what was probably the same polysaccharide.

The mucopolysaccharides (chondroitin sulfate B and heparitin sulfate) are probably produced in excess; a defect in removal is less likely. Furthermore, the mucopolysaccharides are, by any evidence yet available, "normal"; that is, they have all the properties of those identified in certain normal tissues. (These mucopolysaccharides are not found in the urine of normal persons.) Meyer and colleagues[195] point out that the mucopolysaccharides produced by connective tissue in different sites fall into distinct patterns. Chondroitin sulfate B occurs normally in all connective tissue with the exception of cartilage, bone, and cornea, whereas heparitin sulfate has been isolated only from lung and aorta (and—in large amounts—from amyloid liver). It is suggested, therefore, that connective tissue cells each produce only one specific type of product; for example, cells producing hyaluronic acid cannot produce any of the chondroitin sulfates. Tentatively Meyer and co-workers[196] propose that the Hurler syndrome is a genetic error in the chemical differentiation of the fibroblasts—"a chemical metaplasia." The excessive production of polysaccharides results in the accumulation of these substances, not only in the connective tissue cells themselves but also in the cells of many organs, and the excretion of large amounts in the urine. The Hurler syndrome is, in this view, both a generalized disorder of connective tissue and a storage disease ("thesaurosis"). Storage of lipid in the brain and deficiency of glycogen in the liver are probably secondary effects of the derangement of normal cellular function produced by the storage.

As pointed out earlier, hydrocephalus from meningeal involvement is undoubtedly a factor in the progressive impairment of intellect. Furthermore, a biochemical mechanism common to connective tissue and brain may be faulty. Just as in phenylketonuria and galactosemia, the details of how the normal biochemical and functional status of the brain is disturbed in the Hurler syndrome are unknown.

It is possible that the corneal involvement is a primary feature of the syndrome and not a secondary feature due to the deposit of an anomalous polysaccharide. Corneal grafting might settle the question.

The manner in which abnormal deposits occur in the intima and elsewhere is reminiscent of the handling in rabbits of methylcellulose and pectin,[118,119] both of which are macromolecular carbohydrates. Hueper[119] observed ballooning of cells in the liver, spleen, kidney, arterial intima, bone marrow, and anterior pituitary when pectin was administered intravenously in rabbits and dogs. However, "no lesion was found in the cerebral parenchyma, the vascular system of the brain or the choroid plexus."

The clinicopathologic differences between the Hurler syndrome, on the one hand, and the syndromes of Gaucher and of Niemann and Pick, on the other, are suggestive evidence that the storage material in the Hurler syndrome is not lipoid. In neither Gaucher's disease nor Niemann-Pick disease are the parenchymal cells of epithelial organs involved. (Thannhauser[277] refers to Gaucher's disease as "reticular and histiocytic cerebrosidosis" and to Niemann-Pick disease as "reticular and histiocytic sphingomyelinosis.") The bone lesions of Gaucher's disease, such as the Erlenmeyer flask deformity of the long bones, result from the involvement of the marrow and not from the implication of fundamental skeletal building blocks as in the Hurler syndrome.

In reference to the skeletal lesions of the Hurler syndrome, it is noteworthy that chondroitin sulfate B and heparitin sulfate have not been identified in normal bone and cartilage. (See p. 29.)

Prevalence and inheritance

Prior to the first edition of this book (1956), few cases had been described in Negroes and we had not seen the disease in a Negro. Since then several such cases have been reported,[12,64,79,92,130,149,272,278] and we have observed a Negro family with three affected members (Fig. 9-3). The characteristic facies may be more easily overlooked in the Negro child. The syndrome has been reported in Chinese,[41,77] in Oriental Indians,[99,187] and in Egyptians.[11]

MPS I displays features of inheritance consistent with a recessive autosomal trait.[102] Parental consanguinity[25,102] is frequent, and affection of multiple sibs of both sexes without the occurrence of affected individuals in the preceding generation ("familial" characteristics) is often the case. There are no well-documented descriptions of skeletal deformities or other abnormalities in close relatives of patients with full-blown cases to suggest that partial expression of the trait in the heterozygous state may occur. Concordance in identical twin sisters has been described.[216] Craig[51] described the disorder in a twin brother and sister.

In 1950, Jervis[133] reviewed the information on 103 families described in the literature. When the ratio of affected to unaffected sibs was corrected by the method of Bernstein and that of Lenz, statistically significant agreement with the expected 1:3 ratio was obtained. (Jervis did not recognize the possibility of a second genotype, the sex-linked recessive form—see below. If sex is not taken into account, a sex-linked recessive disorder will fulfill satisfactorily certain of the criteria for an autosomal recessive trait: both parents are phenotypically normal and one fourth of all children are affected. In the group analyzed by Jervis there were ninety-three affected males and fifty-two affected females.) Cousin marriages are *known* to have occurred in eleven of the 103 families and probably actually occurred in more. Using Hogben's formula, Jervis calculated that a 10% consanguinity rate would correspond to a phenotype frequency of 1 in 40,000.

MUCOPOLYSACCHARIDOSIS II (MPS II, Hunter syndrome)

Clinical manifestations

Usually MPS II is in all respects less severe than MPS I. But here, as in MPS I, leading features are stiff joints (with, for example, clawhands), dwarfing, hepatosplenomegaly, and gross facial appearance responsible for the designation "gargoylism." However, mental deterioration progresses at a slower rate, lumbar gibbus does not occur, and progressive deafness is a frequent feature. Nodular skin lesions are sometimes present on the posterior thorax or arms. Clouding of the cornea of clinically evident degree has not been observed;* this is

*The only possible exception to this statement is represented by one of twelve affected males in a kindred reported by van Pelt.[291,292] The patient was a 3¼-year-old boy who was said to have "weakly positive" corneal clouding. However, van Pelt did not examine the patient personally, slit-lamp examination was not done, and by the time of report the patient had died as a result of complications of surgery for umbilical hernia.

the clearest difference between MPS I and MPS II. In older patients with MPS II, slight corneal clouding may be evident on the slit-lamp examination, but the involvement is minimal. (The features distinguishing MPS I and MPS II are outlined in Table 11.) Atypical retinitis pigmentosa occurs in cases of MPS II.[114] Some of the oldest survivors in the kindred (Fig. 9-11) reported by Beebe and Formel[15] are blind as a result of the retinal changes.[76] The patient often survives to his thirties; the oldest known patient with MPS II died at the age of 60 years.[76]

Changes in the head of the femur with precocious osteoarthritis are usually present in older patients. The foot is of the pes cavus type. The fifth toe is often overlapping. Hooper's patient[114] was operated upon for talipes equinovarus at the age of 17 years.

Changes in the skin[154] in the form of grooving and either ridged[47] or nodular[7] thickening, especially over the upper arms and thorax, have been described. In two of the reports[7,47] the changes were strikingly similar, especially as to location—"symmetrically distributed in an area of about 6 by 10 cm., extending from the angle of the scapula towards the axillary line." (See Fig. 9-8.) This distribution is probably the characteristic one.[100] Hypertrichosis is usually striking.

The occurrence of papilledema in these patients (Figs. 9-7 and 9-10) has suggested hydrocephalus, or at least increased intracranial pressure. The patient shown in Fig. 9-7 retained the fundus picture of "papilledema" for at least ten years. Optic atrophy was described in two sibs by Davis and Currier.[58] Consistent with the development of atypical retinitis pigmentosa,[114] the electroretinogram becomes "extinguished."[93]

Petit mal seizures developed in the patient shown in Fig. 9-7. The deafness in this patient, when tested at age 24 years, appeared to be of the perceptive type.

Despite long-standing hepatosplenomegaly, manifestations of hepatic dysfunction are usually minimal. In a 29-year-old patient[261] with fairly marked hepatosplenomegaly, cephalin flocculation, thymol turbidity, serum proteins, prothrombin time, and Bromsulphalein excretion were all unequivocally normal.

In Hunter's historic report[120] he remarked on the occurrence in one of his patients of cardiomegaly and both systolic and diastolic murmurs. As noted on p. 325, follow-up suggests that one and possibly both brothers died cardiac deaths in their late teens. Pulmonary hypertension is frequent in patients with MPS II (Fig. 9-9).

Death from "heart failure" (either congestive or coronary artery in type) often occurs before the age of 20 years. Of the patients described by Smith and associates,[261] one died at the age of 28 years and another was "reasonably well" at 29 years of age. Hooper[114] described a 37-year-old patient who was still living. In two of his other patients, death occurred at 20 and 30 years of age, respectively. The oldest patient in my series is now 34 years old, and another died at age 32. (See Fig. 9-7 for one of these.) Beebe and Formel[15] described nine well-documented cases of the Hurler syndrome in one family. Five had died at an age in excess of 40 years. There were four survivors—45, 43, 17, and 14 years of age, respectively. Follow-up[76] showed that one affected male had died at the age of 60 years. (See Fig. 9-11.)

Murray[208] described a 43-year-old patient with MPS II and marked respiratory

A

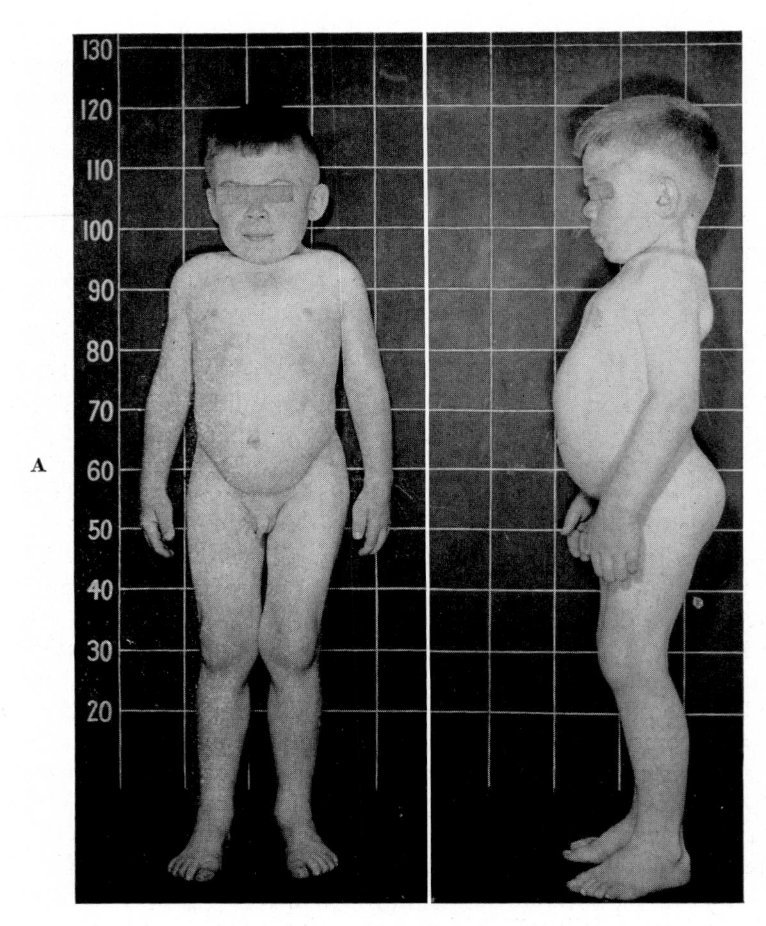

Fig. 9-7. Typical case of the Hunter syndrome, or MPS II (I. S. 204375). **A,** At the age of 10 years. This patient, 22 years old in **B,** had dysostosis multiplex, deafness, "chronic rhinitis," exertional dyspnea, hepatomegaly, restricted joint mobility, hydrocele, and hernia, but no splenomegaly or corneal opacification. Mentality was retarded. The patient graduated from high school because of courtesy promotions. He read voluminously, especially Ellery Queen novels! No inclusions could be demonstrated in the white cells. The testes were small and soft. However, the patient shaved daily and erections and nocturnal emissions occurred. Vision was 20/100 in the right eye, 20/30 in the left. A startling finding was bilateral papilledema, probably long-standing, with "bone corpuscle" pigmentary degeneration of both fundi, especially the right. A peculiar feature was the subjective response to administration of thyroid extract (p. 386). The patient died at age 32 years. Autopsy showed cerebral atrophy with internal hydrocephalus, extensive involvement of the heart valves, and in the cornea (which was not grossly cloudy but had a "deep haze" on biomicroscopy) accumulations of material with the staining properties of mucopolysaccharide.

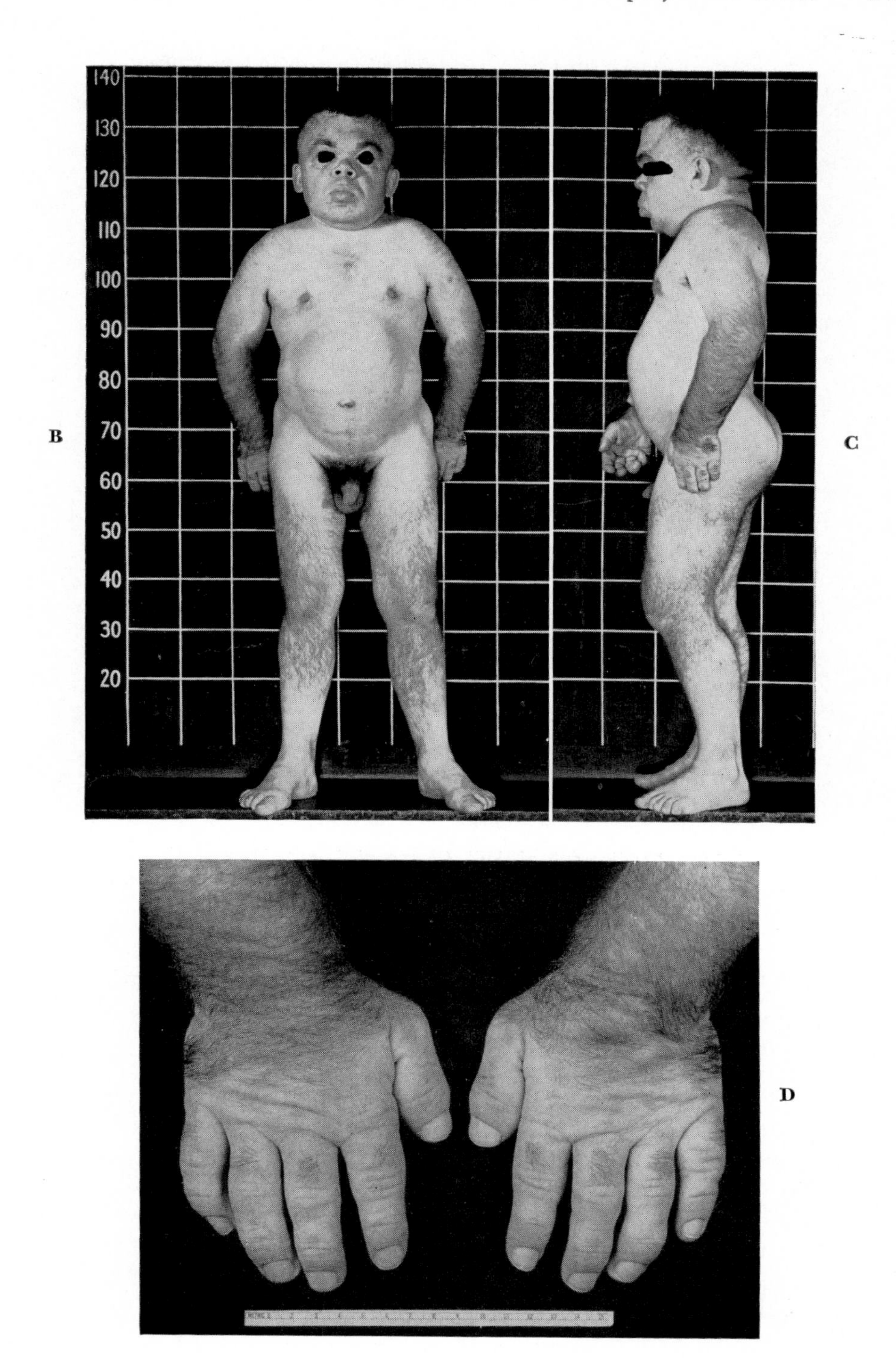

Fig. 9-7, cont'd. B and **C,** Same patient as in **A,** at the age of 22 years. **D,** Hands of same patient.

Continued.

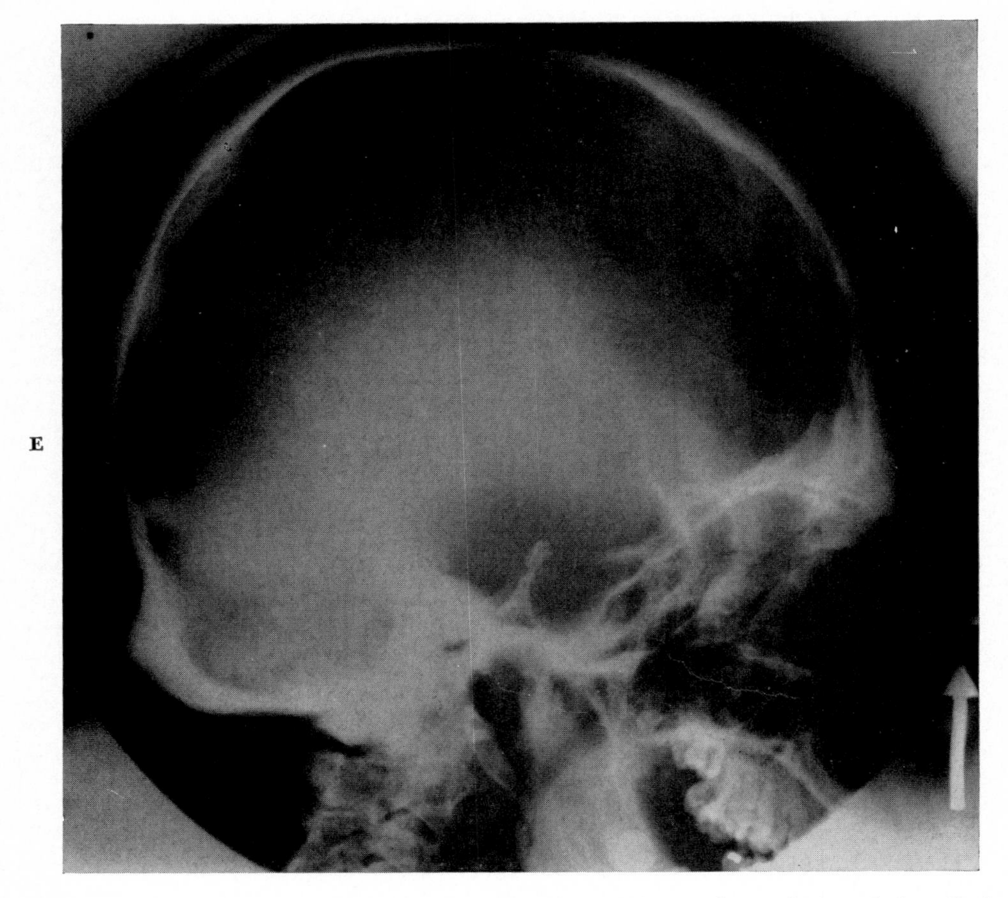

Fig. 9-7, cont'd. E, Lateral radiograph of skull. Characteristic anterior pocketing of the sella is present. There are obvious frontal and occipital areas of hyperostosis. The mastoid air cells are underdeveloped and in general the mastoid is more dense than normal.

disability. The man had sufficient intelligence to do defense work during World War II and to work as a flagman on construction jobs thereafter. Clinical features were stunting of growth, limitation of joint mobility, deafness, coarse facies, short neck, kyphoscoliosis with mild pectus excavatum, hernias, hepatosplenomegaly, and pallor of the optic discs with visual impairment. Deformity of the larynx and nasopharynx and enlargement of the tongue seemed to be responsible for airway obstruction. This impression was supported by the marked relief afforded by tracheostomy, which the patient had for over ten years. Kyphoscoliosis, restriction of chest movement, upper airway obstruction, chronic respiratory infection, and abnormalities of diffusion from parenchymal involvement in the basic process are mechanisms in the respiratory disability of the mucopolysaccharidoses.

Case 3. W. B. (605145), age 33 years, has typical clinical and chemical features of MPS II. As is often the case in X-linked recessive states in which affected males do not have children, the family history is negative.

Skeletal features common to several of the mucopolysaccharidoses are demonstrated by

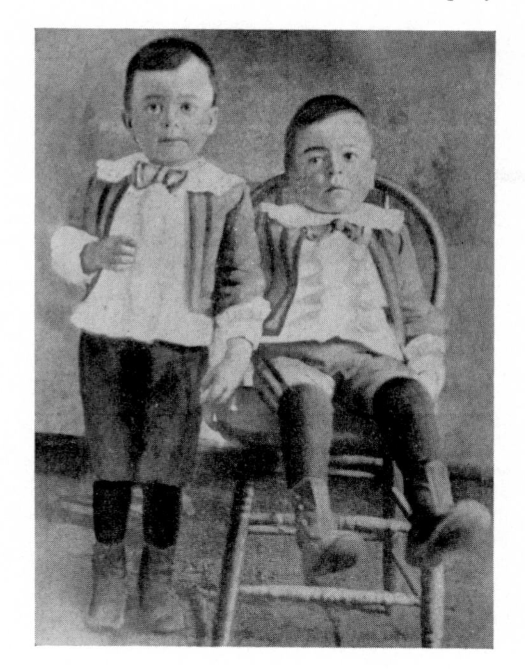

F

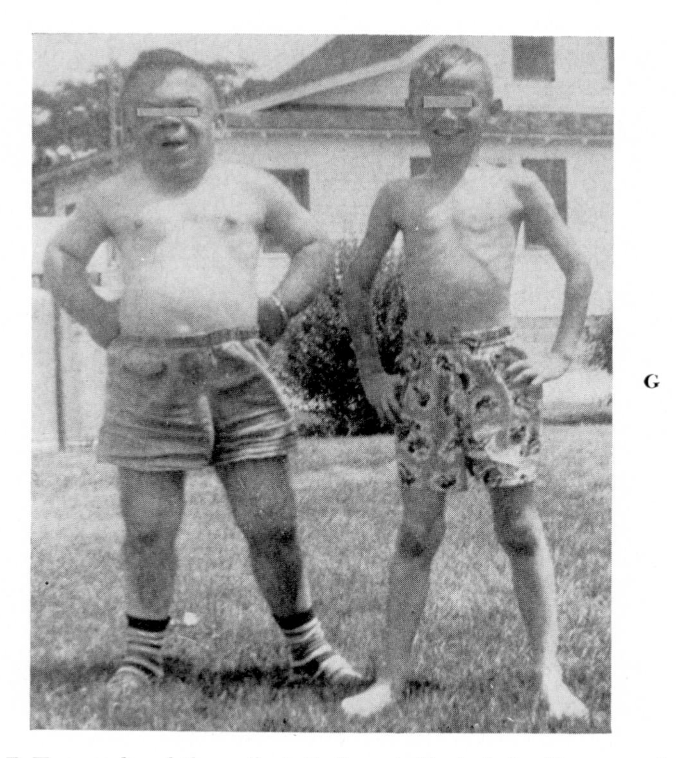

G

Fig. 9-7, cont'd. F, Two uncles of the patient. Both probably had the Hunter syndrome. **G,** The propositus (on left), 22 years of age, and his unaffected brother (on right), 8 years of age.

Continued.

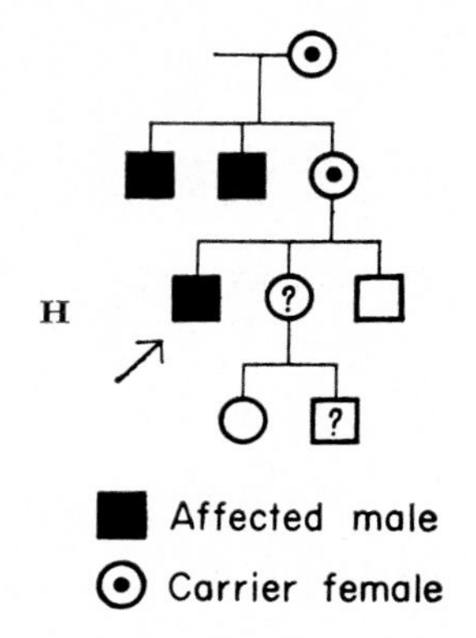

Fig. 9-7, cont'd. H, Pedigree. The propositus is indicated by the arrow.

Two maternal uncles, **F,** had the Hunter syndrome with characteristic skeletal features, deafness, and symptoms of cardiac incompetence. They died at the ages of 12 nd 17 years, one having been found dead in bed. The patient's parents are normal and he has two normal siblings. A young nephew of the patient may have the disease; I have not had an opportunity to examine the child but the descriptions are suggestive.

The possible occurrence in four males in three generations is consistent with, and at least mildly indicative of, inheritance of the trait as a sex-linked recessive. Lamy and associates[151] have also presented a pedigree with affected males in three generations.

Meyer[194] was able to demonstrate relatively large amounts of chondroitin sulfate B and heparitin sulfate in the urine of the propositus. No chemical difference from the autosomal recessive form of the disease was demonstrated by these studies.

clinical and x-ray examination. However, he is 66 inches tall—unusual in this disease (Fig. 9-9). His parents are tall and he has had exceptionally good care throughout his life. Although intellect is clearly affected, the impairment is not uniform. He attended a topnotch private school and, although he did not graduate, he received advanced instruction in economics. He works in his father's stock exchange office and reads the *Wall Street Journal.*

Hernias were repaired at ages 6 and 14 years. Splenectomy for suspected Banti's disease was performed at age 8 years and operations for knock-knees at ages 12 and 14. A hearing aid has been worn from age 7 years.

Episodic faintness beginning about age 29 was interpreted as due to hypoglycemia and was helped by a high-protein diet. The mild breathlessness present for most of his life he attributed to limitation in chest expansion. Several episodes of heart failure were precipitated by respiratory infections.

Examination revealed the facial features of "gargoylism," some limitation of motion in all joints, clawhands, and peculiar high-arched feet with the fifth toe overlapping the side of the foot. By slit-lamp view the cornea showed a slight haze, deep in the stroma and more pronounced in the lower third. By direct inspection, however, the corneas were perfectly clear. The second sound in the pulmonary area was markedly accentuated. The liver was five fingerbreaths below the right costal margin.

Laboratory studies showed bilirubin of 1.4 mg.%, 30% BSP retention in 45 minutes, glucose tolerance tests with glucose levels of 32 and 46 mg.% at 4 and 5 hours, respectively, and uric acid consistently above 7 mg.%

Chest x-ray films showed prominent pulmonary arteries and generalized enlargement of the heart (Fig. 9-9). Cardiac catheterization showed pulmonary artery pressure to be 109/45 mm. Hg, with moderate elevation of end-diastolic pressure in the right ventricle and mild elevation in the left ventricle. Electrocardiogram showed the changes of right ventricular hypertrophy. Respiratory function studies showed marked reduction in vital capacity (37% of predicted) and, by spirogram, there was evidence of moderate airway obstruction. Isuprel produced no change.

Both chondroitin sulfate B and heparitin sulfate were present in the urine in excess. In

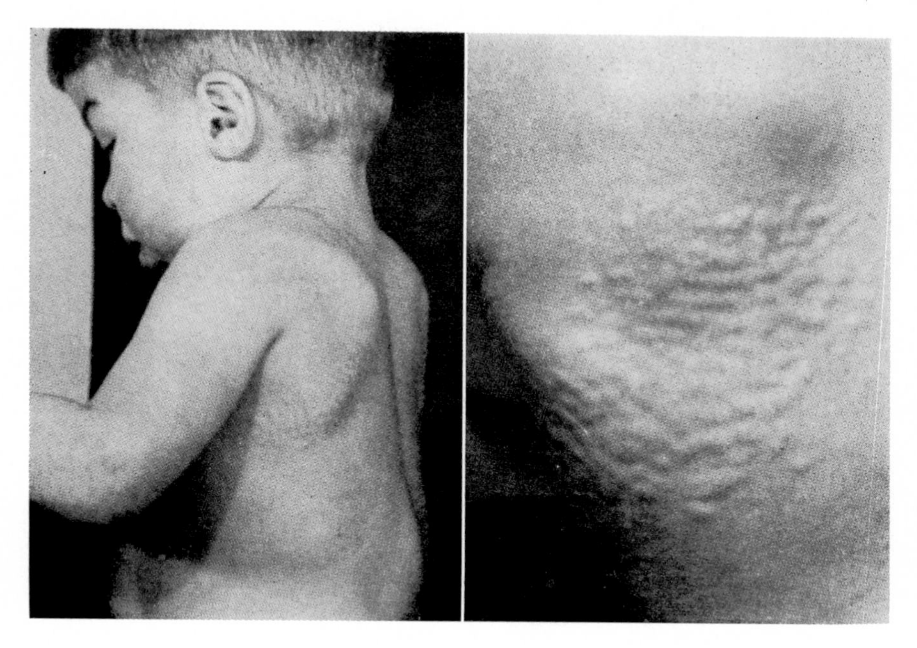

Fig. 9-8. Skin changes in MPS I and MPS II (From Andersson, B., and Tandberg, O.: Acta Paediat. **41**:162, 1952.)

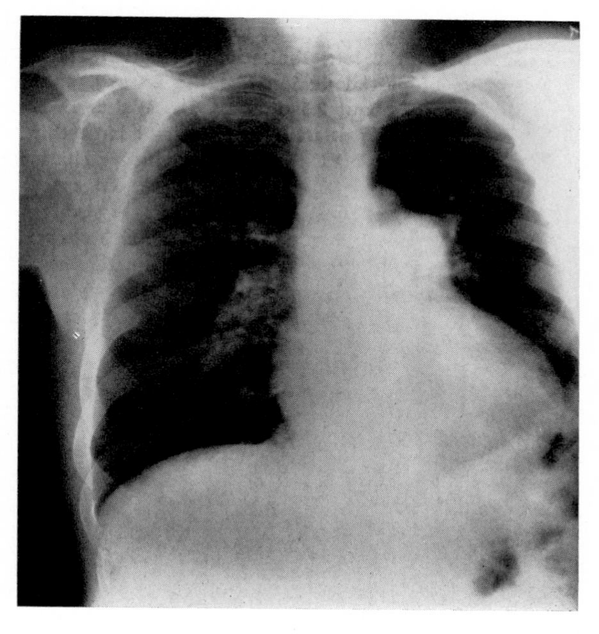

Fig. 9-9. MPS II. Chest x-ray film in W. B. (see text), 33-year-old patient with severe pulmonary hypertension.

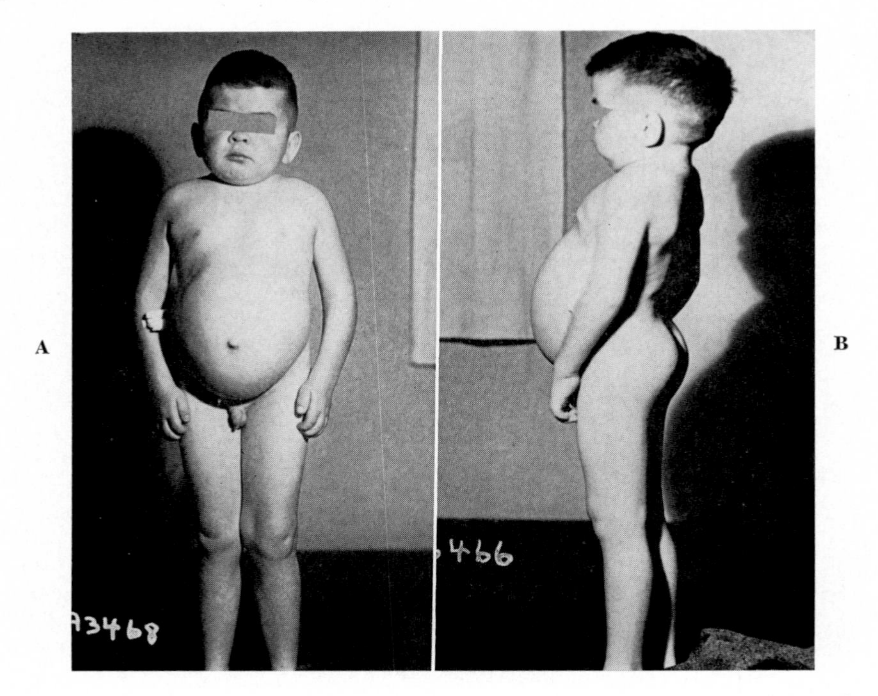

Fig. 9-10. J. M. J. (U53195), 10 years old, was noted to have a short neck, and large head at birth, had frequent colds and trouble in breathing, because of a "low bridge" of the nose, and had noted limitation of joint movement. However, he had always done well in school and was in the fifth grade. In a school examination he was found to "need glasses," and papilledema was discovered by the ophthalmologist consulted. There had been no headache or vomiting and no impairment of vision so far as the patient was concerned. Examination revealed, in addition to the features obvious in the photographs, the liver to be enlarged 4 cm. below the right costal margin and the spleen 2 cm. below the left; limitation of motion of the elbows, wrists, toes (which were fixed in a position of partial flexion like the fingers), ankles, knees, and spine; height of 44½ inches; papilledema of about 2.5 diopters. Dr. Walter E. Dandy performed ventriculograms which showed "symmetrically dilated ventricles and large third ventricle, aqueduct of Sylvius and fourth ventricle, and air in all the cisternae, including chiasmatis and interpeduncularis, and, curiously, the large main trunks of the subarachnoid spaces but no air in the branches. The main trunks were terminated in large bulbous ends. It was, therefore, communicating hydrocephalus with congenital absence of the terminal branches of the subarachnoid space." (The quotation is from Dr. Dandy's operative note.) Choroid plexectomy was performed in an effort to relieve the hydrocephalus. Histologically, the excised choroid plexus appeared atrophic. The patient died two weeks after operation, of an infectious complication. Autopsy was not performed. This patient resembles closely the one pictured in Fig. 9-7, who also had papilledema that has, however, not been progressive. The photographs, **A** and **B,** demonstrate the general skeletal changes, prominent abdomen, and clawhands. In **C** and **D** is displayed the bilateral papilledema.

the circulating blood, 20% of the lymphocytes had metachromatic granules in the cytoplasm when stained with toluidine blue.

Pathology

In general the changes are identical to those described for MPS I. Histologically, even the cornea may show qualitatively the same changes as in MPS I (Fig. 9-7), even though clouding is not evident grossly.

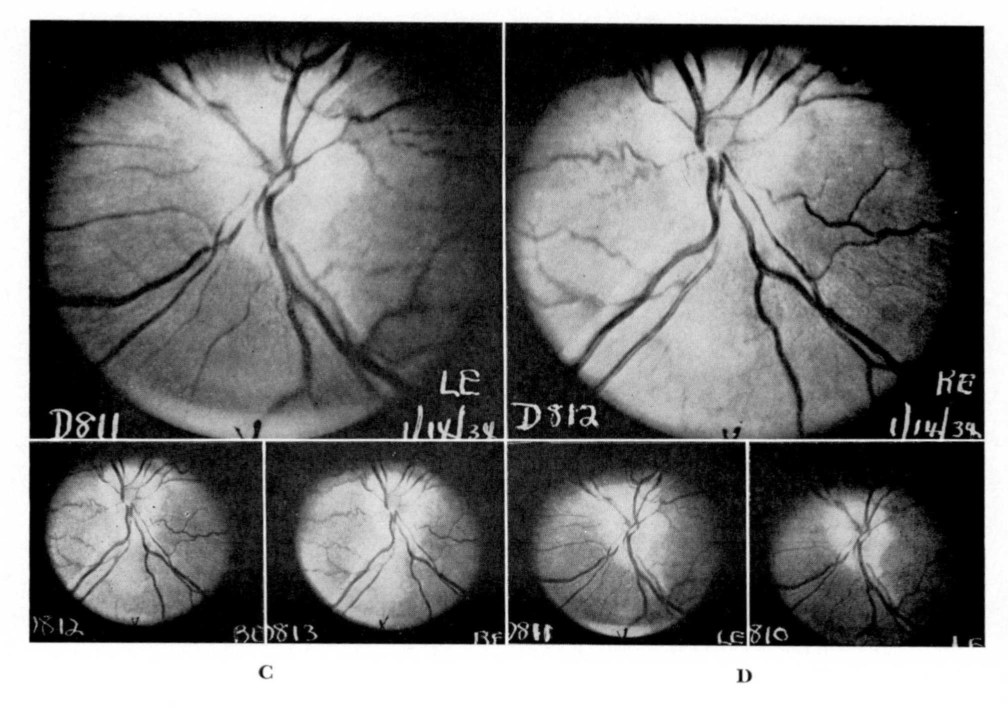

C D

Fig. 9-10, cont'd. For legend see opposite page.

Multiple abnormalities of the middle and inner ear were discovered in one twice-reported case.[261,304]

The fundamental defect

Patients with MPS II excrete excessive amounts of chondroitin sulfate B and heparitin sulfate in the urine. Although some[276] have claimed that the proportions of the two mucopolysaccharides differ in MPS I and MPS II, others[179] have been unable to demonstrate a quantitative or qualitative difference in the mucopolysacchariduria of the Hurler and Hunter syndromes. Such is not a contradiction to the conclusion that MPS I and MPS II are genetically distinct and must have different fundamental defects. The fact that two mucopolysaccharides are excreted suggests that the derangement in mucopolysaccharide metabolism in these disorders is at some step shared in common by them. It is likely that several such steps, each under separate genetic control, exist.

Prevalence and inheritance

The Hunter syndrome appears to be only about one fifth as frequent as the Hurler syndrome.

So far as is known, no patient with any of the six types of mucopolysaccharidosis discussed here has procreated. A few mature spermatozoa were seen on testis histology in one case of MPS II.[261] The patients with MPS II and those with the Scheie syndrome (MPS V) may be capable of reproduction. Because of the low gene frequency, it is statistically unlikely that the spouse would be a

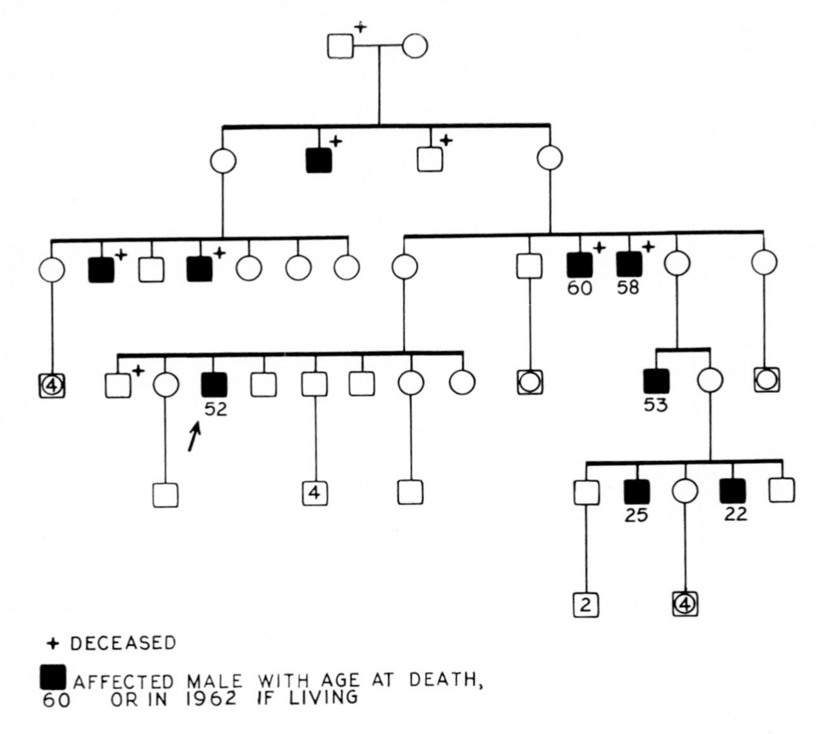

Fig. 9-11. MPS II. Updated (1963) pedigree of kindred reported by Beebe and Formel.[15] (Courtesy Dr. A. E. H. Emery, now of Manchester, England.)

carrier of the gene, unless, of course, the mating is consanguineous. In the X-linked Hunter syndrome, all sons of an affected male would be unaffected and all daughters would be carriers.

In the case of an X-linked trait which is of such a nature that the affected males do not reproduce, it can be shown that one third arise by new mutation in the X chromosome which is given to the affected son by his mother and that two thirds are inherited from the mother through an X chromosome in which the mutation occurred in an early generation.[175] If the mutation occurred in the maternal grandfather or grandmother no second case might occur in the family. Thus, a typical X-linked pedigree pattern is expected in only a minority of cases. There are, nonetheless, numerous reports of an X-linked pedigree pattern for the Hunter syndrome,[15,37,55,114,169,203,214,275,291,292,304] and in many other instances[47,61,75,120,134,169,170] this theory of inheritance is consonant with the known facts. Njå[214] first proposed that cases without corneal opacity are most likely to show X-linked recessive inheritance. Lamy's analysis[151] corroborated Njå's suggestion. Whereas about 90% of all reported patients with "gargoylism" had cloudy cornea, only about 60% of male patients showed the sign.

In the report by Beebe and Formel[15] nine cases were described, occurring in four generations of a family of Dutch extraction that has resided in the Catskill Mountains for about 250 years. Of nineteen males, nine were affected. Of sixteen female sibs of affected males, none was affected. All nine affected males were related through their mothers, who were presumably carriers. Furthermore, they were all descended from the same female ancestor, who was almost certainly likewise a carrier or who perhaps started the disease (by mutation), just as Queen Victoria probably initiated hemophilia[268] in the royal houses of Europe. Five other females could be identified as carriers by reason of affected brothers and sons. Six females had borne only normal children. (See Fig. 9-11.)

Most of the patients with "gargoylism" who survived beyond the age of 20 years were male. In Jervis' survey,[133] which concerned "gargoylism" generally and probably included cases of MPS I, MPS II, and MPS III, of which only MPS II is X-linked, the sex was stated in 145 cases. Of these, ninety-three (64%) were male. Of 112 sibships, sixty-five could, by reason of the fact that all affected individuals were male, represent the hypothesized sex-linked variety of the disease. There were twenty-seven sibships with more than one affected individual; of these, twelve had only males affected, four had only females affected, and in eleven both males and females were affected. The average age of the affected in dividuals in the sibships with more than one affected individual, all males, was 6.65 years. The comparable value for the sibships containing both male and female affected individuals was 10.02 years. Although this appears to contradict the rough impression that the patients with the sex-linked variety are older when they come to medical attention and when they die, it must be remembered that these collected sibships may contain some in which the trait was inherited as an autosomal recessive; these may weigh down the average. It is likely that some females with the Sanfilippo syndrome (MPS III), an autosomal recessive, survive beyond age 20.

Again following Jervis' survey,[133] the cornea was analyzed (1) in the isolated female cases plus the sibships with affected persons of both sexes and (2) in the isolated male cases plus the sibships with affected persons all male. In the case of multiple affected sibs all affected persons in that sibship were counted as having cloudy cornea if one was said to show it. In sibships of the first type, the cornea was described in sixty-nine individuals, of whom fifty-one (74%) had corneal clouding. In category 2, the cornea was described in seventy individuals, of whom thirty-nine (55.6%) had corneal clouding.

Parents of the subjects with the Hunter syndrome (and the other five mucopolysaccharidoses) have been invariably unaffected. Study of urinary mucopolysaccharides has provided no sure method for identifying the heterozygous female.[37] Study of skin fibroblasts may, however, be such a method. In skin fibroblasts from males with the Hunter syndrome, Danes and Bearn[56] have demonstrated intracellular accumulation of mucopolysaccharides, by staining with toluidine blue. In the fibroblasts of mothers in such cases a proportion of cells have a normal appearance with this stain, whereas the remainder show mucopolysaccharide accumulations identical to those in the hemizygous affected males. The fathers show no abnormality. The observations provide strong proof of X-linked inheritance; they also support the Lyon hypothesis (p. 19).

MUCOPOLYSACCHARIDOSIS III

(MPS III, Sanfilippo syndrome, polydystrophic oligophrenia, heparitinuria)

Although it is inherited as an autosomal recessive, as is MPS I, MPS III is distinct clinically and biochemically from MPS I and MPS II.[185a]

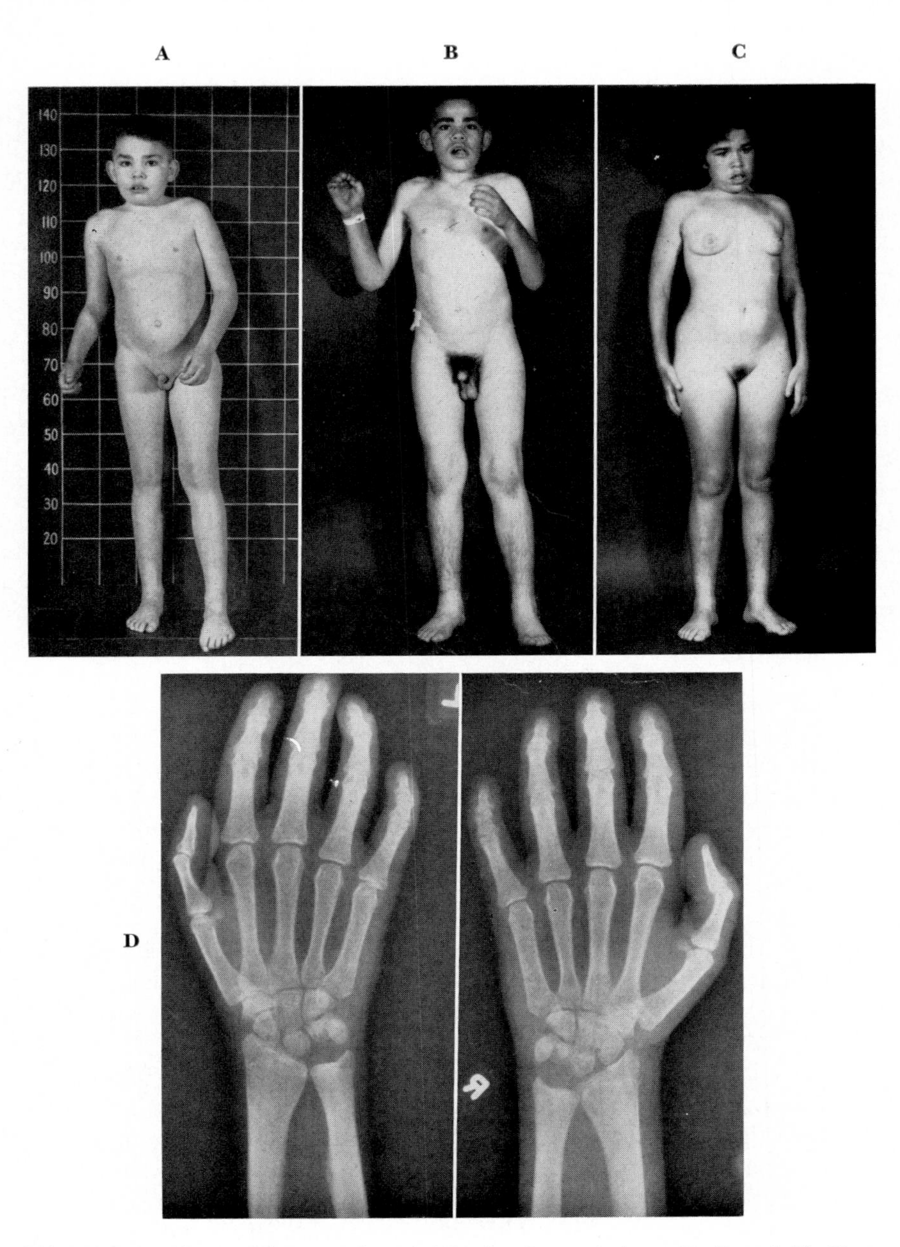

Fig. 9-12. MPS III (the Sanfilippo syndrome). The brother and sister (D. F. and M. F.) are described in detail in the text. **A,** D. F., age 10. **B,** D. F., age 16. **C,** M. F., age 15. **D,** Hands in M. F. at age 15. **E,** Spine in D. F., age 16. Minimal changes are present at the anterior surfaces of the lumbar vertebrae. **F,** Spine in M. F., age 15. Other than possible straightening of the vertebral column, no abnormalities are seen. **G,** Skull in M. F., age 15. Thickening of the calvarium, especially in the occipital area, is striking. (From McKusick, V. A., Kaplan, D., Wise, D., Hanley, W. B., Suddarth, S. B., Sevick, M. E., and Maumenee, A. E.: Medicine **44:**445, 1965.)

Clinical manifestations

In brief the clinical characteristics are severe mental retardation and relatively less severe somatic changes.[246] Intellect deteriorates so that by school age mental retardation is evident and by the teens is outspoken. Because good bodily strength is combined with severe mental defect, management is often a problem. Clouding of the cornea does not occur. (In the patients of Sanfilippo and associates[246] corneal changes were detected in one of five patients subjected to slit-lamp examination.) Hepatosplenomegaly is only slight or moderate. Stiffness of

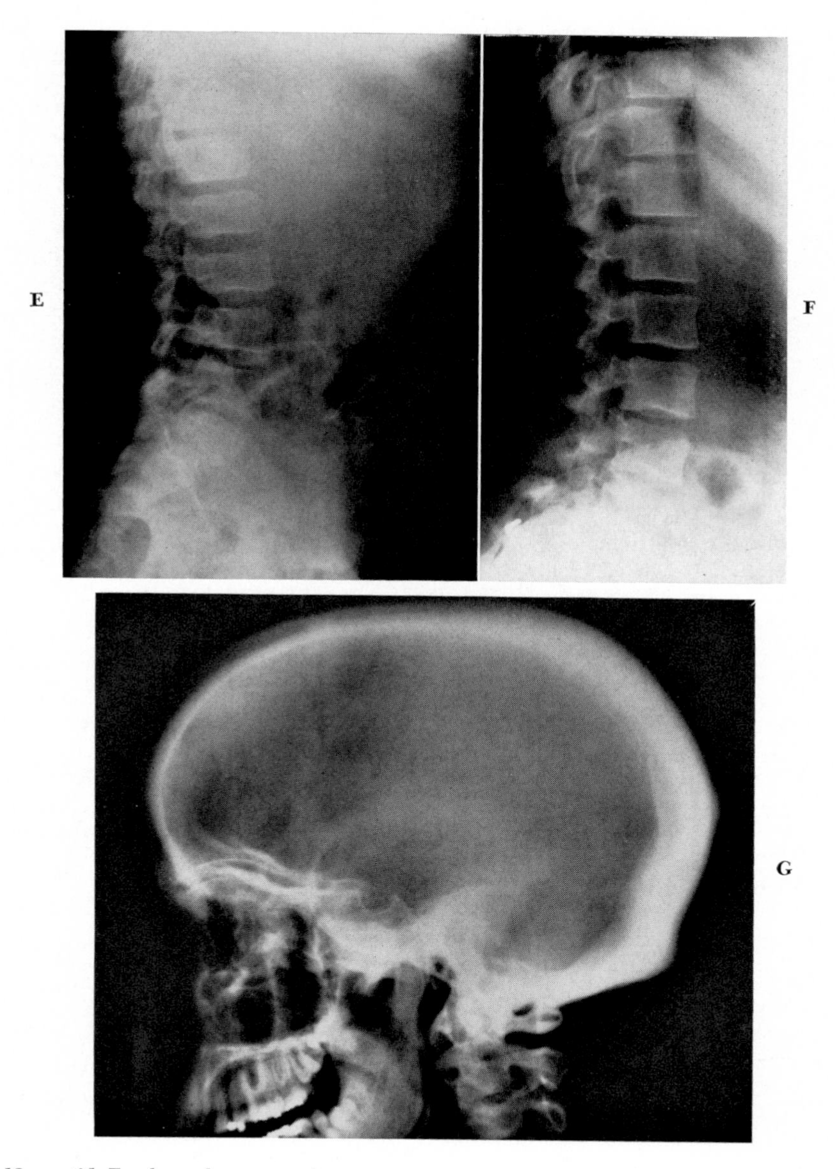

Fig. 9-12, cont'd. For legend see opposite page.

all joints occurs, as in MPS I and MPS II, but is less severe. Dwarfing also is only moderate, and radiologically the skeleton shows minor changes only. The calvarium is dense and the ribs are moderately thickened. Changes in the anterior surface of the bodies of the lumbar vertebrae (Fig. 9-12*E*) are present in some cases; the corners are beveled.

Cardiac abnormalities have not been described in these patients. This disorder is probably compatible with survival to the third or fourth decade.

The following patients are sibs:

Case 4. D. F. (799359), born July 20, 1947, was first seen in February, 1958 (Fig. 9-12). The parents are apparently unrelated. Both are of German ancestry, but several generations separate them from the ancestors who immigrated to this country. For the first four years of life the boy was not considered abnormal. In the latter part of his fourth year an increase in aggressive behavior was noted. Thereafter, agitation increased markedly. He started school at age 6 years but was able to attend only about six weeks because he would not sit still in class or follow instructions. His speaking ability deteriorated rapidly in the seventh and eighth years. The patient was at that time noted to have a "potbelly." At the age of 9 years, as part of his agitated behavior, he acquired the habit of clapping his hands as he walked around and of pounding the walls with the flat of the hands. The diagnosis of the Hurler syndrome was first made at the age of 10 years.

The appearance in 1958 is well illustrated by Fig. 9-12*A*. All features are consistent with mild Hurler syndrome: coarse facial features, short neck, suggestively clawhands, and prominent abdomen. He was of normal height, however, and had no enlargement of the liver and spleen. Examination of the eyes under anesthesia showed no abnormality. X-ray films showed the long bones of the extremities and the ribs to be somewhat enlarged. The vertebrae were judged normal. Dr. Karl Meyer of Columbia University found mucopolysaccharide in the urine, 36 mg. per liter, most of which was heparitin sulfate; there was no chondroitin sulfate B.

At the age of 12 years the patient stopped talking altogether and made only animal-like sounds. He also became totally incontinent, requiring the wearing of diapers. A stiff manner of walking was noted and the patient stopped growing. At age 14 years a left inguinal hernia was repaired but recurred six months later. "Curling of the fingers" and inability to extend the elbows fully were noted at the age of 15 years. During that year also, puberty occurred with development of pubic hair and a deeper voice and enlargement of the phallus. He was always a mouth breather and had frequent respiratory infections. Whereas the first teeth were normal, the second teeth were widely and irregularly spaced and small. During the fifteenth year, severe generalized seizures had their onset.

Examination at the age of 16 years showed an agitated, severely retarded boy (Fig. 9-12*B*). Fine lanugo-like hair covered the back and buttocks. The bridge of the nose was depressed, the nares were patulous, and the lips were large. The mouth was held open constantly. The neck was strikingly short and thick. The liver edge was 4 cm. below the right costal margin. The spleen was not felt. The elbows and fingers could not be fully extended. No cardiac abnormality was detected by physical examination, electrocardiogram, or chest x-ray study.

X-ray films showed thickened calvarium and distal tapering of the radius and ulna bilaterally. Again the cornea was clear by slit-lamp examination.

In 1963 the patient was found to excrete heparitin sulfate, 123 mg. per liter, in the urine. (Urine volumes were, however, rather small. Three days were required to collect about one liter.)

Case 5. M. F. (1084542), born July 25, 1948, was first seen in August, 1963, at the age of 15 years (Fig. 9-12*C*). She was more intelligent than her brother, used some words and phrases, and was toilet-trained. Menses began at the age of 12 years.

The patient began school at age 6 years and for two years apparently performed satisfactorily. In her third year she began to be inattentive and agitated and refused to sit still in class. She became excited and aggressive when with other children. Hearing loss was first noted at age 7 and was progressive thereafter. At age 10 or 11 years limitation of motion of the elbows and fingers was noted. Speech deteriorated, and repetition of words or phrases when she was agitated became a feature. She would bite her fingernails until bleeding occurred.

The permanent teeth were late in developing and were irregularly spaced. Unlike her brother, she would sit quietly and watch television. She was a mouth breather and snored.

Examination revealed, as in the brother, depressed nasal bridge, patulous lips, crowded, irregular teeth, short neck, enlargement of the liver 3 cm. below the costal margin, and limitation in extension of the elbows and fingers. Unlike the brother, she had a flat abdomen. The skin showed lanugo-like hair generally. Examinations of the eyes (including slit-lamp examination) and heart revealed no abnormality.

When the patient was studied in 1963, heparitin sulfate was excreted in the urine in large amounts—about 83 mg. per liter. (As in the brother, urine volumes were small and about three days were required for collection of one liter.)

In the brother and sister, 20 and 28%, respectively, of the peripheral lymphocytes contained metachromatic granules on staining with toluidine blue.

The father (H. F. F., 1084513) and the mother (S. F., 1084544) showed no abnormality in the physical examination, skeletal x-ray films, or urine mucopolysaccharide excretion. The mother has no other children.

Pathology

No reports of postmortem findings in recognized cases of the Sanfilippo syndrome are available.

The fundamental defect

Patients with MPS III excrete large amounts of heparitin sulfate in the urine. Only this mucopolysaccharide is excreted in excess.

Prevalence and inheritance

MPS III is inherited as an autosomal recessive. An estimate of its frequency is even more of a guess than in the cases of MPS I and MPS II. Some patients are probably institutionalized and not recognized as cases of the Hurler syndrome because of the relatively inconspicuous somatic features. The disorder may occur appreciably more often than "one out of every 100,000 to 200,000 people" as estimated by Terry and Linker.[276] It has been reported in the American Negro.[255]

MUCOPOLYSACCHARIDOSIS IV (MPS IV, Morquio syndrome, keratosulfaturia)

Probable cases of the Morquio syndrome were reported as cases of achondroplasia by Osler[219] and by Voisin and Voisin.[294] (See Fig. 9-13.) Simultaneously and independently in 1929 Morquio,[206] of Uruguay, and Brailsford,[27] of Birmingham, England, gave definitive descriptions. Thereafter it became known as the Morquio syndrome or, less frequently, as the Morquio-Brailsford syndrome. Other designations used in the literature include chondro-osteodystrophy and eccentro-osteochondrodysplasia.

In the last few years other features of this disorder, in addition to merely the orthopedic ones, have come to attention. During a thirty-year-period after the publication of Morquio and Brailsford's descriptions, a wide variety of cases found their way into the literature under the Morquio sobriquet.[224,228,258] Many of these, with our increased knowledge of hereditary skeletal disease, are not now considered to have been the same disorder as that described by Morquio. Cases pigeonholed with the Morquio syndrome include what we would now classify as X-linked spondylo-epiphyseal dysplasia,[124] multiple epiphyseal dysplasia,[262] diastrophic dwarfism,[150,180] or other entities.[34,108,239] Robinow[234] included under the "Morquio syndrome" a considerable number of entities clearly dis-

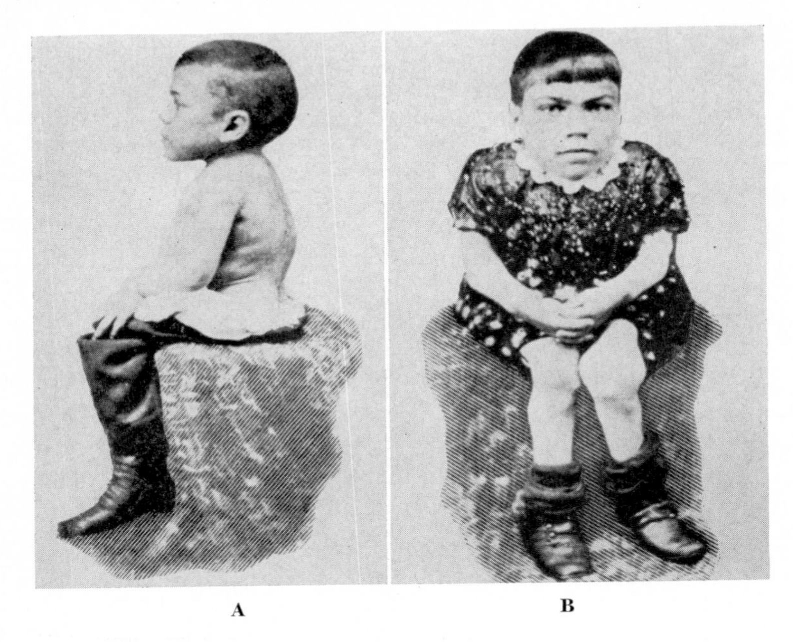

Fig. 9-13. MPS IV (the Morquio syndrome). Brother, **A,** and sister, **B,** in a French Canadian family reported by Osler in 1897. (From Osler, W.: Trans. Cong. Amer. Phys. **4**:169, 1897.)

tinct from that described by Morquio and Brailsford and stated that inheritance could be dominant, recessive, or X-linked. Partly because of the "trashcan" state of the nosography of the Morquio syndrome, it was proposed, when corneal abnormalities were discovered in the Morquio syndrome, that a new entity was involved, deserving a new name. Wiedemann,[301] followed by Zellweger and colleagues,[309] gave the name Morquio-Ullrich syndrome to the disorder in cases having the typical skeletal features described by Morquio and Brailsford but also with corneal changes. This, despite the fact that Ullrich[285] probably did not describe personal cases of this type!

It is my impression that the entity described by Morquio and Brailsford was precisely that in which we now recognize extraskeletal involvement. (An attempt should be made to establish this by follow-up of the cases resported by these workers.) It is contended that *no* patients with skeletal changes identical to those described by Brailsford and Morquio fail to develop ocular (and usually cardiac) manifestations if they survive to adolescence. This is the view advanced also by Maroteaux and Lamy[184] and by Robins and associates[235] Although a view opposite to the above has been expressed,[95] it is not established, I feel, that any "residual Morquio syndrome" exists after the "Morquio-Ullrich" cases have been removed. It must be kept in mind that the extraskeletal manifestations have appeared relatively late in some cases. The discovery of a characteristic type of mucopolysacchariduria in these cases has provided a further basis for definition of the Morquio syndrome. In view of the above considerations, the entity is here called simply *the Morquio syndrome.*

Clinical manifestations

Differences of the Morquio syndrome (MPS IV) from MPS I will be emphasized. These patients are strikingly dwarfed (Fig. 9-14), and in older children the skeletal findings are quite distinctive. In the first year or two of life, however, the lumbar spine may show beaking similar to that of the Hurler syndrome; for other reasons, as well, MPS I and MPS IV are difficult to distinguish, at that stage, by any means except the urinary pattern of mucopolysaccharide excretion. This point is well illustrated by the cases described below. See also Fig. 5 of Robins and co-workers[235] Later, the radiologic changes in MPS IV are different from those of MPS I, flat vertebrae being particularly characteristic of the MPS IV. All the bones are markedly osteoporotic. Drastic changes in the femoral heads are present, from an early age (Fig. 9-14). Knock-knees are usual.

The wrists are enlarged and the hands misshapen. However, the joints are usually not stiff. Indeed some, such as the wrists, may be hyperextensible. A barrel chest with pigeon breast ("sternal kyphos") is surmounted by a short neck. The stance is semi-crouching (Fig. 9-14). The facies is characteristic, with broad mouth, prominent maxilla, short nose, and widely spaced teeth. The corneas become diffusely opacified,[295] but this process progresses more slowly than in MPS I. Clouding obvious to the unaided eye is usually not evident until after the age of 10 years. Grossly it has the appearance of a filmy haze rather than a ground glass appearance as seen in MPS I and MPS V. Hernia probably occurs with increased frequency; inguinal hernia was present in Brailsford's case.[27] Neurologic symptoms frequently result from spinal cord and medullary compression. Spastic paraplegia is frequent (Plate 1, *A*), and respiratory paralysis occurs in late stages.[6] Intelligence is normal or only mildly impaired.

In our series[179] aortic regurgitation was present in three teen-age patients from three unrelated families. Most patients with MPS IV die before 20 years of age. Two affected brothers known to us (E. J. J. and R. E. J.) died at ages 37 and 40 years; both had aortic regurgitation.* This cardiac abnormality has not been noted in previous reports of the Morquio syndrome.

Garn and Hurme[90] described abnormality of both the deciduous and the permanent teeth in three sibs out of nine. The six unaffected sibs had normal dental enamel. The evidence of defect consisted of thinness of enamel, shown by x-ray film, tendency of the enamel to fracture and flake off, and a dull grayish appearance of the crowns of the teeth. The diagnosis of MPS IV was supported by the description of corneal opacities in a follow-up report.[234] Cases reported by Ruggles,[241] by Whiteside,[300] and by Gasteiger and Liebenam[91] were probably also instances of MPS IV.

Cases 6 and 7. The patients shown in Fig. 9-14 were 5 and 15 years old at the time of this study. However, x-ray films covering the entire life span were available for review. Five sibs were normal. Another sib, male, died at 33 hours. He may have been affected. The father and mother were of English and English-Irish ancestry, respectively, and were not known to be related.

The elder brother had clubbed feet at birth. The diagnosis of Morquio syndrome was made at the age of 13 months. In the younger brother the diagnosis was made at birth because his facial appearance was like his brother's and because motion at the elbows was limited. An inguinal hernia was repaired at the age of 14 months in the younger brother.

*Information courtesy Dr. John J. Rick, Coldwater, Mich.

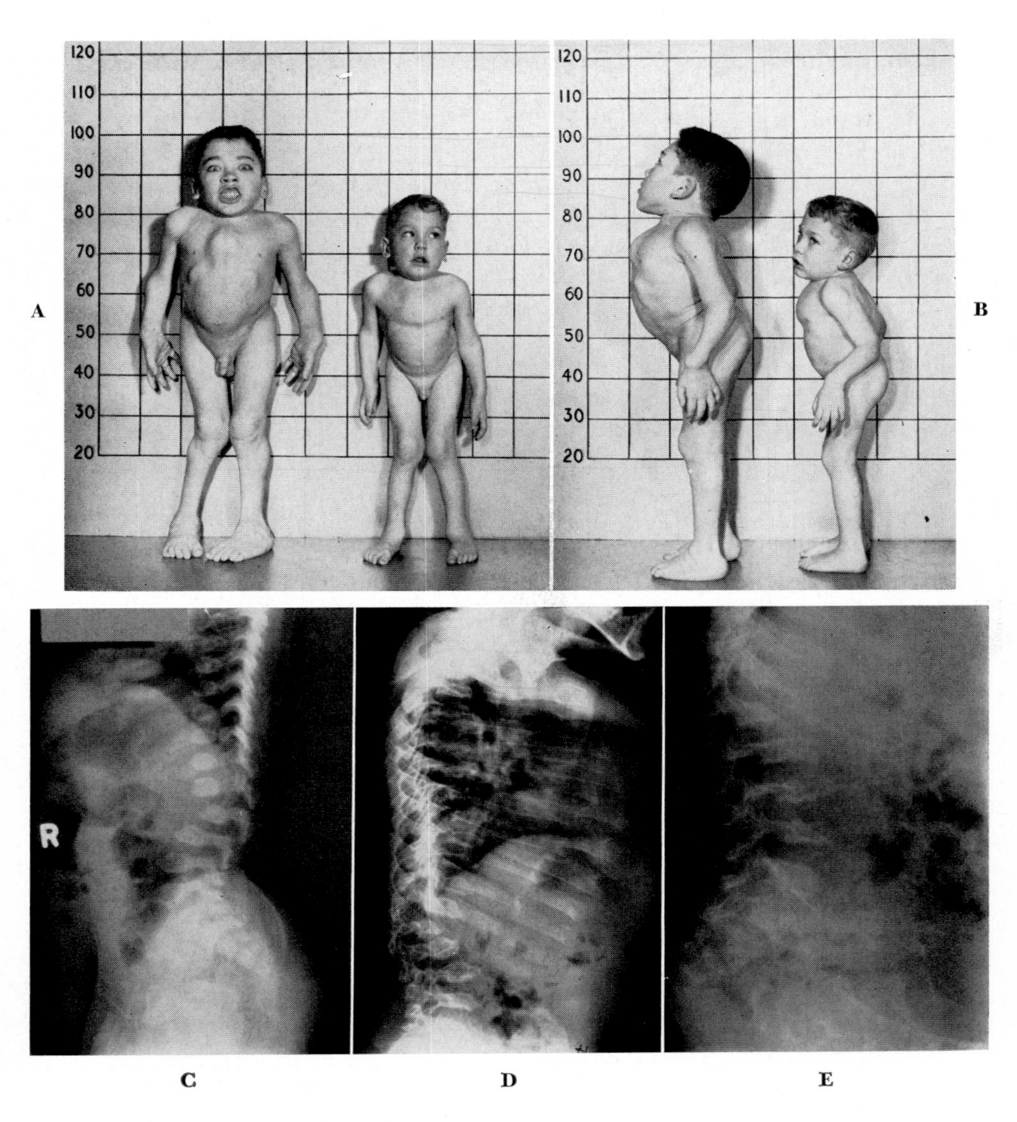

Fig. 9-14. MPS IV (the Morquio syndrome). These brothers (J. G. and M. G.) are described in detail in the text. **A,** and **B,** General appearance. **C** to **E,** Spine in J. G. at ages 13 months, 8 years, and 15 years, respectively. The early changes are indistinguishable from those of MPS I (cf. Fig. 9-2*C*). Marked osteoporosis and platyspondyly are later developments. **F** and **G,** Hands in J. G., age 15, **F,** and in M. G., age 5, **G.** Osteoporosis and abnormal shapes of all bones are demonstrated. **H,** Spinal curvature in M. G., age 5. **I,** Left hip in M. G., age 5. See Plate 1, *B,* for corneal clouding in older boy. (From McKusick, V. A., Kaplan, D., Wise, D., Hanley, W. B., Suddarth, S. B., Sevick, M. E., and Maumenee, A. E.: Medicine **44**:445, 1965.)

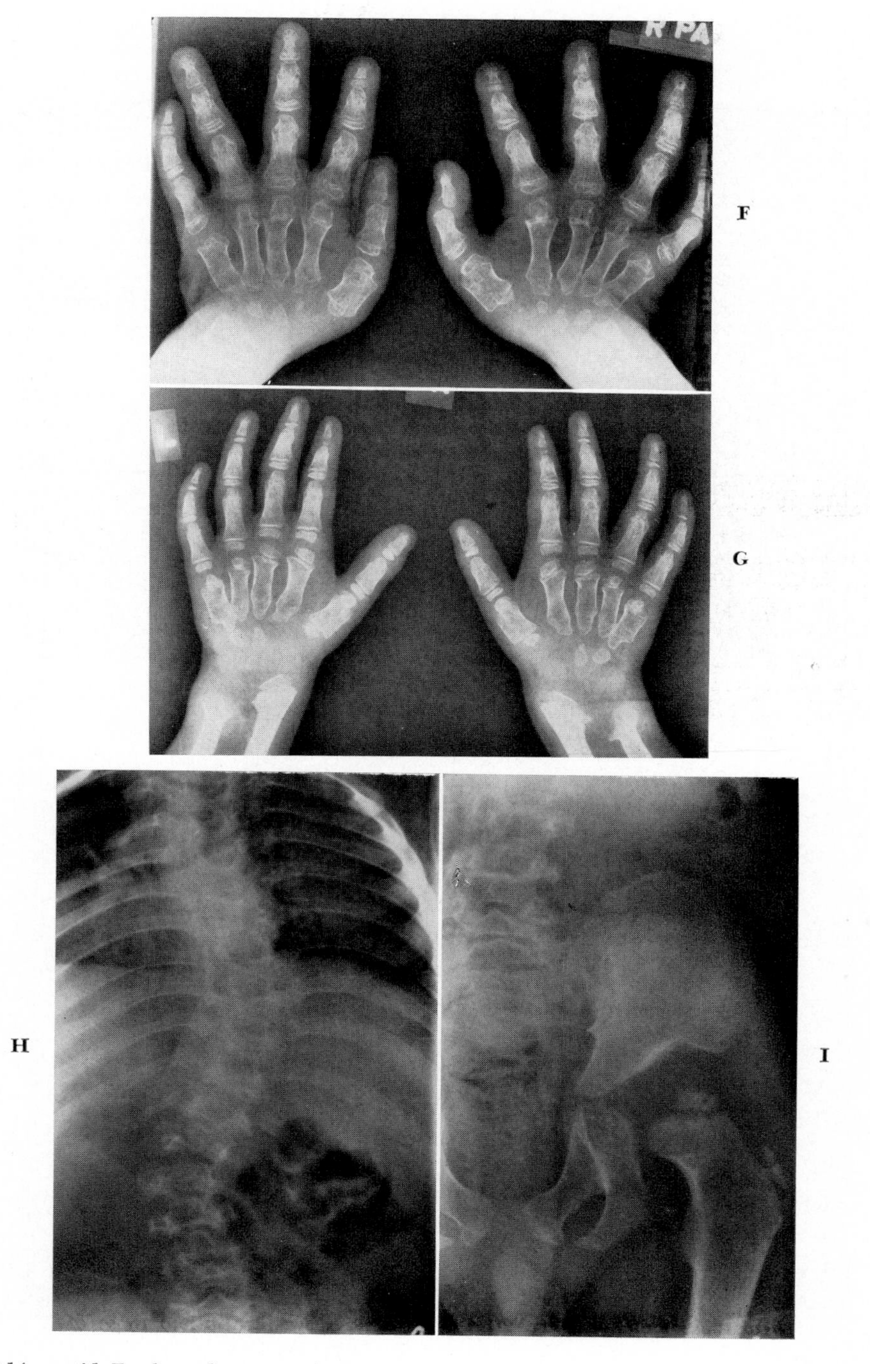

Fig. 9-14, cont'd. For legend see opposite page.

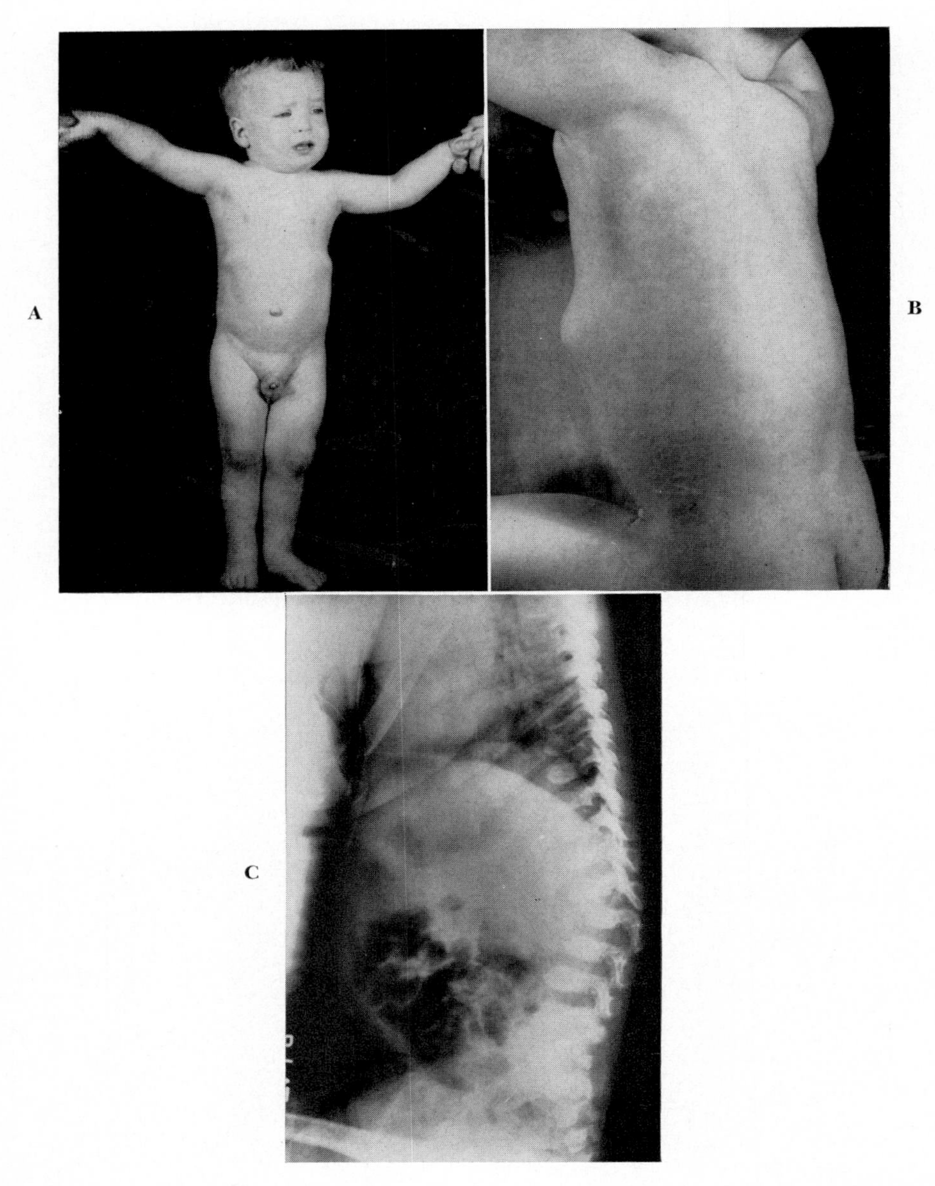

Fig. 9-15. MPS IV (the Morquio syndrome) in a 21-month-old boy, J. J., described in detail in the text. **A,** General appearance. **B,** Lumbar gibbus and flared lower ribs are demonstrated. **C,** X-ray view of the spine. As in Fig. 9-14*C,* the findings are identical to those of MPS I. **D,** Hands. **E,** Feet. (From McKusick, V. A., Kaplan, D., Wise, D., Hanley, W. B., Suddarth S. B., Sevick, M. E., and Maumenee, A. E.: Medicine **44**:445, 1965.)

A diffuse corneal haze was noted when the elder brother, then age 8, was first seen by an ophthalmologist. Examination four years later showed little change.

The findings of the physical and radiologic examinations are well shown in Fig. 9-14. Intelligence was normal. The older brother (age 15 years) had lax wrists, the murmur of aortic regurgitation, and diffuse grayish clouding of the cornea bilaterally. Slit lamp showed the corneal changes to be primarily in the posterior stroma and to be uniformly distributed. The 5-year-old brother had slight but definite clouding of the cornea demonstrable by slit lamp only. A granular appearance of the fundus in the macular area was observed. Urine from only the younger boy has been studied so far, and 60 to 70 mg. of keratosulfate per liter were found. Peripheral blood films for both boys revealed no lymphocytic metachromatic granules, but the majority of the polymorphonuclear leukocytes showed varying numbers of small clusters of clearly defined metachromatic granules within the cytoplasm, i.e. Reilly granulation.

Case 8. J. J. (1106668) is the only child of parents who are not known to be related. No similarly affected persons are known in the family of either parent.

The child was first studied at the age of 21 months (Fig. 9-15) because of skeletal abnormalities, which had been noted first at the age of 4 months: flaring of the lower rib cage and a lump on the lumbar spine. Mental and physical development had been normal, otherwise. His first tooth erupted at the age of 4 months, and he stood with support at 8 months, walked at 17 months, and spoke two-word sentences at 19 months. At the age of 6 weeks he had been hospitalized for two weeks with vomiting, jaundice, and mild enlargement of the liver. Neonatal hepatitis was diagnosed. A right hydrocele was found at that time.

Main features of the examination at the age of 21 months are shown in the illustrations. The flaring of the lower ribs and the lumbar gibbus are striking. The hands are stubby and less extensible than one would expect for a child of this age. The liver was palpated 3 cm. below the right costal margin, the tip of the spleen was palpable, and a small umbilical hernia and right hydrocele were present.

The child was initially thought to show a typical instance of MPS I, i.e. the autosomal recessive variety of Hurler syndrome.

Significant investigations included the following. Slit-lamp examination revealed fine gray stippling in the corneal stroma bilaterally, most marked in the periphery. X-ray films showed a gibbus at L1, a slight reduction in height of the vertebral bodies, and an anteroinferior lipping of the lumbar vertebral bodies. The metacarpals and phalanges showed swelling of the shafts with slight tapering distally. Coxa valga was present. No lymphocyte inclusions were found in the peripheral blood but, as in the previous two cases, the cytoplasm of approximately 50% of the polymorphonuclear leukocytes contained clusters of small but clearly defined metachromatic granules.

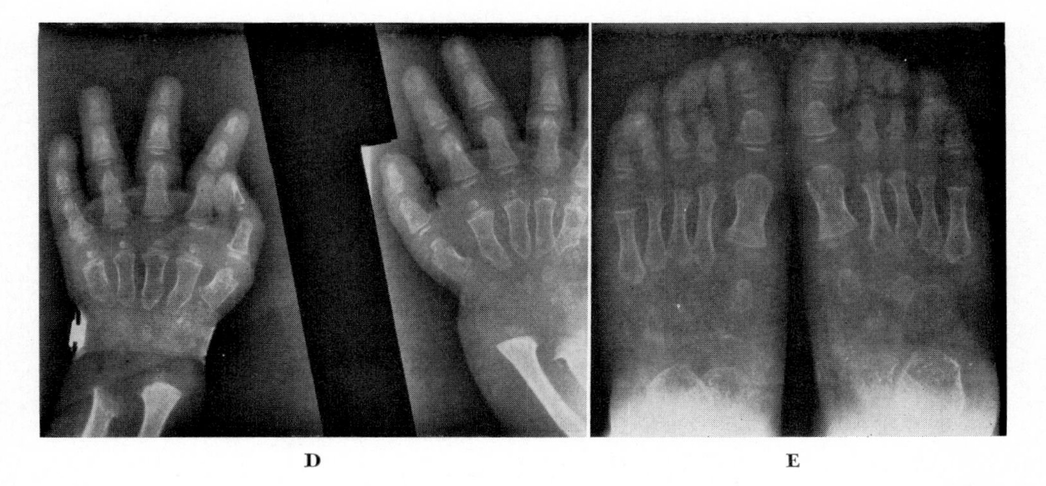

D E

Fig. 9-15, cont'd. For legend see opposite page.

On study of the urine, 92.7 mg. of acid mucopolysaccharide per liter was recovered, most of it being keratosulfate. A second study two months after the first yielded similar results. The cetylammonium bromide screening test[231,232] was strongly positive.

Pathology

An autopsy has been reported by Einhorn and colleagues[70]; and bone biopsies were presented by Aegerter and Kirkpatrick,[2] by Shelling,[257] and by Anderson and colleagues.[6] Zellweger and colleagues[309] found Reilly granules in the leukocytes of their cases. These may be absent in early stages, however. (See reference 248a.)

The fundamental defect

Patients with the Morquio syndrome excrete large amounts of keratosulfate in the urine.[14,183,184,222,267]

(Robins and associates[235] concluded that one group of patients with the Morquio syndrome excrete, during childhood at least, excessive amounts of chondroitin sulfate A in the urine. The clinical characterization of this group will be important. Such patients may not be properly considered illustrative of the Morquio syndrome.)

Prevalence and inheritance

The Morquio syndrome is inherited as an autosomal recessive (Fig. 9-16). It appears to be quite rare, probably no more frequent than 1 in 40,000 births.

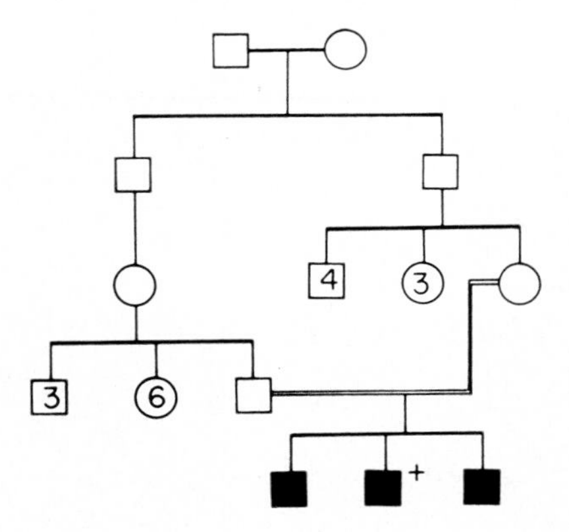

Fig. 9-16. MPS IV (the Morquio syndrome) in all three offspring (black squares) of the marriage of first cousins once removed. The second son, the proband, indicated by the cross, died suddenly at age 9 with acute breathlessness attributed to heart failure. The surviving sons were 21 and 16 years old at the time of study. Both appeared normal at birth. In the older, spinal curvature was noted as the first abnormality at age 2. In the younger, the disorder was anticipated and spinal curvature and prominent chest were detected by the age of 8 months. In both, examination revealed skeletal features typical of the Morquio syndrome. Their heights were 40 inches and 37 inches. The wrists were excessively mobile. Both had diffusely cloudy corneas. Respiratory movements were restricted in both, and the younger had the murmur of aortic regurgitation. Both had mildly spastic legs with sustained ankle clonus and extensor plantar response. The younger had difficulty in initiating micturition. The elder surviving brother is shown in Plate 1, *A*.

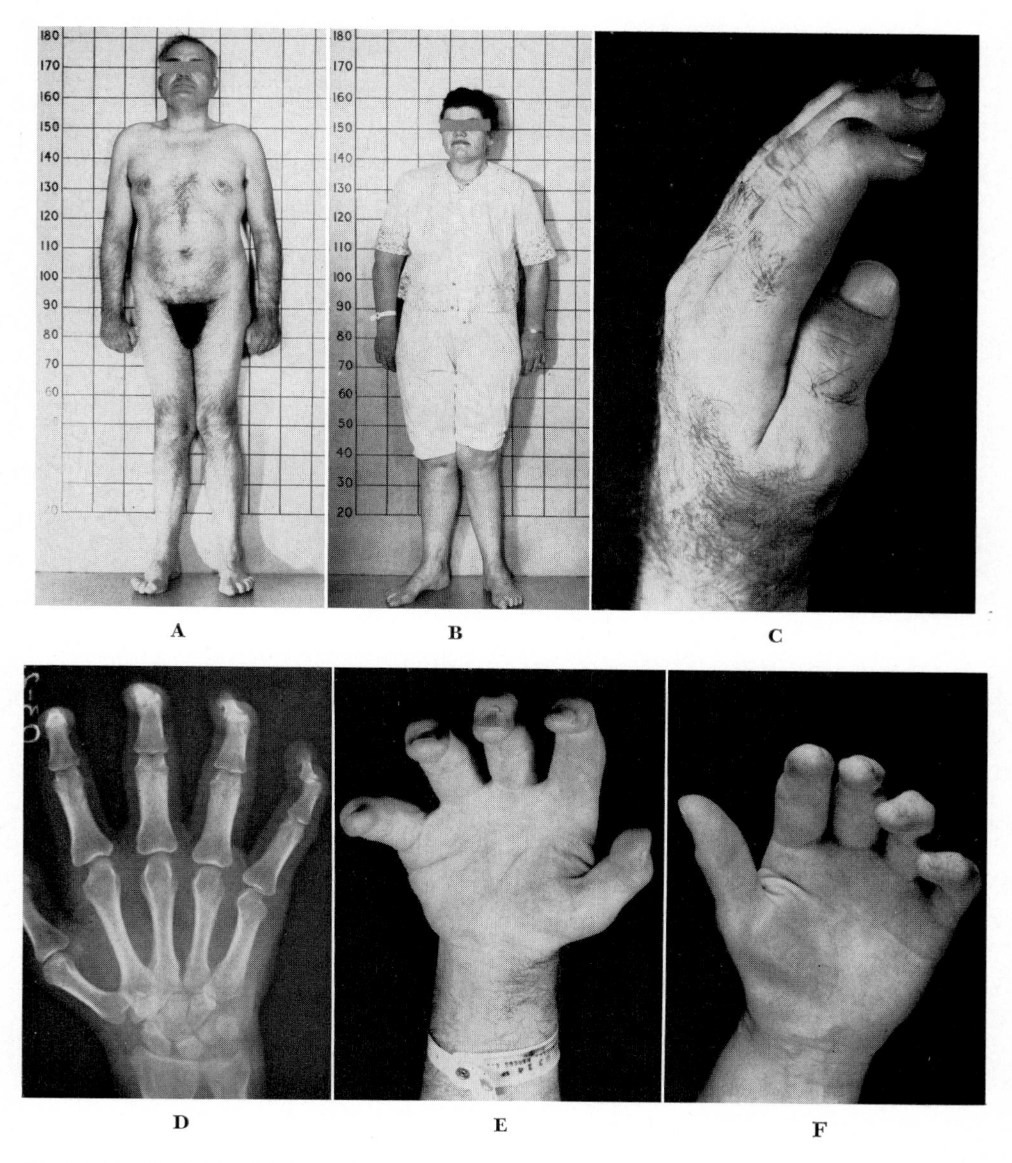

Fig. 9-17. MPS V (the Scheie syndrome). This brother and sister (M. E. McC. and M. McC.) are described in detail in the text. **A** and **B,** General appearance. Hypertrichosis, genu valgum, misshapen foot and "broad-mouthed" facies are noteworthy features. **C,** Clawhand in brother. **D,** X-ray film of hand in **C. E** and **F,** Atrophy of abducens pollicis brevis muscle, due to carpal tunnel compression of the median nerve, in brother, **E,** and sister, **F.** See Plate 1, *C,* for corneal clouding in the brother.

MUCOPOLYSACCHARIDOSIS V (MPS V, Scheie syndrome)

This condition was described by Scheie and colleagues[248] as a variant of the Hurler syndrome.

Clinical manifestations

The intellect is impaired little or not at all. Scheie's patients were of "near genius" intelligence, and one of ours (Case 9, below) is an attorney of at least average intelligence. Stiff joints, clawhands, excessive body hair, and "retinitis pigmentosa" occur, as in MPS II; but in this, unlike that condition, corneal clouding is a striking feature. The clouding is most dense peripherally in some patients, although in others, particularly in the earlier stages, involvement is uniform. Corneal grafts become opacified.[148,248] Stature is usually in the normal or low-normal range. The facies is characteristically "broad-mouthed." Median nerve compression in the carpal tunnel ("carpal tunnel syndrome") is frequently present.

It is clear from the patients we have studied that aortic valve disease is a feature of the syndrome. Most have aortic regurgitation. One patient 47 years of age, however, has remained asymptomatic in this respect. (See Case 9.) Experience is still too limited to know to what extent life-span is abbreviated in this disorder.

Psychosis was a feature in two (Cases 10 and 11) of the four adults we have studied.

The following two patients are brother and sister (Fig. 9-17*A* and *B*):

Case 9. M. E. McC. (1050314), the proband, is a white male attorney, born in 1917. Deformed feet and stiff fingers were noted at age 7 years. He was considered the most intelligent member of his family and more intelligent than his unaffected brother. He was class valedictorian in high school, for example. Progressive difficulty with night vision began at the age of 27 years, with restriction of the fields of vision in daylight. "Steamy corneas" were first noted by his ophthalmologist, at age 13 years.* Right inguinal herniorrhaphy was performed at age 42 years. Hearing deficit was noted in the right ear at age 46 years. Intellect may have deteriorated somewhat in recent years.

The findings when investigated in 1962 and again in 1964 included height of 175 cm. ($68\frac{9}{10}$ inches); short neck and coarse features, with broad mouth and jaw and fleshy tongue; stiff, clawlike hands with carpal tunnel syndrome and stiff wrists; short feet with high arches and overlapping fifth toe; marked clouding of the cornea, more dense peripherally; extensive retinitis pigmentosa bilaterally; and the diastolic murmur of aortic regurgitation (blood pressures, 145/65 mm. Hg). The aortic second sound was exceptionally ringing. The distal phalanges were flexed at about 90 degrees with the rest of the fingers but could be straightened passively. The wrists could not be extended beyond the neutral position. He could not supinate the forearms more than about 60 degrees. Except for the foot abnormalities, all other peripheral joints had normal range of motion. The liver was palpable and probably somewhat enlarged.

X-ray films showed spatulate ribs, and cystic and other changes in the bones of the wrists and hands.

The presence of carpal tunnel syndrome was indicated by numbness of the fingers supplied by the median nerve, marked wasting of the abducens pollicis brevis muscle, and characteristic nerve conduction changes†: stimulation at the elbow evoked no thumb movement or muscle action potential. Antidromic sensory velocity (stimulating at the wrist and recording at the elbow) was estimated at 26.8 M. per second as compared with a velocity of 63.6 M. per second in the unaffected ulnar nerve.

---

*Courtesy of the late Dr. Harvey B. Searcy, Tuscaloosa, Ala.

†These studies were performed by Dr. Michael P. McQuillan, Johns Hopkins Hospital.

The hearing loss was largely limited to the right ear, and audiologic findings suggested a cochlear location of the lesion. The electroretinogram was almost completely extinguished, consistent with neuroepithelial degeneration.

The urine showed excessive excretion of chondroitin sulfate B (about 60 mg. per liter). Bone marrow and circulating leukocytes showed no definite mucopolysaccharide inclusions.

Case 10. M. McC. (1119314), white female, sister of M. E. McC., was born in 1930. Stiff hands and wrists and deformed feet were first noted at the age of 5 years. As early as age 7 an appearance suggesting mongolism was noted by her ophthalmologist. Clouding of the cornea was first noted by him at about age 20 years. She was regarded by her parents as a slow learner. However, she succeeded in completing a four-year college course, of which the last year was spent in a southern teachers college. She attempted to teach school but had a "nervous breakdown" for which she was hospitalized and given electroshock therapy. Other treatments have been necessary since that time. She cares for her aged parents. She has noted numbness and anesthesia of the fingers.

Physical examination in 1964 showed height of 160.5 cm. (63⅕ inches), the same facial characteristics as in her brother (Fig. 9-12*B*), and similar hand and foot deformities, which were less severe, however. There was bilateral genu valgum. Grossly the corneal clouding seemed more diffuse than in the brother; however, slit-lamp examination showed possible peripheral concentration. The fundi showed retinal pigmentation and the electroretinogram was almost completely extinguished. The heart had a harsh systolic murmur with characteristics of aortic stenosis. The abducens pollicis brevis muscle was strikingly atrophied.

In the peripheral blood approximately 1 to 3% of the lymphocytes showed indistinct, poorly formed metachromatic granules in the cytoplasm. The Rebuck skin window demonstrated metachromatic inclusions in macrophages. The urine contained about 100 mg. of chondroitin sulfate B per liter.

No other similarly affected persons are known in this family. One other sib is completely normal. Interestingly, he is slightly shorter than the affected brother, M. E. McC., and in the past has been considered less competent intellectually.

Cases 11 and 12. Through the courtesy of Dr. Scheie it was possible to examine the brother and sister (T. L. and R. L.) in whom he described the entity to which we assign his name. The facial resemblance to the cases reported here and shown in Fig. 9-17 was so striking that they could all pass for sibs. The other clinical features were also similar. It is specifically to be noted that both of Scheie's patients—a male, age 33, and his sister, age 31 years—have aortic regurgitation. The brother has had a psychotic episode. Leukocyte studies reveal no obvious metachromatic granules. Urine mucopolysaccharide analyses show large amounts of chondroitin sulfate B.

Pathology

The skin[103] and the cornea and conjunctiva[248] show the same histologic changes as have been observed in MPS I (p. 341). In those instances in which the carpal tunnel has been explored for relief of nerve compression[299] an excess of collagenous tissue has been found. No autopsy observations are available. The nature of the aortic valve lesion is not known; in no case of MPS V has an autopsy been performed.

The fundamental defect

These patients excrete excessive amounts of chondroitin sulfate B in the urine.

Prevalence and inheritance

MPS V is almost certainly inherited as an autosomal recessive. Both Scheie and colleagues[248] and we[179] have observed affected brother and sister. The frequency of the disorder is unknown.

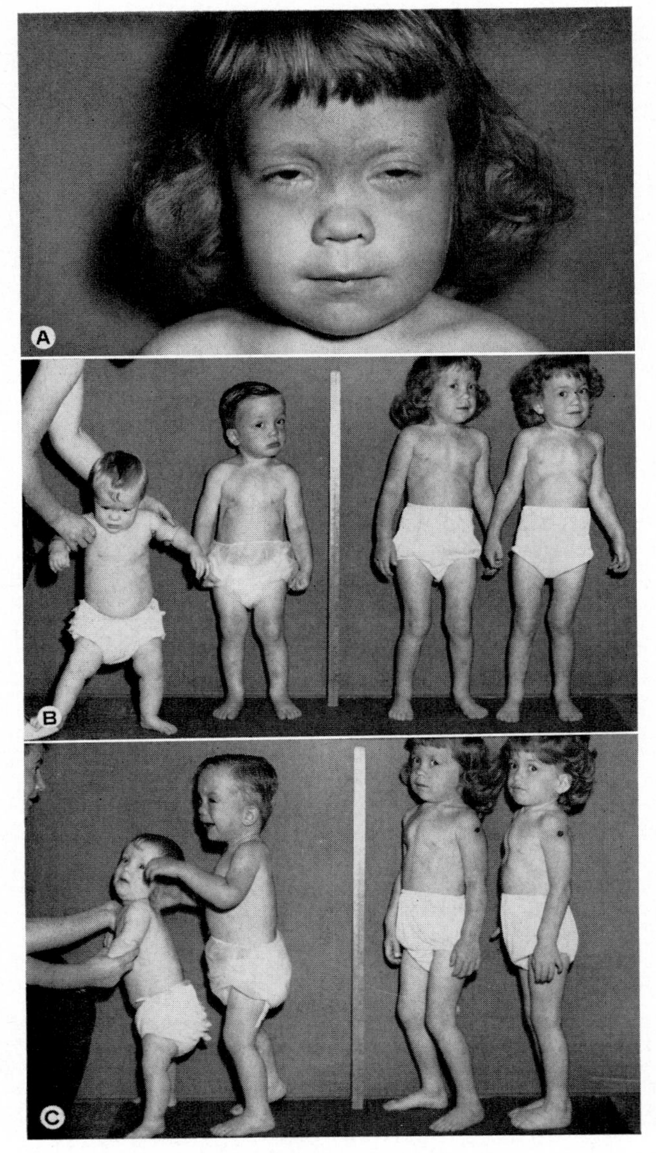

Fig. 9-18. MPS VI (the Maroteaux-Lamy syndrome). The four sibs shown in this series of photographs are described in detail in the text. **A,** Facial appearance in the proband, K. S., age 5½ years. **B** and **C,** Four affected sibs. Left to right: L. S., age 6 months; S. S., age 2½ years; K. S., age 5¼ years; D. S., age 4 years. **D** and **E,** Four affected sibs, in order of age, two years after views shown in **B** and **C.** The progressive changes are particularly striking in the two youngest children. Semiflexion at the knees is evident. **F,** Clawhands in proband, K. S., age 5½ years. **G,** Hands and forearms in D. S. The radius and ulna are short, thickened, and somewhat bowed. The metacarpals and phalanges have an abnormal configuration. **H,** Spine in L. S., age 2½ years. **I,** Spine in D. S., age 4 years. In this and the preceding figure, beaking and posterior displacement of the upper lumbar vertebrae are evident. The ribs are abnormally broad. **J,** Skull in L. S., showing shoe-shaped sella. **K,** Pelvis and hips in K. S., age 5½ years. Note irregularity of the epiphyseal ossification centers and coxa valga. (From McKusick, V. A., Kaplan, D., Wise, D., Hanley, W. B., Suddarth, S. B., Sevick, M. E., and Maumenee, A. E.: Medicine 44:445, 1965.)

MUCOPOLYSACCHARIDOSIS VI

(MPS VI, Maroteaux-Lamy syndrome, polydystrophic dwarfism)

MPS VI is a condition that was first delineated on clinical and chemical grounds by Maroteaux, Lamy, and their colleagues.[185a,186] They pointed to several previously reported cases which may represent the same entity.

Clinical manifestations

Abnormality, namely growth retardation, is first noted at the age of 2 or 3 years. Stunting of both the trunk and the limbs is usually present, as well as genu valgum, lumbar kyphosis, and anterior sternal protrusion. The face is abnormal, as shown in Fig. 9-18*A*. Although the facial features are not pathognomonic and are not as striking as in MPS I, they suggest that the patient's ailment falls in the category of mucopolysaccharidoses. Restriction of articular movement is present, as in several of the other entities.

Hepatosplenomegaly is present in most cases. Cardiac manifestations have not been noted. Corneal opacities develop fairly early. Deafness is present in some patients and may be due in part to recurrent otitis media.

Points of central importance to the differentiation from MPS I and MPS V are (1) that intellectual development is normal and (2) that the osseous ab-

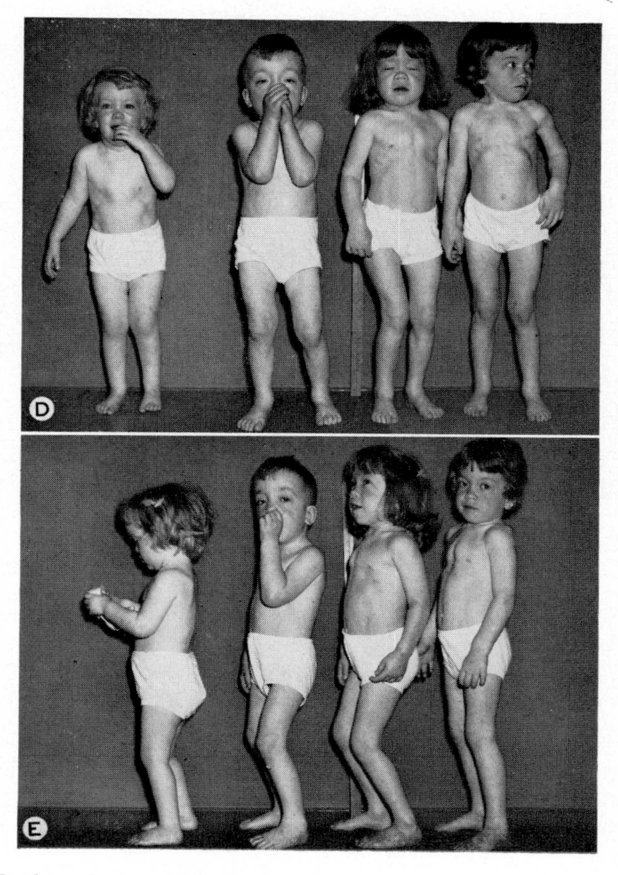

Fig. 9-18, cont'd. For legend see opposite page.

Continued.

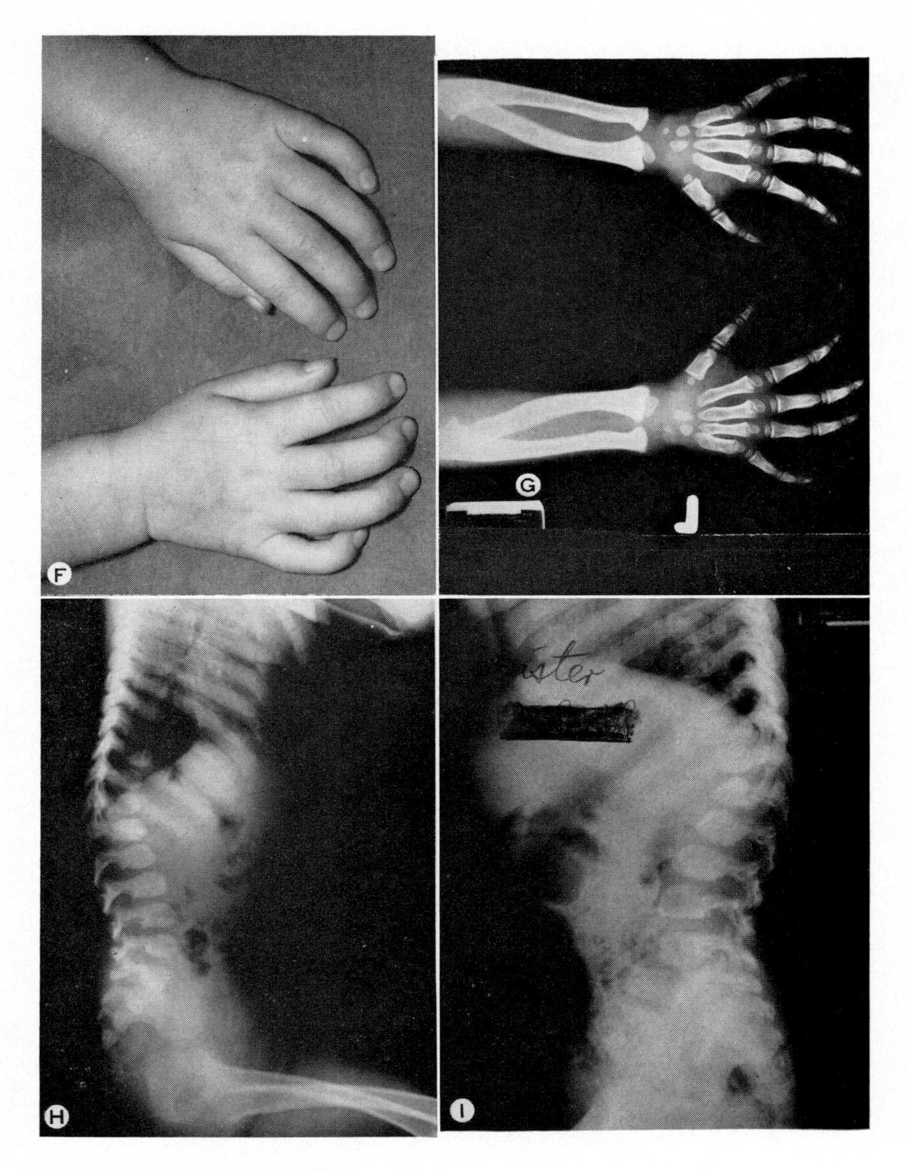

Fig. 9-18, cont'd. For legend see p. 372.

normality is severe, being qualitatively similar to that of MPS I. In the long bones of the extremities the metaphyses are of irregular structure and the epiphyses are slightly deformed—particularly the head of the femur, which may be fragmented, and the upper end of the humerus, which is hatchet-shaped. The distal end of the radius and ulna is oblique. The carpal and tarsal ossification centers are hypoplastic. The vertebral bodies have reduced height. The first lumbar and last dorsal vertebrae are wedged-shaped and posteriorly displaced. The ribs are flattened.

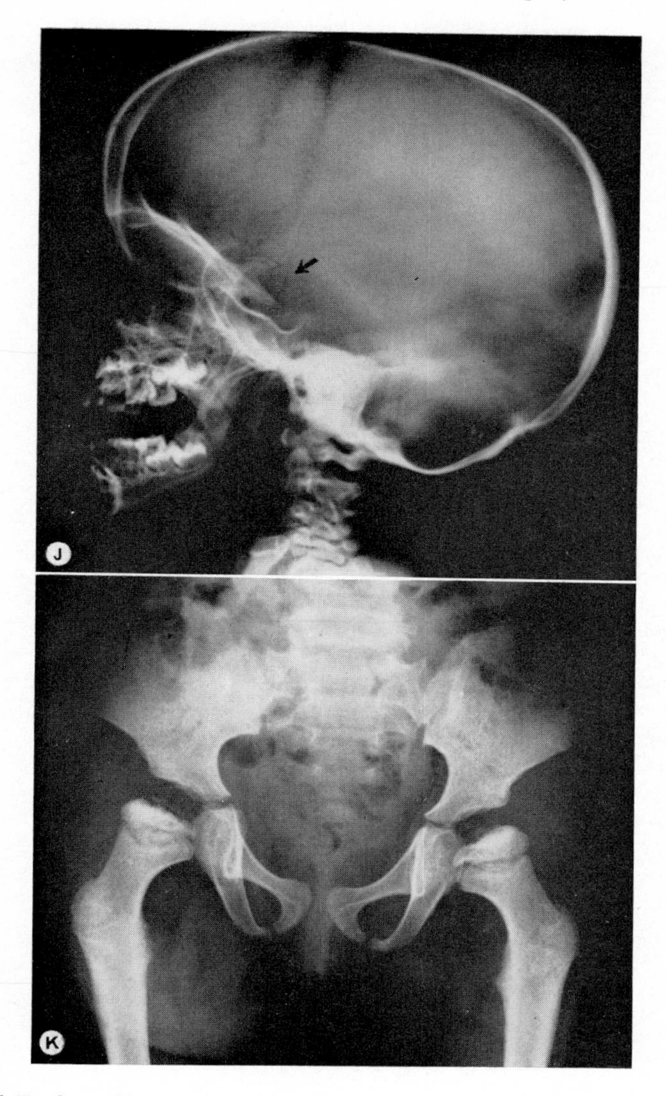

Fig. 9-18, cont'd. For legend see p. 372.

The blood shows both polymorphonuclear inclusions[185a] and lymphocytic inclusions.

The four sibs* described below (Fig. 9-18) are thought to have the Maroteaux-Lamy syndrome:

Cases 13 to 16. The eldest, K. S. (G.M.C. 307-966), a daughter of apparently unrelated parents, had been noted since infancy to have noisy breathing, a wobbly gait, and stiff joints. Hip pain, beginning at about 5 years of age, prompted medical attention. Mental development has progressed normally and she remains in the highest section of her class. The gross facies

*These cases[179] were studied by S. D. Suddarth and M. E. Sevick of the Geisinger Medical Center, Danville, Pa., and are presented here with their permission.

is shown in Fig. 9-18*A*, and the broad hands with stubby fingers and flexion contractures are seen in Fig. 9-18*F*. Other evident features are an elongated large head, corneal cloudiness, macroglossia, lower dorsal kyphosis, and a prominent sternum. Examination shows hepatosplenomegaly and a vibratory systolic murmur. The roentgenograms showed "bullet-shaped" phalanges and "wedge-shaped" vertebrae.

After these features were pointed out to the parents, they suggested that all four of their children may be affected. Fig. 9-18 illustrates their similarities. There are also noteworthy differences: the features of D.S. have remained fine and her corneal opacities are only faintly visible; S. S. has a head size that is disproportionately large. The skeletal changes are illustrated in Fig. 9-18*G* to *K*.

The two older girls (now 6 and 8 years of age) are performing superiorly in the first and third grades despite recurrent catarrhal otitis with intermittent gross hearing loss, recurrent and persistent bronchitis, increased deformity and stiffness of the fingers in K. S., and the constant need for a body jacket in D. S. to prevent progressive scoliosis. Both have systolic murmurs, prominent second sounds, and normal blood pressures. K. S. may have early clubbing of the fingers. Adenoidectomy and tonsillectomy helped the noisy respirations, but apparently not the recurrent otitis and bronchitis.

S. S. has changed the most during 2½ years of observation. His head size has increased only from 52.5 to 54 cm., but his eyes are much more prominent and grossly cloudy. He limps, with apparent shortening of the right limb, and has much louder breathing and more frequent otitis media and bronchitis. There is a persistent small umbilical hernia and he had an inguinal hernia repaired in infancy. Both S. S. and L. S. have developed soft systolic murmurs with a prominent second sound. Both have grown 6 to 7 inches, speak well, and are toilet-trained.

No abnormality of the electroretinogram was detected.[93]

All four children show Reilly granulations of the polymorphonuclear leukocytes and metachromatic cytoplasmic inclusions in 10 to 25% of lymphocytes. Large amounts of mucopolysaccharide, almost exclusively chondroitin sulfate B, were identified in the urine. Values, expressed as milligrams per liter, were as follows: K. S., age 7½ years, 250 mg.; D. S., age 6, 185 mg.; S. S., age 4½, 90 mg.; and L. S., age 2½ years, 180 mg. per liter.

Pathology

No information is available on cases in whom the diagnosis of MPS VI is certain.

The fundamental defect

Patients with MPS VI excrete large amounts of chondroitin sulfate B; only this mucopolysaccharide is excreted in excess.

Prevalence and inheritance

Although no worthwhile estimates are available, in part because the Maroteaux-Lamy syndrome has only recently been delineated, the disorder must be quite rare. I have firsthand knowledge of only one family, that which is described above.[179] It is inherited as an autosomal recessive. In Maroteaux and Lamy's family, the parents were related.

DIAGNOSIS OF THE MUCOPOLYSACCHARIDOSES

The amount of mucopolysaccharides excreted normally in the urine ranges from 3 to 15 mg. per 24 hours.[233] Chondroitin sulfate A comprises about 80% of the excreted mucopolysaccharide, with chondroitin sulfate B and heparitin sulfate accounting, in about equal parts, for the remainder.[160]

Simple tests for excessive acid mocopolysaccharides in the urine have been devised by Dorfman, using the turbidity produced with acidified bovine serum albumin,[63,267] and by Berry and Spinanger,[21] using metachromasia produced with toluidine blue.* A simple procedure, the cetyltrimethylammonium bromide test† of urine, adapted from Meyer's preparative method for mucopolysaccharides,[199,218] promises to be particularly useful.[40,231,232] A procedure requiring preliminary dialysis of urine and based on Dische's carbazole reaction for uronic acid was proposed by Segni and co-workers.[254] Dorfman[66] urges caution in use of the screening tests in infants and young children because mucopolysaccharide excretion may normally be greater early in life.

Since the report of Reilly in 1941,[230] the demonstration of metachromatic granules in circulating polymorphonuclear leukocytes and in bone marrow cells has been used by many workers as a diagnostic approach.[131,238] Although the bone marrow was more often positive (p. 378), Reilly granulation‡ (of the circulating polymorphs) was frequently not demonstrable.[231] However, Muir and co-workers[207] demonstrated a good correlation between the lymphocytic findings and the urinary excretion of mucopolysaccharide in the Hurler syndrome.

The method used to demonstrate metachromatic granules in the cytoplasm of circulating lymphocytes is that of Muir and co-workers.[207] The toluidine blue stain after methyl alcohol fixation has been found[179] completely satisfactory and, in contrast to the May-Gruenwald stain which the above workers also used, is specific for mucopolysaccharide. (See Fig. 9-19, Plate 1, *D* to *G*, and Plate 2.)

We[179] have found no metachromatic granules in the cytoplasm of lymphocytes from normal persons or in patients with a variety of disorders such as achondroplasia, Marfan's syndrome, and multiple epiphyseal dysplasia. Occasionally, however, isolated clusters of a few very small, clearly defined pink granules have been found in the cytoplasm of polymorphonuclear leukocytes from normal persons.

The circulating leukocytes were studied[179] in eight cases of MPS I, two of MPS II, and five of MPS III. In all, obvious metachromatic granules have been found in from 10 to 60% of the lymphocytes, thus confirming the findings of Muir and associates.[207] On the other hand, Reilly granulations have been found infrequently and with no apparent relation to one or more of the entities. They were present in only one case of the Sanfilippo syndrome (MPS III). Possibly the

*The following is the simplified "filter paper test" devised by Berry[20,21]: Place 5, 10, and 25 μl. of urine as separate spots on a piece of Whatman No. 1 filter paper. Use a micropipette to add 5 μl. at a time, allowing each increment to dry before adding another. Dip paper in an aqueous solution of 0.04 toluidine blue (buffered at pH 2.0) for about 1 minute, drain, and rinse in 95% ethanol. (The toluidine blue solution is prepared by dissolving 30 mg. of dye in 100 ml. of Coleman certified buffer solution, pH 2.0.)

†The following is the CTAB test as used by Renuart[231]: The reagent consists of a 5% solution of cetyltrimethylammonium bromide (hexadecyltrimethylammonium bromide) in one molar buffer, pH 6.0. One milliliter of CTAB reagent is added to 5 ml. of clean, fresh urine at room temperature. (Any cold urine gives a positive test.) The mixture is agitated by swirling and then allowed to stand at room temperature for 30 minutes. Increased urinary mucopolysaccharide concentration is indicated by a heavy, flocculent precipitate. The reaction is almost immediate in cases of MPS I, but may be more delayed and less striking in others of the mucopolysacchridoses. A control urine should be tested simultaneously. In addition to a chilled urine, pyuria can produce a false positive test.

‡Reilly granulations are probably indistinguishable from the Alder granulations of the polymorphonuclear leukocytes, which occur as a dominantly inherited trait without associated manifestations.[3,135,302]

appearance of Reilly granulations depends on a quantitative phenomenon, but it may well be that other, unrecognized factors are involved. (Table 10.)

In four cases of the Morquio syndrome (MPS IV), scattered irregular aggregations of metachromatic granules, distinct from Reilly granules, have been noted in the cytoplasm of the majority of the polymorphs. Possibly this difference in form reflects the fact that in the Morquio syndrome it is a different mucopolysaccharide, namely keratosulfate, which accumulates.

In four cases of the Scheie syndrome (MPS type V) lymphocytic granules either have been absent or have been present in a very ill-defined form in only a small proportion of cells; this probably represents a quantitative phenomenon, since patients in these cases excrete less mucopolysaccharide than do those in cases of MPS types I, II, and III. Reilly granulations of the polymorphs were found in none of the four subjects.

Pearson and Lorincz[221] demonstrated mucopolysaccharide granules in bone marrow cells of seventeen of eighteen consecutive patients with "the Hurler syndrome" seen in a two-year period. The patient without such findings was a 7-year-old boy thought to have the X-linked form (MPS II). Presumably, the other cases were MPS I. Some X-linked cases do show bone marrow inclusions, however, as we were able to demonstrate (Plate 1, *F*) in the 31-year-old male shown in Fig. 9-7. All twelve patients studied by Jermain and associates[131] showed granulated bone marrow cells that they considered to be phagocytic clasmatocytes.

With the Rebuck skin window technique[229,248] one can detect metachromatic granules in both macrophages and polymorphonuclear leukocytes.[29] (See Plate 1, *G*.)

Definitive differential diagnosis sometimes requires refined studies of urinary mucopolysaccharides with precise identification of the substance (s) excreted. For example, in young children with MPS IV the differentiation from MPS I may be possible only by identifying the mucopolysaccharide present in excess in the urine as keratosulfate. Study of serum mucopolysaccharides in the mucopolysaccharidoses are now under way. Elevated plasma levels of acid mucopolysaccharide in the Hurler syndrome were found by Sanfilippo and Good,[245] using the Bollet method.

Plate 1. A, MPS IV (the Morquio syndrome). The elder surviving brother in the kindred diagrammed in Fig. 9-16. There are signs of spastic paraplegia. **B,** MPS IV (the Morquio syndrome). Steamy corneal clouding in elder brother pictured in Fig. 9-14. **C,** MPS V (the Scheie syndrome). Corneal clouding, most dense peripherally, in male shown in Fig. 9-17. **D** to **G,** Inclusions in white blood cells. **D,** Specific lymphocytic inclusions, in case of MPS III. **E,** Reilly granulations of polymorphonuclear leukocytes, in case of MPS III. **F,** Metachromatic cytoplasmic inclusions in macrophage in bone marrow of case of MPS II, shown also in Fig. 9-7. **G,** Metachromatic granules in cytoplasm of inflammatory cells elicited by the Rebuck skin window technique in a case of MPS II, also shown in Fig. 9-7. (From McKusick, V. A., Kaplan, D., Wise, D., Hanley, W. B., Suddarth, S. B., Sevick, M. E., and Maumenee, A. E.: Medicine **44**:445, 1965.)

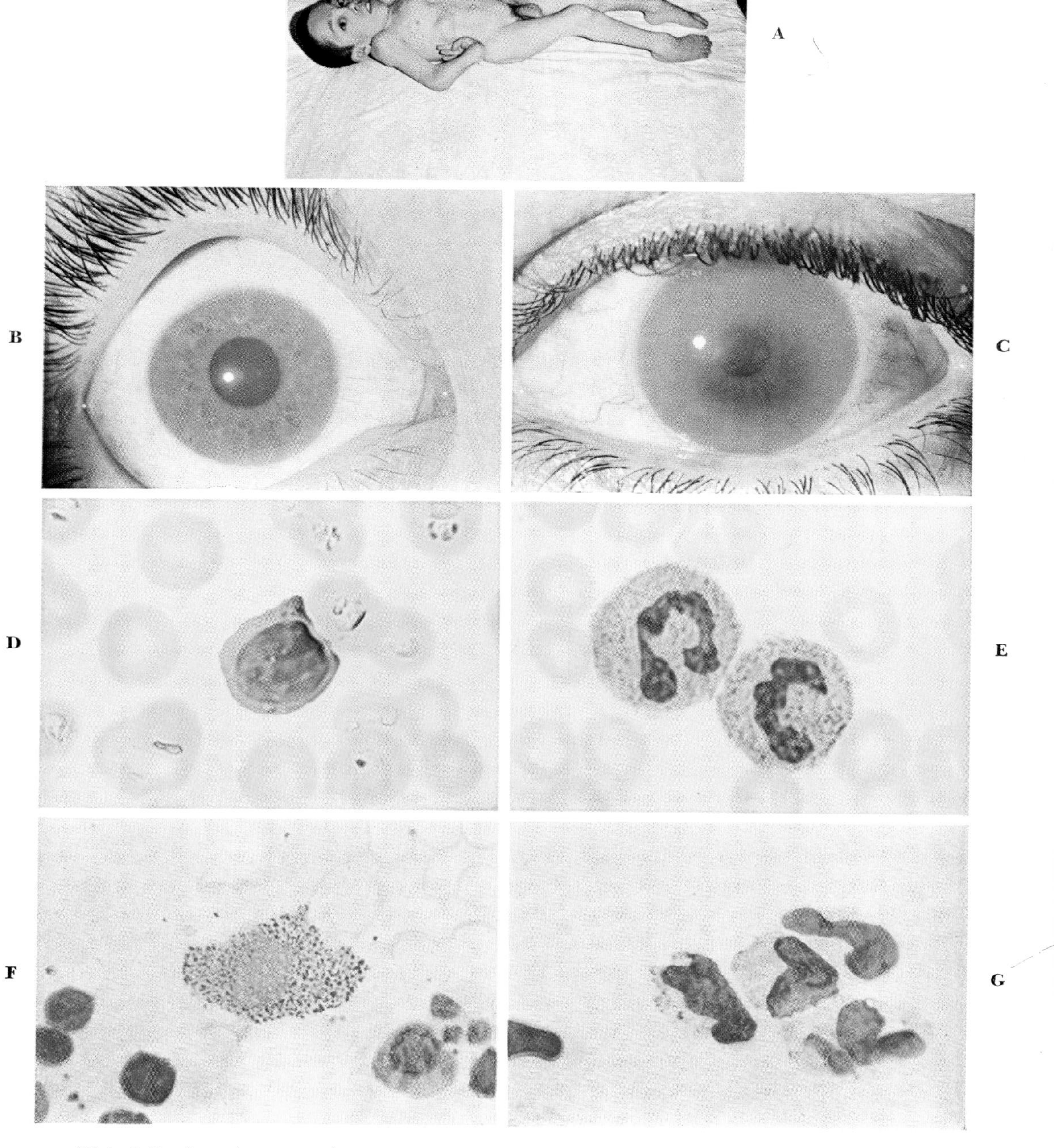

Plate 1. For legend see opposite page.

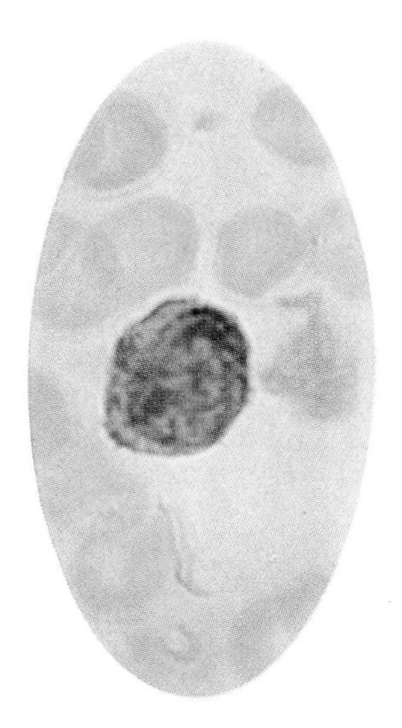

Plate 2. Metachromatically staining cytoplasmic inclusions in a circulating lymphocyte. Stained with toluidine blue. (From J.A.M.A., Jan. 18, 1965.)

Table 10. Metachromatic cytoplasmic inclusions

	Cases	*Lymphocytes*	*Polymorphs*
MPS I (Hurler syndrome)	8	All positive in 10 to 60% of cells (MPS I, II, III)	+/−
MPS II (Hunter syndrome)	2		+/−
MPS III (Sanfilippo syndrome)	5		Only 1 positive
MPS IV (Morquio syndrome)	4	0	Atypically + in all 4
MPS V (Scheie syndrome)	4	+/−	+/−
MPS VI (Maroteaux-Lamy syndrome)	4	All positive in 10 to 25% of cells	All positive

OTHER GENETIC MUCOPOLYSACCHARIDOSES?

It is more than likely that the six entities described earlier in this chapter are not the only genetic defects of mucopolysaccharide metabolism. The following discussion concerns conditions in which such a disturbance is suspected.

In 1928, from Freiburg, Germany, Schinz and Furtwängler[249] described a sibship of eleven, the offspring of a first-cousin marriage, in which a man then 29 years old and three of his sisters were identically affected by a disorder in which the most striking feature was stiff joints. Flexion deformity and reduced mobility in the fingers and toes were combined with limited mobility in the ankles, wrists, knees, elbows, hips, shoulders, and spine. The face was described as red, with somewhat prominent forehead, broad nose, and fleshy ("fleischig") tongue. Umbilical hernia was present in the brother, whose eyes were said then to be normal. He worked as a bookkeeper and was considered of normal intelligence. Height was 156 cm. (61⅖ inches). X-ray films in this man showed thick skull, shortened posterior cranial fossa, and prominent external and internal occipital protruberances. A striking feature was extensive disturbance in the development of (or a destruction of) the carpal and tarsal bones. (See Fig. 9-20*C*.)

In 1934 Horsch[116] described a sister from the same sibship. The features were identical, including those in the carpal and tarsal bones. The brother described in the earlier report[249] was restudied; cysts in the head of the humerus and epiphyses of the radius were described. Cysts were also observed in the digital epiphyses of these patients, and secondary subluxation of the phalanges was noted.

In 1938 Schmidt,[251] ophthalmologist in Freiburg, reported corneal abnormality in the same four sibs: "Both corneas appear finely clouded in their totality. Slit-lamp examination shows that the diffuse clouding is composed of numerous

A

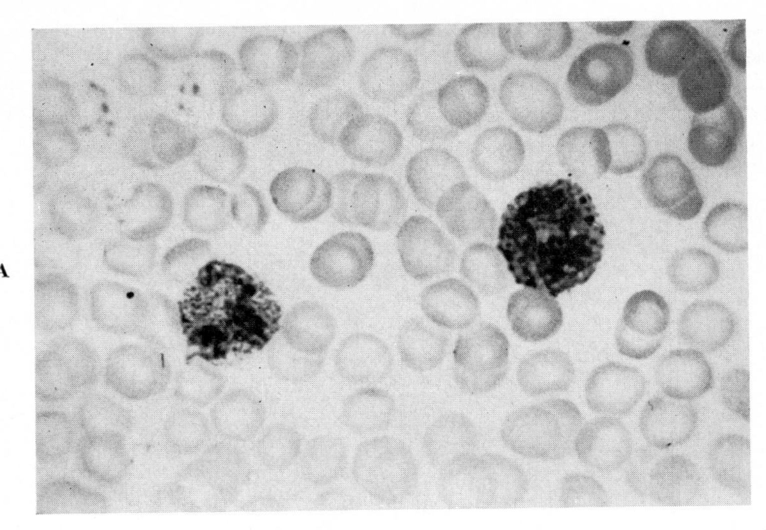

Fig. 9-19. Cytoplasmic inclusions in the Hurler syndrome. **A,** Peripheral blood. The lighter cell is a polymorphonuclear leukocyte of the type described by Reilly[230] (Type I polymorph). There are small lilac-staining granules of relatively uniform size in the cytoplasm. The darker cell, which superficially resembles a basophil, has large lilac-blue granules of nonuniform size (Type II polymorph). **B,** Peripheral blood. Lymphocyte with lilac and blue granules. **C,** Bone marrow myelocytes. The darker cell in the center is probably the precursor of the Type II polymorph in the peripheral blood. The other two cells with lilac granules are probably the precursors of the similar cells in the peripheral blood (Type I polymorph). The patient was a 3½-year-old boy with typical manifestations of the Hurler syndrome. The total white cell count was 17,400 per cubic millimeter with the following differential:

28% Type I polymorph
6% Type II polymorph
55% lymphocytes without granules
9% lymphocytes with granules
2% monocytes
——
100%

Formalin was found to dissolve the granules. After basic lead acetate fixation the granules were stained by toluidine blue. (Wright-Giemsa stain; ×1,600; reduced ¼.) (Courtesy Dr. Ralph L. Engle, Jr., New York City.)

very fine gray specks which are located mainly in the middle parenchymal layers. In the deep and superficial portions they are less numerous. A difference is noted between the center and periphery of the cornea, the granules being coarser in the center than at the periphery. They are grayish white in color. Otherwise the cornea has no alteration. The surface is smooth and fluorescein-negative. No defect in Descemet's membrane is detected. Surface sensibility is reduced. The other reflecting media, the iris and the fundus of the eye are free of pathologic changes."*

These may have been cases of MPS V. The greater changes in the carpal and tarsal bones than in the cases in our series may be only a matter of degree.

---

*Translation from Schmidt, R.: Klin. Msbl. Augenheilk. **100:**616, 1938.

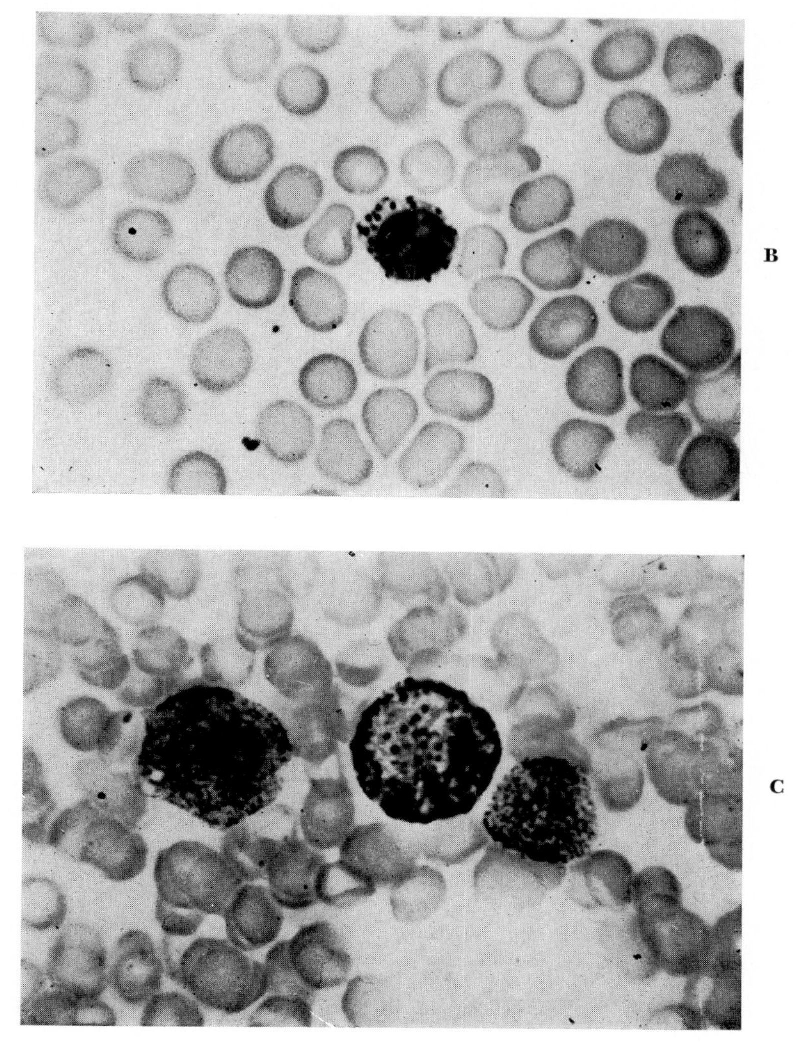

Fig. 9-19, cont'd. For legend see opposite page.

Scharf[247] described an isolated case similar to the patients of Schinz and others; the parents were first cousins.

Lahdensuu[148] described four affected sibs, three girls and a boy, the oldest being 19 years of age, with joint contractures, corneal clouding, most dense in the periphery, coarse facies, bony changes, and normal intelligence. The carpal bones were small with irregular contours. Corneal transplants became opacified. Again, these resemble most closely the cases of Scheie syndrome but may represent the Maroteaux-Lamy syndrome, as was suggested by Maroteaux and colleagues.[185a]

Abul-Haj and coworkers[1] proposed that Farber's lipogranulomatosis (Fig. 9-21) is a mucopolysaccharidosis. This disorder is characterized by onset in the first weeks of life and the following features: irritability, hoarse cry, nodular,

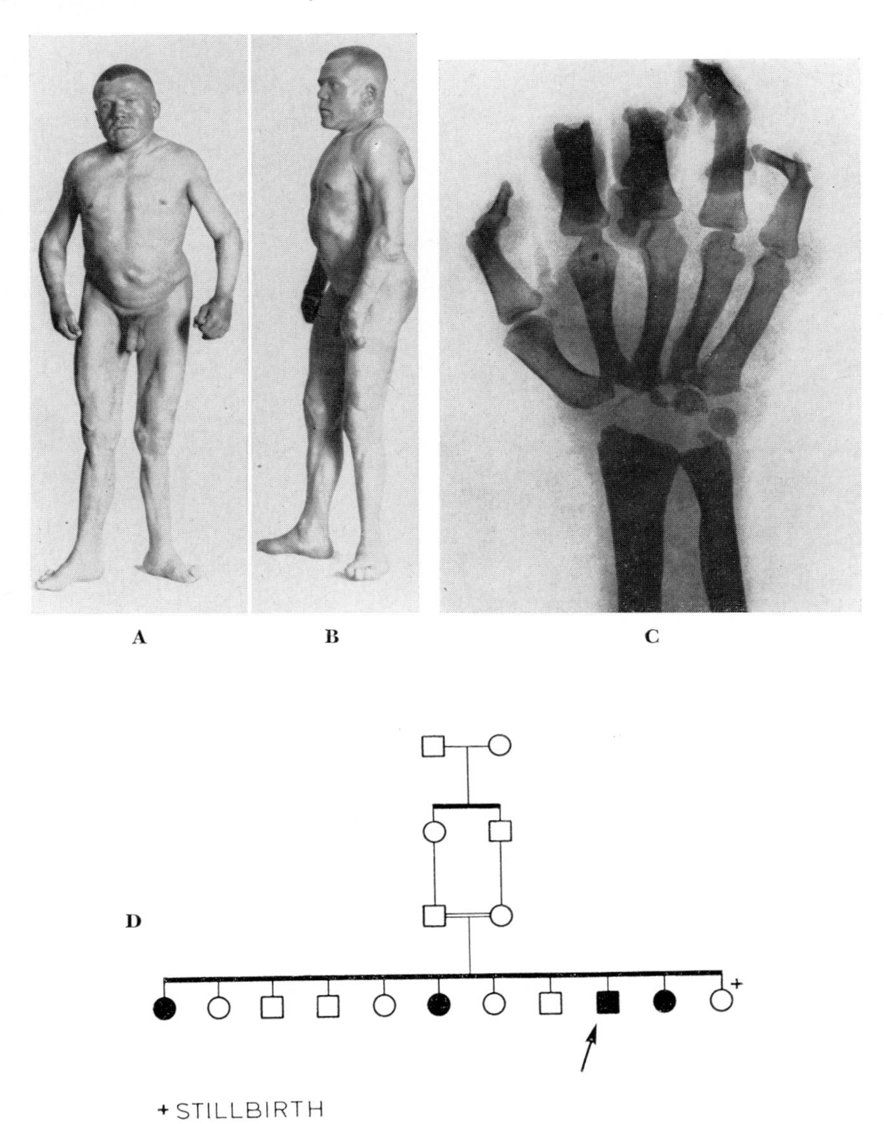

Fig. 9-20. Family reported by Schinz and by others.[116,249,251] Diagnosis: possibly MPS V, possibly a separate mucopolysaccharidosis. **A** and **B,** General appearance. **C,** X-ray film of the hand. Both wrists showed more drastic changes than in any of the cases reported here. **D,** The pedigree.

erythematous swellings of the wrists and other sites, particularly those subject to trauma, and severe motor and mental retardation. Death occurs by 2 years of age. The histologic appearance of the nodules is granulomatous. In the nervous system both neurons and glial cells are swollen with stored material having the characteristics of a nonsulfonated acid mucopolysaccharide.[1] Urinary excretion of mucopolysaccharides has apparently not been studied in any of these cases. Autosomal recessive inheritance is likely. Two of Farber's patients were sibs.[80]

Puretić and colleagues[225] described a newly recognized form of connective tissue disorder in an 11-year-old boy. Three sibs died in infancy with painful flexural contractures of the elbows, shoulder joints, and knees, which developed at about 3 months of age. Other features included deformity of the skull and face, stunted growth, osteolysis of the terminal phalanges, and multiple subcutaneous nodules.

The case reported by Rocher and Pesme[236] as an instance of "pleonosteosis (Léri's disease) with opalescent corneas" was probably MPS IV or MPS VI. As pointed out by Rukavina and colleagues,[242] others of the reported cases of Léri's pleonosteosis were probably in fact instances of a mucopolysaccharidosis, especially MPS II or MPS V. True Léri's disease[156,299] is a rare entity characterized by dominant inheritance, flexion contractures of the fingers, enlarged thumbs and first toes, limited joint motion, short stature, mongoloid facies, and normal intelligence. The hand looks much like that in MPS II or MPS V, but fixed finger flexion occurs only at the first interphalangeal joint. Carpal tunnel syndrome is said[299] to occur in Léri's pleonosteosis, as in MPS V (Fig. 9-17*E* and *F*). However, it is likely that Watson-Jones' patient with this complication (his Case 4) indeed had MPS V; only his first family appears to have had Léri's pleonosteosis with dominant inheritance. "Pleonosteosis," the term suggested by Léri because he thought overproduction of bone was the nature of the disorder, is a misnomer because the main abnormality seems to reside in ligaments. Mucopolysaccharide metabolism has apparently not been studied.

François' syndrome (dermo-chondro-corneal dystrophy) is characterized[86,87,129] by skeletal deformity of the hands and feet, "xanthomatous" nodules on the pinnae, dorsal surface of the metacarpophalangeal and interphalangeal joints, posterior surface of the elbows, nose, etc., and by corneal dystrophy. Mucopolysaccharide metabolism has apparently not been studied in this disorder.

The genetic determination of macular corneal dystrophy is clearly established.[188,296] Both autosomal dominant and autosomal recessive inheritance has been observed. On the basis of nine cases of macular corneal dystrophy Klintworth and Vogel[142] concluded that this disorder is a localized acid mucopolysaccharide storage disease of the corneal fibroblast. The cutaneous fibroblasts of one patient were structurally unaltered, and the urine did not contain an excess of acid mucopolysaccharide.

"Acquired" disturbances in mucopolysaccharide metabolism do not concern us here. For example, Ultmann and colleagues[286] described a 58-year-old man with systemic mastocytosis, in whose urine Dr. Karl Meyer of Columbia University found 24 mg. per liter per day of a mucopolysaccharide identified as heparitin sulfate. We found no excess mucopolysacchariduria in a 68-year-old man with long-standing severe systemic mastocytosis. Zimmer and associates[311] found normal 24-hour urine mucopolysaccharide excretion in twenty-one patients with mastocytosis, and in seven patients studied in this way serum mucopolysaccharides were not increased.

In search for a disturbance of mucopolysaccharide metabolism in clinically delineated genetic disorders of the skeleton and/or cornea, urines were assayed for mucopolysaccharide content, in collaboration with Dr. David Kaplan.[179] No

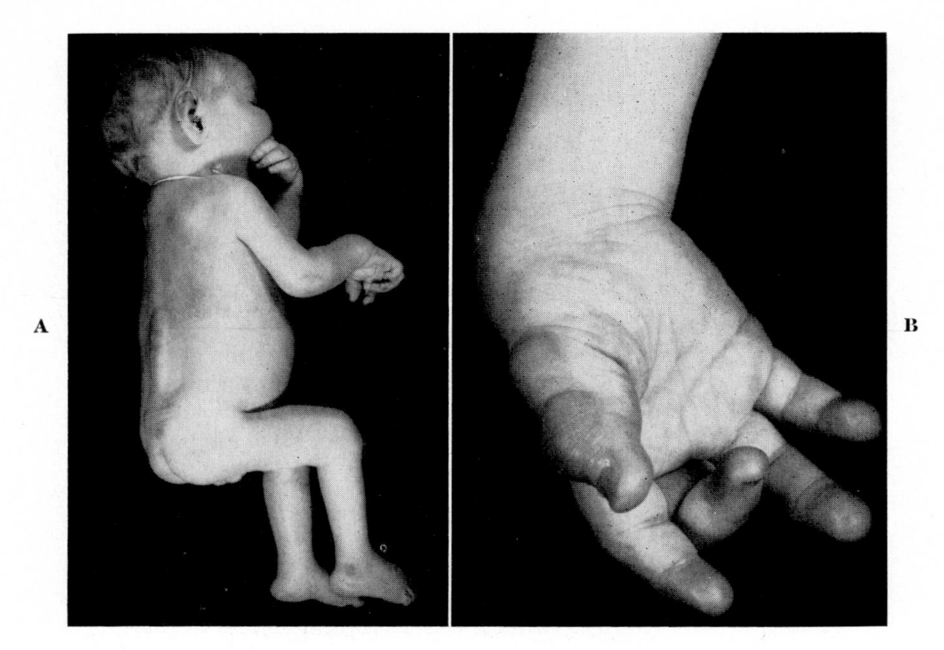

Fig. 9-21. Farber's lipogranulomatosis. J. R. C. (J.H.H. 932852), 5 months old at the time of these photographs, was apparently well until the age of 10 weeks. Thereafter, hoarseness, stridor, and the joint and skin changes demonstrated here developed. Motor and intellectual development was severely retarded. Persistent neutrophilic leukocytosis (15,000 to 20,000/mm.^{3}) was a feature. X-ray films showed joint destruction. He died at the age of 20 months. In addition to the changes shown in the photographs, nodular thickenings of the heart valves, especially the aortic and mitral, were found. Histologically the nodular lesions at many sites showed polymorphous granulomatous infiltration, with vacuolated cells. The spleen, lymph nodes, and bone marrow were minimally involved and the liver not at all. The intestinal changes resembled those of Whipple's disease. In the central nervous system both neuronal and glial cells were ballooned by cytoplasmic storage material. The additional finding of gliosis and granuloma formation distinguished it from Tay-Sachs or Niemann-Pick disease. (The above patient was referred to by Ford[81] and was reported in detail by Abul-Haj and colleagues.[1] **A,** General appearance. Note swellings over pressure points such as the spine and ischial tuberosities. **B,** Swellings of the thumb and wrist. **C,** Biopsy of granuloma showing ballooned cells. (Hematoxylin and eosin; ×430.) A biopsied lymph node showed cells of the same type. **D** and **E,** PAS-positive inclusion material in cells of lymph node. (PAS stain; **D,** ×380; **E,** ×1400.)

abnormality of mucopolysaccharide excretion was detected in the following patients:

1. Two sibs with isolated recessively inherited congenital corneal dystrophy[95a,188]
2. Two sibs and a third child from an unrelated family, with diastrophic dwarfism[151,180]
3. Members of two families with dominantly inherited multiple epiphyseal dysplasia[176]
4. Several patients with the Ellis-van Creveld syndrome[177]
5. Several patients with cartilage-hair hypoplasia[178]
6. Several patients with the X-linked spondyloepiphyseal dysplasia[124]
7. Mother and two daughters (1081594, 1081595, and 1081596) with domi-

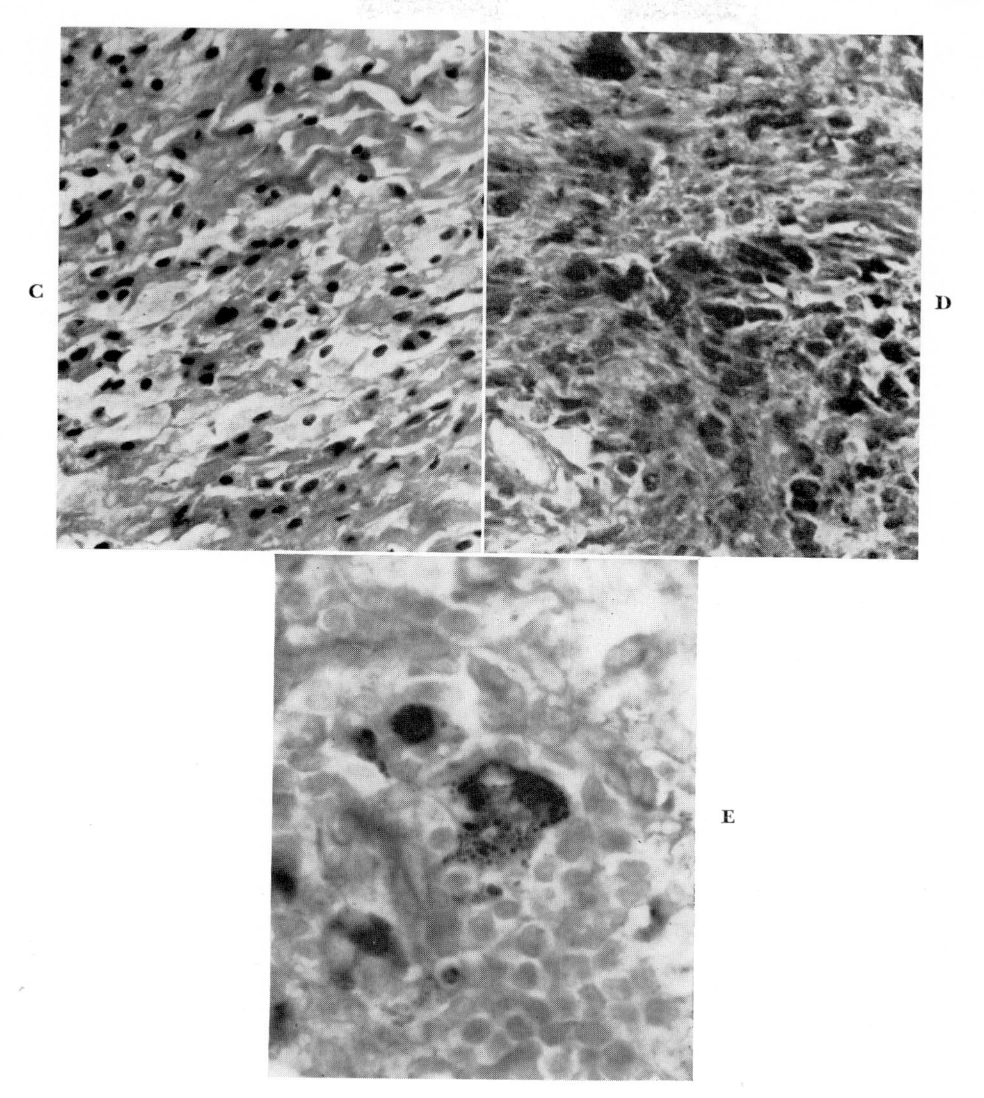

Fig. 9-21, cont'd. For legend see opposite page.

nant spondyloepiphyseal dysplasia, "pseudo-achondroplastic" type[82]

8. A 14-year-old boy (R. C., 1076991) with an undiagnosed disorder manifested by ectopic cartilage and bone formation
9. Two brothers with osteochondritis dissecans (W. M., 495606; E. M., 625295)
10. Two sisters (D. S., 1073527; T. S., 1073528) with epiphyseal dystrophy with cataracts (? chondrodystrophia calcificans congenita[4])
11. Several patients with classic achondroplasia
12. Several patients with the nail-patella syndrome[164,166]
13. Several patients with multiple exostoses[164,263]

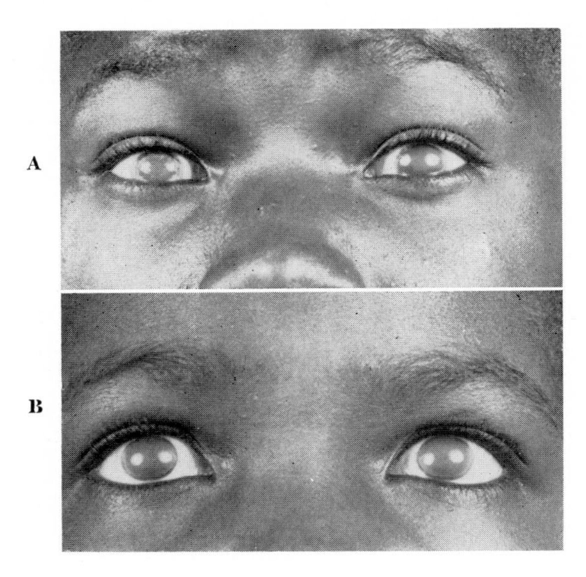

Fig. 9-22. A localized mucopolysaccharidosis? Congenital corneal dystrophy in brother, **A,** and sister, **B,** ages 11 and 10 years, respectively. The parents were second cousins. Two sibs were unaffected. Urinary mucopolysaccharide excretion was normal. No abnormality was detected on general physical examination and radiographic study of the skeleton. "Steamy cornea" was detected in the first weeks of life in both sibs. The change appears to be in the corneal stroma with no epithelial change. In the brother (644879) right corneal transplantation was performed before this photograph. The transplant remained clear for the first two weeks after operation and then gradually became edematous and after three to four months completely opaque. (These cases were called to my attention by Dr. A. E. Maumenee, who reported them, together with similar ones, in 1960.)

OTHER CONSIDERATIONS

No definitive treatment for the mucopolysaccharidoses is known. Hurler,[121] in one of her original cases,[123] observed that thyroid extract, while having no measurable effect, produced subjective improvement in the patient. We have observed the same phenomenon (Fig. 9-7). Large doses of prednisone had no effect on urinary excretion of mucopolysaccharide.[101]

Differential diagnosis

The differentiation of the six mucopolysaccharidoses has been discussed *in extenso* already and is summarized in Table 11. Some simulating conditions are discussed, furthermore, in the section on other possible genetic mucopolysaccharidoses, above.

It is worthwhile mentioning the simulation of the changes in the lumbar spine, as well as some of the other features of MPS I, by *congenital hypothyroidism.*[273a] I had the opportunity to see one such case (C. D., U.S.P.H.S. 235041). Modern methods for the laboratory diagnosis of hypothyroidism easily resolve the problem of differentiation.

Furthermore, Landing and colleagues[153] described a form of neurovisceral lipidosis that previously was reported as "Hurler variant," "pseudo-Hurler disease," or "Tay-Sachs disease with visceral involvement." O'Brien and colleagues[218a] suggested that a logical designation for the condition is *generalized gangliosidosis.* Again the changes in the lumbar spine are strikingly similar to those in MPS I.

Corneal transplants

In cases of MPS V reported by Scheie and colleagues[248] transplants became opacified, suggesting that the corneal clouding in this mucopolysaccharidosis and perhaps in the others as well is a consequence of deposition of mucopolysaccharide. It is possible that the opacification was a graft reaction, however, because it occurred within a few weeks after surgery. Lahdensuu,[148] of Helsinki, noted opacification of corneal transplants in one of four sibs who were labelled "Pfaundler-Hurlerschen Krankheit" but, as noted earlier, more likely suffered from MPS V.

In a case of MPS I King[141] performed a lamellar corneal graft in one eye and a penetrating graft in the other. Whereas the first resulted in improved vision, the second never healed, with resulting loss of all vision. Lamellar grafts may, therefore, be the treatment of choice. Results are, of course, limited not only by severity of the generalized disease but also by the progressive retinal degeneration, which is now recognized as a feature of these disorders.

Retinal degeneration

Retinal degeneration of pigmentary type has often escaped attention in cases of mucopolyaccharidosis, in large part because of the difficulties in observing the changes in the presence of corneal clouding. Changes of this type were found in the case of MPS II shown in Fig. 9-7. They were observed, furthermore, in cases of MPS III and MPS V described here. The electroretinogram was strikingly abnormal, being "nearly extinguished." Franceschetti and co-workers[84] gave a full review of the retinal changes in the mucopolysaccharidoses, together with personal observations. It is clear from the electroretinograms,[93] as well as from histologic studies, that retinal changes occur in MPS types I, II, III, and V.

The biochemical basis of phenotype

Why do mental retardation, corneal clouding, stiff joints, and aortic regurgitation occur in some and not in others of the six mucopolysaccharidoses? To a considerable extent the presence or absence of these extraskeletal features is a matter of degree. All six entities may show them at some stage. The relation between heparitin sulfate and mental retardation is most suggestive of a clinical-chemical correlation. In our experience heparitin sulfate is absent in MPS V and MPS VI, in which mental retardation is mild at the most, and is excreted in large amounts in MPS III, in which the clinical picture is dominated by mental retardation. However, the biochemical findings of Terry and Linker[276] are in disagreement with ours and would not indicate a particular association between heparitin sulfate excretion and mental retardation.

Stiff joints and the carpal tunnel syndrome imply involvement of collagen. Several observations made by using in vitro systems suggest that mucopolysaccharides exert an influence on collagen fiber formation.[210,305] The role of mucopolysaccharide-protein complexes in the rigidity of hyaline cartilage is demonstrated by the drooping ears of rabbits injected with papain.[280] The absence of stiff joints in the Morquio syndrome (limitation of motion may result from joint deformity in this entity) is unique among the six types of MPS. The marked bone rarefaction of Morquio syndrome may bear some relationship to the observation that mucopolysaccharides inhibit nucleation of apatite crystals by collagen fibrils.[211]

Meyer and associates[200] reported that injection of certain acid mucopolysaccharides stimulates the regrowth of hair of shaved areas in rabbits. The findings are of obvious note in connection with the excessive growth of body hair which is characteristic of all six mucopolysaccharidoses with the probable exception of MPS IV.

Nature of the basic defect

Perplexing features of MPS I and MPS II are (1) the excretion of excessive amounts of *two* mucopolysaccharides in the urine and (2) the excretion of the same two mucopolysaccharides in the two entities, which are clearly distinct both clinically and genetically. This dual problem is, however, not a unique one in biochemical genetics, and may mean simply that the basic defect resides in a metabolic step shared by the two mucopolysaccharides. In this connection it may be significant that iduronic acid, a component of chondroitin sulfate B (Table 3, p. 30), has been identified also in heparitin sulfate.[42]

Normally, acid mucopolysaccharides are tightly bound to protein. Dorfman[65,66] has suggested that the basic disorder in the Hurler syndrome concerns the binding protein. Possibly because of change in the amino acid sequence, binding is less effective. The mechanisms for normal control on synthesis of mucopolysaccharides may not be operative, with the result that excessive mucopolysaccharides continue to be produced. Some support for this suggestion comes from the unusual ease of extraction of mucopolysaccharides from tissues of patient with the Hurler syndrome. (An alternative explanation of the last finding is that mucopolysaccharides are produced in excess of the normal capacity of the binding protein.) A deficiency of serine, which there is reason to think is important in the linkage between chondroitin sulfate and protein,[6] might account for imperfect binding of mucopolysaccharide. On theoretical grounds one might, however, expect the disorder resulting from a defect in the binding protein to show dominant inheritance (p. 16). The recessive inheritance of all the mucopolysaccharidoses weighs against Dorfman's suggestion. There might, of course, be a deficiency in an enzyme responsible for linking mucopolysaccharide to the binding protein.

An animal homolog?

The clinical, biochemical, and pathologic features of snorter dwarfism of Hereford cattle[281] have been studied by Lorincz and colleagues[163,164,166,168] as a possible animal homolog of the Hurler syndrome. The disorder is inherited as autosomal recessive. Clinical features include short nose with labored breathing (from which the term "snorter" is derived), rounded forehead, widely spaced eyes, large tongue, short neck, hydrocephalus, beaked lumbar vertebrae, dwarfism, rough hair, and thickened hide. The abnormalities are progressive. Differences from MPS I include absence of corneal clouding, significant hepatosplenomegaly, characteristic changes in the long bones, and typical "gargoyle" cells in the liver and other tissues. Mucopolysacchariduria was demonstrated by Lorincz and

Table 11. The genetic mucopolysaccharidoses

MPS	*Clinical*	*Genetic*	*Biochemical*
I (Hurler syndrome)	Early clouding of cornea, grave manifestations	Autosomal recessive	Chondroitin sulfate B Heparitin sulfate
II (Hunter syndrome)	No clouding of cornea, milder course	X-linked recessive	Chondroitin sulfate B Heparitin sulfate
III (Sanfilippo syndrome)	Mild somatic, severe central nervous system effects	Autosomal recessive	Heparitin sulfate
IV (Morquio syndrome)	Severe bone changes of distinctive types, cloudy cornea, intellect +/−, aortic regurgitation	Autosomal recessive	Keratosulfate
V (Scheie syndrome)	Stiff joints, coarse facies, cloudy cornea, intellect +/−, aortic regurgitation	Autosomal recessive	Chondroitin sulfate B
VI (Maroteaux-Lamy syndrome)	Severe osseous and corneal change, normal intellect	Autosomal recessive	Chondroitin sulfate B

confirmed by McIlwain and Eveleth.[173] Tyler and co-workers[283] on the other hand recovered only chondroitin sulfate A and no chondroitin sulfate B or heparitin sulfate. They concluded that this and the absence of gargoyle cells from the tissues make it unlikely that the bovine disease is comparable to gargoylism in man. (See also Mayes and associates.[190])

SUMMARY

At least six distinct forms of primary genetic disturbance of mucopolysaccharide metabolism can be delineated by combined clinical, genetic, and biochemical studies. The distinguishing features of these six entities are outlined in Table 11. It is virtually certain that other distinct entities exist in the heterogeneous group of heritable disorders of connective tissue.

REFERENCES

1. Abul-Haj, S. K., Martz, D. G., Douglas, W. F., and Geppert, L. J.: Farber's disease. Report of a case with observations on its histogenesis and notes on the nature of the stored material, J. Pediat. **61**:221, 1962.
2. Aegerter, E. E., and Kirkpatrick, J. A., Jr.: Orthopaedic diseases: physiology, pathology and radiology, Philadelphia, 1958, W. B. Saunders Co., p. 99.
3. Alder, A. von: Konstitutionell bedingte Granulationsveränderungen der Leucocyten und Knochenveränderungen, Schweiz. Med. Wschr. **80**:1095, 1950.
4. Allansmith, M., and Senz, E.: Chondrodystrophia congenita punctata (Conradi's disease), Amer. J. Dis. Child. **100**:109, 1960.
5. Anderson, B., Hoffman, P., and Meyer, K.: A serine-linked peptide of chondroitin sulfate, Biochim. Biophys. Acta **74**:309, 1963.
6. Anderson, C. E., Crane, J. T., Harper, H. A., and Hunter, T. W.: Morquio's disease and dysplasia epiphysalis multiplex, J. Bone Joint Surg. **44-A**:295, 1962.

7. Andersson, B., and Tandberg, O.: Lipochondrodystrophy (gargoylism, Hurler snydrome) with specific cutaneous deposits, Acta Paediat. **41**:162, 1952.
8. Asboe-Hansen, G.: Bullous diffuse mastocytosis with urinary hyaluronate excretion, Acta Dermatovener. **42**:211, 1962.
9. Ashby, W. R., Stewart, R. M., and Watkins, J. H.: Chondro-osteo-dystrophy of the Hurler type (gargoylism); a pathological study, Brain **60**:149, 1937.
10. Astaldi, G., and Strosselli, E.: Histochemische Untersuchungen an den Leukoblasten und Leukocyten der konstitutionellen Alderschen Anomalie, Schweiz. Med. Wschr. **88**:989, 1958.
11. Awwaad, S.: Dysostosis multiplex—review of literature and report of two cases with unusual manifestations, Arch. Pediat. **78**:184, 1961.
12. Aycock, E. K., and Paul, J. R., Jr.: Gargoylism; a report of two cases in Negroes, J. S. Carolina Med. Ass. **53**:128, 1957.
13. Barnett, E. J.: Morquio's disease, J. Pediat. **2**:651, 1933.
14. Bartman, J., Mandelbaum, I. M., and Gregoire, P. E.: Mucopolysaccharides of serum and urine in a case of Morquio's disease, Rev. Franç. Étud. Clin. Biol. **8**:250, 1963.
15. Beebe, R. T., and Formel, P. F.: Gargoylism: sex-linked transmission in nine males, Trans. Amer. Clin. Climat. Ass. **66**:199, 1954.
16. Beradinelli, W.: Gargoylisme chez un petit noir, Presse Méd. **64**:1757, 1956.
17. Berggård, I., and Bearn, A. G.: The Hurler syndrome: a biochemical and clinical study, Amer. J. Med. **39**:221, 1965.
18. Berkhan, O.: Zwei Fälle von Skaphokephalie, Arch. Anthrop. **34**:8, 1907.
19. Berliner, M. L.: Lipin keratitis of Hurler's syndrome (gargoylism or dysostosis multiplex); clinical and pathologic report, Arch. Ophthal. **22**:97, 1939.
20. Berry, H. K.: Procedures for testing urine specimens dried on filter paper, Clin. Chem. **5**:603, 1959.
21. Berry, H. K., and Spinanger, J.: A paper spot test useful in study of Hurler's syndrome, J. Lab. Clin. Med. **55**:136, 1960.
22. Bindschedler, J. J.: Polydystrophie du type Hurler chez un frére et une soeur, Bull. Soc. Pédiat. Paris **36**:571, 1938.
23. Binswanger, E., and Ullrich, O.: Ueber die Dysostosis multiplex (Typus Hurler) und ihre Beziehungen zu anderen Konstitutionsanomalien, Z. Kinderheilk. **54**:699, 1933.
24. Bishton, R. L., Norman, R. M., and Tingey, A.: The pathology and chemistry of a case of gargoylism, J. Clin. Path. **9**:305, 1956.
25. Böcker, E.: Zur Erblichkeit der Dysostosis multiplex, Z. Kinderheilk. **63**:688, 1943.
26. Boldt, L.: Beitrag zur Dysostosis multiplex (von Pfaundler-Hurler), Z. Kinderheilk. **63**:679, 1943.
27. Brailsford, J. F.: Chondro-osteo-dystrophy, roentgenographic and clinical features of child with dislocation of vertebrae, Amer. J. Surg. **7**:404, 1929; The radiology of bones and joints, ed. 5, Baltimore, 1953, The Williams & Wilkins Co.
28. Brante, G.: Gargoylism: a mucopolysaccharidosis, Scand. J. Clin. Lab. Invest. **4**:43, 1952.
29. Bridge, E. M., and Holt, L. E., Jr.: Glycogen storage disease; observations on the pathologic physiology of two cases of the hepatic form of the disease, J. Pediat. **27**:299, 1945.
30. Brown, D. H.: Tissue storage of mucopolysaccharides in Hurler-Pfaundler's disease, Proc. Nat. Acad. Sci. **43**:783, 1957.
31. Brown, David H. (St. Louis): Personal communication.
32. Brown, D. O.: Morquio's disease, Med. J. Aust. **1**:598, 1933.
33. Burke, E. C., and Teller, W. M.: Snorter dwarfism in cattle related to gargoylism in children, J. Amer. Vet. Med. Ass. **139**:1211, 1961.
34. Butterworth, T., and Strean, L. P.: Clinical genodermatoses, Baltimore, 1962, The Williams & Wilkins Co.
35. Caffey, J.: Gargoylism (Hunter-Hurler disease, dysostosis multiplex, lipochondrodystrophy); prenatal and neonatal bone lesions and their early postnatal evaluation, Amer. J. Roentgen. **67**:715, 1952.
36. Cameron, J. M., and Gardiner, T. B.: Atypical familial osteochondrodystrophy, Brit. J. Radiol. **36**:135, 1963.
37. Campbell, T. N., and Fried, M.: Urinary mucopolysaccharide excretion in the sex-linked form of the Hurler syndrome, Proc. Soc. Exp. Biol. Med. **108**:529, 1961.
38. Carlisle, J. W., and Good, R. A.: The inflammatory cycle—a method of study in Hurler's disease, Amer. J. Dis. Child. **99**:193, 1960.

39. Chadwick, D. L.: In Fishbein, M., editor: First Inter-American Conference on Congenital Defects, Philadelphia, 1963, J. B. Lippincott Co., p. 147.
40. Chadwick, D. L. (Los Angeles): Personal communication, 1964.
41. Chou, Yi-Che: Ocular signs in gargoylism, Clin. Med. J. **78**:130, 1959.
42. Cifonelli, J. A., and Dorfman, A.: The uronic acid of heparin, Biochem. Biophys. Res. Commun. **7**:41, 1962.
43. Clauson, J., Dyggve, H. V., and Melchior, J. C.: Mucopolysaccharidosis, Arch. Dis. Child. **39**:364, 1963.
44. Cocchi, U.: Polytope erbliche enchondrale Dysostosen, Fortschr. Roentgenstr. **72**:435, 1950.
45. Cocchi, U.: Hereditary diseases with bone changes. In Schinz, H. R., Baensch, W. E., Friedl, E., and Uehlinger, E.: Roentgen-diagnostics, New York, 1951, Grune & Stratton, Inc., p. 728.
46. Cockayne, E. A.: Gargoylism (chondro-osteodystrophy, hepatosplenomegaly, deafness in two brothers), Proc. Roy. Soc. Med. **30**:104, 1936.
47. Cole, H. N., Jr., Irving, R. C., Lund, H. Z., Mercer, R. D., and Schneider, R. W.: Gargoylism with cutaneous manifestations, Arch. Derm. Syph. **66**:371, 1952.
48. Cordes, F. C., and Hogan, J. J.: Dysostosis multiplex (Hurler's disease); lipochondrodystrophy; gargoylism; report of ocular findings in five cases, with a review of the literature, Arch. Ophthal. **27**:637, 1942.
49. Cottier, H.: Infantile kardiovaskuläre Sklerose bei Gargoylismus, Schweiz. Z. Allg. Path. **20**:745, 1957.
50. Coward, N. R., and Nemir, R. L.: Familial osseous dystrophy (Morquio's disease), Amer. J. Dis. Child. **46**:213, 1933.
51. Craig, W. S.: Gargoylism in a twin brother and sister, Arch. Dis. Child. **29**:293, 1954.
52. Crawford, T.: Morquio's disease, Arch. Dis. Child. **14**:70, 1939.
53. Crigler, J. F., Jr., and Najjar, V. A.: Congenital familial nonhemolytic jaundice with kernicterus, Pediatrics **10**:169, 1952.
54. Crome, L.: Epiloia and endocardial fibro-elastosis, Arch. Dis. Child. **29**:136, 1954.
55. Cunningham, R. C.: A contribution to the genetics of gargoylism, J. Neurol. Neurosurg. Psychiat. **17**:191, 1954.
56. Danes, B. S., and Bearn, A. G.: Hurler's syndrome: demonstration of an inherited disorder of connective tissue in cell culture, Science **149**:987, 1965.
57. David, B.: Ueber einen dominanten Erbgang bei einer polytopen enchondralen Dysostose Typ Pfaundler-Hurler, Z. Orthop. **84**:657, 1954.
58. Davis, D. B., and Currier, F. P.: Morquio's disease. Report of two cases, J.A.M.A. **102**:2173, 1934.
59. Dawson, I. M.: The histology and histochemistry of gargoylism, J. Path. Bact. **67**:587, 1954.
60. Debré, R., Marie, J., and Thieffry, S.: La polydystrophie de Hurler: le "gargoylisme" d'Ellis (á l'occasion des trois observations nouvelles), Sem. Hôp. Paris **22**:309, 1946.
61. De Lange, C.: Dysostosis multiplex of the Hurler type (gargoylism), Psychiat. Neurol. (Basel) **1-2**:2, 1942.
62. De Lange, C., Gerlings, P. G., de Kleyn, A., and Lettinga, T. W.: Some remarks on gargoylism, Acta Paediat. **31**:398, 1944.
63. Denny, W., and Dutton, G.: Simple urine test for gargoylism, Brit. Med. J. **1**:1555, 1962.
64. Dorfman, A.: Studies on the biochemistry of connective tissue, Pediatrics **22**:576, 1958.
65. Dorfman, A.: The Hurler syndrome. In Fishbein, M., editor: First Inter-American Conference on Congenital Defects, Philadelphia, 1963, J. B. Lippincott Co., pp. 41-52; also 146-149.
66. Dorfman, A.: Metabolism of acid mucopolysaccharides, Biophys. J. (supp.) **4**:155, 1964.
67. Dorfman, A., and Lorincz, A. E.: Occurrence of urinary acid mucopolysaccharides in the Hurler syndrome, Proc. Nat. Acad. Sci. **43**:443, 1957.
68. Eichenberger, K.: Kann die Dysostosis Morquio als selbständiges Krankheitsbild vom Gargolyismus abgetrennt werden? Ann. Paediat. **182**:107, 1954.
69. Einhorn, N. H., Moore, J. R., Ostrum, H. W., and Rountree, L. G.: Osteochondrodystrophia deformans (Morquio's disease). Report of three cases, Amer. J. Dis. Child. **61**:776, 1941.
70. Einhorn, N. H., Moore, J. R., and Rountree, L. G.: Osteochondrodystrophia deformans (Morquio's disease). Observations at autopsy in one case, Amer. J. Dis. Child. **72**:536, 1946.
71. Ek, J. I.: Cerebral lesions in arthrogryposis multiplex congenita, Acta Paediat. **47**:302, 1958.
72. Ellis, R. W. B.: Gargoylism (chondro-osteodystrophy, corneal opacities, hepatosplenomegaly and mental deficiency), Proc. Roy. Soc. Med. **30**:158, 1936.

73. Ellis, R. W. B., Sheldon, W., and Capon, N. B.: Gargoylism (chondro-osteo-dystrophy, corneal opacities, hepatosplenomegaly and mental deficiency), Quart. J. Med. **5**:119, 1936.
74. Ellman, P.: A rare primary osseous dystrophy, Brit. J. Child. Dis. **30**:188, 1933.
75. Emanuel, R. W.: Gargoylism with cardiovascular involvement in two brothers, Brit. Heart J. **16**:417, 1954.
76. Emery, A. E. H.: Unpublished observations on the kindred reported by Beebe and Formel.[15]
77. Engel, D.: Dysostosis multiplex (Pfaundler-Hurler syndrome), two cases, Arch. Dis. Child. **14**:217, 1939.
78. Engle, R. L., Jr. (New York City): Personal communication.
79. Epps, R. P., and Scott, R. B.: Gargoylism (Hurler's syndrome; lipochondrodystrophy dysostosis multiplex); report of 2 cases in Negro children, J. Pediat. **52**:182, 1958.
80. Farber, S., Cohen, J., and Uzman, L. L.: Lipogranulomatosis, a new lipo-glyco-protein "storage" disease, J. Mount Sinai Hosp., N.Y. **24**:816, 1957.
81. Ford, F. R.: Diseases of the nervous system in infancy, childhood and adolescence, ed. 4, Springfield, Ill., 1960, Charles C Thomas, Publisher, p. 828.
82. Ford, N., Silverman, F. N., and Kozlowski, K.: Spondylo-epiphyseal dysplasia (pseudo-achondroplastic type), Amer. J. Roentgen. **86**:462, 1961.
83. Franceschetti, A., and Forni, S.: The heredo-familial degenerations of the cornea, Acta 16th Internat. Cong. Ophthal. London, July 17-22, 1950, pp. 157-193.
84. Franceschetti, A., François, J., and Babel, J.: Les hérédodégénérescences chorio-rétiniennes (dégénérescences tapeto-rétiniennes), vol. 2, Paris, 1963, Masson et Cie, pp. 998-1000.
85. François, J.: Dystrophie dermo-chondro-cornéenne familiale, Bull. Acad. Roy Med. Belg. **14**:135, 1949.
86. François, J.: Dystrophie dermo-chondro-cornéenne familiale, Ann. Oculist (Paris) **182**:409, 1949.
87. François, J., and Detrait, C.: Dystrophie dermo-chondro-cornéenne familiale, Ann. Paediat. **174**:145, 1950.
88. François, J., and Rabaey, M.: Examen histochimique de la dystrophie cornéenne et étude de l'hérédité dans un cas de gargoylisme (maladie de Hurler), Ann. Oculist (Paris) **185**:784, 1952.
89. Garn, S. M. (Yellow Springs, Ohio): Personal communication.
90. Garn, S. M., and Hurme, V. O.: Dental defects in three siblings afflicted with Morquio's disease, Brit. Dent. J. **93**:210, 1952.
91. Gasteiger, H., and Liebenam, L.: Beitrag zur Dysostosis multiplex unter besonderer Berüchsichtigung des Augenbefundes, Klin. Mbl. Augenheilk. **99**:333, 1937.
92. Gilbert, E. F., and Guin, G. H.: Gargoylism; a review including two occurrences in the American Negro, J. Dis. Child. **95**:69, 1958.
93. Gills, J. P., Hobson, R., Hanley, W. B., and McKusick, V. A.: Hurler's disease and allied mucopolysaccharidoses, Arch. Ophthal. **74**:596, 1965.
94. Glegg, R. E., Eidinger, D., and Leblond, C. P.: Some carbohydrate components of reticular fibers, Science **118**:614, 1953.
95. Goidanich, I. F., and Lenzi, L.: Morquio-Ullrich disease. A new mucopolysaccharidosis, J. Bone Joint Surg. **46-A**:734, 1964.
95a. Goldberg, M. F., Maumenee, A. E., and McKusick, V. A.: Corneal dystrophies: mucopolysaccharide metabolism, Arch. Ophthal. **74**:516, 1965.
96. Grebe, H.: Die Chondrodysplasia, ihre Klinik, Differentialdiagnose und Erbpathologie, Habilitationsschrift, Frankfurt, 1942. Cited by Ullrich.[285]
97. Green, M. A.: Gargoylism (lipochondrodystrophy), J. Neuropath. Exp. Neurol. **7**:399, 1948.
98. Greenfield, J. G., and others: Neuropathology, London, 1958, Edward Arnold & Co., p. 468.
99. Griffiths, S. B., and Findlay, M.: Gargoylism: clinical, radiological and haematological features in two siblings, Arch. Dis. Child. **32**:229, 1958.
100. Grumbach, M. M. (New York City): Personal communication.
101. Grumbach, M. M., and Meyer, K.: Urinary excretion and tissue storage of sulfated mucopolysaccharides in Hurler's syndrome, Amer. J. Dis. Child. **96**:467, 1958.
102. Halperin, S. L., and Curtis, G. M.: The genetics of gargoylism, Amer. J. Ment. Defic. **46**:298,
103. Hambrick, G. W., and Scheie, H. G.: Studies of the skin in Hurler's syndrome: mucopolysaccharidosis, Arch. Derm. **85**:455, 1962.

104. Harvey, R. M.: Hurler-Pfaundler syndrome (gargoylism). Review of the literature with report of an additional case, Amer. J. Roentgen. **48**:732, 1942.
105. Hässler, E.: Die Beziehungen der Hurlerschen Krankheit (Dysostosis multiplex-dysostotische Idiotie-Gargolismus) zum Kretinismus, Mschr. Kinderheilk. **86**:96, 1941.
106. Haust, M. D., and Landing, B. H.: Histochemical studies in Hurler's disease: a new method for localization of acid mucopolysaccharide, and an analysis of lead acetate "fixation," J. Histochem. Cytochem. **9**:79, 1961.
107. Helmholtz, H. F., and Harrington, E. R.: Syndrome characterized by congenital clouding of the cornea and by other anomalies, Amer. J. Dis. Child. **12**:793, 1931.
108. Helwig-Larsen, H. F., and Mørch, E. T.: Genetic aspects of osteochondrodystrophy. Silfverskiöld's and Morquio's syndromes, Acta Path. Microbiol. Scand. **22**:335, 1945.
109. Henderson, J. L.: Gargoylism; review of principal features with report of five cases, Arch. Dis. Child. **15**:215, 1940.
110. Henderson, J. L., MacGregory, A. R., Thannhauser, S. J., and Holden, R.: Pathology and biochemistry of gargoylism; report of three cases with review of literature, Arch. Dis. Child. **27**:230, 1952.
111. Hessburg, P. C.: Hurler's disease, Henry Ford Hosp. Med. Bull. **10**:419, 1962.
112. Hillman, J. W., and Johnson, J. T. H.: Arthrogryposis multiplex congenita in twins, J. Bone Joint Surg. **34-A**:211, 1952.
113. Hochheim, W., Körner, H., and Liebe, S.: Beitrag zur den polytopen, erblichen, enchondralen Dysostosen, Arch. Orthop. Unfallchir. **47**:463, 1955.
114. Hooper, J. M. D.: Unusual case of gargoylism, Guy's Hosp. Rep. **101**:222, 1952.
115. Horrigan, W. D., and Baker, D. H.: Gargoylism: a review of the roentgen skull changes with description of a new finding, Amer. J. Roentgen. **86**:473, 1961.
116. Horsch, K.: Ueber hereditäre degenerative Osteoarthropathie, Arch. Orthop. Unfallchir. **34**:536, 1934.
117. Hubeny, M. J., and Delano, R. J.: Dysostosis multiplex, Amer. J. Roentgen. **46**:336, 1941.
118. Hueper, W. C.: Macromolecular substances as pathogenic agents, Arch. Path. **33**:267, 1942.
119. Hueper, W. C.: Experimental studies in cardiovascular pathology. Pectin atheromatosis and thesaurosis in rabbits and in dogs, Arch. Path. **34**:883, 1942.
120. Hunter, C.: A rare disease in two brothers, Proc. Roy. Soc. Med. **10**:104, 1917.
121. Hurler, G.: Ueber einen Typ multipler Abartungen, vorwiegend am Skelettsystem, Z. Kinderheilk. **24**:220, 1919.
122. Husler, J.: Handbuch der Kinderheilkunde, ed. 4, vol. 1, p. 651.
123. Jackson, W. P. U.: Clinical features, diagnosis and osseous lesions of gargoylism exemplified in 3 siblings, Arch. Dis. Child. **26**:549, 1951.
124. Jacobsen, A. W.: Hereditary osteochondrodystrophia deformans. A family with twenty members affected in five generations, J.A.M.A. **113**:121, 1939.
125. Jacobson, L., Kibel, M. A.: Hurler's syndrome: a clinical report on two cases, Central Afr. J. Med. **4**:193, 1958.
126. James, T.: Multiple congenital articular rigidities: a review of the literature with report of 2 cases, Edinburgh Med. J. **58**:565, 1951.
127. Jelke, H.: Gargoylism; report of a case, Ann. Paediat. **177**:355, 1951.
128. Jelke, H.: Gargoylism. II. Post-mortem findings in an earlier published case, Ann. Paediat. **184**:101, 1955.
129. Jensen, W. J.: Dermo-chondro-corneal dystrophy, Acta Ophthal. **36**:71, 1958.
130. Jermain, L. F., Rohn, R. J., and Bond, W. H.: Studies on the role of the reticuloendothelial system in Hurler's disease, Clin. Res. **7**:216, 1959.
131. Jermain, L. F., Rohn, R. J., and Bond, W. H.: Studies on the role of the reticuloendothelial system in Hurler's disease, Amer. J. Med. Sci. **239**:612, 1960.
132. Jervis, G. A.: Familial mental deficiency akin to amaurotic idiocy and gargoylism, Arch. Neur. Psychiat. **47**:943, 1942.
133. Jervis, G. A.: Gargoylism: study of 10 cases with emphasis on the formes frustes, Arch. Neur. Psychiat. **63**:681, 1950.
134. Jewesbury, R. C., and Spence, J. C.: Two cases: (1) oyxcephaly and (2) acrocephaly, with other congenital deformities, Proc. Roy. Soc. Med. **14**:27, 1921.
135. Jordans, G. H. W.: Hereditary granulation anomaly of leucocytes (Alder), Acta Med. Scand. **129**:348, 1947.

136. Josephy, H.: Lipoidosis of the brain combined with glycogenosis of the liver, J. Neuropath. Exp. Neurol. **8**:214, 1949.
137. Kaplan, D., and Fisher, B.: The effect of methylprednisolone on mucopolysaccharides of rabbit vitreous humor and costal cartilage, Biochem. Biophys. Acta **93**:102, 1962.
138. Kaplan, D., and Meyer, K.: The fate of injected mucopolysaccharides, J. Clin. Invest. **41**:741, 1962.
139. Kennealy, E. V.: The ocular manifestations of gargoylism, Amer. J. Ophthal. **36**:663, 1953.
140. Kibel, M., and Jacobson, L. (South Rhodesia): Personal communication.
141. King, J. H., Jr. (Washington, D. C.): Personal communication, 1964.
142. Klintworth, G. K., and Vogel, F. S.: Macular corneal dystrophy. An inherited acid mucopolysaccharide storage disease of the corneal fibroblast, Amer. J. Path. **45**:565, 1964.
143. Kny, W.: Zur Kenntnis der Dysostosis multiplex Typ Pfaundler-Hurler, Z. Kinderheilk. **63**:366, 1942.
144. Kobayashi, N.: Acid mucopolysaccharide granules in the glomerular epithelium in gargoylism, Amer. J. Path. **35**:591, 1959.
145. Krovetz, L. J., Lorincz, A. E., and Schiebler, G. L.: Cardiovascular manifestations of the Hurler syndrome. Hemodynamic and angiocardiographic observations in 15 patients, Circulation **31**:132, 1965.
146. Kressler, R. J., and Aegerter, E. E.: Hurler's syndrome (gargoylism); summary of literature and report of case with autopsy findings, J. Pediat. **12**:579, 1938.
147. Lagunoff, D., Ross, R., and Benditt, E. P.: Histochemical and electron microscopic study in a case of Hurler's syndrome, Amer. J. Path. **41**:273, 1962.
148. Lahdensuu, S.: Fälle der sogenannten Pfaundler-Hurlersche Krankheit (Dysostosis multiplex), Mschr. Kinderheilk. **92**:340, 1943.
149. Lahey, M. E., Lomas, R. D., and Worth, T. C.: Lipochondrodystrophy (gargoylism), J. Pediat. **31**:220, 1947.
150. Lamy, M., and Maroteaux, P.: La nanisme diastrophique, Presse Méd. **68**:1977, 1960.
151. Lamy, M., Maroteaux, P., and Bader, J. P.: Étude génétique du gargoylisme, J. génét. hum. **6**:156, 1957.
152. Lamy, M., Maroteaux, P., and Frézal, J.: Les chondrodystrophies genotypiques. Définition et limites, Sem. Hôp. Paris **34**:1675, 1958.
153. Landing, B. H., Silverman, F. N., Craig, J. M., Jacoby, M. D., Lahey, M. E., and Chadwick, D. L.: Familial neurovisceral lipidosis, Amer. J. Dis. Child. **108**:503, 1964.
154. Lausecker, H.: Zur Symptomatologie der Dysostosis multiplex (Pfaundler-Hurler), Hautarzt **5**:538, 1954.
155. Léri, A.: Une maladie congénitale et héréditaire de l'ossification: la pléonostéose familiale, Bull. Soc. Méd. Hôp. Paris **45**:1228, 1921.
156. Léri, A.: Pléonostéose familiale (dystrophie osseuse genéraliseé, congénitale et héréditaire), Presse Méd. **2**:13, 1922.
157. Levin, S.: A specific skin lesion in gargoylism, Amer. J. Dis. Child. **99**:444, 1960.
158. Lindsay, S.: The cardiovascular system in gargoylism, Brit. Heart J. **12**:17, 1950.
159. Lindsay, S., Reilly, W. A., Gotham, Th. J., and Skahen, R.: Gargoylism. II. Study of pathologic lesions and clinical review of twelve cases, Amer. J. Dis. Child. **76**:239, 1948.
160. Linker, A., and Terry, K. D.: Urinary acid mucopolysaccharides in normal man and in Hurler's syndrome, Proc. Soc. Exp. Biol. Med. **113**:743, 1963.
161. Lipton, E. L., and Morgenstern, S. H.: Arthrogryposis multiplex congenita in identical twins, Amer. J. Dis. Child. **89**:233, 1955.
162. Lorincz, A. E.: Acid mucopolysaccharides in the Hurler syndrome, Fed. Proc. **17**:266, 1958.
163. Lorincz, A. E.: "Snorter" dwarf cattle, a naturally occurring heritable disorder of acid mucopolysaccharide metabolism which resembles the Hurler syndrome, Amer. J. Dis. Child. **100**:488, 1960.
164. Lorincz, A. E.: Heritable disorders of acid mucopolysaccharide metabolism in humans and in snorter dwarf cattle, Ann. N.Y. Acad. Sci. **91**:644, 1961.
165. Lorincz, A. E.: Mucopolysacchariduria in children with hereditary arthro-osteo-onychodysplasia (Abstract), Fed. Proc. **21**:173, 1962.
166. Lorincz, A. E.: Hurler's syndrome in man and snorter dwarfism in cattle. Heritable disorders of connective tissue acid mucopolysaccharide metabolism, Clin. Orthop. **33**:104, 1964.
167. Lorincz, A. E. (Chicago): Personal communication.

168. Lorincz, A. E., and colleagues: Mucopolysaccharidosis in snorter dwarf cattle, J. Anim. Sci. **19**:1216, 1960.
169. Lunström, R.: Gargoylism; three cases, Nord. Med. **33**:41, 1947.
170. Lurie, L. A., and Levy, S.: Gargoylism, Amer. J. Med. Sci. **207**:184, 1944.
171. McCormick, W. F.: Rupture of the stomach in children. Review of the literature and a report of seven cases, Arch. Path. **67**:416, 1959.
172. MacGillivray, R. C.: Gargoylism (Hurler disease), J. Ment. Sci. **98**:687, 1952.
173. McIlwain, P., and Eveleth, D. F.: Urinary mucopolysaccharides of dwarf cattle, Vet. Med. **57**:508, 1962.
174. McKusick, V. A.: Hereditary disorders of connective tissue, Bull. N.Y. Acad. Med. **35**:143, 1959.
175. McKusick, V. A.: On the X chromosome of man, Quart. Rev. Biol. **37**:69, 1962; also Washington, D. C., AIBS, 1964.
176. McKusick, V. A., and colleagues: Medical genetics 1958-1960, St. Louis, 1961, The C. V. Mosby Co., Figs. 64 and 65, pp. 476-479.
177. McKusick, V. A., Egeland, J. A., Eldridge, R., and Krusen, D. E.: Dwarfism in the Amish. I. The Ellis-van Creveld syndrome, Bull. Hopkins Hosp. **115**:306, 1964.
178. McKusick, V. A., Eldridge, R., Hostetler, J. A., and Ruanguit, U.: Dwarfism in the Amish. II. Cartilage-hair hypoplasia, Bull. Hopkins Hosp. **116**:285, 1965.
179. McKusick, V. A., Kaplan, D., Wise, D., Hanley, W. B., Suddarth, S. B., Sevick, M. E., and Maumenee, A. E.: The genetic mucopolysaccharidoses, Medicine **44**:445, 1965.
180. McKusick, V. A., and Milch, R. A.: The clinical behavior of genetic disease: selected aspects, Clin. Orthop. **33**:22, 1964.
181. Magee, K. R.: Leptomeningeal changes associated with lipochondrodystrophy (gargoylism), Arch. Neur. Psychiat. **63**:282, 1950.
182. Maroteaux, P., and Lamy, M.: Les dysplasies spondylo-épiphysaires génotypiques, Sem. Hôp. Paris **34**:1685, 1958.
183. Maroteaux, P., and Lamy, M.: Opacités cornéennes et trouble metabolique dans la maladie de Morquio, Rev. Franc. Étud. Clin. Biol. **6**:481, 1961.
184. Maroteaux, P., and Lamy, M.: La maladie de Morquio. Étude clinique, radiologique et biologique, Presse Méd. **71**:2091, 1963.
185. Maroteaux, P., and Lamy, M.: Achondroplasia in man and animals, Clin. Orthop. **33**:91, 1964.
185a. Maroteaux, P., and Lamy, M.: Hurler's disease, Morquio's disease and related mucopolysaccharidoses, J. Pediat. **67**:312, 1965.
186. Maroteaux, P., Lévêque, B., Marie, J., and Lamy, M.: Une nouvelle dysostose avec elimination urinaire de chondroitine-sulfate B, Presse Méd. **71**:1849, 1963.
187. Mathur, P. S.: Gargoylism, Indian J. Pediat. **24**:372, 1957.
188. Maumenee, A. E.: Congenital hereditary corneal dystrophy, Amer. J. Ophthal. **50**:1114, 1960.
189. Mauri, C., and Soldati, M.: Les caracteristiques cytochimiques des granulations cellulaires de Alder. Definition de la dysostose enchondrale multiple en tant que polysaccharidose, Schweiz. Med. Wschr. **88**:992, 1958.
190. Mayes, J. S., Hansen, R. G., Gregory, P. W., and Tyler, W. S.: Mucopolysaccharide excretion in dwarf and normal cattle, J. Anim. Sci. **23**:833, 1964.
191. Meyer, H. F., and Brennemann, J.: A rare osseous dystrophy (Morquio), Amer. J. Dis. Child. **43**:123, 1932.
192. Meyer, K.: Chemistry of ground substance: In Asboe-Hansen, G., editor: Connective tissue in health and disease. Copenhagen, 1954, Ejnar Munksgaard, p. 54.
193. Meyer, K.: Abstracts of 130th Amer. Chem. Soc. Meetings, Sept., 1956, p. 150.
194. Meyer, K. (New York City): Personal communication.
195. Meyer, K., Davidson, E., Linker, A., and Hoffman, P.: The acid mucopolysaccharides of connective tissue, Biochim Biophys. Acta **21**:506, 1956.
196. Meyer, K., Grumbach, M. M., Linker, A., and Hoffman, P.: Excretion of sulfated mucopolysaccharides in gargoylism (Hurler's syndrome), Proc. Soc. Exp. Biol. Med. **97**:275, 1958.
197. Meyer, K., and Hoffman, P.: Hurler's syndrome, Arth. Rheum. **4**:552, 1961.
198. Meyer, K., Hoffman, P., and Linker, A.: Chondroitin sulfate B and heparitin sulfate (Abstract), Ann. Rheum. Dis. **16**:129, 1957.

199. Meyer, K., Hoffman, P., Linker, A., Grumbach, M. M., and Sampson, P.: Sulfated mucopolysaccharides of urine and organs in gargoylism (Hurler's syndrome). II. Additional studies, Proc. Soc. Exp. Biol. Med. **102**:587, 1959.
200. Meyer, K., Kaplan, D., and Steigleder, G. K.: Effect of acid mucopolysaccharides on hair growth in the rabbit, Proc. Soc. Exp. Biol. Med. **108**:59, 1961.
201. Meyer, K., Linker, A., Davidson, E. A., and Weissman, B.: The mucopolysaccharides of bovine cornea, J. Biol. Chem. **205**:611, 1953.
202. Meyer, S. J., and Okner, H. B.: Dysostosis multiplex with special reference to ocular findings, Amer. J. Ophthal. **22**:713, 1939.
203. Millman, G., and Whittick, J. W.: A sex-linked variant of gargoylism, J. Neurol. Neurosurg. Psychiat. **15**:253, 1952.
204. Mittwoch, V.: Nuclear segmentation of the neutrophils in heterozygous carriers of gargoylism, Nature **193**:1209, 1962.
205. Mittwoch, V. (London): Personal communication, 1964.
206. Morquio, L.: Sur une forme de dystrophie osseuse familiale, Bull. Soc. Pédiat. de Paris **27**:145, 1929.
207. Muir, H., Mittwoch, V., and Bitter, T.: The diagnostic value of isolated urinary mucopolysaccharides and of lymphocytic inclusions in gargolyism, Arch. Dis. Child. **38**:358, 1963.
208. Murray, J. F.: Pulmonary disability in the Hurler syndrome (lipochondrodystrophy). A study of two cases, New Eng. J. Med. **261**:378, 1959.
209. Naidoo, D.: Gargoylism (Hurler's disease): neuropathological report, J. Ment. Sci. **99**:74, 1953.
210. Nemeth-Csoka, M.: Untersuchungen über die kollagen Fasern. I. Ueber die submicroscopische Struktur der in vitro präzipitierten kollagen Fasern und die stabilisierende Rolle der sauren Mukopolysaccharide, Acta Histochem. **9**:282, 1960.
211. Neuman, W. F.: Chemical dynamics of bone mineral. In Rodahl, K., Nicholson, J. T., and Brown, E. M., editors: Bone as a tissue, New York, 1960, McGraw-Hill Book Co., Inc.
212. Newell, F. W., and Koistinen, A.: Lipochondrodystrophy (gargoylism); pathologic findings in five eyes of three patients, Arch. Ophthal. **53**:45, 1955.
213. Nisbet, N. W., and Cupit, B. F.: Gargoylism; report of a case, Brit. J. Surg. **41**:404, 1954.
214. Njå, A.: A sex-linked type of gargoylism, Acta Paediat. **33**:267, 1946.
215. Noller, F.: Dysostosis multiplex (Hurler) und verwandte Krankheitsbilder, Deutsch. Z. Chir. **258**:259, 1943.
216. Nonne, M.: Familiäres Verkommen (3 Geschwister) einer Kombination von imperfekter Chondrodystrophie mit imperfekten Myxoedema infantile, Deutsch. Z. Nervenheilk. **83**:263, 1925.
217. Norman, R. M., Tingey, A. H., Newman, C. G. H., and Ward, S. P.: Tay-Sachs disease with visceral involvement and its relation to gargoylism, Arch. Dis. Child. **39**:634, 1964.
218. O'Brien, D., and Ibbott, F. A., editors: Laboratory manual of pediatric micro- and ultramicro-biochemical techniques, ed. 3, New York, 1962, Harper & Row, Publishers.
218a. O'Brien, J. S., Stern, M. B., Landing, B. H., O'Brien, J. K., and Donnell, G. N.: Generalized gangliosidosis, another inborn error of ganglioside metabolism? (Abstract), J. Pediat. **67**:949, 1965.
219. Osler, W.: Sporadic cretinism in America, Trans. Cong. Amer. Phys. **4**:169, 1897.
220. Park, E. A., and Powers, G. F.: Acrocephaly and scaphocephaly with symmetrically distributed malformations of the extremities, Amer. J. Dis. Child. **20**:235, 1920.
221. Pearson, H. A., and Lorincz, A. E.: A characteristic bone marrow finding in the Hurler syndrome, Pediatrics **34**:280, 1964.
222. Pedrini, V., Lenuzzi, L., and Zambotti, V.: Isolation and identification of keratosulfate in urine of patients affected by Morquio-Ullrich disease, Proc. Soc. Exp. Biol. Med. **110**:847, 1962.
223. Pfaundler, M.: Demonstrationen über einen Typus kindlicher Dysostose, Jahrb. Kinderheilk. **92**:420, 1920.
224. Pohl, J. F.: Osteodystrophy (Morquio's disease): progressive kyphosis from congenital wedge-shaped vertebrae, J. Bone Joint Surg. **21**:187, 1939.
225. Puretić, S., Puretić, B., Fiser-Herman, M., and Adamčić, M.: A unique form of mesenchymal dysplasia, Brit. J. Derm. **74**:8, 1962.

226. Putnam, M. C., and Pelkan, K. F.: Scaphocephaly with malformations of skeleton and other tissues, Amer. J. Dis. Child. **29**:51, 1925.
227. Rainer, S., and Böök, J. A.: Genetics and blood morphology in amaurotic idiocy, Lancet **1**:1077, 1958.
228. Rask, M. R.: Morquio-Brailsford osteochondrodystrophy and osteogenesis imperfecta: report of a patient with both conditions, J. Bone Joint Surg. **45-A**:561, 1963.
229. Rebuck, J., and Crowley, J.: A method of studying leukoctye functions in vivo, Ann. N.Y. Acad. Sci. **59**:757, 1955.
230. Reilly, W. A.: The granules in the leucocytes in gargoylism, Amer. J. Dis. Child. **62**:489, 1941.
231. Renuart, A. W.: Screening procedures in mentally retarded and/or neurologically abnormal children, Unpublished paper.
232. Renuart, A. W. (Butner, N. C.): Personal communication.
233. Rich, C., Di Ferrante, N., and Archibald, R. M.: Acid mucopolysaccharide excretion in the urine of children, J. Lab. Clin. Med. **50**:686, 1957.
234. Robinow, M.: Morquio's disease, Clin. Orthop. **11**:138, 1958.
235. Robins, M. M., Stevens, H. F., and Linker, A.: Morquio's disease: an abnormality of mucopolysaccharide metabolism, J. Pediat. **62**:881, 1963.
236. Rocher, H.-L., and Pesme, P.: Un cas de pléonostéose (maladie de Léri) avec cornées opalescentes, J. Méd. Bordeaux **123**:121, 1946.
237. Rose, J. R., Hawke, W. A., and Brown, A.: Gargoylism, Arch. Dis. Child. **16**:71, 1941.
238. Royer, P.: La cellule de Buhot et le diagnostic du gargoylisme, Sang **30**:37, 1959.
239. Rubin, P.: Dynamic classification of bone dysplasias, Chicago, 1964, Year Book Medical Publishers, Inc.
240. Rudder, B. de: Ueber "Phosphatiddiathese" und ihr Verhältnis zur Dysostosis multiplex und Dysostosis Morquio, Z. Kinderheilk. **63**:407, 1942.
241. Ruggles, H. C.: Dwarfism due to disordered epiphyseal development, Amer. J. Roentgen. **25**:91, 1931.
242. Rukavina, J. G., Falls, H. F., Holt, J. F., and Block, W. G.: Léri's pleonosteosis, a study of a family with review of the literature, J. Bone Joint Surg. **41-A**:397, 1959.
243. Russell, D. S.: Observations on the pathology of hydrocephalus. Special report series, Med. Res. Counc. No. 265, London, 1948, p. 52.
244. Salam, M., and Idriss, H.: Infantile amaurotic family idiocy and gargoylism in siblings, Pediatrics **34**:658, 1964.
245. Sanfilippo, S. J., and Good, R. A.: A laboratory study of the Hurler syndrome (Abstract), Amer. J. Dis. Child. **102**:140, 1964.
246. Sanfilippo, S. J., Podosin, R., Langer, L. O., Jr., and Good, R. A.: Mental retardation associated with acid mucopolysacchariduria (heparitin sulfate type), J. Pediat. **63**:837, 1963.
247. Scharf, J.: Ein Beitrag zur Kenntnis der Dysostosis multiplex (Hurler) unter besonderer Berücksichtigung der Erbverhältnisse, Gräefe Arch. Ophthal. **143**:477, 1941.
248. Scheie, H. G., Hambrick, G. W., Jr., and Barness, L. A.: A newly recognized forme fruste of Hurler's disease (gargoylism), Amer. J. Ophthal. **53**:753, 1962.
248a. Schenk, E. A., and Haggerty, J.: Morquio's disease, a radiologic and morphologic study, Pediatrics **34**:839, 1964.
249. Schinz, H. R., and Furtwängler, A.: Zur Kenntnis einer hereditären Osteoarthropathie mit rezessivem Erbgang, Deutsch. Z. Chir. **207**:398, 1928.
250. Schmidt, M. B.: Die anatomischen Veränderungen des Skeletts bei der Hurlerschen Krankheit, Zbl. Allg. Path. **79**:113, 1942.
251. Schmidt, R.: Eine bischer nicht beschriebene Form familiäres Hornhautentartung in Verbindung mit Osteoarthropathie, Klin. Msbl. Augenheilk. **100**:616, 1938.
252. Schwarz, H., and Gagne, R.: A case of gargoylism, Canad. Med. Ass. J. **66**:375, 1952.
253. Sears, H. R., and Maddox, J. K.: A case of Hurler's disease, Med. J. Aust. **1**:488, 1945.
254. Segni, G., Romano, C., and Tortorolo, G.: Diagnostic test for gargoylism (Letter), Lancet **2**:420, 1964.
255. Shands, A. R., Raney, R. B., and Brashear, H. R.: Handbook of orthopaedic surgery, ed. 6, St. Louis, 1963, The C. V. Mosby Co.
256. Shelling, D. H.: Osteochondrodystrophia deformans (Morquio's disease). In Brennemann's practice of pediatrics, vol. 4, Hagerstown, 1948, W. F. Prior Co., Inc., chap. 29.

257. Shelling, D. H.: In McQuarrie, Irvine, and Kelley, Vincent C., editors: Brennemann's practice of pediatrics, Hagerstown, 1959, W. F. Prior Co., Inc., chap. 29.
258. Singh, S., Petrie, J. G., and Pirozynski, W. J.: Clinicopathological review of ten cases of Morquio's disease, Canad. J. Surg. **5**:404, 1962.
259. Sjolin, S., and Skoog, T.: The clawhand in gargoylism, its pathology and treatment, Acta Paediat. **41**:563, 1952.
260. Slot, G., and Burgess, G. L.: Gargoylism, Proc. Roy. Soc. Med. **31**:1113, 1937.
261. Smith, E. B., Hempelmann, T. C., Moore, S., and Barr, D. P.: Gargoylism (dysostosis multiplex): two adult cases with one autopsy, Ann. Intern. Med. **36**:652, 1952.
262. Smith, R., and McCort, J. J.: Osteochondrodystrophy (Morquio-Brailsford type): occurrence in three siblings, Calif. Med. **88**:55, 1959.
263. Solomon, L.: Hereditary multiple exostosis, Amer. J. Hum. Genet. **16**:351, 1964.
264. Sorsby, A.: Hereditary affections of the retina and choroid, Acta Genet. Med. (Roma) **13**:20, 1964.
265. Stacey, M., and Baker, S. A.: Chemical analysis of tissue polysaccharides, J. Clin. Path. **9**:314, 1956 (appendix to paper of Bishton et al.[24]).
266. Steen, R. E.: A family consisting of three cases of Hunter's polydystrophy (gargoylism) with cardiac lesions (Abstract), Brit. Heart J. **19**:585, 1957; Hunter's polydystrophy (gargoylism) with cardiac lesions and some formes frustes, Brit. Heart J. **21**:269, 1959.
267. Steiness, I.: Acid mucopolysaccharides in urine in gargoylism, Pediatrics **27**:112, 1961.
268. Stern, C.: Principles of human genetics, San Francisco, 1950, W. H. Freeman & Co., Publishers, p. 406.
269. Stern, W. G.: Arthrogryposis multiplex congenita, J.A.M.A. **81**:1507, 1923.
270. Straus, R., Merliss, R., and Reiser, R.: Gargoylism. Review of the literature and report of the sixth autopsied case with chemical studies, Amer. J. Clin. Path. **17**:671, 1947.
271. Strauss, L.: The pathology of gargoylism. Report of a case and review of the literature, Amer. J. Path. **24**:855, 1948.
272. Strauss, L., and Platt, R.: Endocardial sclerosis in infancy associated with abnormal storage (gargoylism). Report of a case in an infant, age 5 months, and review of the literature, J. Mount Sinai Hosp. N.Y. **24**:1258, 1957.
273. Summerfeldt, P., and Brown, A.: Morquio's disease: Report of two cases, Arch. Dis. Child. **11**:221, 1936.
273a. Swoboda, W.: Anguläre dorsolumbale Kyphose als unbekanntes skelettzeichen beim kongenitalen Myxöedem, Fortschr. Röentgenstrahl. **73**:740, 1950.
274. Taylor, H. E.: The role of mucopolysaccharides in the pathogenesis of intimal fibrosis and arteriosclerosis of the human aorta, Amer. J. Path. **24**:871, 1953.
275. Teller, W. M., Rosevear, J. W., and Burke, E. C.: Identification of heterozygous carriers of gargoylism, Proc. Soc. Exp. Biol. Med. **108**:276, 1961.
276. Terry, K., and Linker, A.: Distinction among four forms of Hurler's syndrome, Proc. Soc. Exp. Biol. Med. **115**:394, 1964.
277. Thannhauser, S.: Lipoidoses: diseases of the cellular lipid metabolism, New York, 1950, Oxford University Press.
278. Thomas, J. E.: Gargoylism in the African: report of a case, Cent. Afr. J. Med. **4**:112, 1958.
279. Thomas, L.: Reversible collapse of rabbit ears after intravenous papain, and prevention of recovery by cortisone, J. Exp. Med. **104**:245, 1956.
280. Thomas, L., McCluskey, R. T., Potter, J. L., and Weissmann, G.: Comparison of the effects of papain and vitamin A on cartilage. I. The effects in rabbits, J. Exp. Med. **111**:705. 1960.
281. Turman, E. J.: Methods for controlling hereditary defects, Polled Hereford World, p. 10, Sept. 1960.
282. Tuthill, C. R.: Juvenile amaurotic idiocy, Arch. Neurol Psychiat. **32**:198, 1934.
283. Tyler, W. S., Gregory, P. W., and Meyer, K.: Sulfated mucopolysaccharides of urine from brachycephalic bovine dwarfs, Amer. J. Vet. Res. **23**:96, 1962.
284. Ullrich, O.: Die Pfaundler-Hurlersche Krankheit. Ein Beitrag zum Problem pleiotroper Genwirkung in der Erbpathologie des Menschen, Ergebn, Inn. Med. Kinderheilk. **63**:929, 1943.
285. Ullrich, O., and Wiedemann, H. R.: Zur Frage der konstitutionellen Granulationanomalien der Leukocyten in ihrer Beziehung zu enchondralen Dysostosen, Klin. Wschr. **31**:107, 1953.

286. Ultmann, J. E., Mutter, R. D., Tannenbaum, M., and Warner, R. R. P.: Clinical, cytologic and biochemical studies in systemic mast cell disease, Ann. Intern. Med. **61:**326, 1964.
287. Uzman, L. L.: Chemical nature of the storage substance in gargoylism, Arch. Path. **60:**308, 1955.
288. Uzman, L. L.: Personal communication, March 9, 1956.
289. Valentin, B.: Pleonosteosis familiaris (Léri). In Schwalbe-Gruber: Die Morphologie der Missbildungen des Menschen und der Tiere, Part 3, Jena, Gustav Fischer, p. 502.
290. Vanace, P. W., Friedman, S., and Wagner, B. M.: Mitral stenosis in an atypical case of gargoylism: a case report with pathologic and histochemical studies of the cardiac tissues, Circulation **21:**80, 1960.
291. Van Pelt, J. F.: Gargoylism, Thesis, Nijmegen University, 1960.
292. Van Pelt, J. F., and Huizinga, J.: Some observations on the genetics of gargoylism, Acta Genet. (Basel) **12:**1, 1962.
293. Veasy, C. A.: Ocular findings associated with dysostosis multiplex and Morquio's disease, Arch. Ophthal. **25:**557, 1941.
294. Voisin, J., and Voisin, R.: Un cas d'achondroplasie, Encephale (Paris) **4:**221, 1909.
295. Von Noorden, G. K., Zellweger, H., and Ponseti, I. V.: Ocular findings in Morquio-Ullrich's disease, Arch. Ophthal. **64:**585, 1960.
296. Waardenburg, P. J., Franceschetti, A., and Klein, D.: Genetics and ophthalmology, vol. 1, Springfield, Ill., 1961, Charles C Thomas, Publisher.
297. Wagner, R.: Glycogen content of isolated white blood cells in glycogen storage disease, Amer. J. Dis. Child. **73:**559, 1947.
298. Washington, J. A.: Lipochondrodystrophy. In Brennemann's practice of pediatrics, vol. 4, Hagerstown, 1937, W. F. Prior Co., Inc., chap. 30.
299. Watson-Jones, R.: Léri's pleonosteosis, carpal tunnel compression of the median nerves and Morton's metatarsalgia, J. Bone Joint Surg. **31-B:**560, 1949.
300. Whiteside, J. D., and Cholmeley, J. G.: Morquio's disease; review of literature with description of 4 cases, Arch. Dis. Child. **27:**487, 1952.
301. Wiedemann, H. R.: Ausgedehnte und allgemeine erblich bedingte Bildungs- und Wachstumsfehler des Knochengerüstes, Mschr. Kinderheilk. **102:**136, 1954.
302. Wolf, H. G.: Zur Frage der Alder-Anomalie der Leukocyten, Z. Kinderheilk. **75:**27, 1954.
303. Wolfe, H. J., Blennerhasset, J. B., Young, G. F., and Cohen, R. B.: Hurler's syndrome. A histochemical study. New techniques for localization of very water-soluble acid mucopolysaccharides, Amer. J. Path. **45:**1007, 1964.
304. Wolff, D.: Microscopic study of temporal bones in dysostosis multiplex (gargoylism), Laryngoscope **52:**218, 1942.
305. Wood, G. C.: The formation of fibrils from collagen solutions. III. The effect of chondroitin sulphate and some other naturally occurring polyanions on the rate of formation, Biochem. J. **75:**605, 1960.
306. Woodin, A. M.: The corneal mucopolysaccharide, Biochem. J. **51:**319, 1952.
307. Zeeman, W. P. C.: Gargoylismus, Acta Ophthal. **20:**40, 1942.
308. Zellweger, H., Giaccai, L., and Firzli, S.: Gargoylism and Morquio's disease, Amer. J. Dis. Child. **84:**421, 1952.
309. Zellweger, H., Ponseti, I. V., Pedrini, V., Stamler, F. S., and von Noorden, G. K.: Morquio-Ullrich's disease, J. Pediat. **59:**549, 1961.
310. Zierl, F.: Ueber Skelettveränderungen bei der juvenilen Form der amaurotischen Idiotie, Z. Ges. Neurol. Psychiat. **131:**400, 1930.
311. Zimmer, J. G., McAllister, B. M., and Demis, D. J.: Mucopolysaccharides in mast cells and mastocytosis, J. Invest. Derm. **44:**33, 1965.

10

Other genetic disorders of connective tissue

In addition to the entities discussed in detail earlier in this book, a considerable number deserve at least brief mention. Some, e.g. fibrodysplasia ossificans progressiva and osteopoikilosis, may qualify as generalized heritable disorders of connective tissue. A large number of others have involvement apparently limited to the osseous skeleton.

FIBRODYSPLASIA OSSIFICANS PROGRESSIVA

Historical note

The name *myositis ossificans progressiva* is said[46] to have been assigned to this condition by von Dusch in 1868. The designation in which fibrositis is substituted for myositis has been used more frequently in recent decades,[18,35,54] since the primary change is in the connective tissues—specifically aponeuroses, fasciae, and tendons—and the muscles are only secondarily affected. (Rosenstirn[46] suggested "fibrocellulitis.") It is not entirely improper to refer to it as fibrositis, since the lesions may appear to be quite inflammatory during early stages. However, "fibrodysplasia," the term suggested by Bauer and Bode,[2] impresses me (as it has Falls[10]) as most valid. "FOP" is the abbreviation that will be used in this discussion.

In a review of the subject, to which little has since been added, Rosenstirn[46] in 1918 abstracted 119 cases and added his own. The first case may have been described in Guy Patin in 1692. Extraordinarily clear descriptions of the end stages of the disease were provided in the *Philosophical Transactions of the Royal Society of London* in the first half of the eighteenth century by John Freke and others. John Freke (1688-1756), a London surgeon and man of wide culture, was a friend of Fielding, who mentions him twice in *Tom Jones*. Freke saw his case of FOP at St. Bartholomew's Hospital[13]:

> April 14, 1736, there came a Boy of a healthy Look and 14 Years of Age, to ask of us at the Hospital, what should be done to cure him of many large Swellings on

> his Back, which began about 3 Years since, and have continued to grow as large on many Parts as a Penny-loaf, particularly on the left side. They arise from all the *vertebre* of the Neck, and reach down to the *Os sacrum;* they likewise arise from every Rib of his Body, and joining together in all Parts of his Back, as the Ramifications of Coral do, they make, as it were, a fixed bony Pair of Bodice.*

Abernethy, Caesar Hawkins, Jonathan Hutchinson,[26] Volkmann, Kronecker, Virchow, Stephen Paget, Rolleston,[45] Garrod, F. Parkes Weber, Eugene L. Opie, and many others added cases. Since Rosenstirn, other reviews have appeared.[33,34,40] Lutwak estimated that about 260 cases had been reported up to 1963.

Helferich[23] is generally credited with having first described (in 1879) the important association of microdactyly with FOP. The distinctive type of deformity seen in these cases (monophalangy of the great toe) had been described as an isolated anomaly by Fränkel[11] in 1871.

In 1901 Rolleston[45] expressed the opinion that the disease is a defect of the mesoblast. This was probably one of the earliest statements of this idea. It has been stated by many others since that time. For example, Hirsch and Löw-Beer[24] called it an "exceedingly unusual anomaly of the mesenchyme."

Clinical manifestations

The onset of the process in the fasciae and tendons may be in fetal life[26,35,46] or rarely not until after the age of 20 years.[12,24] Usually, however, evidences of the disorder appear in the early years of life, before the age of 10 years.

Typically, localized swellings appear first in the region of the neck and back and later in the limbs. They are sometimes painful. These lumps come and go in a matter of days. Someimes injury appears to be involved in their inception. The lumps may or may not be attached to deep fascia. Sometimes the tumors are cystic and appear to contain blood. Discharge may occur. At times fever is associated with the development and/or absorption of the tumor. In fact, acute rheumatic fever may be simulated.[47] As the disorder progresses, wryneck deformity may develop. The masseter may also be affected, but the tongue, heart, larynx, diaphragm, and sphincters enjoy immunity from the process. The dorsal aspect of the trunk and the proximal (but usually only the proximal) portions of the extremities may be affected. The plantar and palmar fascia may be involved. At the attachments of fibrous structures to bones it is not uncommon for exostoses to develop—for instance, in the occipital area of the skull or as an anterior calcaneal spur.

Eventually, columns and plates (Fig. 10-2) of bone replace the tendons, fasciae, and ligaments. The spine may become completely rigid and the victims converted into columns like Lot's wife at Sodom. Koontz'[29] patient "was completely unable to sit down . . . she either had to lie down or stand up. She had enough motion in one of her knee joints so that she could walk with a very halting, mincing step. She was of slight build, weighing very little, and it was simple to carry this plank-like girl around."[28] Fairbank[9] presents drawings of skeletons showing extensive changes. Often a ridge of bone on the back appears like a handle by which the patient can literally be lifted.[51]

The skin is usually exempt as are the muscles of abdominal well,† perineum,

---

*From Freke, J.: Philos. Trans. Roy. Soc., London, 1740.

†Case 8, below, is an exception to this statement.

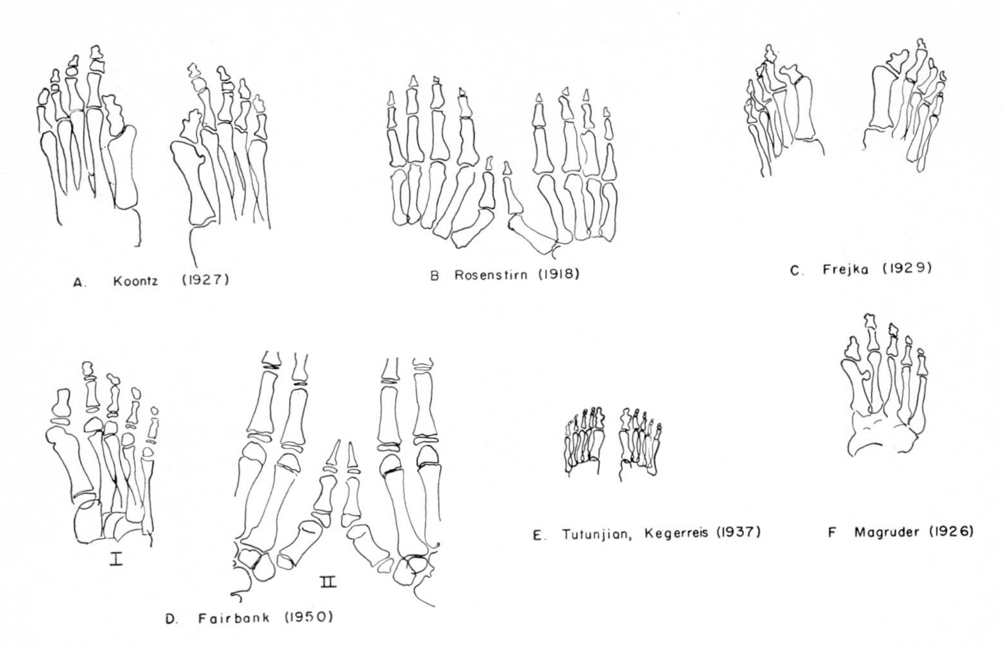

Fig. 10-1. Tracings of x-ray films of hands and feet in selected reported cases (these are not reproduced to the same scale). **A,** Koontz[29]: Hands little affected. In feet, monophalangic first digit and biphalangic fifth digit. On the right the fourth toe is also biphalangic. There are an exostosis on the first right metatarsal and a bone bridge between metatarsals on the left. **B,** Rosenstirn[46]: The short, pointed terminal phalanx of the thumb is typical. The first metacarpal on the left is abnormal in shape. (Frequently the first metacarpal and metatarsal have a disorganized trabecular pattern.) The terminal phalanges of the other digits, especially the second and third, also short and pointed. **C,** Frejka[12]: The fingers were not commented on. The first toe is monophalangic and the others biphalangic at the most. Typical hallux valgus is present. **D,** Fairbank[8]: **I,** 7 years of age. First metatarsal appears to have been lengthened by fusion with the proximal phalanx. The other toes are all biphalangeal. **II,** 10 years of age. The characteristic short, pointed terminal phalanx is seen. There was also microdactyly of the great toes. **E,** Tutunjian and Kegerreis[51]: No comment on the state of the hands. It is interesting to note that monophalangic first toe can be present without microdactyly or hallux valgus. **F,** Magruder[34]: Typical monophalangy of first toe and biphalangy of others. Note exostosis like that in Koontz's patient. **G,** Griffith[19]: Typically short, pointed terminal phalanx of thumbs and of other fingers. Clinically the fifth fingers were curved (clinodactylous). The great toes were monophalangic. **H,** Michelsohn[38]: First toes monophalangic; fifth toes biphalangic. Typical thumbs. **I,** Vastine, Vastine, and Arango[53]: Identical twins. Monophalangy of first toes. Biphalangy of fourth and fifth toes. **J,** van Creveld and Soeters[52]: 5 years of age. Typical thumb. **K,** Mather[36]: Monophalangic first toe. Biphalangic fifth toe. It is noteworthy that in the feet of many of the patients in the illustrated cases of FOP, sesamoid bones have been conspicuous by their absence. In their place, projections like exostoses occur, particularly at the distal end of the first metatarsal. It is likely that these "exostoses" are synostoses of sesamoid bones with the metatarsal.

and eye. The heart is not affected. Remissions and exacerbations are characteristic of the disease. Hernias may occur with increased frequency.[46]

In spite of marked involvement, patients have survived to fairly advanced years, e.g. 61 years in Case 73 described by Fairbank.[9] The patient who was 17½ years old when studied by Koontz[29] was still living and reasonably well, although severely disabled, at the age of 51 years.[28] She died at the age of 56 years.

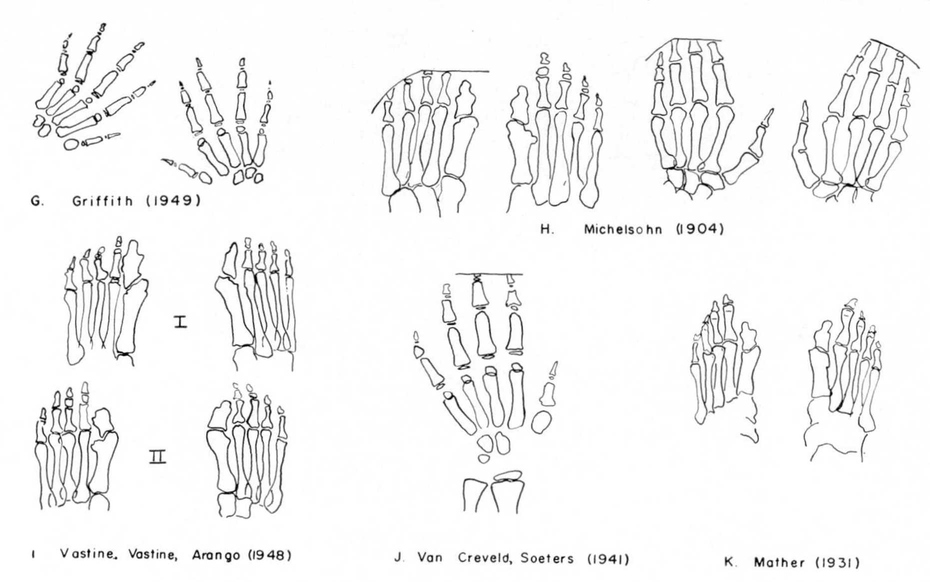

Fig. 10-1, cont'd. For legend see opposite page.

Obviously, microdactyly can be a valuable diagnostic sign in the earlier stages of the process of ossification or before calcification has appeared. The great toe (Fig. 10-1) is affected in the great majority of cases, the thumb less frequently (in less than half of cases), and at times other digits. Hallux valgus frequently results and is often what impresses the observer rather than shortening of the digit (Fig. 10-2). Fairbank[9] states that all the fingers were shortened in two cases. The shortening is the result of change in the phalangeal bones, rarely in the metatarsals. The proximal phalanx may be completely suppressed. A synostosis of the phalanges of the great toe is perhaps the most typical change. Rosenstirn[46] believed that microdactyly is present in all true cases of FOP. Furthermore, the classic review of digital anomalies by Pol[43] indicates that the changes in FOP (Fig. 10-1) are in all likelihood unique to this condition and, for practical purposes, absolutely pathognomonic. Clinodactyly, radial curvature of the fifth finger, may occur in these cases.

The only other skeletal change that has been seen at all frequently is an abnormally broad neck of the femora[19,53] (Figs. 10-2 and 10-5). In children the epiphyseal ossification centers may be large for the patient's age (Fig. 10-5).

Occasionally there is tendency to bruise with negligible trauma.[19] No defect of coagulation is demonstrable in these instances, however.

Review of cases

To my knowledge only nine patients with FOP have been seen in Johns Hopkins Hospital during the past forty years.* All but one are still living. One was reported by Koontz.[29] Two were briefly referred to by Geschickter and Ma-

*Barker's[1] case was porbably calcinosis universalis and not FOP.

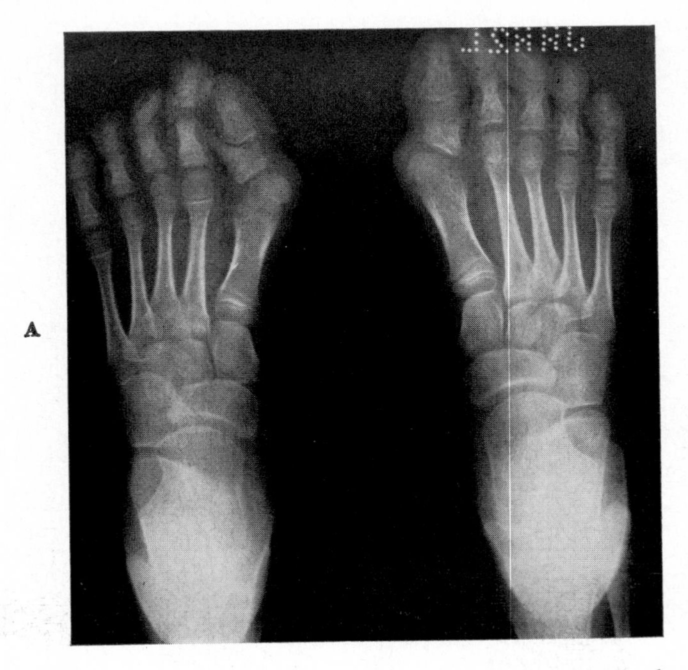

A

Fig. 10-2. X-ray studies in Case 2 of FOP (see text). As demonstrated in **A,** there was distortion of the contour of the distal tip of the first metatarsal and of the proximal phalanges resulting in the hallux valgus deformity seen clinically. It is of note that in this case a normal number of phalangeal bones are present in all the toes. This is, as will be seen from inspection of Fig. 10-1, the exception; as a rule, monophalangy of the great toes is at least present. It will be interesting to see if synostosis occurs in the future as was observed to occur in Michelsohn's patient.[38] The hands were normal. As demonstrated in **B,** the neck of the right femur is slightly widened and blunted; immediately adjacent to the epiphyseal line the left femur is normal. Anomalous bone is seen on each side of the lower lumbar spine, especially the left. The ossification in the axillary areas, **C,** has the appearance of cortical bone. In places, it resembled the ribs in contour. At least one false joint was identified. In the lateral view of the lumbar spine, **D,** plates of bone are clearly demonstrated on the back. **E** and **F,** Although all other features of Case 2 are typical of FOP, the hands do not show the usual changes. The thumbs are normal. Osteoporosis and unusually slender radius and ulna bones are demonstrated in the x-ray films taken at age 19. (The x-ray films shown in **A** to **D** were made at age 8.) **G** and **H,** At age 19, the patient shows relatively fixed position of the arms, involvement of the anterior abdominal musculature by ossification, and short great toes. (By age 19, fusion of the phalanges of the great toe was complete, creating monophalangy!)

seritz.[16] In none of these nine families has another case of FOP been known. All the patients have deformity of the toes and/or fingers. In at least two instances (Cases 1 and 2) digital deformity was also present in other members of the family. One patient (Case 5) did not notice any abnormality until the age of 25 years, when lumps appeared above one knee. In another patient (Case 3) torticollis was noted at 1 month of age, and advanced FOP was present when he was seen at the age of 16 months. Biopsies have been made in at least the last six patients. In the literature there is a slight and nonsignificant predominance of males affected; four of the nine are female. Serum alkaline phosphatase values are available in six patients and are not in excess of values anticipated on the basis of age.

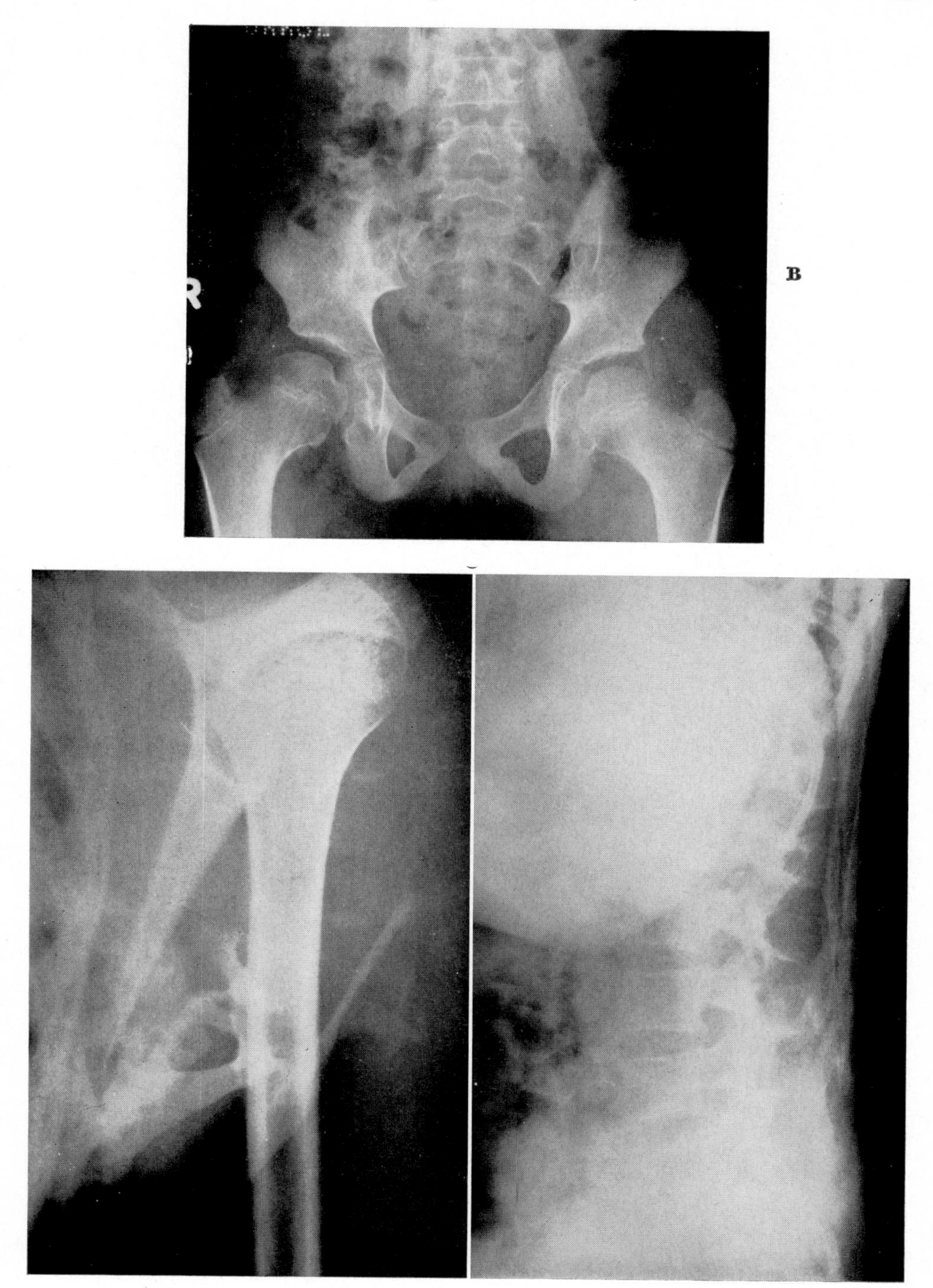

Fig. 10-2, cont'd. For legend see opposite page.

Continued.

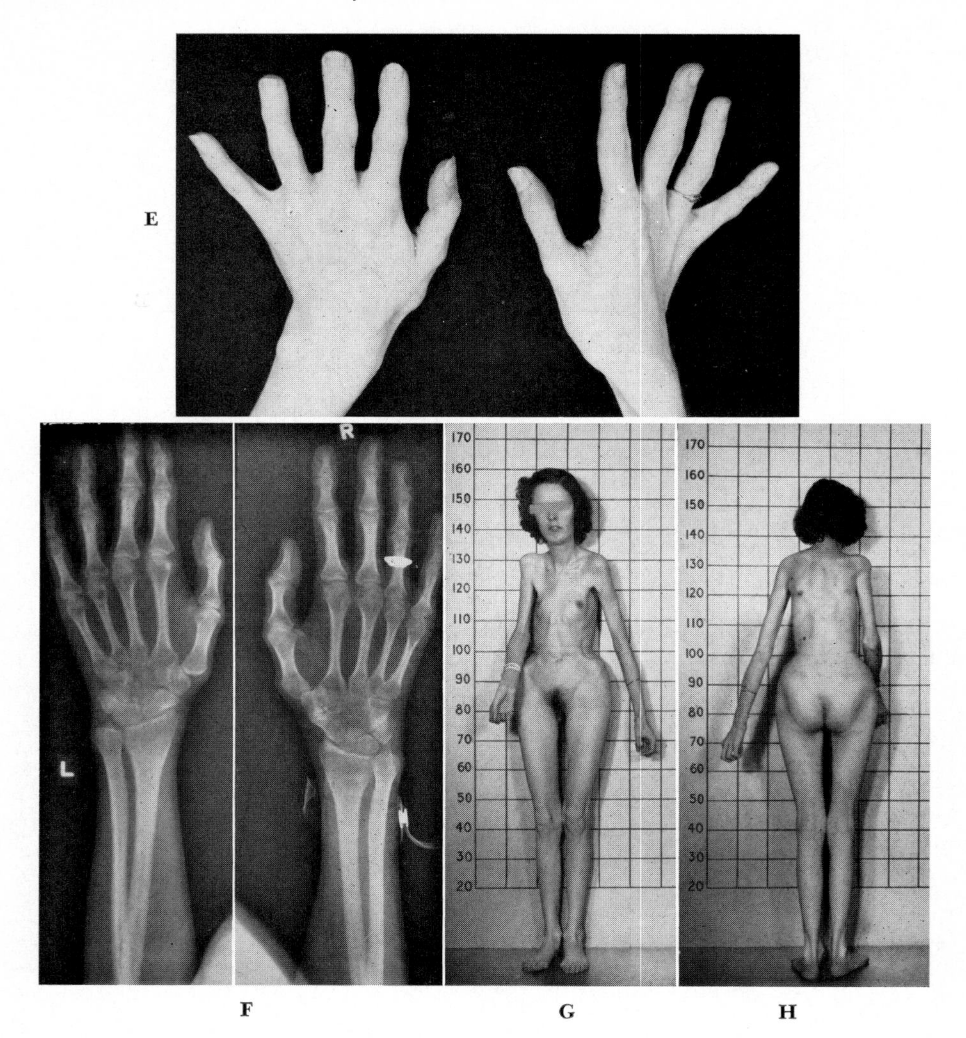

Fig. 10-2, cont'd. For legend see p. 404.

Abstracts of these nine cases follow:

Case 1. The case of N. J., born in 1908, was reported by Koontz[29] in 1927, with excellent illustrations of the gross appearance and radiologic changes, including those of the thumbs and great toes. The maternal grandfather and his two brothers developed late in life what apparently were Dupuytren contractures. A cousin on the maternal side apparently had a deformity of the toes similar to the patient's. The patient's first symptom was stiffness at the age of 9 years. Menstruation never occurred. Both great toes and thumbs were short and malformed. Concentrations of calcium and phosphorus in the blood were normal. I examined the patient in April 1956. She was then 48 years of age. The disease had progressed slowly but steadily. The jaw was partially fixed, she could not sit, and the arms were in an absolutely fixed position with a minimum of wrist motion present. Using a long-handled fork and standing up, the patient was able to feed herself. This patient died in 1964 (age, 56 years) of heart failure. Autopsy showed moderate coronary arteriosclerosis and pulmonary fibrosis. The mechanism of the heart failure was not entirely clear.

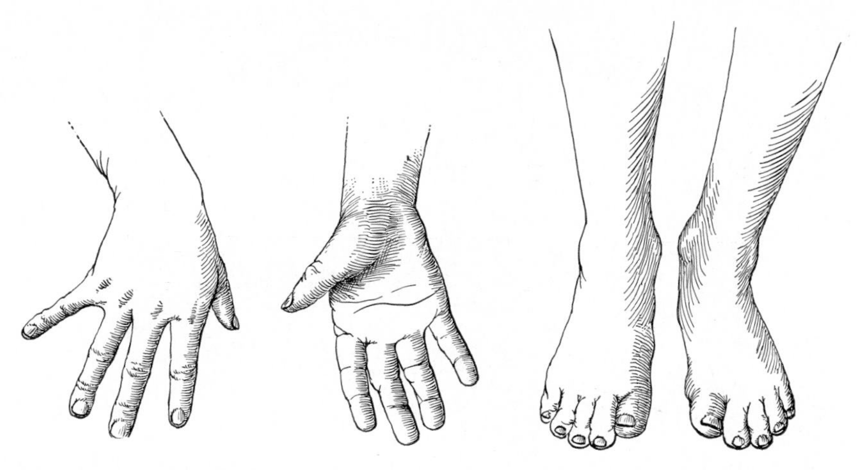

Fig. 10-3. Drawings of the hands and feet of Patient 4 of the FOP series (see text). Microdactyly of the thumbs and toes is strikingly demonstrated.

Case 2. B. W. (A85874), a 7½-year-old white girl, has a normal brother and sister. The father had stunting of the great toes similar to the patient's but no other instance of FOP is known in the family. At 10 months, when the patient began to sit up, the head leaned to the left. At the age of 6½ years, she developed an exostosis on the right knee after trauma. However, she remained apparently well otherwise until the age of about 7 years, when she began to complain of pain in the left side of her neck, and firmness and tenderness were discovered there. Thereafter, swelling and induration developed on the back, abdomen, and shoulder. There was marked limitation of motion of the neck, arms, and spine, and the head was held to the left. Dermatomyositis was the initial diagnosis. See Fig. 10-2 for x-ray studies of this patient.

Case 3. R. W. (A62462) was found at birth to have hallux valgus and short thumbs. At 1 month the head was noted to be bent to the left and there was a firm mass in the sternomastoid muscle. Thereafter asymmetry of the face developed. Lumps appeared in many areas over the back and scalp. These masses never appeared inflamed. There were, however, frequent bouts of unexplained fever. Examination revealed atrophy of the left side of the face. The sternomastoid muscle on the left was converted into a stony hard mass. The ligamentum nuchae was similarly affected. Extensive involvement about the scapulae (which were attached to the ribs) and the trapezius muscles formed a yoke on the back.

Case 4. V. W. (U52691) has seven siblings, but none has either microdactyly or FOP. She was presumably well until the age of 6 years, when she fell from a swing, striking her back. Swelling and discoloration resulted. X-ray films at that time revealed "a spider's web on the spine." Thereafter, there was steadily progressive increase in stiffness and limitation of motion of joints. The thumbs and toes had always been small. It is of note that the facial muscles were involved in this case. By the age of 25 years the jaws became locked and the upper teeth had to be removed to permit alimentation. (See Fig. 10-3 for drawings of this patient.)

Case 5. F. K. (U52689) was well until the age of 25 years, when he developed a "bump" above one knee following trauma. During the following year there were several episodes of soreness and swelling in the left side of the neck, with difficulty in swallowing. There are six siblings. No other members of the family had microdactyly or ossification. The patient's thumbs were small, with fusion of the interphalangeal and metacarpophalangeal joints. All the terminal phalangeal joints of the second and fourth fingers were fused. Hearing was impaired bilaterally. As long as the patient could remember, he had had restriction of motion of the head, mandible, both shoulders, right elbow, both thumbs, both hips, left knee, left ankle, and toes of the left foot. Supposedly, poliomyelitis affecting mainly the left leg had occurred at 5 years of age, but suspicion is cast on the diagnosis by later developments. When restudied in 1963 this patient was found to be remarkably little changed from the state described and photographed thirty years previously. Review of the history indicated that in childhood he was never very active and that severe incapacitation probably began in his teens. As had been true thirty years earlier, he was rendered almost immobile by his disease and showed striking changes in the thumbs and great toes. The thumb was monophalangic. The distal two phalanges of the index fingers were also fused, as were some of the proximal row of the carpal bones. In the feet a single blocklike bone replaced the first metatarsal and phalanges of the first toe. The second, third,

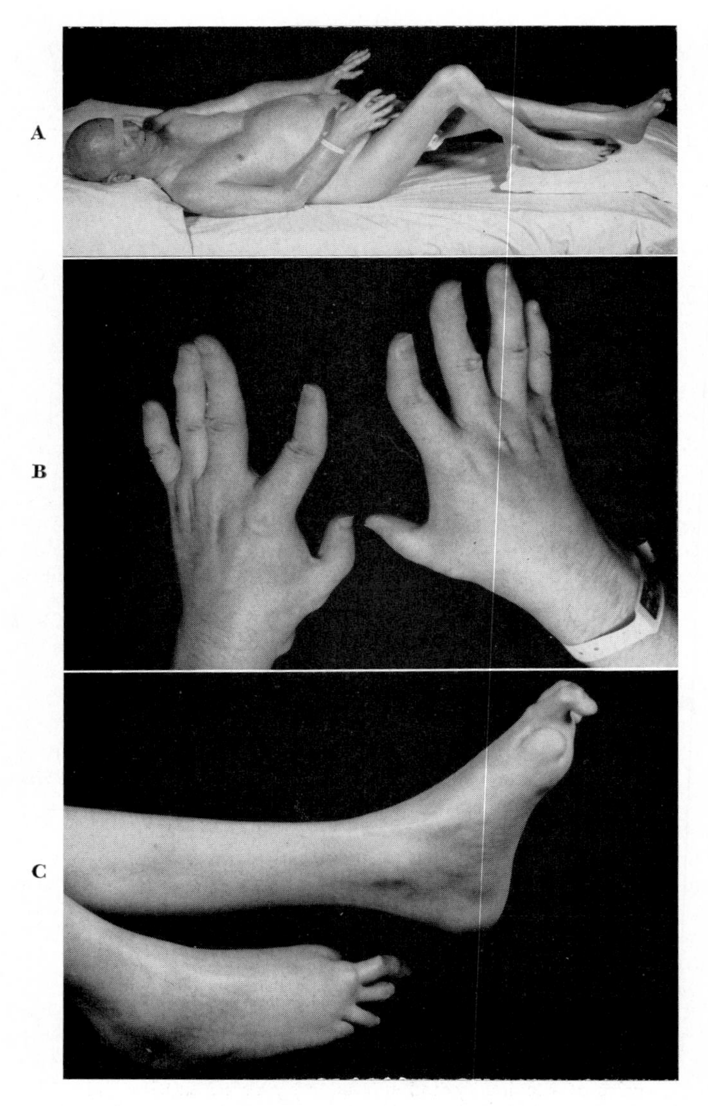

Fig. 10-4. Case 5 at age of 55 years. The patient is almost immobile in the position shown, **A.** Short thumbs, **B,** and short great toes, **C,** are shown. The great toes never had a nail. As shown in **D,** the thumb has a single bone mass comprising fused metacarpal and phalanges. The two distal phalanges of the index and little fingers are also fused. In the foot, **E,** the great toe likewise has a single bone mass comprising fused metatarsal and phalanges. **F,** Bony bridges between lumbar vertebrae and the wing of the ilium and between the femur and pelvis are shown. These x-ray films were made in 1933. X-ray studies made in 1963 showed no change.

and fourth metatarsals were fused with the proximal phalanges. The tarsal bones showed striking fusion with one another and with the metatarsals. The ankle joints were completely fused, as was also the spine, both the vertebral bodies and the apophyseal joints being affected. This is the most severe instance of bony fusions in this series. The deafness was of mixed conductive and nerve type. Although old otitis media was proposed as the cause, ossicle fusion seems possible.

Case 6. M. W. (422628) was seen at the age of 14 years, and a diagnosis of calcinosis of the muscles of both hips was rendered. However, in retrospect there can be no question but that FOP was actually present. The boy had always been stiff, and following a blow on the back at the age of 5 years a lump on the left scapula was noted. The mass was biopsied and called sarcoma. The boy was given only three months to live; he is still alive, although disabled, at

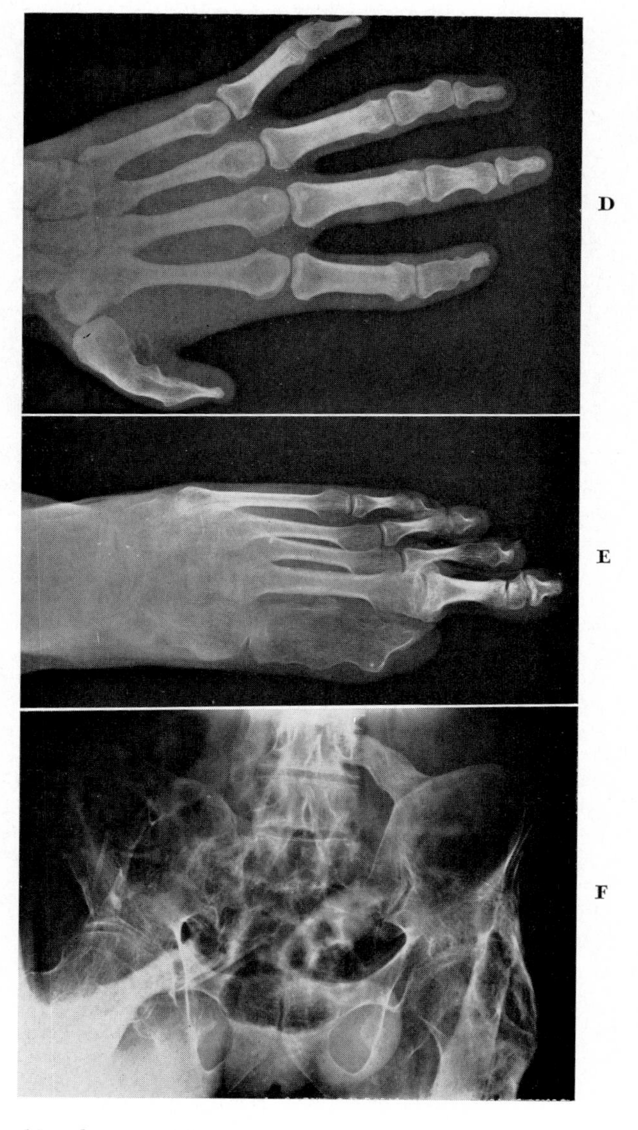

Fig. 10-4, cont'd. For legend see opposite page.

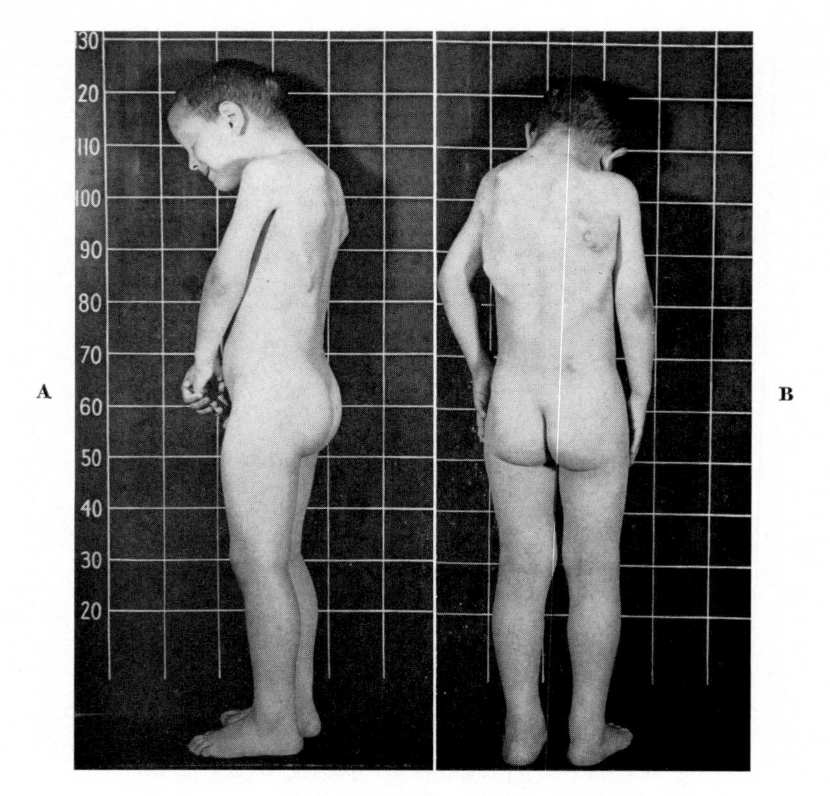

Fig. 10-5. Case 7. **A,** Lateral view (June, 1958). **B,** Rear view (June, 1958). **C,** Feet. **D,** X-ray film of feet (April, 1957). **E,** Occiput, showing ossified nodule. Note the ossification in the tissues of the posterior part of the neck. **F** and **G,** The neck of the femur is short and broad (1954 and 1957). **H,** Exostoses of the tibia at site of tendon attachment.

the age of 27 years. Other lumps appeared and flexion contracture of the hips and right knee gradually developed. The left great toe was short and deformed.

Case 7. P. H. (770577), born Oct. 4, 1951, had, as his first manifestation of FOP, the appearance (in 1954) of transient, nontender "bumps" in the posterior part of the scalp. A biopsy diagnosis of neurofibromatosis was made. The correct diagnosis was made in October, 1956, by which time typical ossifying changes in the aponeuroses of the back had developed. A striking feature at that time was local heat over the involved areas of the back. The thumbs and toes were characteristically short. Two older siblings, born in 1947 and 1949, are normal and no definite abnormality has been detected in members of the family. Other features of note include short, broad femoral necks and exostosis-like spurs on the upper end of each tibia at the site of muscle attachments. (See Fig. 10-5.) Steroid therapy undoubtedly suppresses acute inflammatory phases in this patient. It probably had no effect on the ossification process. (See Lutwak[33] for further details on this patient.)

Case 8. C. A. B. (1136294), born May 22, 1960, was noted at birth to have "bunions" on both feet. At approximately 2 weeks of age the mother noted that the infant's head could not be turned to one side. A physician rendered a diagnosis of wryneck. Heat, swelling, and firmness of the sternocleidomastoid and other neck muscles were progressive, and right sternocleidomastoid myomectomy was performed at age 1 year. Between 2 and 3 years of age she began to develop bony protuberances over the posterior chest wall. A characteristic evolution beginning with erythema, swelling, and warmth characterized the lesions. By 4½ years of age marked immobilization of the head and shoulder girdle with restriction of thoracic expansion had de-

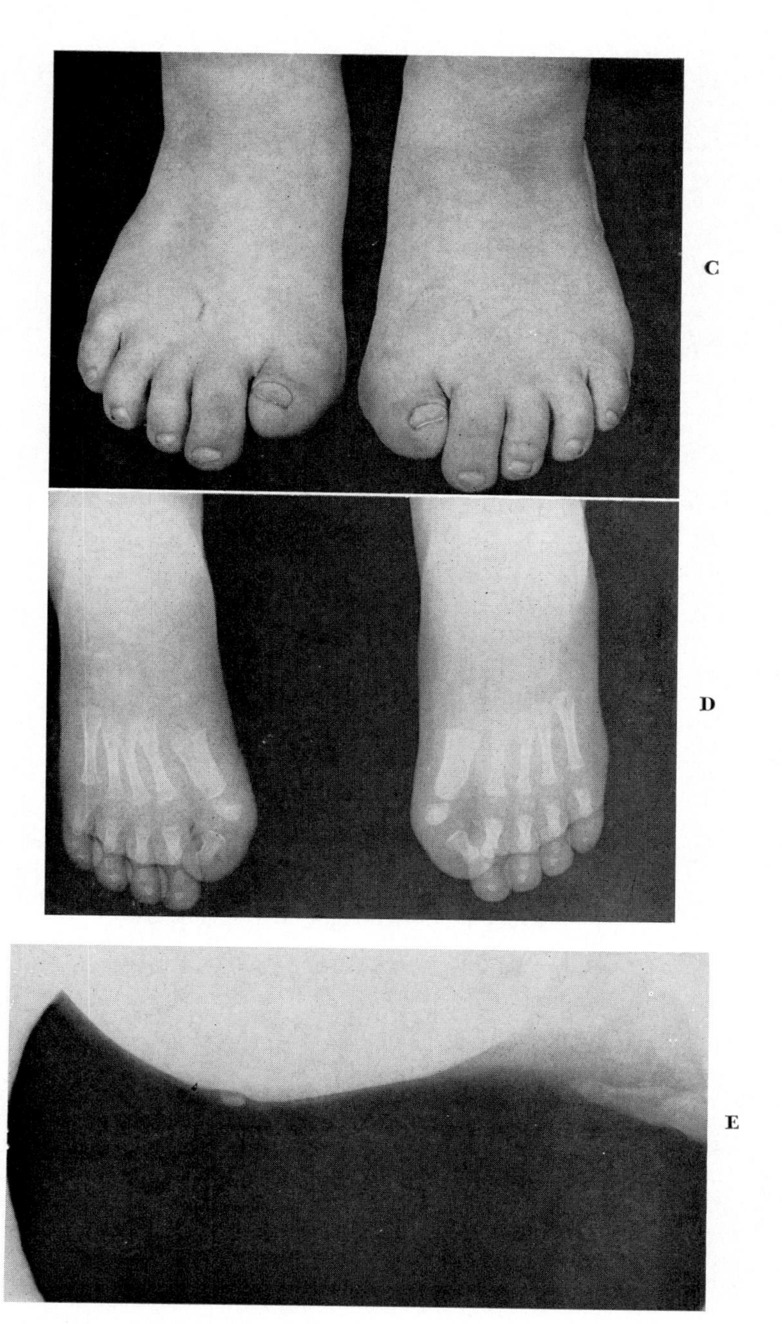

Fig. 10-5, cont'd. For legend see opposite page.

Continued.

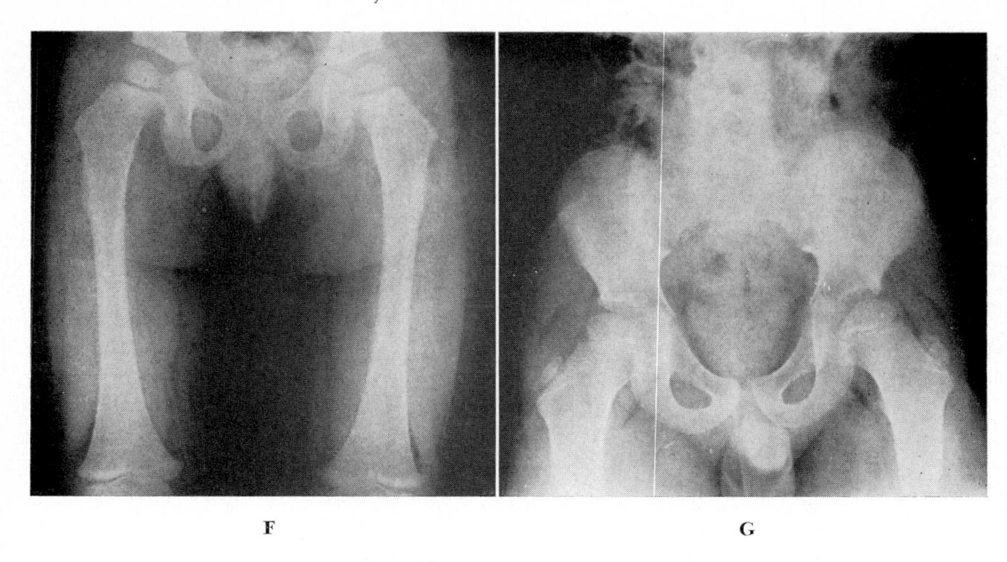

F G

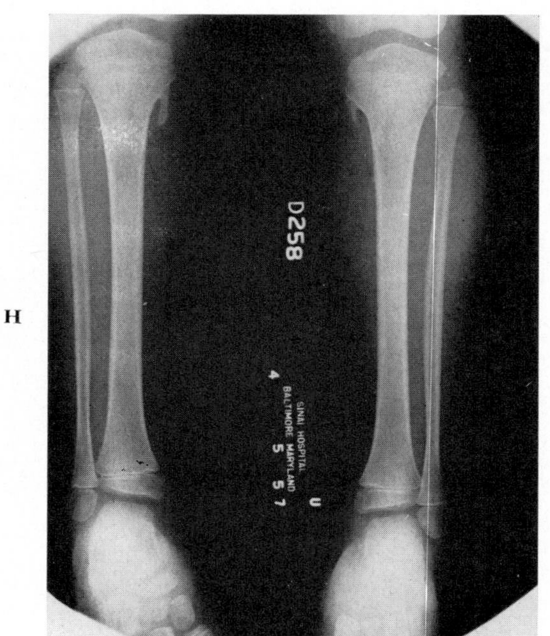

H

Fig. 10-5, cont'd. For legend see p. 410.

veloped. As well as an extensive posterior truncal development of bone, the anterior abdominal wall contained firm lumps and plates. Mobility of the lower extremities was little if any reduced. The great toes were monophalangic and short with hallux valgus. The thumbs appeared normal and were normal by x-ray study. As in Case 7, ossified tendinous insertions suggesting exostoses of diaphyseal aclasis were seen in the distal femur, radius, and ulna and the proximal humerus.

Case 9. J. U. (1011125), born December, 1949, first developed "lumps" in the scalp above the ears at 18 months of age. The thumbs and first toes were noted to be small at birth. Progressive involvement of the back, axillae, and arms led to complete immobility of the upper trunk, neck, shoulders, and elbows. At age 5½ years, he was still able to feed himself and, because of relatively little involvement of the legs, to play actively. The arms were small. The knees and ankles were prominent. No new lesions had appeared for over a year, the last one being on the bottom of the left foot. Lesions on the back had ulcerated with extrusion of calcific material but then healed satisfactorily. The patient is the youngest of four children of normal parents who were 41 (father) and 35 years old at the time of his birth. The oldest of the four children died of brain tumor at age 6.

Prevalence and inheritance

In 1918 Rosenstirn,[46] in reviewing this disorder, could find 119 cases in the literature. In later reviews[35,40] other cases have been added. Lutwak[33] found about 260 well-documented cases. The disease is appreciably more frequent in males, in a ratio of 4:1 according to some[47] but 3:2 by the statement of others. In Rosenstirn's collection of cases, 62% were male (sixty-eight males and forty-two females, of cases clearly described as to diagnosis and sex).

Sympson[50] reported microdactyly in father and son, with FOP in the son, and Stonham[49] reported the same situation. Drago[6] observed the same situation in a mother and son. Koontz[29] described "contractures of two fingers" in four relatives of the patient. The anomaly apparently developed later in life, however, and may have been Dupuytren's contracture. Burton-Fanning and Vaughan[5] described FOP (the full syndrome) in both father and son. Gaster[15] observed the disorder, including phalangeal deformity, in five male members of three generations—three brothers, the father, and the paternal grandfather. Vastine and coworkers[54] and Eaton and associates[7] each saw FOP in both of a pair of identical twins. It may be that this disease trait is dominant, with a particularly wide range of expressivity. Many of the cases may be new dominant mutations; very few of the patients have children to whom the disease can be transmitted. There seems to be no increase in consanguineous marriages among the parents. Multiple affected sibs, except for identical twins, are rare. Viparelli[55] pointed out increased parental age in sporadic cases, suggesting that these represent new dominant mutations.

Pathology

The early histologic changes are not known. Obviously it is these which are of most significance in reference to the basic abnormality. It is clear[20] that the skeletal muscle is fundamentally normal. Geschichter and Maseritz[16] picture cartilage and also "young osteoid tissue surrounded by osteoblasts." The surgical pathologist may find it difficult to distinguish FOP from osteogenic sarcoma. In the case described by Paul[42] both were thought to have been present.

The basic defect

That the fundamental disorder resides in connective tissue seems indisputable. Isolated bone tissue may be found in the skin,[46] well removed from muscles. No aberration of calcium metabolism has been demonstrated. In one case (P. H., 770577) ossification began in the galea aponeurotica. The serum transaminase activity was normal during stages of activity of the disease, as manifested by fever, leukocytosis, and local heat. Because of the similarities of behavior to the calcification and ossification that occur after traumatic and other injury which involves necrosis of tissue, one suspects that this is fundamentally a dystrophy of connective tissue, with secondary calcification. Rosenstirn believed that the fundamental defect resides in the small blood vessel and that the initial lesion is a hemorrhage that is followed by organization and ossification.

The observations of Wilkins and associates[57] are important and point the way to an area for possibly productive investigation by other techniques, such as tissue culture of fibroblasts from these patients. Specifically they found a very high level of alkaline phosphatase activity in the areas of heterotopic cartilage and bone formation. The activity was, in fact, higher than in normal rib. Lins and Abath[31] also found high alkaline phosphatase activity in biopsy material.

Emphasizing that the proposal is merely hypothesis, Lutwak[33] cautiously suggested that a congenital deficiency of an inhibitor material or a relative excess of an inhibitor-destroying mechanism may be present in FOP. The hypothesis was based on the suggestion of the Neumans[39] and Glimcher.[17] Collagen everywhere in the body exists in a crystalline configuration conforming to that of calcium hydroxyapatite. Bone mineral crystallization occurs on collagen fibers, probably by a mechanism of epitaxy (crystal seeding). Calcium and phosphate are present in tissue fluids in concentrations adequate for crystallization. It has been postulated that normally a circulating inhibitor of crystallization is present, preventing mineral deposition. At sites of bone formation, the inhibitor is thought to be destroyed, permitting mineralization to occur.

An alternative hypothesis in FOP is the presence of an abnormal collagen capable of supporting ossification at abnormal sites.

An enigmatic feature of this syndrome has been the association of an anomaly of the conventional congenital type, microdactyly, with the other cardinal component, ectopic ossification, which behaves more like a hereditary weakness of some element of connective tissue. Previously, in discussing the explanation for the association of congenital anomalies of conventional types with hereditary disorders that behave more like abiotrophies, it was proposed that the presence of a basic tissue defect results in an abnormal environment for embryologic development so that specific congenital defects occur predictably with increased incidence. Such may be the case with the microdactyly of FOP. Certainly, a disorder of normally ossified tissues is not too farfetched an association. However, a more straightforward explanation is possible. There is an intriguing set of observations reported by Michelsohn,[38] suggesting that in connection with the abnormality of growth of the first digits in FOP there is no sharp distinction between antenatal and postnatal developments. The patient in question was a 17-year-old girl when seen. In the first months of life the mother noted pronounced shortening and stiffening of the great toes, with no morphologic or functional abnormality of the thumbs. At the age of 7 years when the changes in the muscles were beginning, the thumbs became painfully swollen and later stiff, then ankylosed. By definition the change in the great toes was synostosis and that in the thumbs, ankylosis. However, it may be that the same basic process was operating in both instances. The predominant and usually unique involvement of the first digit may be related to the difference in the growth pattern of the first digit as compared with the others.

The malformation of the digits appears to occur in the fairly regular manner of a Mendelian autosomal dominant trait; ossification occurs in less predictable fashion. The factors determining whether ossification will occur in a given case of microdactyly are entirely obscure. Rosenstirn[46] reported that both FOP and microdactyly occurred in a setter dog. It is a pity that breeding and other experiments were not undertaken on this valuable animal.

Other considerations

In the differential diagnosis, calcinosis universalis, dermatomyositis, Weber-Christian disease, and other conditions must come in for consideration. The picture suggests torticollis in the early stages.[35] Calcinosis universalis is probably basically a "collagen vascular" disease with secondary calcification.[56] It is certainly not a heritable disorder. The patient described by Barker,[1] a Negro male who was for many months on the wards of the Johns Hopkins Hospital, probably had calcinosis universalis and not FOP. Actually there must be very few descriptions of FOP in Negroes.

Beryllium has been used in the treatment of FOP.[51] Since beryllium suppresses alkaline phosphatase activity,[21,27] there might be some rationale for this therapy. This effect of beryllium was, however, unknown in 1937 when it was used; furthermore, its benefit was, at the most, doubtful. Adrenocortical hormones were used in Case 2 and in patients reported in the literature.[32,44] Again, benefit is, at the most, dubious. Somewhat encouraging results in an early and active case were described by Riley and Christie,[44] but no benefit was noted in an old, probably static case. In other instances[198] steroids did no good even when given early. X-ray therapy may aggravate the condition. Lutwak[33] found that the course of the disease was unaffected by treatment with hydrocortisone, dexamethasone, triiodothyronine, propylthiouracil, or disodium ethylenediaminetetraacetate (EDTA).

Summary

The cardinal manifestations of fibrodysplasia ossificans progressiva are microdactyly and progressive ossification of fasciae, aponeuroses, and other fibrous structures related to muscles. Microdactyly is always most striking in the thumb and great toes. It probably represents fundamentally the same disorder occurring usually, although not exclusively, during antenatal development. There is usually a synostosis with resulting monophalangic great toe.

This disorder is probably inherited as a Mendelian dominant with irregular penetrance.

OSTEOPOIKILOSIS (Osteo-dermato-poikilosis)

Osteopoikilosis, like osteopetrosis, was first described in a definitive manner (earlier references[86] can be found) by the German radiologist, H. Albers-Schönberg (1915).[58] It is sometimes referred to as "spotted bones," an appropriate designation as seen from Fig. 10-6. "Osteopoikilosis" (variations: "osteopoecilia," "osteopecilia," "osteopoicilosis," "osteopoikilie") is derived from Greek words meaning "mottled bones." The bone lesion is also referred to as "osteitis condensans generalisata" or "osteosclerosis disseminata." Bauer and Bode[2] called it "osteodysplasia enostotica." The skin lesions were first described in 1928 by Buschke and Ollendorff[63] (and later by Curth[68]) as "dermatofibrosis lenticularis

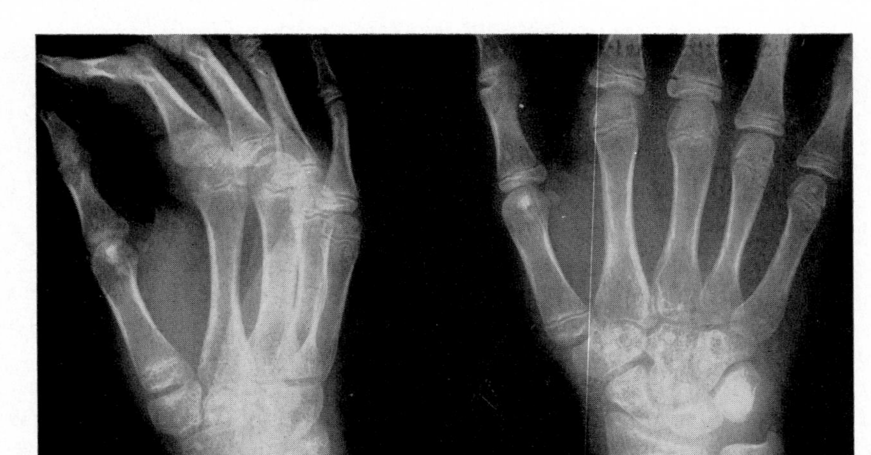

Fig. 10-6. Typical osteopoikilosis discovered incidentally when radiologic studies for a wrist injury were performed (J.H.H. 644704) in a 13-year-old white boy.

disseminata." Osteo-dermato-poikilosis might be a satisfactory designation for the entire syndrome.

Neither the osseous nor the cutaneous lesions are of any known clinical significance whatever. They are usually discovered incidentally, since the bone lesions are asymptomatic and the skin lesions inconspicuous. One reason why the clinician should be familiar with this condition is that he may avoid confusing the condition for osteoblastic metastases to the skeleton.[82]

The bone lesions are circumscribed, round areas of increased bone density, usually less than 1 cm. in diameter, situated particularly at the ends of the bones of the extremities (but not necesarily in the epiphyses) and in the small bones of the feet and wrists (Fig. 10-7). The lesions may or may not be bilaterally symmetric. At times the lesions are linear (striate) in distribution.[92] For example, Voorhoeve[90] found vertical striae parallel to the long axis of the bones and as a fan in the wings of the ilia, but no spots, in two children whose father had typical spots and no striae. (See Fig. 10-8 for a demonstration of the distribution of lesions.) The skull has been spared in most cases. Bistolfi[60] described involvement of the occipital bone. All three cases of Funstein and Kotschiew[71] had skull involvement and indeed the calvarial lesions dominated the picture in Erbsen's[70] case. In the case of Martinčić[77] unusual involvement of the lumbar spine was present.

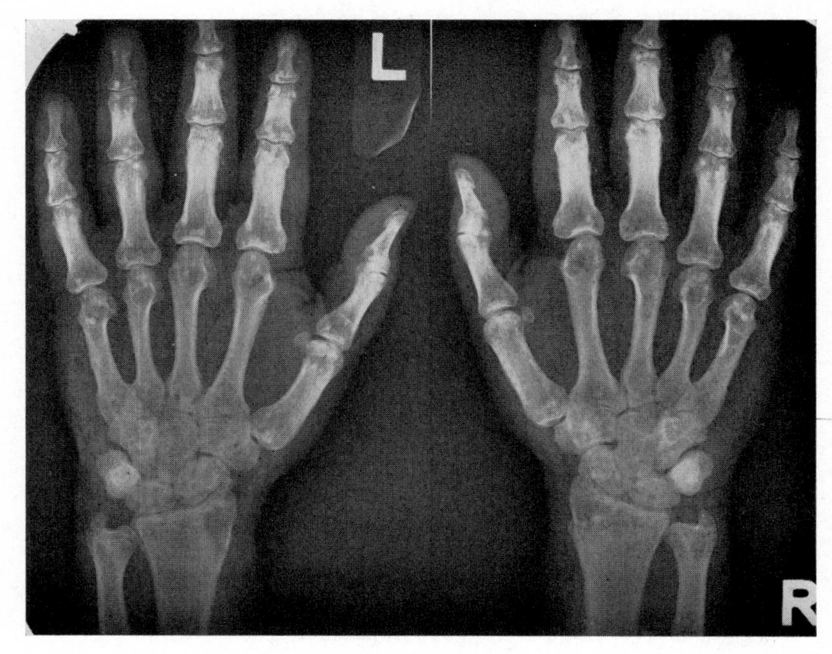

Fig. 10-7. Osteopoikilosis in M. M. (644555), 47 years of age. Asymptomatic. No skin manifestations. Family not available for study.

As was nicely demonstrated by Funstein and Kotschiew[71] the islands tend, in pronounced cases, to be oriented along the "traction and pressure lines,"[77] especially at points of crossing of these lines.

The skin lesions, always inconspicuous, are most often located on the posterior aspect of the thighs and buttocks, occasionally on the arms and trunk, but never on the face. Their location bears no constant relation to that of the bone lesions, although it is noteworthy that the head is usually affected neither by skin nor by bone lesions. They are closely situated, slightly elevated, whitish yellow, and usually oblong or oval in outline. Like the bone lesions, they have been described as occurring in longitudinal streaks. They are usually about the size of a lentil or pea, from which the name of the skin lesions (dermatofibrosis lenticularis disseminata) is in part derived. Most of the cases of bone lesions that have been subjected to careful inspection have been found to show skin lesions as well. Busch[62] described skin changes in six patients, Buschke and Ollendorff[63] in one, and Šváb[87] and Windholz[92] in two each.

Information on the age of appearance and evolution of both the osseous and cutaneous changes is meager. It is clear that lesions may be present at both sites in the first years of life. Furthermore, it appears that once formed, the bone lesions remain static for many years. The longest reported follow-up, seventeen years, was in a female first observed at the age of 14 years.[78]

Keloids may occur with increased frequency in these patients.[68] The only internal medical ramification that has even been suggested is that of fibrous nodules of the peritoneal lining discovered at laparotomy in a 13-year-old patient who complained of severe abdominal pains.[85] It can fairly be stated that this was

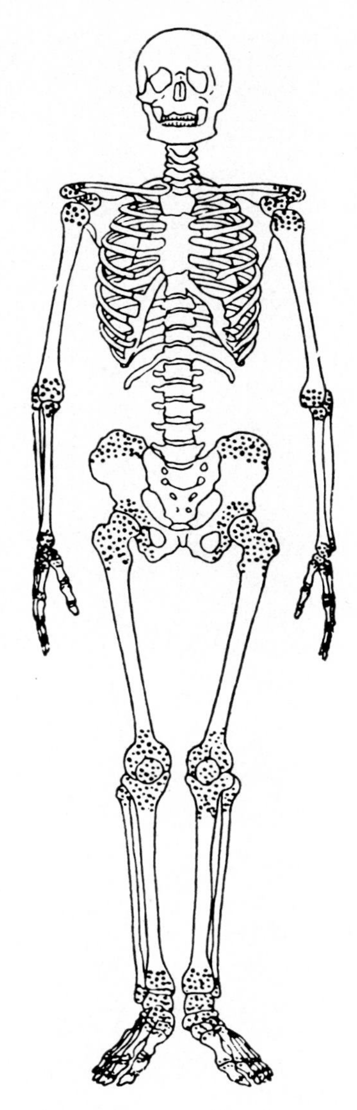

Fig. 10-8. Typical location of bone lesions in osteopoikilosis.[22]

not a "clear case," however. Grossly the nodules suggested tubercles. Scleroderma beginning at the age of 7 months was described in association with osteopoikilosis by von Bernuth.[89] However, I doubt seriously that the bone condition described and pictured was the same as that under discussion here. In a case reported by Nichols and Shiflett[78] an obscure generalized skeletal disease was present in addition to osteopoikilosis; the authors thought there was no connection. There were exostoses in the cases of Albers-Schönberg,[58] Risseeuw,[81] and Albronda.[59] Copeman[65] saw osteopoikilosis in association with rheumatoid arthritis. In general, one seems justified in considering this situation as incapable of producing symptoms and as prognostically insignificant.

The bone lesions were examined histologically by Schmorl[83] in an 18-year-old boy who died of seemingly unrelated cause. He found that each "island" is a clump of osseous trabeculae that are thicker at the periphery than at the center. The trabeculae at the center form a complex network with ordinary marrow in the space between. The skin lesions consist of collagenous fibrosis with preservation of the elastic fiber elements.[62,63]

From the point of view of inheritance this disorder behaves as a Mendelian autosomal dominant. Busch[62] found fourteen cases in three generations of one family, and the condition probably extended further back in the ancestry, since there were three affected siblings in the first generation studied. Hinson[73] studied it in two generations. In x-ray films of the entire skeleton Bloom[61] found only a single spot in the sister of a patient with widespread involvement. Wilcox[91] saw the bone condition in father and daughter; Voorhoeve,[90] in father, son, and daughter. Risseeuw[81] saw the disorder in a man, six of his children, and a grandson. Albronda[59] saw the bone condition in a woman and one son and daughter; there was no skin change.

The basic defect appears to be a spotty hyperplasia of collagen in the corium and bone matrix. This is, however, little more than a restatement of the histologic findings. What is basically involved in this defect and why there is the peculiar spotty distribution are obscure. Voorhoeve[90] thought the bone lesions arise in cartilage. He based this theory on the fact that in two children he observed striate lesions extending a variable distance into the diaphysis from the epiphyseal line. The relative immunity of the skull and clavicle ("membranous bones") may be supporting evidence for enchondral origin.

In a paper entitled "Follicular Atrophoderma and Pseudopelade Associated With Chondrodystrophia Calcificans Congenita," Curth[69] has written about an interesting familial and almost certainly hereditary disorder involving bone and skin. As indicated in her references to the literature, others have reported cases. In the case of the skin involvement it may be connective tissue that is primarily affected and not the epidermis. However, studies to date leave the nature of the basic defect in question. It is certainly distinct from osteo-dermato-poikilosis. There is probably no fundamental kinship between so-called "stippled epiphyses" (chondrodystrophia calcificans congenita[66]) and osteopoikilosis. Traub[88] has described mottling of the epiphyses, superficially resembling osteopoikilosis, in cases of pituitary gigantism, and a vaguely similar picture is associated with cretinism.[80]

LÉRI'S PLEONOSTEOSIS

In 1921 André Léri,[97] Parisian orthopedist, described a previously unrecognized condition in a 35-year-old man and his children by a second wife, a daughter 4 years and a son 3 weeks of age. The child by his first wife was normal. The disorder was not present at birth and became evident sooner or later in extrauterine life. The father was only 62 inches tall and had short, broad hands and feet with thickened palmar pads and accentuated creases, with limitation of motion in the wrists, elbows, hips, and knees. The toes, and presumably the thumbs as well, were broad and stiff. Fairly numerous cases have since been described in the French literature,[96,99,102,104,105] including one report from Russia,[96] and some in the German literature (see reference 100 for list of German reports);

there have also been reports in journals of Brazil and Argentina (see reference 107), but there appears to be only one article in British journals[107] and none at all in the periodical American medical literature.

The term "pleonosteosis" suggested by Léri was based on his impression, probably inaccurate, that the basic abnormality is one of excessive ossification.

The clinical characteristics of Léri's pleonosteosis are broadening and deformity of the thumbs and great toes, flexion contractures of the interphalangeal joints, and limitation of motion in other joints, including even those of the spine. A form of "hammertoe" may develop. Mongoloid facies has been described[107] but is by no means an invariable feature (see Case 1 of reference 107). Furthermore, in the majority of cases of Mongoloid features, the patients are normally intelligent, e.g. Watson-Jones'[107] Patient 2 who was a university graduate. However, there are at least two reports of impairment of the intellect.[101,105]

There is usually semifixed internal rotation of the upper limbs and external rotation of the lower limbs. In general the limbs are short. The joints of the hands in particular may appear to be swollen. The hands are short, square, and thick. Changes in the lower extremities seem to be less striking, but this may be a function of the fact that less intricate movements are required of the feet and ankles.

A complication of the fibrous hyperplasia in the hands and feet can be nerve compression: carpal tunnel syndrome involving the median nerves and Morton's metatarsalgia from involvement of the digital nerves of the feet.

Watson-Jones[107] described the dense fibrous tissue removed from the wrist and consisting essentially of a highly hyperplastic anterior carpal ligament. The specimen consisted of greatly increased, dense collagenous tissue which in portions was actually fibrocartilage. Elastic fibers were conspicuous in their absence. Mucinous material was present, and in tissue removed from the foot, numerous "tissue mast cells" were described.

The fundamental abnormality was thought by Léri to be one of excessive and perhaps precocious ossification of the epiphyses. It seemed more likely to Watson-Jones[107] that the joint deformities are due to capsular contractures, that in general the abnormality resides in the fibrous tissues, and that the "thickening of the bones may be due to periosteal traction at their metaphyseal attachments."

All evidence suggests that pleonosteosis is inherited as a Mendelian autosomal dominant trait.

Although uncommon, Léri's pleonosteosis almost certainly occurs more frequently than the rarity of reports in American publications would suggest. In their monograph *Human Heredity*, Neel and Schull[101] describe a 34-year-old woman with progressive loss of joint mobility and moderately severe contractures beginning in adolescence. Movements of the hands in particular were awkward and clumsy. The mother, 58 years of age, was affected and by this time of life was unable to perform most fine movements of the hands and the rest of the body. A brother of the proposita and a half-brother of her mother were also affected. A feature of all affected persons was a broad thumb. The proposita sought information on whether her two sons would be affected. Since one of them already displayed broad thumbs, the inquirer was advised that a vocation requiring manual dexterity would be inadvisable. Rukavina and colleagues[106] have reported the family in full.

The nosography of this disorder is far from fully established. Cocchi[93] includes this condition in the group of "polytopic enchondral dysostoses" in which he also includes the Morquio snydrome and the Hurler syndrome. In a detailed clinicopathologic study based on two brothers, Materna[100] described what he called Léri's pleonosteosis, which differs radically from the condition in the four patients reported by Watson-Jones.[107] There was no mention of limitation of joint mobility. The entire skeleton revealed extensive changes with "innumerable microfractures," fish vertebrae, a wedge vertebra, and coarsening and widening of the tubular bone, among other changes. The father was thought to have the same disorder as his two sons. One of the sons died at the age of 42 years of heart failure; no autopsy was performed. In the other, heart disease believed to be rheumatic was discovered at autopsy. This brother had had repair of bilateral inguinal hernias at the age of 14 months.

In the differential diagnosis, a mucopolysaccharidosis and arthritis, either rheumatoid or degenerative, come in for consideration. One would be suspicious that the case thought by Rocher and Pesme[102] to be one of pleonosteosis with corneal opacification was, in fact, a mucopolysaccharidosis. Sometimes thoracic outlet syndrome (compression of components of the cervical plexus) is suspected.[107]

PAGET'S DISEASE OF BONE

Is Paget's disease of bone a generalized disorder of connective tissue? The evidence that Paget's disease of bone can legitimately be considered a heritable abiotrophy, probably of the collagen matrix of bone, can be summarized in the way indicated below. None of the pieces of evidence is by itself conclusive, but taken together they make a rather convincing argument.

1. The hereditary nature of the process appears to be established. However, it is worth while to examine the evidence for this, since one review,[150] which is otherwise comprehensive, makes no mention of the genetic factor in discussing etiology. In 1889 Paget[145] himself wrote: "I have tried in vain to trace any hereditary tendency to the disease. I have not found it twice in the same family." However, the observations of familial aggregation reported from even before that time (beginning with Pick[147] in 1883) are fairly numerous. (See Fig. 10-9.)

In 1946 Koller[133] could find in the literature twenty-eight families in which more than one case was described. Since then other reports[109,110,116,129,131,139,143,153,159] of familial aggregation have appeared. Stemmermann[159] identified it in members of three successive generations. It appears to have occurred in four generations of a Jewish family known to me and also in two other kinships, as indicated in Fig. 10-9. Aschner and associates[109] described it in monozygous twin brothers and claimed that by 1952 a total of fifty-seven families with multiple cases had been described. Martin[137] and others (Fig. 10-9) also described the disease in both of identical twins.

When one undertakes to study the heredity of a condition such as Paget's disease, one encounters several difficulties. In the first place, the disease has some of the earmarks of an abiotrophy. That it is an abiotrophy remains, of course, to be established. At any rate the disease usually has its onset late in life, by which

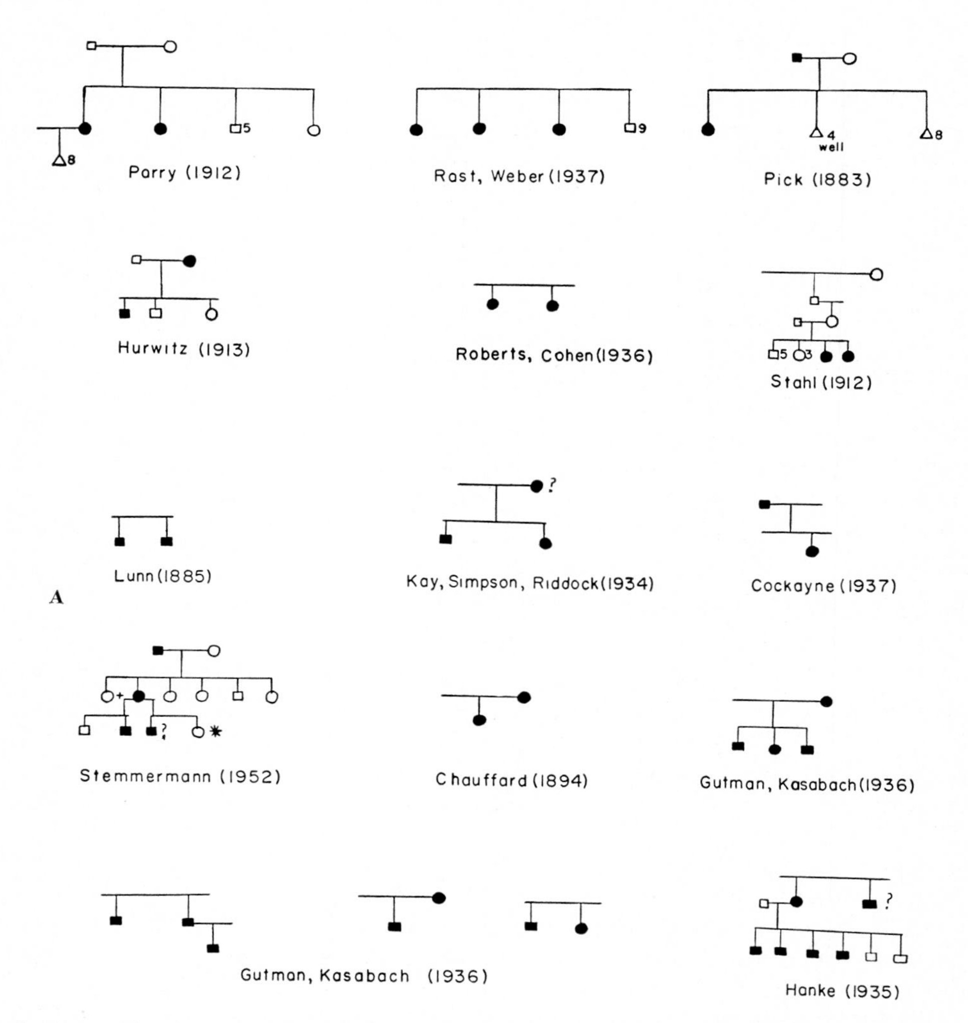

Fig. 10-9. Thirty-five pedigrees from the literature and two from the unpublished experience of Brayshaw and McKusick, showing familial aggregation of Paget's disease. Moehlig[139] and Ashley-Montagu[110] and probably others reported Jewish pedigrees. Concordance in identical twins was reported by Koller,[133] by Mozer,[142] and by Dickson and associates.[118] In the last instance there was a striking similarity of distribution in the twins, both having, for example, tibial involvement. In the twins observed by Mozer[142] onset of the clinically evident abnormalities occurred at the age of 48 years in both. In Irvine's[129] pedigree the affected male died of a malignant osteoclastoma of the jaw, and both daughters had the onset of Paget's disease of the skull and jaw at the age of 18 years. In the pedigree of Brayshaw and McKusick in Fig. 9-2*B*, the first individual in the second generation, a female (A. H., 511948), had so-called osteitis pubis and changes in the skull compatible with Paget's disease. The alkaline phosphatase, however, was always normal. The other two affected individuals (C. T., 502845; W. T., 620032) had Paget's disease in entirely typical form. These patients were discovered on study of the records of the hospital; if a more detailed study of the family were made, other members would probably be found to be affected.

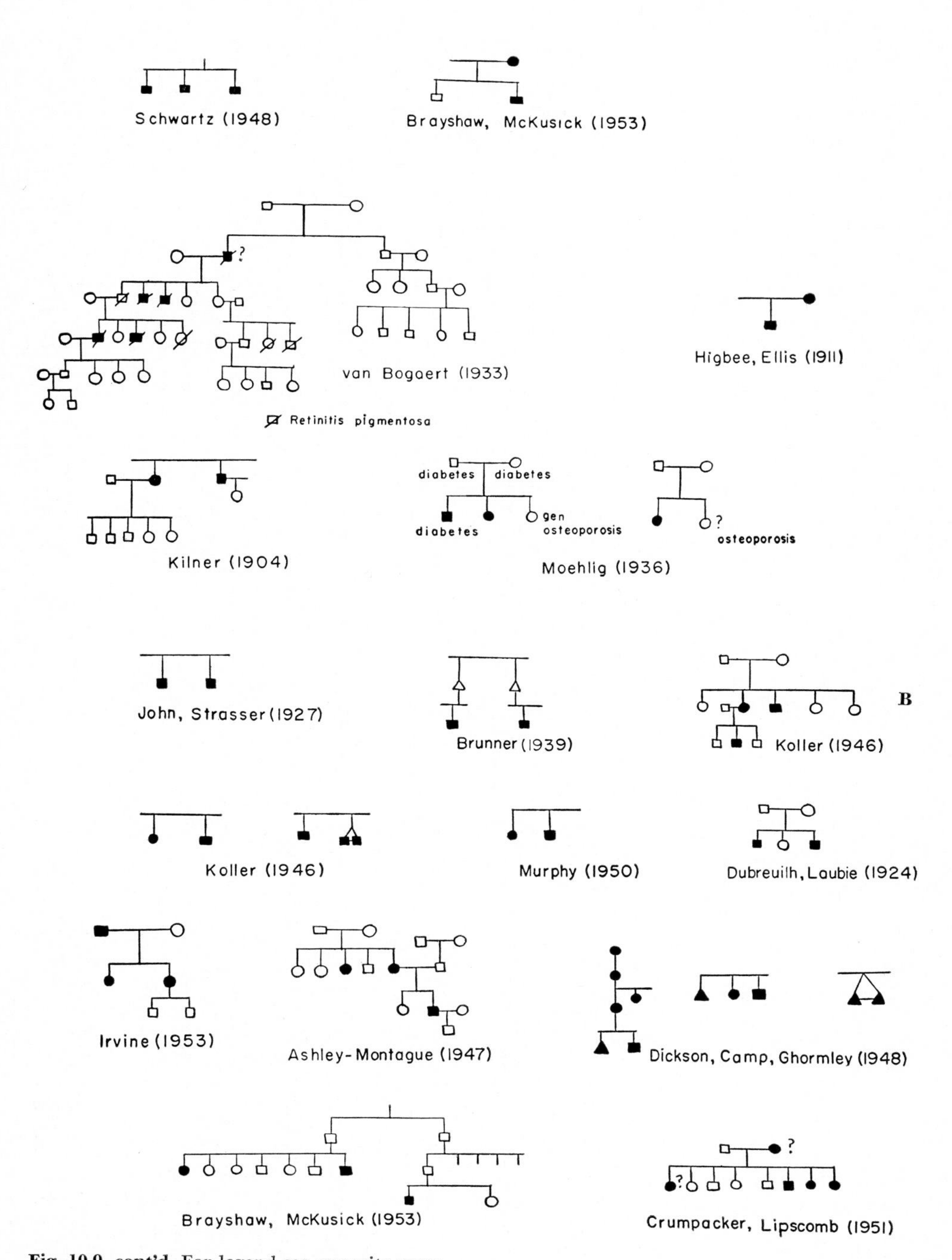

Fig. 10-9, cont'd. For legend see opposite page.

time the parents are likely to have died, the siblings may be widely scattered geographically, and the children will probably not yet be old enough to have developed the disease. In the second place, Paget's disease is often subtle in its manifestations. A very high proportion of affected persons are asymptomatic, and the change in bone is discovered only incidentally on radiologic examination made for unrelated purposes or possibly in search for an explanation of an otherwise obscure elevation of serum alkaline phosphatase activity. In the course of a detailed study of 7,941 individuals over 61 years of age, eighty-five cases of Paget's disease were found, but of these cases only three had complaints referable to the disorder of bone.[140] In connection with the last difficulty it may be that a study of families, using alkaline phosphatase determinations as a screening procedure, would be productive. The first type of difficulty—the age factor—would not, to be sure, be circumvented.

In general, the data accumulated are consistent with the view that the trait for Paget's disease is controlled by a simple autosomal Mendelian dominant gene. However, Ashley-Montagu[110] suggested that it is inherited as a sex-linked recessive.

Considering how frequently Paget's disease occurs in at least mild form (3% of all persons over 40 years of age, according to Schmorl[152]), one might say that it would be extraordinary if thirty or forty families with more than one case could *not* be discovered. Along the same line it may be noted that Sabatini[151] found Paget's disease in two married couples in which the marital partners were unrelated. Actually I believe there is a significant familial aggregation of cases. Particularly in the pedigrees with more than two cases is the evidence convincing. The incidence of Paget's disease in the general population is roughly 0.013%.[133] It can be estimated that the chance of two or more cases occurring in the same family by random distribution alone is very slight indeed.

2. Angioid streaks of the retina are associated with only two conditions with any regularity. These are pseudoxanthoma elasticum and Paget's disease of bone.[141,161] Angioid streaks of the fundus of the eye, pseudoxanthoma elasticum in the skin, and Paget's disease in the bones have been observed in the same patient.[166] There may be reasons for believing there is no fundamental relationship between Paget's disease and pseudoxanthoma elasticum: the first may be inherited as a Mendelian dominant and the second as a Mendelian recessive; the first occurs more frequently in men and the second in women. (Paget's disease seems to occur more commonly in men but in more severe form in women.)

Although Paget's disease and pseudoxanthoma elasticum may be basically distinct entities, the fact that angioid streaks, which are an integral part of a definite disorder of connective tissue (PXE), occur also in Paget's disease suggests that Paget's disease may likewise be a disorder of connective tissue with abnormalities much more widespread than the bone lesions alone would suggest.

Also in Paget's disease, there occur other ocular abnormalities such as corneal degeneration,[163] cataract,[134] and choroiditis[114] independent of angioid streaks, which raise further the question of whether a generalized abiotrophy of connective tissue may be present.

3. A quality of reasonableness, although not constituting proof, makes it attractive to persons familiar with bone and with the clinical behavior of Paget's disease to speculate that the disease is fundamentally an abiotrophy of the col-

lagen matrix of bone, which breaks down with the passage of years. Albright[108] presents evidence that Paget's disease is primarily a destruction or, perhaps it is permissible to say, a degeneration of bone with secondary reparative overproduction of bone.

In general, the involvement of the skeleton follows a pattern of localization consistent with the view that "wear-and-tear" is a contributing factor in the development of the lesions. Weight-bearing structures are usually involved primarily. The bones of the upper extremity are, for example, much less often involved than those of the legs. The victims of Paget's disease in severe form are often obese. The high incidence of obesity and tallness in the families of patients with Paget's disease was emphasized by Moehlig.[138,139]

The femur[152] is one of the most commonly affected bones (over 30% of cases) and the humerus, one of the least (less than 5%).* The most frequently affected bone is the sacrum (57% of cases). The vertebrae are affected in half of cases and the incidence of involvement in descending frequency is lumbar, thoracic, and cervical spine. In brief, beginning with the sacrum there is a progressive decrease in frequency of involvement as one progresses craniad. An amazing finding[152] is that the right femur is involved by Paget's disease over twice as often as the left femur (31% as against 15%). Undoubtedly, people are right-legged or left-legged just as they are right-handed or left-handed. In the skull Albright and Reifenstein[108] picture an instance of predominant involvement laterally at the attachment of the masseter and temporal muscles. Involvement of other areas of the skull, often a striking feature, is more difficult to explain on a "wear-and tear" basis. However, it must be remembered that "wear-and-tear" is probably only a contributing factor in the development and localization of the disorder, the primary factor being perhaps a hereditary weakness. The situation with Paget's disease may be like that of pseudoxanthoma elasticum in which "wear-and-tear" appears to be responsible for the site of principal localization of the skin changes. Schmorl[152] noted that changes tend to be most pronounced at the attachments of tendons and ligaments to bones. Kay and co-workers[131] made the important observation that in a brother and sister (Fig. 10-9*A*) with Paget's disease, both with unilateral involvement of the radius, the left radius was involved in the left-handed individual and the right radius in the right-handed one! This appears to be a nice demonstration of the cooperation of genetic and postnatal factors.

The significance of localized trauma preceding the onset of monostotic Paget's disease is difficult to evaluate (p. 332 of reference 158). The reported cases may represent coincidence.

4. Vascular disease has been thought to occur prematurely and with increased incidence in these patients.[156] This has been thought to be independent of the "high output" heart failure, which may occur as a result of the vascular peculiarities that functionally resemble arteriovenous fistulae.[120,160] Medial sclerosis of the Mönckeberg type has been thought to occur especially often in these persons. Harrison and Lennox[125] found valvular calcification in 39% of their patients with Paget's disease, an incidence five times that in a control group of comparable age distribution. Vascular calcification may be related merely to the

*The statistics listed here are derived from the classic necropsy study of Schmorl.[152]

periodic hypercalcemia to which these persons are subjected. The elevation of circulating alkaline phosphatase may contribute. Extraskeletal calcification occurs commonly in these patients,[144,154,164] possibly for the reasons listed, possibly because of an abnormality of connective tissues. Urinary calculi, which are frequent, would seem to be explained by the high urinary excretion of calcium. Salivary calculi, which were identified in twenty of 111 cases,[150] may have a somewhat similar basis.

This fourth bit of evidence is by far the weakest of the points bearing on the possible nature of Paget's disease as an abiotrophy of the collagen matrix of bone.

Hitherto, a principal view of the pathogenesis of Paget's disease has implicated vascular changes. This view would consider that intimately related to the primary defect is the increased vascularity of the bones, which (1) may represent a significant and at times intolerable burden to the heart similar to that of arteriovenous fistulae,[156] (2) is a problem in hemostasis to surgeons, for instance the neurosurgeon performing craniotomy in instances of involvement of the skull,[117] and (3) results in the fact that the skin overlying bones severely affected by Paget's disease may be warmer than elsewhere. In the present state of ignorance it is probably at least equally valid to suspect that Paget's disease of bone may be an abiotrophy of the collagen matrix and that the vascular phenomena are secondary developments.

OTHER POSSIBLE HEREDITARY AND GENERALIZED DISORDERS OF CONNECTIVE TISSUE

Christiaens and associates[171] have described (with clinical photographs and autopsy findings) the association of pronounced *cutis laxa* with bilateral and severe pulmonary emphysema. The latter was the cause of death in the 18-month-old infant. No mechanical factor to account for the emphysema was discovered. A generalized defect of elastic fibers was hypothesized and seemingly found support in the results of histologic studies. The cutis laxa present in this infant was appropriately named, as indicated by photographs that show the skin hanging, from the trunk in particular, in large loose folds. This disorder is not to be confused with either the Ehlers-Danlos syndrome or pseudoxanthoma elasticum; there is no evidence of fundamental alliance with either. Cutis laxa may be inherited as an autosomal dominant, many of the severe cases being fresh mutants. Sestak[200] reported two families with multiple cases: a father and daughter in one; a brother and sister and their great-grandmother in the second family.

Reported in the literature and occasionally encountered in practice are cases of generalized abnormality suggestive of a disorder of connective tissue but not clearly classifiable in any of the categories discussed in this book. Fittke[179] describes such a situation under the title "On an Unusual Form of 'Multiple Congenital Degeneration' (Chalodermia and Dysostosis)." The proband, a 10½-month-old female, had shown, from birth, that the skin of her entire body, with the exception of the face, fell in loose, redundant folds. On stretching, it returned to its original position very slowly. The skeletal system showed widely persistent fontanelles, slight oxycephaly, and dislocation of one hip with flattening of the other acetabulum. There was no known consanguinity, but the family lived in an area of Europe where most persons were related. The mother, 25 years of age, had long been under treatment for "weak knee joints." A first cousin of the proband, 7¾ years of age, showed the same type of loose skin, which was restored only slowly to its original position after stretching. Noted also were pigeon breast, static scoliosis, and flat feet. The fontanelles did not close until the third year. The case of "cutis laxa" with bone dystrophy reported by Debré and colleagues[175] may be identical.

Gout, like ochronosis (Chapter 7), is an inborn error of metabolism in which connective tissue becomes involved. However, the nature of the basic defect in gout and the genetics of the disorder are much less well understood. Furthermore, the change in connective tissue is probably not of such intimate molecular nature as is the case in alkaptonuria, in which collagen is probably affected. For these reasons, as well as the availability of excellent reviews[198,212] of the subject, gout has not been discussed here in detail.

Generalized arterial calcification of infancy has been noted in multiple sibs[184,192,212] (Fig. 10-10). The justification for mentioning it in a discussion of generalized heritable disorders of connective tissue is provided by the evidence suggesting that fundamentally the disorder is a degeneration of elastic fiber. The calcification shows a remarkable predilection for the internal elastic lamina. Considerable material with the staining properties of mucopolysaccharide accumulates around the elastic laminae.[211] Fine calcium incrustation of the lamina is the minimal lesion. Later the lamina is ruptured and occlusive changes of the intima take place. Death from myocardial infarction usually occurs in the first six months after birth. The clinical diagnosis is suggested by the discovery of calcification in a peripheral vessel in an infant with electrocardiographic evidence of coronary artery disease. Idiopathic infantile hypercalcemia, of which there may be more than one etiologic variety, is probably unrelated; to my knowledge there is not yet evidence of a genetic variety of infantile hypercalcemia.

Clearly there are genetic differences in the tendency to *keloid* formation. Negroes and some Caucasian families are notoriously susceptible.[167]

Certain hereditary syndromes display abnormalities of structures other than connective tissues. Such a syndrome is that which goes by Werner's name.[185,197,203,205] The victim of the *Werner syndrome,* which is usually inherited as an autosomal recessive, displays short stature, with slender limbs and stocky trunk; scleroderma-like changes, especially in the skin of the extremities, with the development of ulcers over the ankle malleoli, Achilles tendons, heels, and toes and with atrophy of the corium demonstrable microscopically; localized soft tissue calcifications; and, finally, premature arteriosclerosis with Mönckeberg calcification. However, the patients also display premature canities and balding, juvenile cataract,* weak high-pitched voice, atrophy of the epidermis as well as the corium, hypogonadism, osteoporosis, and increased incidence of diabetes mellitus. This is an intriguing disorder, as far as definition of the basic defect is concerned. One is reminded of myotonia dystrophica, in which baldness, cataract, and hypogonadism cannot in the present state of ignorance be related to the disorder of muscle.

---

*The internist must keep the Werner syndrome[193] in mind in connection with patients who appear to have a more conventional, acquired variety of scleroderma. Cataracts can be the tip-off to the presence of this hereditary syndrome.

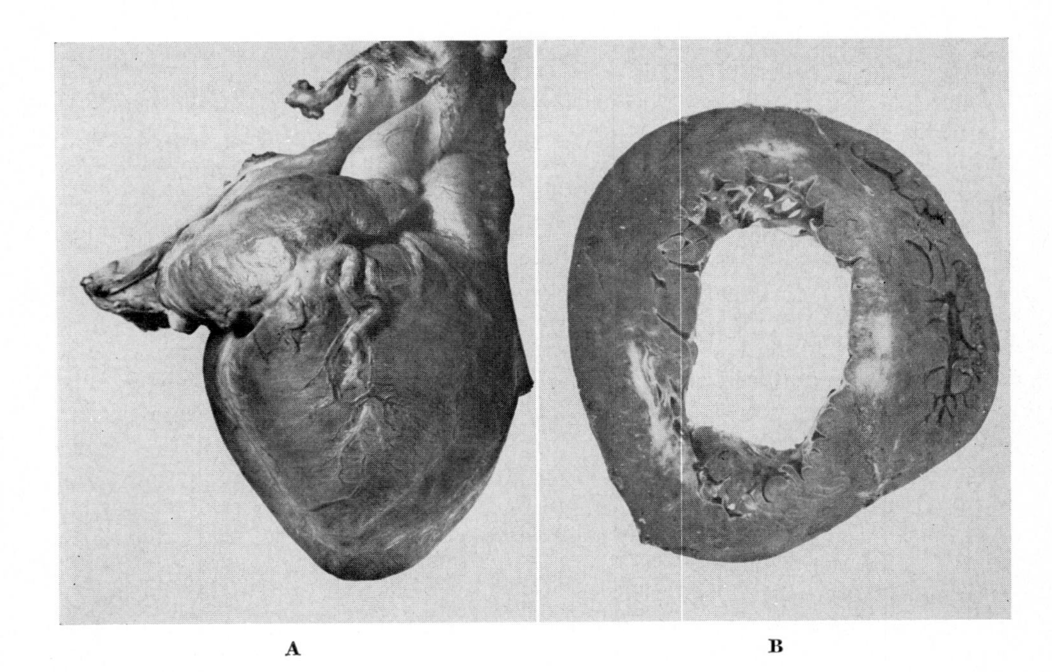

Fig. 10-10. Brothers with generalized arterial calcification of infancy. M. W. died of heart failure at the age of 4 months. Beginning at the age of 3 weeks he appeared to have a respiratory infection, with cough and dyspnea. He was pale and had episodes of sweating. On several occasions he had attacks in which he cried out suddenly and stiffened his body. Peripheral cyanosis, cardiac and hepatic enlargement, and ST segment and T-wave changes in the electrocardiogram were found. The striking feature was the presence of calcified, tortuous coronary arteries, **A.** When the heart was sectioned, evidence of old and recent myocardial infarction was discovered, **B.** Calcification was seen in small arteries of the omentum. Histologically many arteries, including the aorta and pulmonary artery, showed calcification around elastic laminae, which appeared fragmented, **C.** In the outer part of the pulmonary artery, granuloma formation was demonstrated in the area of interruption of the elastic fibers, **D.** The aorta, **E,** stained by the periodic acid-Schiff technique, showed deeply stained margins of abnormal elastic fibers contrasting with the weakly staining edges of normal fibers. In the coronary artery, **F,** after calcium was removed by dilute nitric acid, material staining with periodic acid–Schiff was demonstrated surrounding the elastic lamellae. The association of the calcium deposition with abnormal elastic fibers was demonstrated in the stains of the aorta, **G,** with the von Kossa technique. The above histologic findings suggest that accumulation of mucopolysaccharide is a consequence of degenerative change in elastic fibers. Similar evidence is available in Erdheim's cystic medial necrosis, in the Marfan syndrome, and in experimental lathyrism. That alteration in the mucopolysaccharide of ground substance is followed by deposition of calcium salts is well recognized. In generalized arterial calcification of infants, the "basic defect" may reside in the elastic fibers. Accumulation of mucopolysaccharide and deposition of calcium may be secondary and tertiary phenomena. C. W., brother of M. W., died at the age of 7 months following an illness identical to that in M. W. Serum calcium concentration and alkaline phosphatase activity were normal. Autopsy revealed widespread arterial calcification and myocardial infarction. (Photographs and information courtesy Dr. Alan L. Williams, Melborne, Australia.)

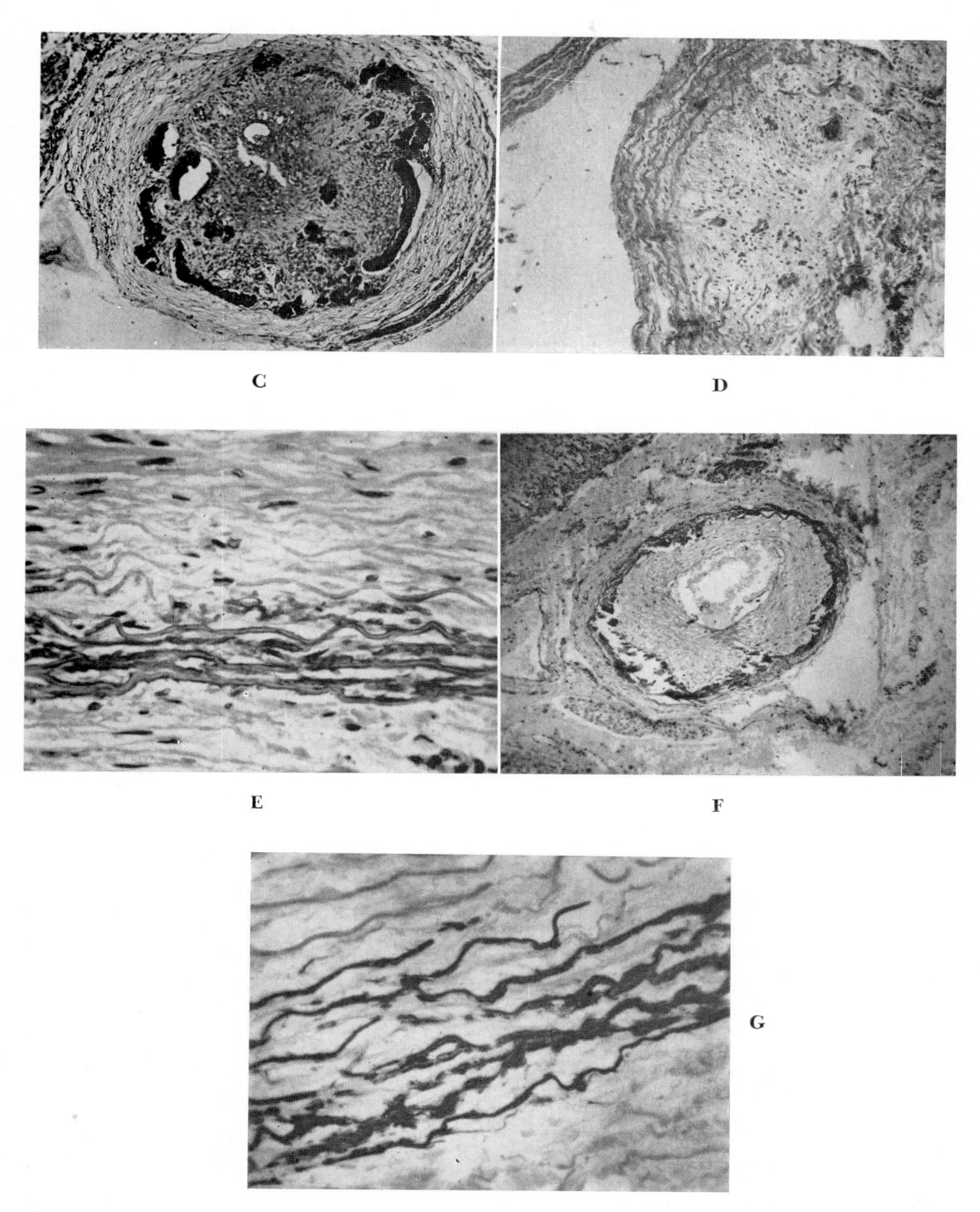

Fig. 10-10, cont'd. For legend see opposite page.

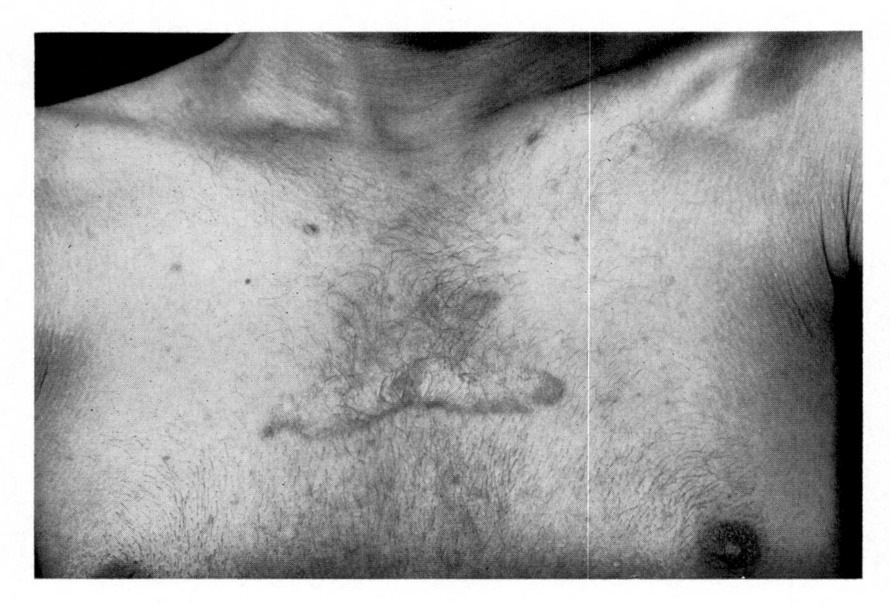

Fig. 10-11. Transverse keloid over sternum in mulatto male (D. C., 835228) whose father has an identical keloid. Trauma at this site preceding development of the keloid is not recalled.

In 1928 Pelger and in 1931 Huët, both of the Netherlands, described an anomaly of the nucleus of the leukocyte that in essence consists of a deficiency in segmentation.[206] It was found to be inherited as a dominant. Nachtsheim[195] found the anomaly in one person in 1,000 in the population of Berlin. What ostensibly is the same anomaly occurs in the rabbit, where again it is inherited as a dominant. When two animals affected with the nuclear anomaly are bred, it is found that those offspring which are presumably homozygous for the Pelger-Huët trait demonstrate a severe form of chondrodystrophy.[187,195] The trait is lethal or sublethal in this homozygous form. At least one instance in man of a presumed homozygous form of *Pelger-Huët anomaly* has been reported.[183] Although the change in the leukocyte was more striking than usually seen, no skeletal abnormality was detected. The basis of the relationship between the nuclear anomaly and the chondrodystrophy in the homozygous rabbits is obscure.

In *Dupuytren's contracture*[170,181,188,190,201,204] and in *Peyronie's disease,*[194,198] convincing evidence of a hereditary basis is available. Furthermore, the two conditions are probably associated more frequently than chance alone would dictate. The occurrence of knuckle pads[180,181,191,201,208,210] and plantar nodules[173] in association with Dupuytren's contracture, together with a possible relationship of the latter condition to epilepsy,[176,191,201] gives reason to think that Dupuytren's contracture is a common manifestation of a generalized disorder affecting connective tissue. Genetic investigation is hampered by its appearance late in life and the overall high frequency in older persons.[177]

Stickler and colleagues[48] described a "new" entity which appears to be a heritable disorder of connective tissue. Inherited as an atuosomal dominant, it is characterized by (1) progressive myopia, beginning in the first decade of life and leading to retinal detachment and blindness, and (2) premature degenerative changes in various joints. The designation suggested by the authors is "hereditary progressive arthro-ophthalmopathy."

There is a large number of members of the epiphysitis or *aseptic necrosis* group of disorders in which, more perhaps than in any other area of medicine, eponyms abound and confound. The following six entities are only a partial enumeration:

Phalangeal epiphyses	Thiemann[169]
Tubercle of tibia	Osgood-Schlatter
Head of femur	Legg-Calvé-Perthes[207]
Spine	Scheuermann
Tarsal scaphoid	Köhler
Semilunar	Kienböck, etc.

All of these probably have a hereditary background, although the evidence in Legg-Perthes' disease is most complete. It is peculiar that each seems to be a distinct genotypic entity. There is, for example, no evidence that more than one of these entities occurs in the same patient or that one member of an affected

Table 12. Rubin's classification of bone disorders*

I. Epiphyseal dysplasias
   A. Epiphyseal hypoplasias
      1. Failure of articular cartilage: spondyloepiphyseal dysplasia
      2. Failure of ossification of center: multiple epiphyseal dysplasia
   B. Epiphyseal hyperplasia
      1. Excess of articular cartilage: dysplasia epiphysalis hemimelica
II. Physeal dysplasia
   A. Cartilage hypoplasia
      1. Failure of proliferating cartilage: achondroplasia
      2. Failure of hypertrophic cartilage: metaphyseal dysostosis; cartilage-hair hypoplasia
   B. Cartilage hyperplasias
      1. Excess of proliferating cartilage: hyperchondroplasia (Marfan's syndrome)
      2. Excess of hypertrophic cartilage: enchondromatosis
III. Metaphyseal dysplasias
   A. Metaphyseal hypoplasias
      1. Failure to form primary spongiosa: hypophosphatasia
      2. Failure to absorb primary spongiosa: osteopetrosis
      3. Failure to absorb secondary spongiosa: craniometaphyseal dysplasia
   B. Metaphyseal hyperplasia
      1. Excessive spongiosa: multiple exostoses
IV. Diaphyseal dysplasias
   A. Diaphyseal hypoplasias
      1. Failure of periosteal bone formation: osteogenesis imperfecta
      2. Failure of endosteal bone formation: idiopathic osteoporosis, congenita and tarda
   B. Diaphyseal hyperplasias
      1. Excessive periosteal bone formation: progressive diaphyseal dysplasia (Engelmann's disease)
      2. Excessive endosteal bone formation: hyperphosphatasemia (including juvenile Paget's disease and van Buchem's disease)

*Adapted from Rubin, P.: Dynamic classification of bone dysplasias, Chicago, 1964, Year Book Medical Publishers, Inc.

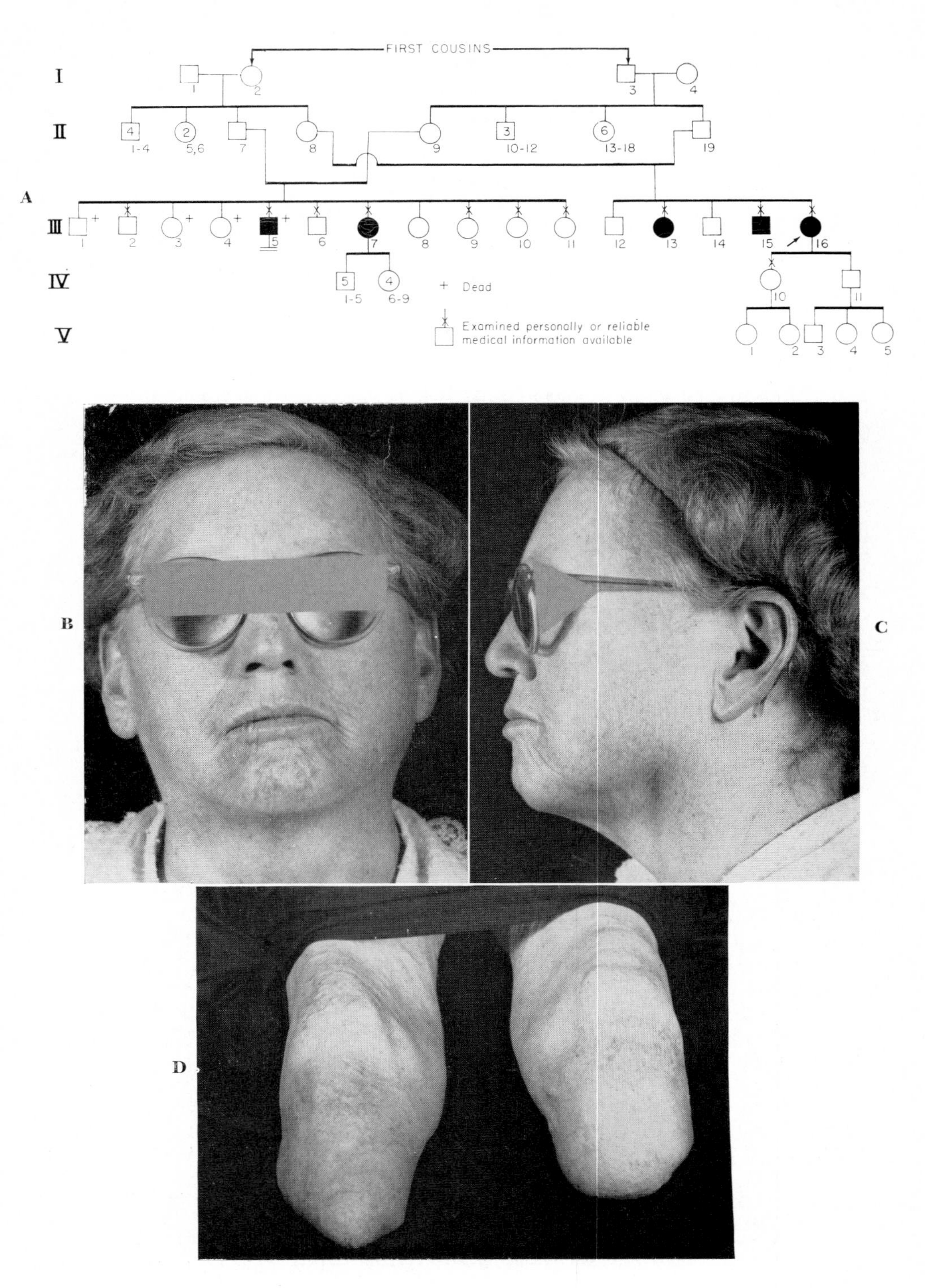

Fig. 10-12. For legend see opposite page.

Fig. 10-12. Werner syndrome. In two sibships of the kindred diagrammed in **A,** five cases of the Werner syndrome were observed. The two sibships are related to each other as double third cousins. The coefficient of relationship of the parents of the affected persons of both sibships is $1/64$, since they are second cousins. Briefly the characteristics of the patients with the Werner syndrome were as follows:

III-5, L. S. (J.H.H. 177405) had bilateral cataract extraction at age 37 years. At the age of 39 years he was noted to have premature graying of the hair, sclerodermatous changes of the extremities with extensive subcutaneous calcification and ulcers about the ankles, testicular atrophy, and short stature (60½ inches) with large torso. Tendons were also calcified, and there was striking crepitus on motion of most joints. It is noteworthy that macular degeneration resembling that usually considered senile in nature was observed at the age of 39 years. The patient died of sarcoma arising in the right thigh. Histologically the appearance of the tumor suggested nerve sheath origin.

III-7, M. S. K. was first discovered to have stigmata of the Werner syndrome when the kindred was restudied in 1962. Diminished vision began at the age of 11 years. Cataracts were removed at the age of 21 years and at 52 years. At the latter time mild diabetes was discovered. By age 25 years she was strikingly gray-haired. She is 62 inches tall, with thin white hair and the characteristic facies of the Werner syndrome. The facial skin was tight and the nose beaked, but the extremities were spared. Three years previously, "central and disseminated patches of healed chorioretinitis" were described and interpreted as an aftermath of toxoplasmosis. However, in view of the retinal changes described in her brother, L. S., it seems possible that these were directly related to the Werner syndrome.

III-13, O. A. was reported by Boatwright and associates.[168] Bilateral cataracts were discovered at age 35 years. Scleroderma of the feet and legs with ulceration and subcutaneous calcification began at the age of 40 years. She was 59 inches tall and the extremities were spindly, especially in comparison with the stocky trunk. The face was birdlike. After the time of the report she was demonstrated by barium swallow to have esophageal changes suggesting scleroderma. Amputation of both legs was performed because of chronic ulcers, and osteogenic sarcoma was discovered in the right first metatarsal and cuneiform bones. The patient died seven months later. Because of the rarity of reported autopsies in the Werner syndrome the findings in this case are of note. Death was the result of widespread metastases of osteogenic sarcoma arising in the leg. In addition, the aorta and coronary arteries showed extensive atherosclerosis. The mitral ring was extensively calcified.

III-15, E. L. R. was first reported by Boatwright and colleagues.[168] Bilateral cataracts were discovered at age 34 years. Soon afterward the hair became gray, and sclerodermatous changes developed in the feet and ankles, with painfully disabling callouses and ulcers. The voice was high pitched. He was found to have diabetes. The case was later reported in more detail, with autopsy findings, by Perloff and Phelps.[199] Autopsy revealed extensive atherosclerosis and vessel calcification but no abnormality of endocrine glands.

III-16, K. E. (459426), our proband, shown in **B** to **D,** was referred to also by Boatwright and his colleagues and by Perloff and Phelps. Changes in the skin of the feet began at age 20 years, and bilateral cataracts were discovered in her thirties. Below-knee amputations, **D,** were performed at the ages of 38 years and 45 years, after sympathectomy and skin grafts had failed. The chest had a barrel configuration and the extremities were spindly. The nose was beaked, **B** and **C.** Radiographic studies showed generalized osteoporosis and calcification at the root of the aorta, extending into the myocardium. A systolic ejection murmur in the aortic area was interpreted as indicative of aortic valve sclerosis with mild stenosis. Esophageal motility was normal. The chromosomes of this patient were found to be normal. X-ray films, e.g. of the hand, showed pronounced osteoporosis. There was subcutaneous calcification over the elbow.

Thus, sarcoma occurred in at least two affected persons in this family. The increased frequency of neoplasia has been noted in the literature. The occurrence of aortic valve sclerosis is illustrated by K. E. (III-16). (Family studied by Dr. R. M. Goodman.)

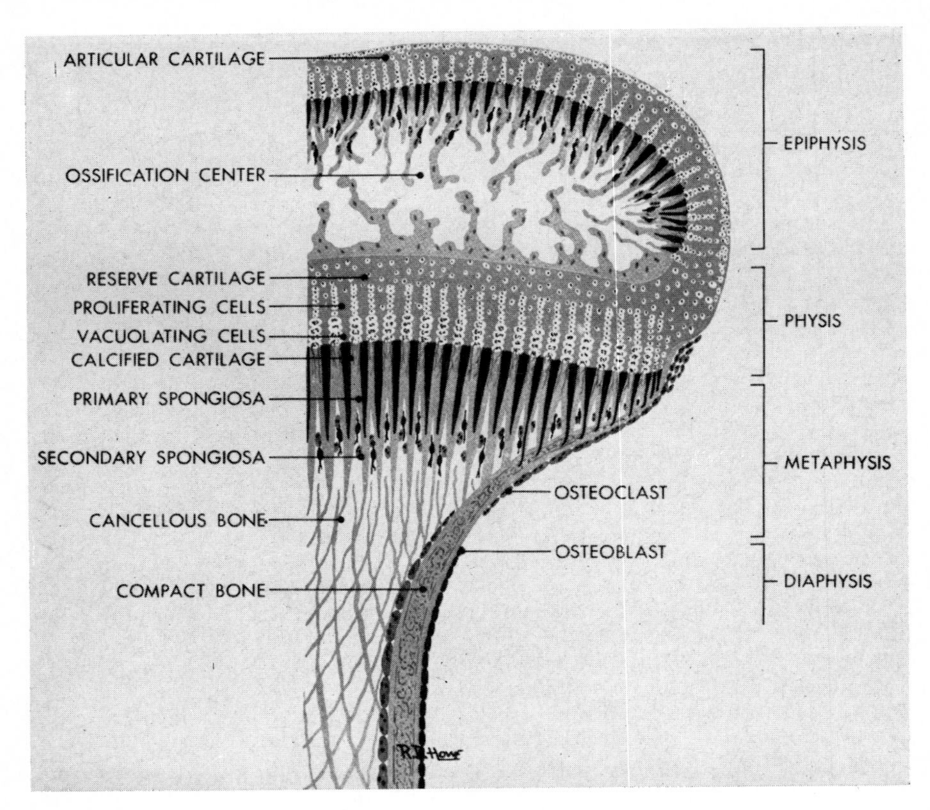

Fig. 10-13. Anatomic-histologic correlation of bone structure. (From Rubin, P.: Dynamic classification of bone dysplasias, Chicago, 1964, Year Book Medical Publishers, Inc.)

family has one variety whereas another member has a different variety. Interestingly, Legg-Perthes' disease probably almost never occurs in bona fide form in the pure Negro, although a simulating condition occurs with sickle cell hemoglobin C disease.[202]

In the case of *epidermolysis bullosa hereditaria* there is a view[178,186,209] of long standing that the basic defect is a deficiency of the elastic fibers of the superficial (papillary) layer of the corium. It is believed by some that normally these fibers bind the epidermis to the corium, and their absence has been thought to explain adequately the bullous lesions of this congenital disorder. Others[174,189] have questioned this theory, mainly on the basis of a failure to confirm the deficiency of elastic fibers on which the theory was predicated. The mucous membranes of the mouth have been involved, but no specific internal lesions have been described in autopsied cases.[174,189]

GENETIC DISORDERS OF THE OSSEOUS SKELETON

The osseous skeleton, the largest specialized connective tissue, participates in many of the generalized heritable disorders of connective tissue discussed here. In addition it is subject to a large number of gene-determined derangements with primary effects apparently limited to bone and cartilage. A review

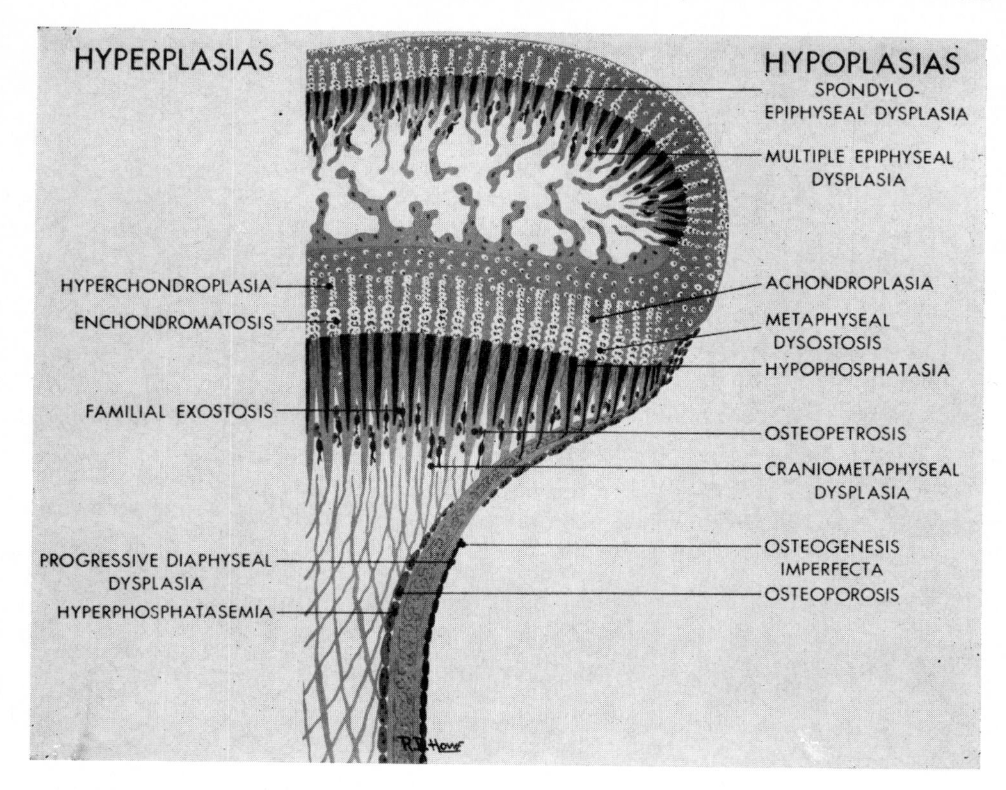

Fig. 10-14. Rubin's "dynamic classification of bone dysplasias." (From Rubin, P.: Dynamic classification of bone dysplasias, Chicago, 1964, Year Book Medical Publishers, Inc.)

of some of these[224,227,243,252,267,306,339] may be helpful in completing the survey undertaken in this book.

Rubin[306] has provided a classification of generalized hereditary dysplasias of the osseous skeleton, which has considerable merit. In this classification the major categories of dysplasia are epiphyseal, physeal, metaphyseal, and diaphyseal. (Rubin's proposal of the term *physis* and its adjective *physeal* to refer to the growth zone seems both useful and logical. See Fig. 10-14.) Each class of dysplasia has hypoplasia and hyperplasia subclasses, and in most of the subclasses more than one genus of disorder is recognized. (See Table 12.) Several of the entities, e.g. cartilage-hair hypoplasia and the Ellis-van Creveld syndrome, have manifestations in nonosseous tissues, also.

Epiphyseal dysplasias

Spondyloepiphyseal dysplasia. At least two varieties are recognized, an autosomal dominant and an X-linked recessive.

The autosomal dominant variety is illustrated by the mother and two daughters described in Fig. 10-15. This is the condition referred to by Maroteaux and Lamy[288] as the pseudo-achondroplastic form of spondyloepiphyseal dysplasia. It is differentiated from classic achondroplasia[244] by the fact that abnormality is

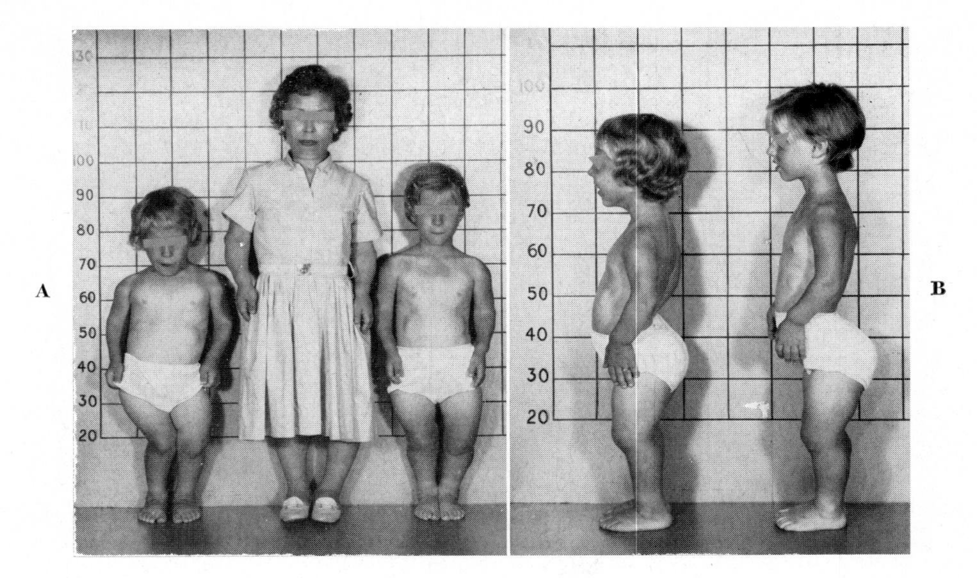

Fig. 10-15. Pseudo-achondroplastic type of spondyloepiphyseal dysplasia. **A,** The mother, age 35, and both children, ages 8 and 11, are affected. (The mother's mother, two of her sisters, and two sons of one of the sisters are also affected. Inheritance is dominant and, although no male-to-male transmission has been observed in this kindred, probably autosomal.) Note the normal size and shape of the head. The skull is radiologically normal. **B,** Both girls show exaggerated lumbar lordosis. **C,** Lumbar spine in the mother showing some flattening, which is, however, not diagnostic. **D,** Lumbar spine in the 11-year-old daughter, showing an anterior projection of the vertebral bodies due to delay in ossification of the annular epiphyses. The lumbar spine, as viewed in frontal projection, does not show caudad narrowing of the interpeduncular distance as is characteristic of achondroplasia. **E,** Hips and pelvis in the mother. **F,** Drastic changes are shown in the hips and knees of the 11-year-old daughter.

usually not evident at birth, by the absence of clinical and roentgenologic abnormality of the face and skull, and by roentgenologic findings of gross abnormalities in the epiphyseal-metaphyseal areas with fragmentation of the epiphyseal ossification centers. The spinal changes are different from those of achondroplasia, and the small sacroiliac notch characteristic of the latter condition is not seen. In children the spinal changes are diagnostic.

Short stature becomes more noticeable in adolescence. The adult height varies from 52 to 62 inches, the dwarfing being of the short trunk variety. Changes in the lumbar vertebrae in the adult are characteristic. These consist of a hump-shaped build-up of eburnated bone in the central and posterior portions of both the superior and inferior plates and a complete lack of visible bone in the distribution of the ring apophyses.[270] At first glance the x-ray appearance suggests extensive calcification of the intervertebral disc, as in alkaptonuria. Precocious osteoarthrosis of the hips, and sometimes of the knees and shoulders, is also a feature of this disorder.

The X-linked variety of spondyloepiphyseal dysplasia was described by Jacobsen[255] as an atypical form of Morquio's syndrome. Occurring only in males, this variety of dwarfism is of the "short trunk" variety. The limbs are long relative to the trunk. The spinal involvement dominates the clinical picture, although

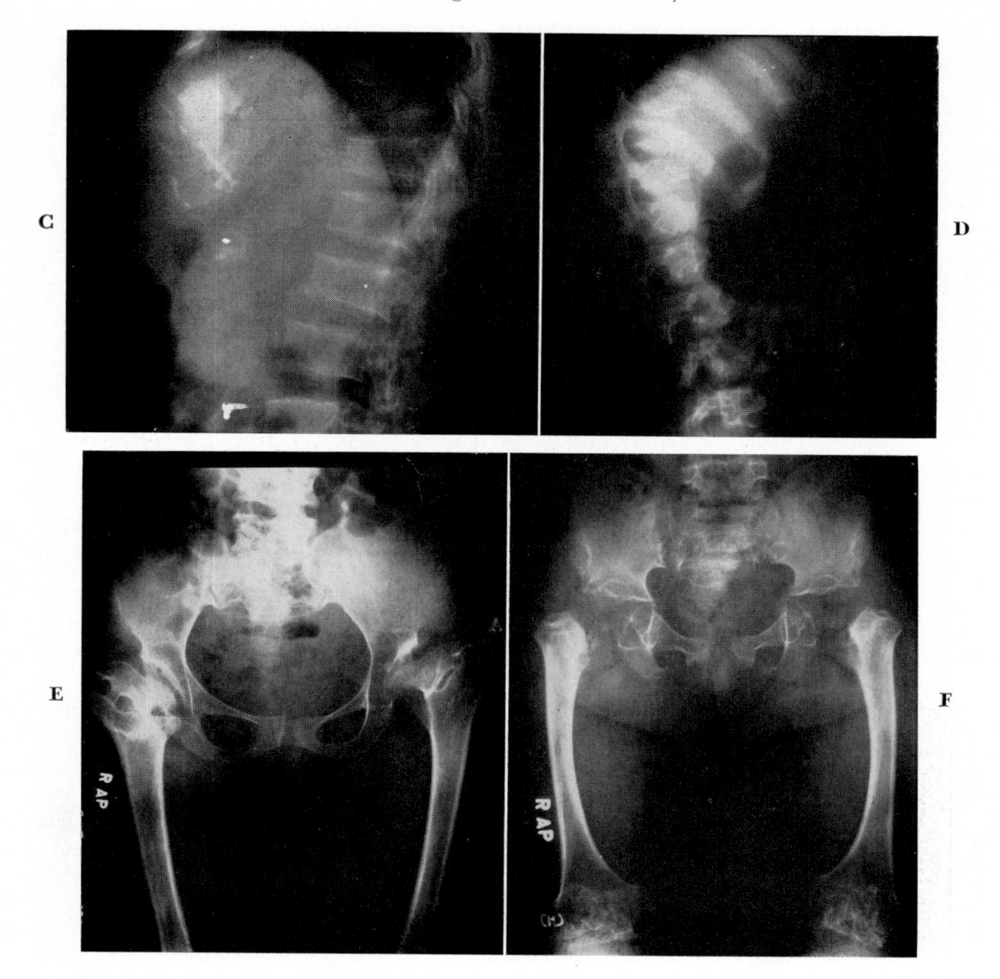

Fig. 10-15, cont'd. For legend see opposite page.

precocious osteoarthrosis occurs in other joints, particularly the hips, knees, and shoulders. Thus, spondyloepiphyseal dysplasia is a particularly appropriate designation. The radiographic changes in the spine are characteristic (Fig. 10-16). The posterior portion of the superior plate of the vertebral bodies, especially the lumbar ones, is "humped." Progressive degenerative changes occur in the same region. The late appearance superficially resembles that of the ochronotic spine (cf. Fig. 7-2). The process is, however, one of the vertebral body and not of the intervertebral disc as in alkaptonuria.

Multiple epiphyseal dysplasia.[218,230,247,274,291,338] One form, inherited as a dominant, is characterized by short stature, brachydactyly, and the development of precocious osteoarthrosis of the hips. The family described in Fig. 10-17 is of this type. Because of involvement of the distal tibial epiphysis, sloping of the tibial joint surface at the ankle is recognizable in the adult. Double patella consisting of a larger anterior part embracing a smaller posterior part

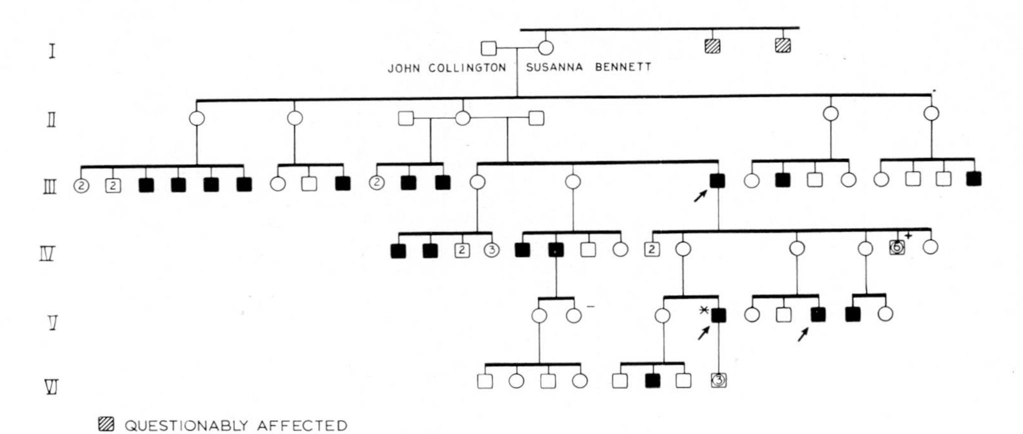

A

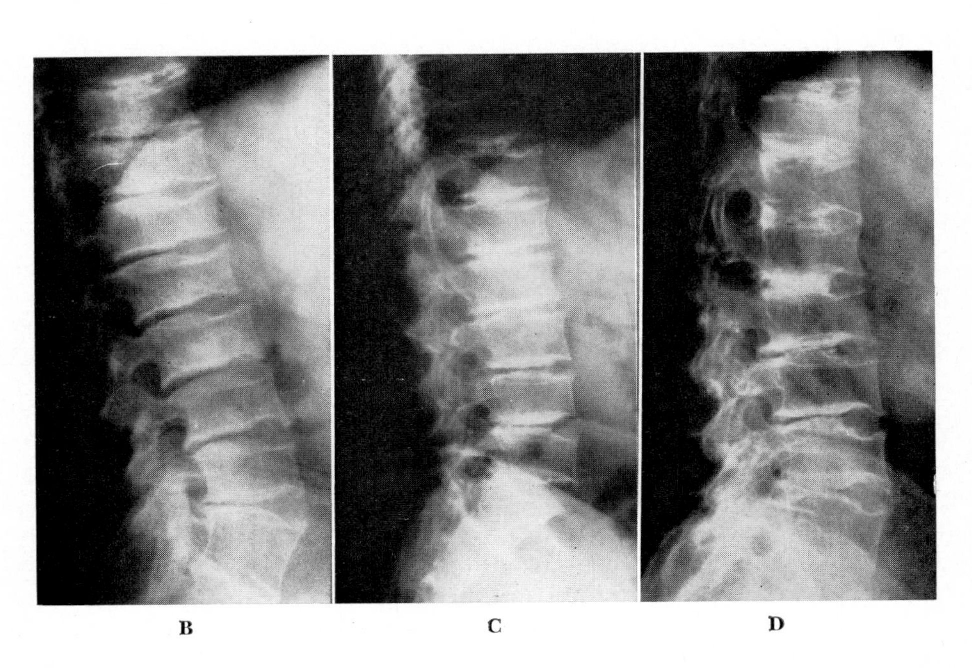

B C D

Fig. 10-16. X-linked spondyloepiphyseal dysplasia. **A,** Partially updated pedigree of family reported by Jacobsen.[255] Radiographic findings shown in **B** to **E. B** to **D,** Graded changes in the lumbar spine. Heaping up of the posterior portion of the superior vertebral plate is pathognomonic, **B.** Progressive degenerative changes are shown in **C** and **D.** At first glance the late changes resemble those of alkaptonuria (cf. Fig. 7-2). However, the changes are in the vertebral plates and not in the intervertebral discs as in alkaptonuria. **E,** Late degenerative "arthritis" of the hips. (Courtesy Dr. Leonard O. Langer, Jr., Minneapolis.)

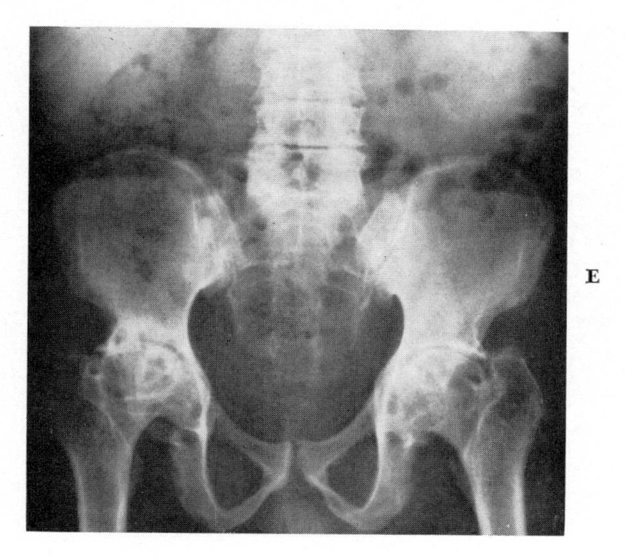

Fig. 10-16, cont'd. For legend see opposite page.

may be demonstrated by lateral radiographs of the knee.[253] Severely affected cases are often mistakenly diagnosed Morquio syndrome. The "cause" of severe precocious osteoarthritis of the hip sometimes is revealed by the discovery of typical changes of epiphyseal dysplasia in a prepubertal child of the patient. Heterogeneity undoubtedly exists in this category. For example, Elsbach's "micro-epiphysial dysplasia" involving mainly but not exclusively the hips, with dominant inheritance, is probably distinct. Chondrodystrophia calcificans congenita is a congenital form of multiple epiphyseal dysplasia.[216,277,304,305]

Physeal dysplasias

Achondroplasia. Achondroplasia is a designation that in the past was often assigned to a hodgepodge of entities. It has now, however, become a well-delineated entity.[290,294] The abnormality is already evident at birth and the diagnosis, suspected clinically, can be confirmed at that stage by the demonstration of characteristic radiologic findings in the spine and pelvis.

The skull and face are involved, with bulging of the head and "scooped-out" nose resulting from exaggerated saddling. The foramen magnum is compressed and small. These changes are the result of impaired development of the chondrocranium—the base of the skull—with unimpaired development of the membranous bones that constitute the calvarium. Internal hydrocephalus frequently results. There is suggestive evidence of true megencephaly in achondroplasia, as a nonskeletal effect of the achondroplasia gene. This factor aggravates the hydrocephalus because of disproportion between the base of the cranium and its contents. Intellect is, on the average, impaired in achondroplastics.

In infants with achondroplasia the spine shows excessive cartilage separating the ossification centers of the vertebrae. In addition, the interpeduncular spaces in the lumbar area, rather than widening caudally,[318] show caudad narrowing. Wedge lumbar vertebra with lumbar gibbus and serious neurologic prob-

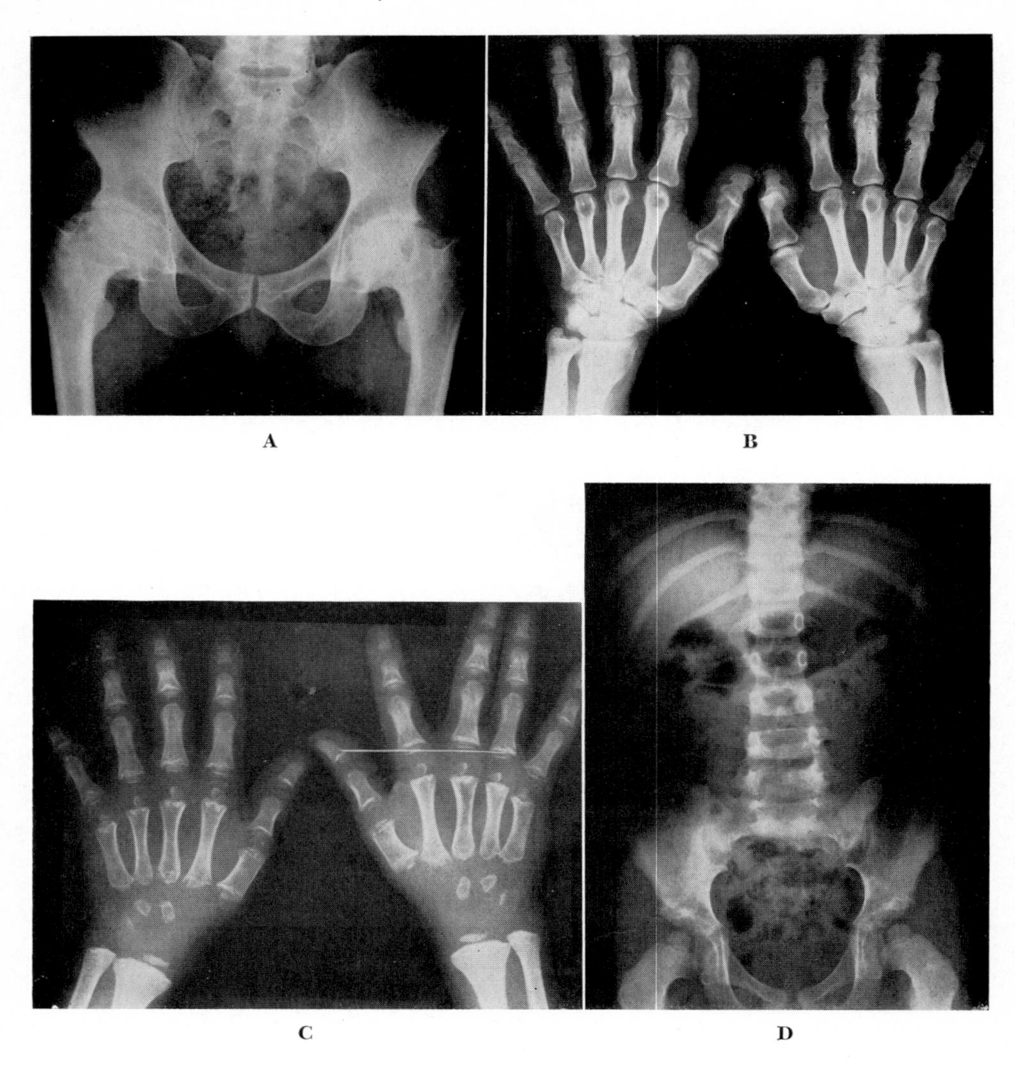

Fig. 10-17. Multiple epiphyseal dysplasia in father and son. The father, **A** and **B,** age 40 years, is moderately short of stature and has short fingers and severe osteoarthrosis of the hips. The son, **C** and **D,** age 9 years, shows the characteristic findings of multiple epiphyseal dysplasia, thus indicating the "cause" of the precocious osteoarthrosis in the father. His sister is also affected. Inheritance is autosomal dominant. The father's father, a brother, and several children of the brother are similarly affected.

lems, particularly paraplegia, develop in the second or third decades in some patients.[241,310,336,337]

In infancy the pelvis shows shortening of the iliac wings and particularly striking changes in the sacroiliac curve, which in achondroplasia is reduced to a small notch.

In the extremities the epiphyseal ossification centers are set into the metaphyseal ends of the bones, creating the circumflex sign or, at an earlier stage, a ball-and-socket appearance. The fingers are pudgy. In the characteristic trident hand *(main en trident)* the fingers cannot be apposed along their entire length because of relatively excessive thickness of the proximal phalangeal portions.

Classic achondroplasia is an autosomal dominant. About seven eighths of cases are new mutations. Reproductive fitness is considerably reduced because of the obstetric problems created by the small pelvis.

Enchondromatosis. Enchondromatosis (Ollier's disease) is manifested by massive proliferation of cartilage in the physeal areas of the extremities.[231,302,307] This condition is included here for comparison with the others. No evidence of a genetic basis has been discovered. Specifically, no familial cases are known and no chromosomal abnormality has been demonstrated. *Maffucci's syndrome*[229] is enchondromatosis with hemangiomata. Brain tumor and malignant tumors of other organs occur rather frequently in patients with Maffucci's syndrome. This condition should not be confused with the *Klippel-Trenaunay-Weber syndrome,*[219,281] in which hemangiomata are associated with asymmetric overgrowth of bones and related soft tissues.

Metaphyseal dysostosis. At least four forms of this disorder are recognized: (1) Jansen type, (2) Schmid type, (3) Spahr type, and (4) cartilage-hair hypoplasia.

The rare *Jansen type* is manifested by drastic changes in the metaphyses.[249] Only about half a dozen cases have been described, and no instance of multiple affected family members is known. Whether genetic or not and—if genetic—whether chromosomal aberration, new dominant mutation, or recessive are unanswered questions.

The *Schmid type of metaphyseal dysostosis,* inherited as an autosomal dominant, has often been confused with achondroplasia.[325] However, the skull is not affected, and the spine and pelvis do not show the changes characteristic of achondroplasia. Affected women have children with little difficulty.[325] The radiologic changes consist particularly of irregularity, with sclerosis and rarefaction in the metaphyseal portions of the long bones.[235,326] Some flaring of the metaphyseal margins occurs. Because of asymmetric involvement at the distal end of the femur with more striking change medially, bowlegs are a frequent problem prompting orthopedic attention. No metabolic defect has been identified. Although curative effects of vitamin D in high dosage have been claimed,[242,299] it seems clear that healing of the radiologically demonstrated changes with immobilization[236] was responsible for the impressions of benefit from vitamin D.

Spahr and Spahr-Hartmann[323] described the *Spahr type,* a form of metaphyseal dysostosis that apparently is autosomal recessive (Fig. 10-20) but otherwise has features similar to the Schmid type.

Cartilage-hair hypoplasia (CHH) is characterized by radiologic changes rather similar to those of the Schmid type, with the following differences: the changes at the knees are more symmetric, and bowlegs rarely a problem. Deformity at the ankle results from excessive length of the distal fibula relative to the tibia. (The fibula is often relatively long in achondroplasia but the projection is at the proximal end.) The fingers are short and the terminal phalanges are particularly short so that the fingernails are relatively broad. Sharply distinguishing this entity are recessive inheritance and the occurrence of fine hair as an integral feature. The caliber of the hair can be shown by micrometry to be abnormally

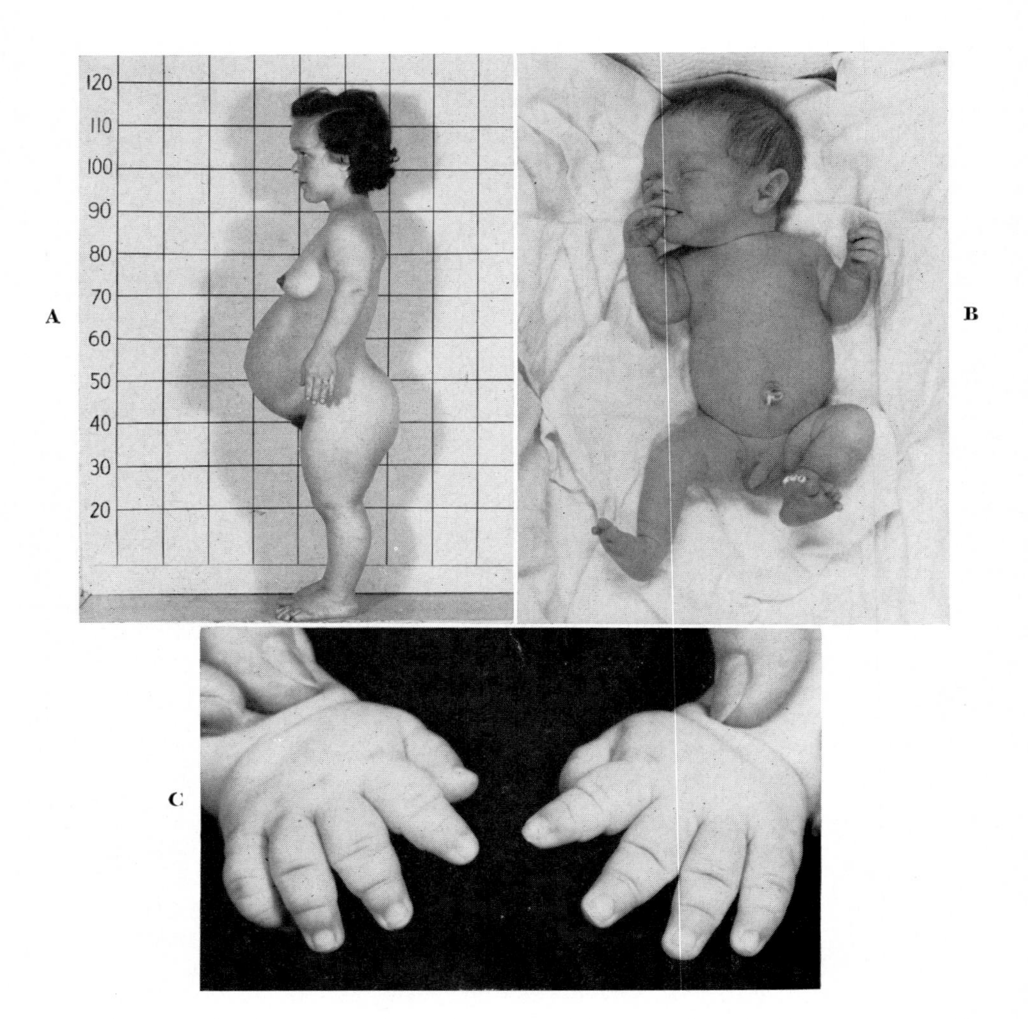

Fig. 10-18. Achondroplasia in mother and in two of three children. **A,** Mother during third pregnancy. Unlike the patients in pseudo-achondroplastic spondyloepiphyseal dysplasia, the bridge of the nose is scooped out and the forehead is bulging. **B,** Newborn achondroplastic son. **C,** Trident hands in 3-year-old daughter. The fingers when opposed do not touch in their entire length. **D,** 3-year-old achondroplastic daughter. **E,** X-ray film of newborn achondroplastic child showing characteristic changes: separation of vertebral ossification centers by excessive cartilage, caudad narrowing of the interpeduncular spaces in the lumbar spine, and small pelvic bones with notchlike sacroiliac groove, in addition to the shortening of the bones of the extremities. **F,** By way of contrast with **E,** the x-ray film of the unaffected sib, taken in the newborn period, is shown. **G,** The pedigree. The mother shown in **A** is in the second generation. Each of her three children, all delivered by Cesarean section, was fathered by a different man. Achondroplasia has not been confirmed in the mother of the mother (I-2). (From McKusick, V. A., and colleagues: Medical genetics 1958-1960, St. Louis, 1961, The C. V. Mosby Co.)

small. Megacolon, a disorder of intestinal absorption suggesting celiac disease, and death from chickenpox may be integral parts of the disorder. No chemical or metabolic defect has yet been identified.

Cartilage-hair hypoplasia was first discovered in an inbred group, the Old Order Amish, living in various parts of the United States and Ontario.[286] However, it has been noted in persons of other national origins. CHH is an autosomal recessive.

Metaphyseal dysplasias

Hypophosphatasia. Hypophosphatasia[234,279,308] is one of the few hereditary generalized disorders of the osseous skeleton in which an enzyme defect has been identified. A ricketslike clinical picture and craniostenosis are leading features. Inheritance is autosomal recessive. The diagnosis is suspected on the basis of

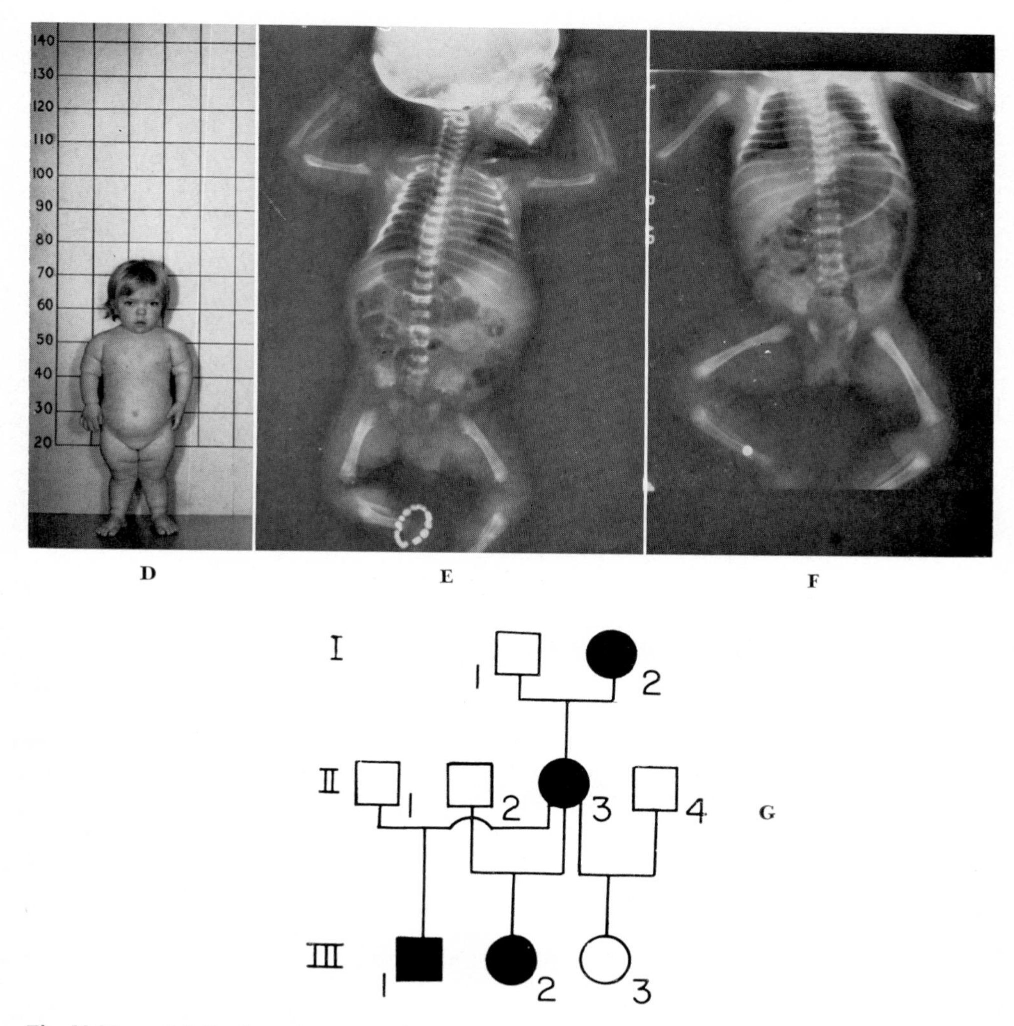

Fig. 10-18, cont'd. For legend see opposite page.

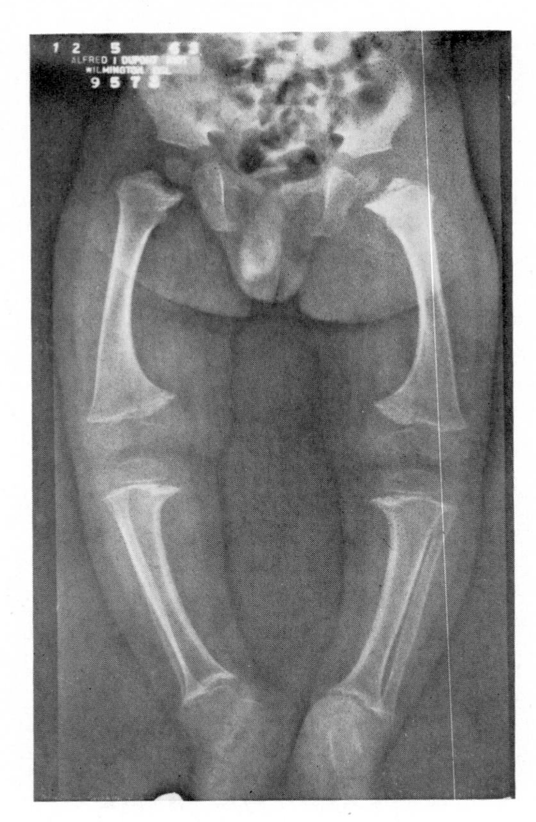

Fig. 10-19. Metaphyseal dysostosis, Schmid type, in 6-year-old boy. Marked changes are seen at both ends of the femora, tibiae, and fibulae. The epiphyseal ossification centers are well formed, however. Asymmetric wedgelike medial involvement of the distal femur results in genu varum. (Courtesy Dr. G. Dean MacEwen, Wilmington, Del.; from McKusick, V. A., Eldridge, R., Hostetler, J. A., Ruangwit, U., and Egeland, J. A.: Bull. Hopkins Hosp. **116:**285, 1965.)

characteristic radiologic changes and is confirmed by demonstration of low alkaline phosphatase in the serum. The leukocytes lack alkaline phosphatase activity,[221] and phosphorylethanolamine is excreted in the urine in excess. Heterozygotes, e.g. parents of affected children, demonstrate reduced white cell alkaline phosphatase. Fraser[246] recognized the following four types depending on the age of onset and severity of manifestations: (1) present at birth or before the age of 6 months, (2) onset in children after 6 months of age, (3) onset in adulthood,[220,223] and (4) an atypical group. The genetic relationship of these is uncertain. A form with dominant inheritance was suggested by Silverman.[317]

Osteopetrosis. Osteopetrosis (likewise called marble bones, osteosclerosis fragilis generalisata, and Albers-Schönberg's* disease) occurs in at least two forms[214,]

---

*Albers-Schönberg[214] was one man; this is not a syndrome named for two persons, like the Ehlers-Danlos syndrome or the Grönblad-Strandberg syndrome. Care should be taken not to confuse osteopetrosis with osteopoikilosis, which was also first described in a definitive manner by Albers-Schönberg; some writers have evidenced this confusion.

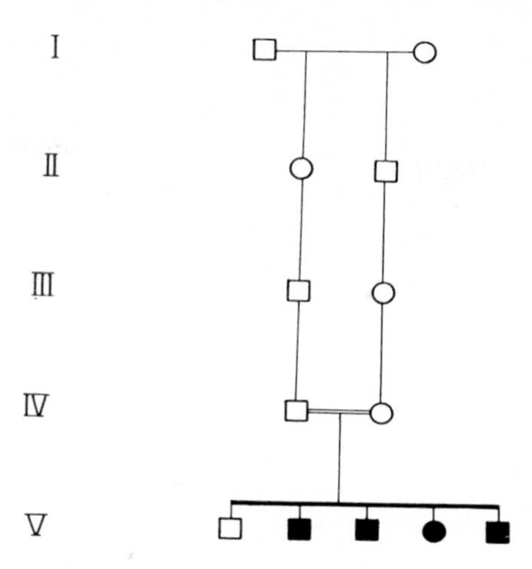

Fig. 10-20. Pedigree of metaphyseal dysostosis, Spahr type, indicating autosomal recessive inheritance. (After Spahr and Spahr-Hartmann[323]; from McKusick, V. A., Eldridge, R., Hostetler, J. A., Ruangwit, U., and Egeland, J. A.: Bull. Hopkins Hosp. **116:**285, 1965.)

[215,260,278,343]: (1) an autosomal recessive form,[280,333] which is also called the malignant form because of early death, and (2) a relatively benign, autosomal dominant form.[248,251,287] In addition, osteosclerosis often termed osteopetrosis is a feature of several entities, including pycnodysostosis, van Buchem's disease (see below), and Engelmann's disease.[240,273,275,292,319]

The recessive, or malignant, form appears very early in life, like osteogenesis imperfecta may be detected *in utero,* involves the entire skeleton, and may result in such encroachment on the hematopoietic space of the bone marrow that pancytopenia is a leading clinical feature.[228,232,262,263,272,300,301] A disorder like that in man has been observed in the rabbit[298] and in domestic fowl.[269]

The main clinical features of the autosomal dominant form of osteopetrosis are fractures and osteomyelitis, especially of the mandible. The bones show dramatic changes radiologically and pathologically. The vertebral bodies have a characteristic "sandwich" appearance because of excessive sclerosis in upper and lower plates with intervening less dense area. Round bones of the extremities have a "bone-within-bone" appearance. The bones are described by some as so hard as to turn the edge of a steel chisel, and by others are claimed to be more like chalk. Usually they are excessively brittle and susceptible to spontaneous fracture. The original patient of Albers-Schönberg[214] was 26 years old and is said to have been living ten years later for re-examination by Reiche. Alexander's patient[215] was 43 years old. The patient illustrated in Fig. 10-22 died at age 45 years of a cause indirectly related to his skeletal disease.

The nail-patella syndrome. Arthro-onycho-dysplasia, the nail-patella syndrome, is manifested by hypoplastic or absent fingernails and patellae, hornlike osseous posterior projections of the ilium ("iliac horns"), and anomaly of the elbows—usually hypoplasia of the head of the radius with dorsal dislocation and limitation of motion.[238,314,331,335,340] Renal abnormality leading to uremia may be an integral feature, having been observed clinically in a number of instances,[309] but has not been well delineated. Inheritance is autosomal dominant. The nail-patella syndrome enjoys the distinction of being caused by one of the few autosomal genes for which a genetic linkage has been identified. The nail-patella locus is on the same chromosome pair as the ABO blood group locus, from which it is separated by about ten recombination units. Which specific pair of autosomes carries these two loci is, however, unknown. The Ellis-van Creveld syndrome (p. 464) is another disorder in which skeletal and ectodermal abnormalities are associated.

Craniometaphyseal dysplasia. Pyle's disease, as this is called, is manifested by changes in the cranial and facial bones leading to characteristic facies[296] and

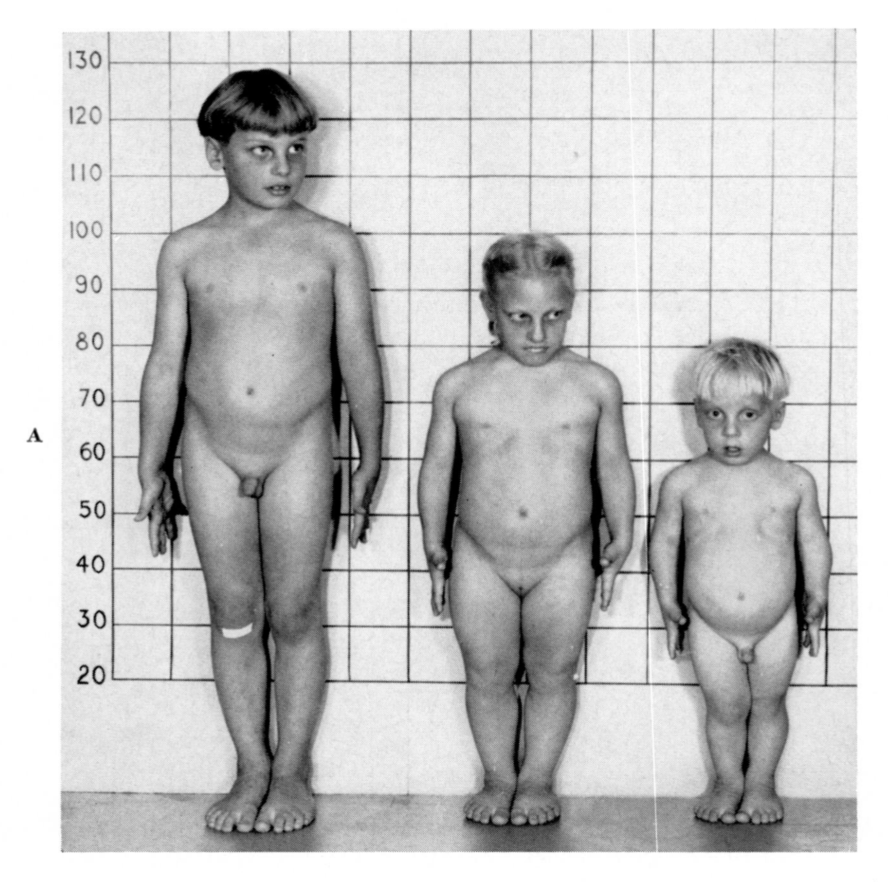

Fig. 10-21. Cartilage-hair hypoplasia (CHH). **A,** Three Amish children: (left-to-right) 7-year-old unaffected boy; 9-year-old affected girl; 5-year-old affected boy. The affected children have Harrison grooves of the chest resembling those of rickets and have thin hair which is lighter in color than that of unaffected sibs. **B,** X-ray changes in 2-year-old child with CHH. **C** and **D,** In rib biopsies, cartilage hypoplasia in a 5-year-old affected child, **D,** is contrasted with the normal findings in a 5-year-old child with congenital heart disease. **E,** Microscopic appearance of hair in six sibs ranging in age from 15 years (at the top) to 3 years (at the bottom). A hair from each of the three sibs in **A** is shown (third, fourth, and fifth from the top). Both small caliber of the hair and deficiency of pigment in the affected 9- and 5-year-old patients are demonstrated. **F,** Hair measurements of a group of CHH cases and their unaffected parents and sibs. (**A** to **E** from McKusick, V. A., Eldridge, R., Hostetler, J. A., and Egeland, J. A.: Trans. Ass. Amer. Phys. **77:**151, 1964; **F** from McKusick, V. A., Eldridge, R., Hostetler, J. A., Ruangwit, U., and Egeland, J. A.: Bull. Hopkins Hosp. **116:**285, 1965.)

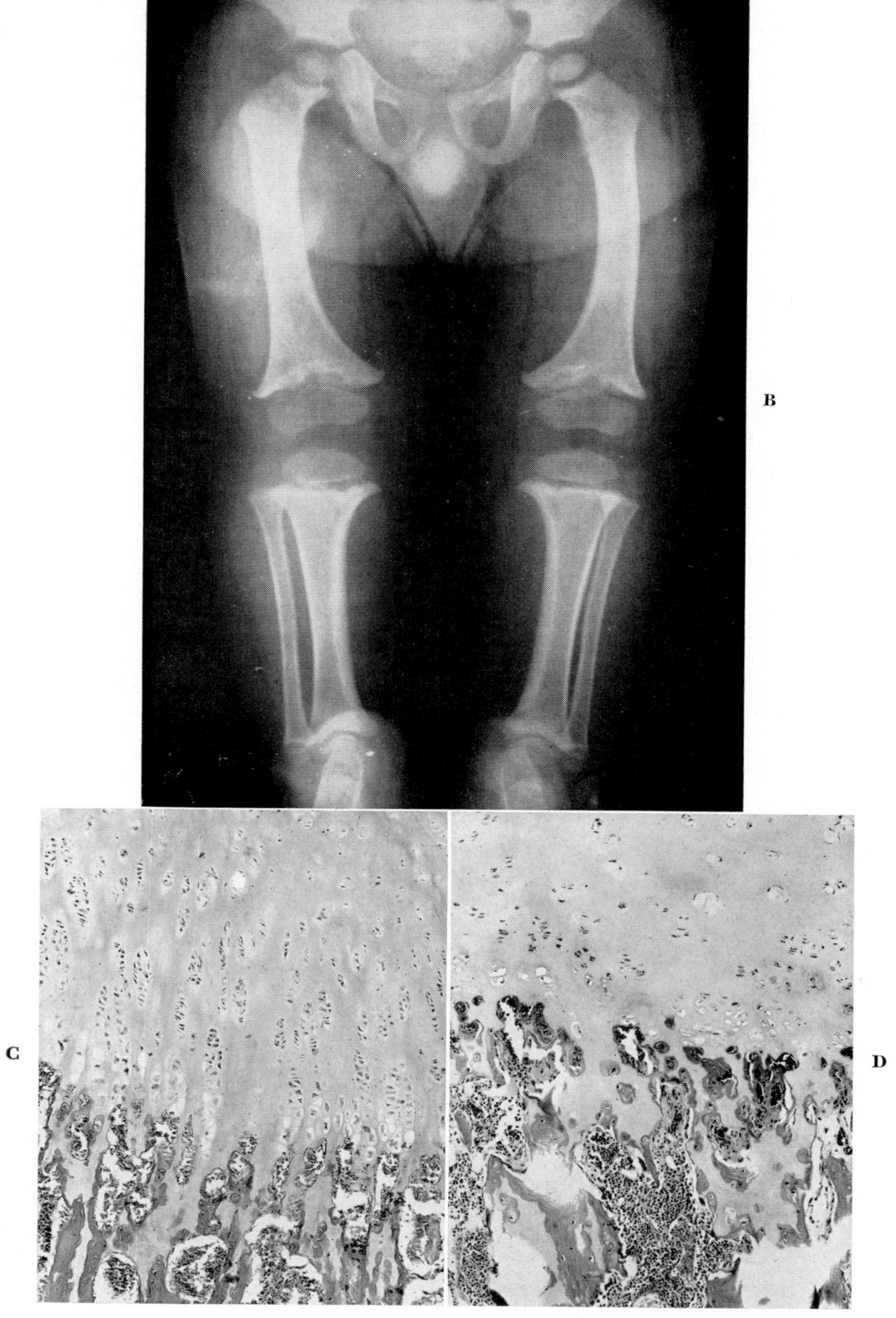

Fig. 10-21, cont'd. For legend see opposite page.

Continued.

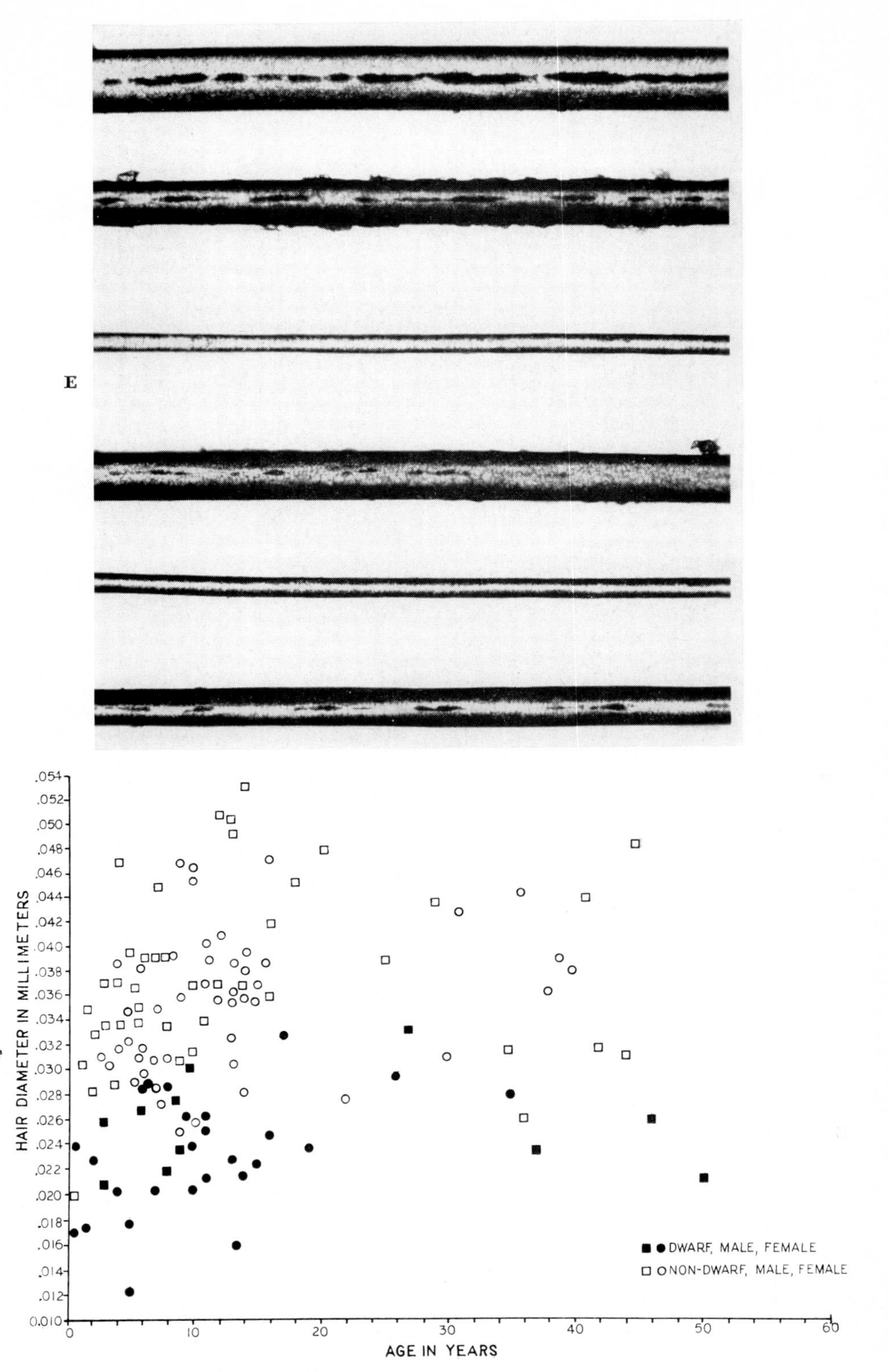

Fig. 10-21, cont'd. For legend see p. 446.

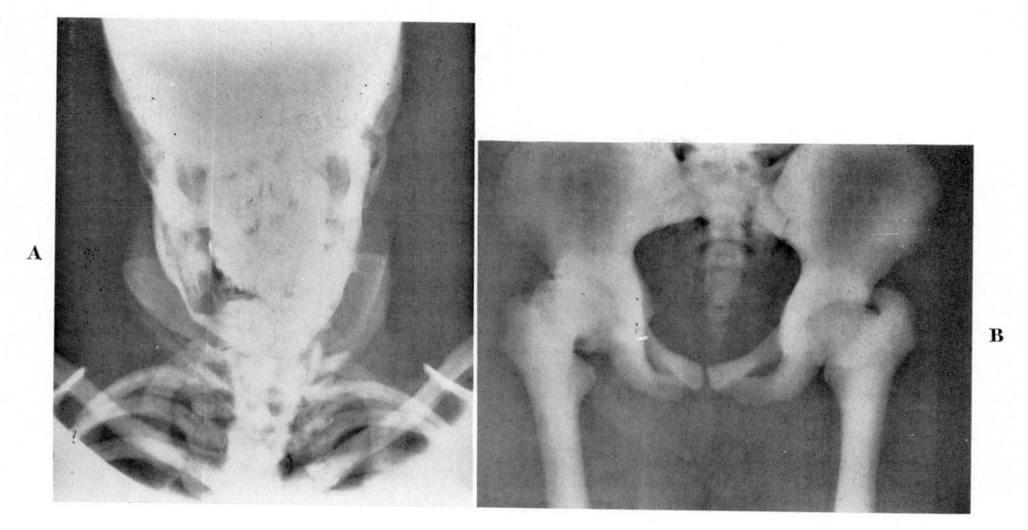

Fig 10-22. Osteopetrosis, "benign" autosomal dominant type. In 1922 the late Dr. Ralph K. Ghormley[248] described "a case of congenital osteosclerosis" in a boy then 9 years old. The father and uncle were similarly affected. The uncle, who subsequently died in his seventies, had much trouble with osteomyelitis of the jaw. The father had a traumatic fracture. The proband sustained fractures whenever he engaged in rough sports. At age 32 he began to have trouble with osteomyelitis of the jaw and progressive stiffening of the hips. Despite his physical handicaps he became an international authority in the field of dielectrics. At the age of 45 years he developed symptoms of a temporal lobe abscess and died from this two days later. The abscess was presumably metastatic from the mandibular infection. **A,** Note the marked sclerotic change in all bones and the surgical defect in the mandible. **B,** Secondary osteoarthrosis of the hips is also demonstrated.

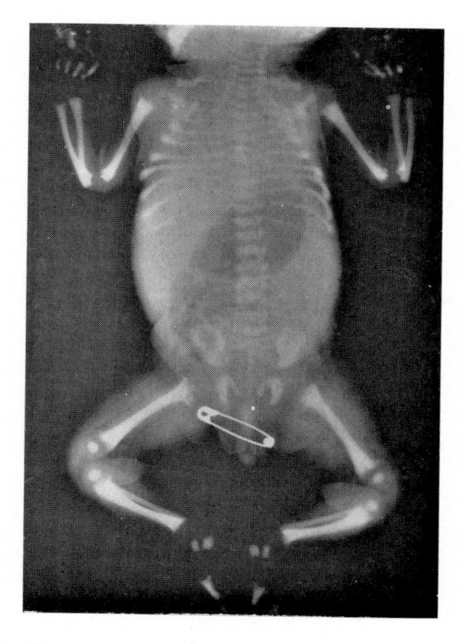

Fig. 10-23. Osteopetrosis, "malignant" autosomal recessive type.

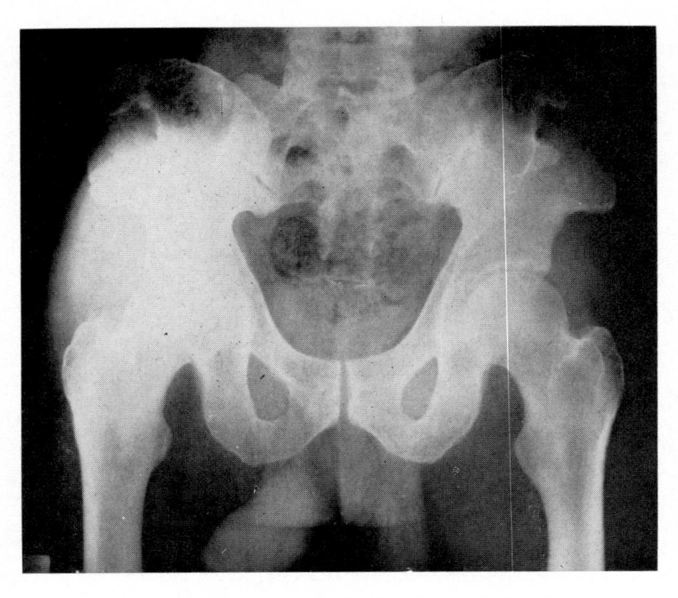

Fig. 10-24. Posterior iliac horns in a man with typical nail-patella syndrome.

enlargement of the metaphyses of the bones of the extremities in the form of an Erlenmeyer flask.[217,265,303,311,312] The disorder is autosomal recessive.

Cleidocranial dysostosis.[245,254,257] In this disorder, development is defective in the skull, which early shows multiple Wormian bones and delay in the closure of sutures, and in the clavicles, which are hypoplastic or absent. Spina bifida occulta in the lower cervical and upper thoracic spine and separation of the symphysis pubis are also frequent. The sacroiliac joints are usually wide, and changes occur in the epiphyses of the phalanges. The acetabulum may be hypoplastic, leading to dislocation of the hip.

Pycnodysostosis. Pycnodysostosis[282,289,316] is another disorder in which both the cranium and other parts of the skeleton are involved. As in cleidocranial dysostosis (with which pycnodysostosis was often confused in the past), multiple Wormian bones and delayed closure of the cranial sutures are features. The ramus of the mandible is hypoplastic so that this bone is essentially straight and the jaw receding. The bones, e.g. ribs and appendicular skeleton, show increased density. As in osteopetrosis, the bones are more fragile than normal and fractures are frequent. Acro-osteolysis (actually hypoplasia) of the terminal phalanges is a characteristic feature that is manifested clinically by short ends of the fingers. Inheritance is autosomal recessive. As stated in Chapter 6, Henri de Toulouse-Lautrec may have suffered from this condition (Fig. 10-28). In addition to a mistaken diagnosis of cleidocranial dysostosis and of osteopetrosis,[313,332] one case was described as a *forme fruste* of gargoylism.[321]

Multiple exostoses. Diaphyseal aclasis is a disorder manifested by cartilaginous excresences near the ends of the diaphyses of bones of the extremities.[256,258,266,327] The ribs and scapulae may also be affected but the skull is not involved. Deformity of the legs, of the arms (resembling Madelung deformity), and of the

Text continued on page 464.

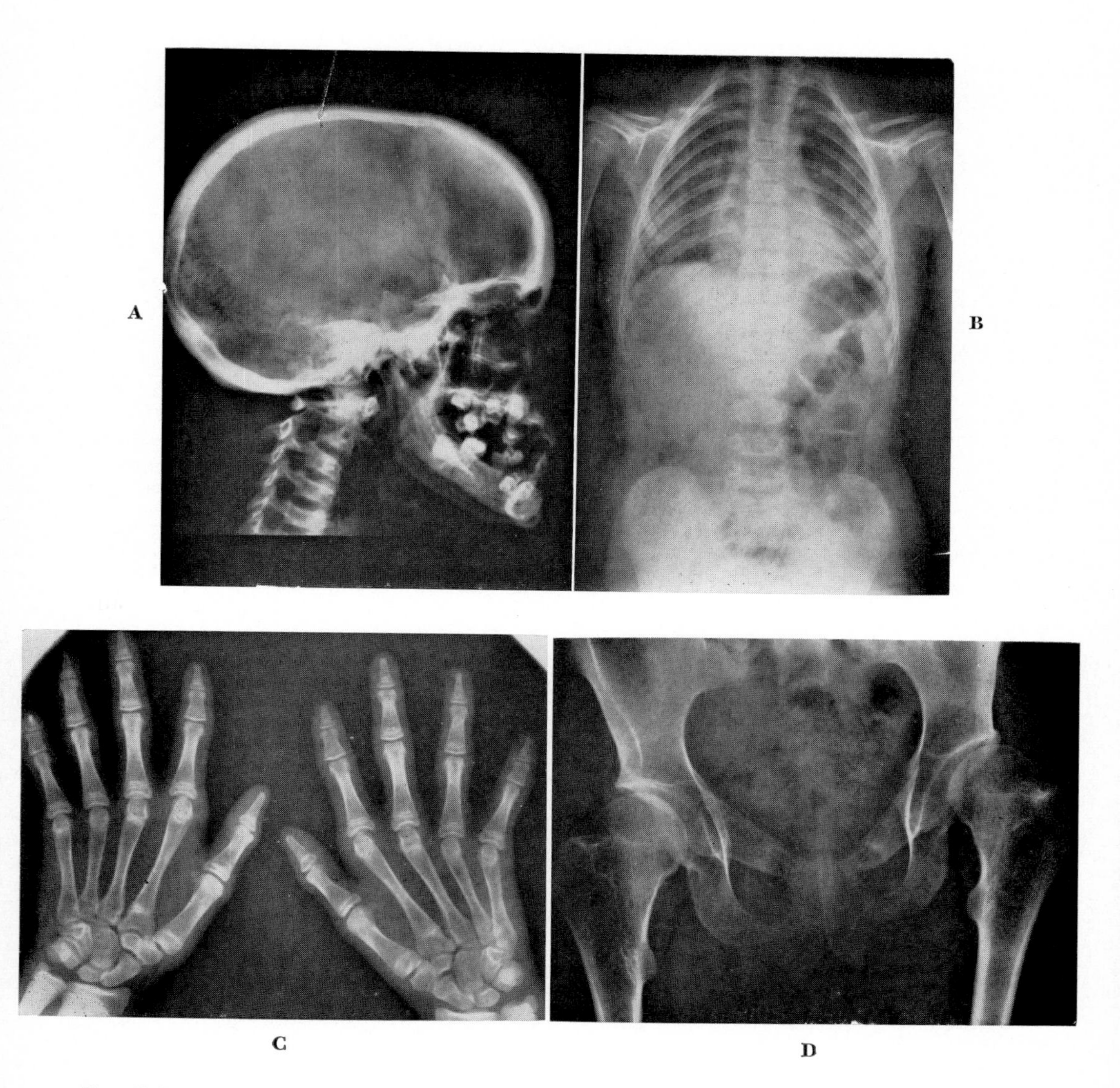

Fig. 10-25. Cleidocranial dysostosis has been observed in many members of at least three generations. **A,** Wide coronal sutures and multiple occipital Wormian bones are demonstrated in K. P., age 25 years. **B,** Hypoplasia of the clavicles, which are in two parts, is evident in D. S., age 7. Some affected members of the family have a severe anomaly of the lower cervical and upper thoracic spine. **C,** Note short middle phalanges in the second and fifth fingers and tapered terminal phalanges in N. S., age 19. **D,** Note the hypoplasia of the pubis and ischium, with separation at the pubic symphysis, in R. S., age 17. The acetabula, especially the left, are shallow. Dislocation of the hip has occurred in several affected members of the family.

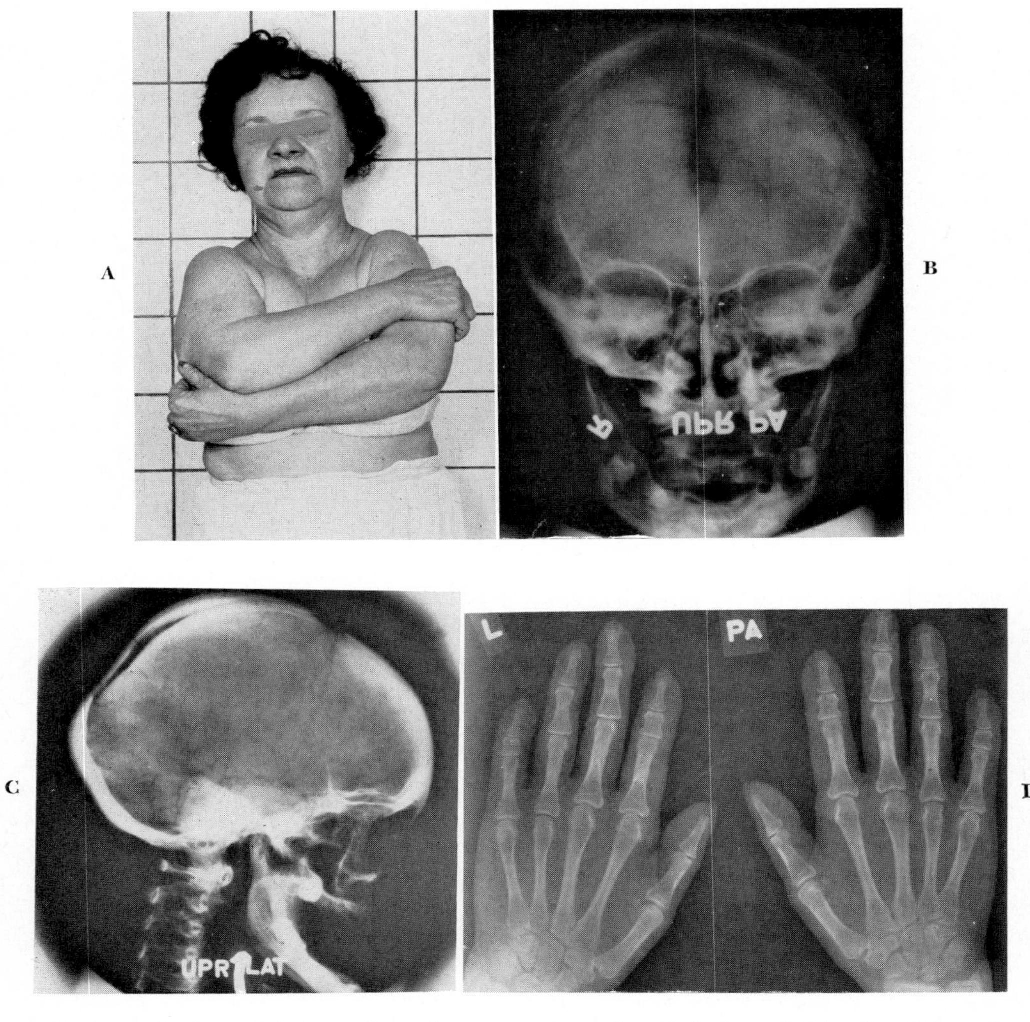

Fig. 10-26. Cleidocranial dysostosis in four generations of a kindred studied by Dr. Raymond Pearl and his colleagues in 1929 (unpublished). Demonstrated here are findings in E. S. (1058205) at the age of 58 years. **A,** Rather prominent forehead and ease of adduction of shoulders are shown. **B** and **C,** Note wide sutures and occipital Wormian bones. She is almost edentulous. **D,** Short second and fifth middle phalanges are shown, as in Fig. 10-25*C*. The mother of this woman, Pearl's proband, was affected, and she has an affected son and grandson. Affected members of this kindred are short of stature. The two members studied most extensively, both females, have adult heights of 59 and 56½ inches.

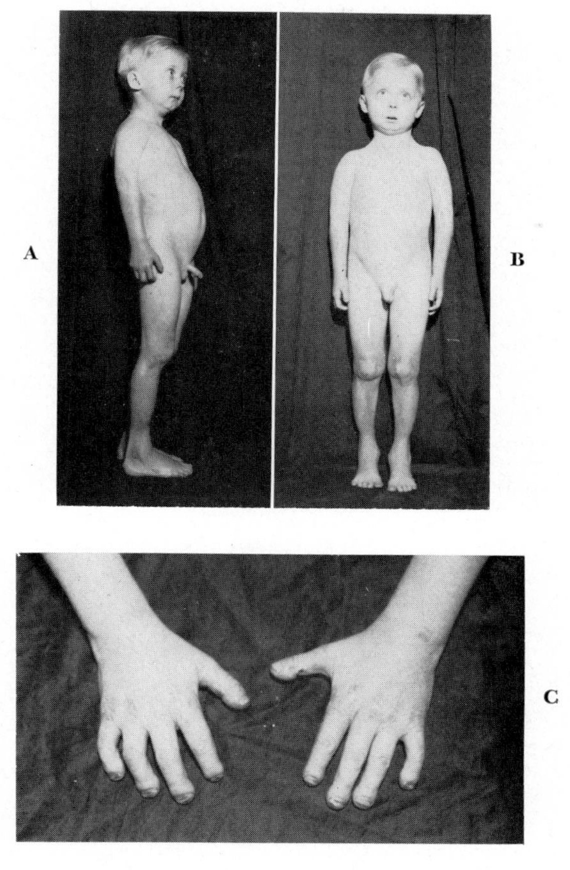

Fig. 10-27. Pycnodysostosis. M. F. (A19633) had all the features of this condition. His appearance was unusual, particularly because of prominent forehead, receding chin, short stature, narrow shoulders, stubby clubbed-appearing terminal phalanges, and mottled rough skin over the chest and back down to the rib margin and over the legs and hands. X-ray films showed open cranial sutures with Wormian bones, increased bone density with longitudinal cortical streaks in the bones of the extremities, and areas of radiolucency in the proximal ends of the humeri, as well as some other bones. The outer end of the left clavicle and the distal phalanges of the fingers and toes showed fragmentation with some calcification in the soft tissues. **A** and **B,** General appearance, age 4¾ years. **C,** Hands. The terminal phalanges are clubbed and stubby with a short, spoonlike fingernail. **D** and **E,** The distal phalanges of all digits show fragmentation of the bone and soft tissue calcification. **F** and **G,** The skull shows widely open sutures and mosaics of multiple Wormian bones. **H,** The bones of the arms show increased density with longitudinal cortical streaking and osteolytic lesions, e.g. at the proximal metaphysis of the humeri. (From McKusick, V. A., and colleagues: J. Chronic Dis. **17**:1077, 1964.)

Continued.

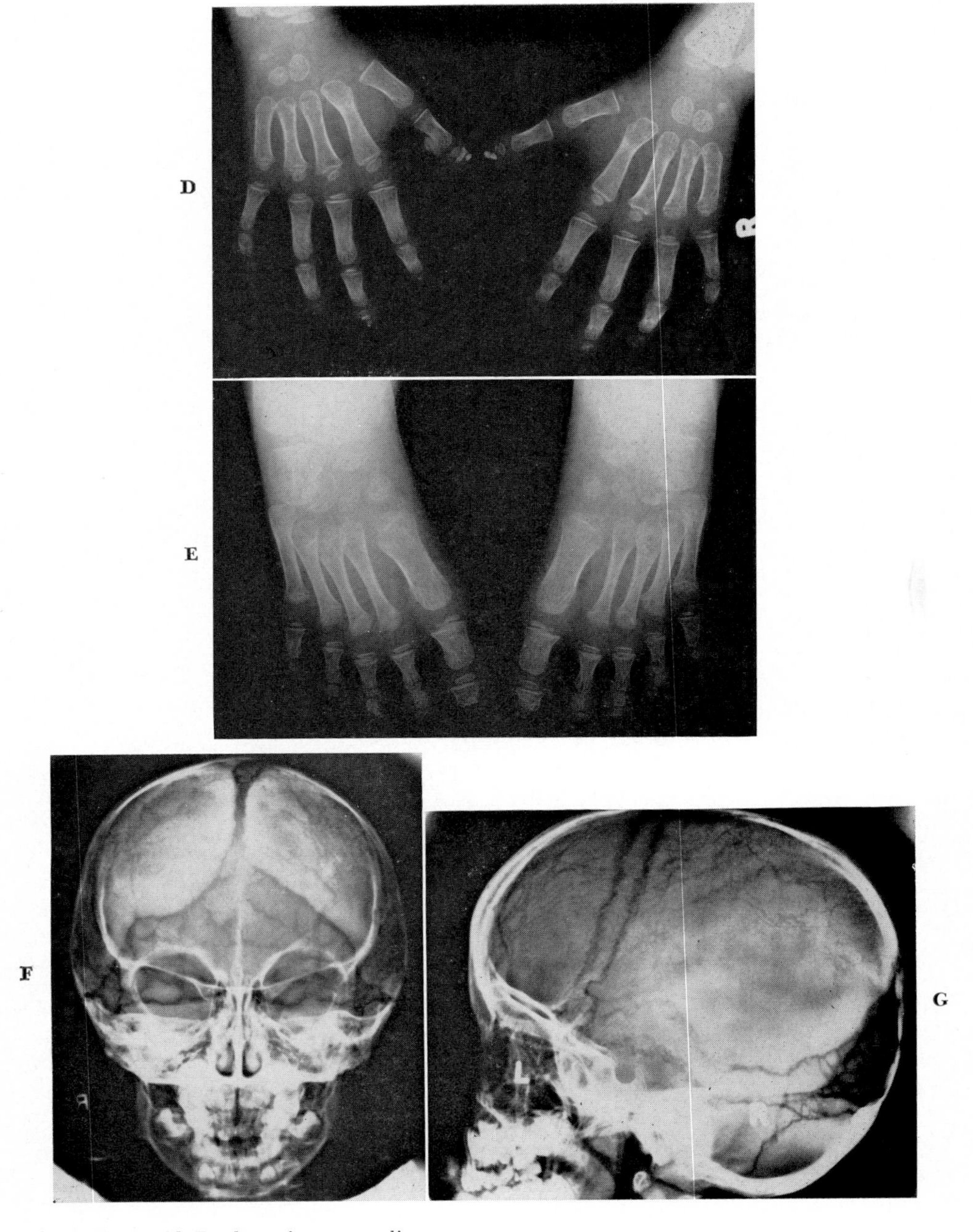

Fig. 10-27, cont'd. For legend see preceding page.

H

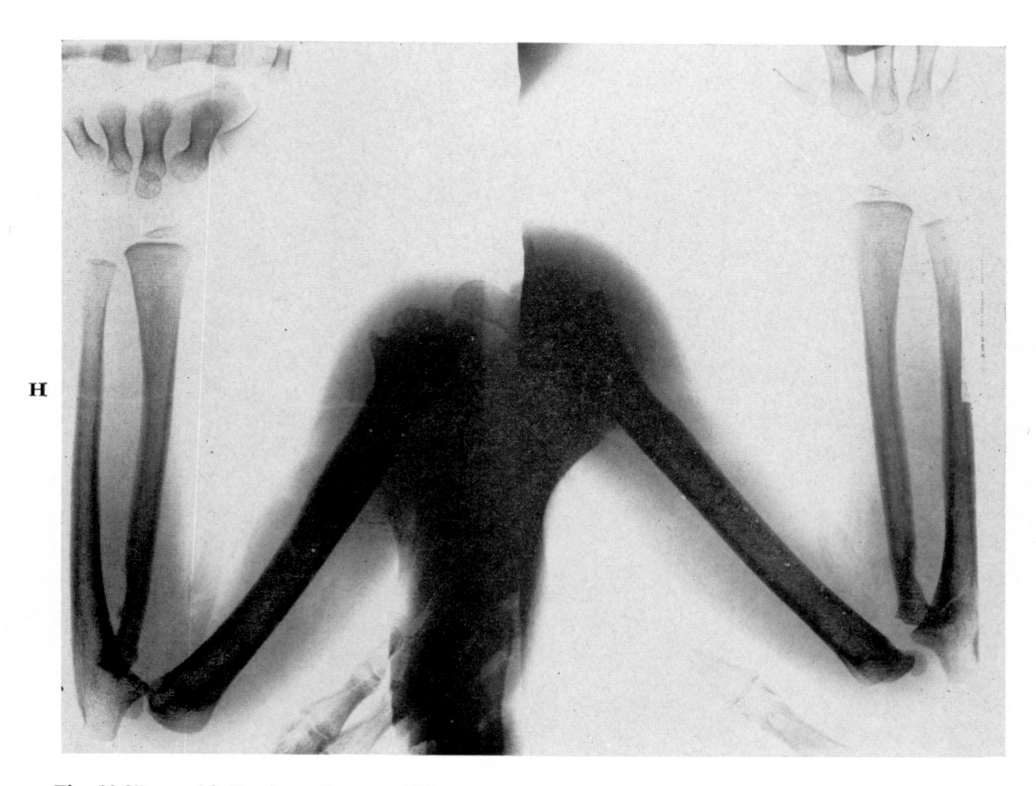

Fig. 10-27, cont'd. For legend see p. 453.

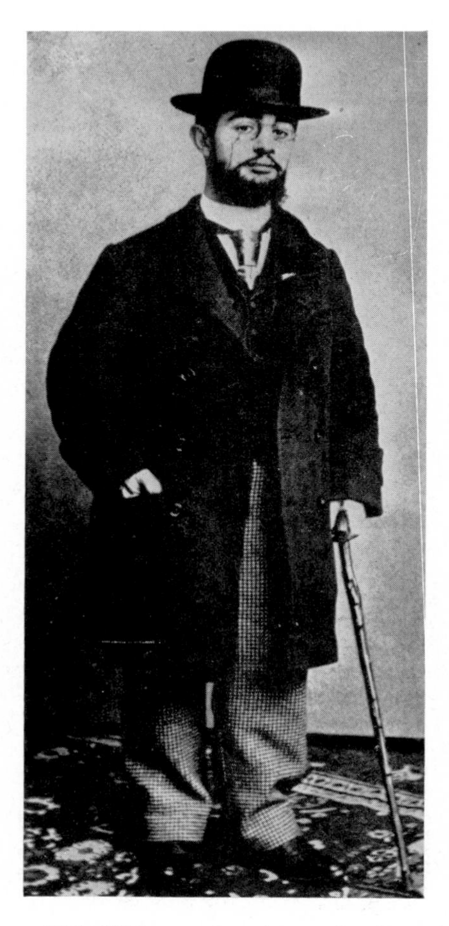

Fig. 10-28. Toulouse-Lautrec (1864-1901) was thought previously to have had osteogenesis imperfecta (p. 261). On review of the evidence in the light of the delineation of the "new" skeletal dysplasia, pycnodysostosis, Maroteaux and Lamy[290a] concluded that this was the condition from which he suffered. Parental consanguinity, fragility of bones leading to fractures with minor trauma, a receding chin and possible open fontanelles, which prompted the artist to wear a hat most of the time, are features pointed out as suggesting pycnodysostosis.

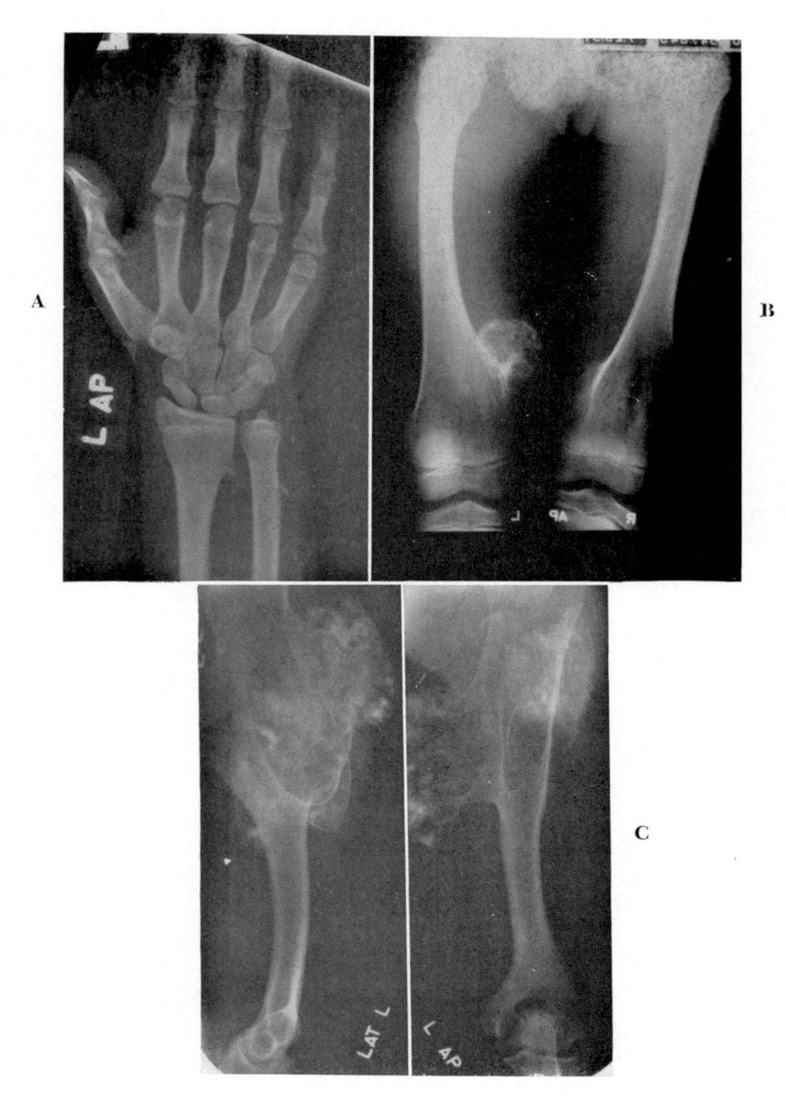

Fig. 10-29. Multiple exostoses. **A,** Small exostoses in 16-year-old girl whose father also has multiple exostoses. **B,** Exostoses of the femur in a 10-year-old boy. That on the right has been partially removed. **C,** Two views of enormous exostoses of left humerus in 40-year-old man.

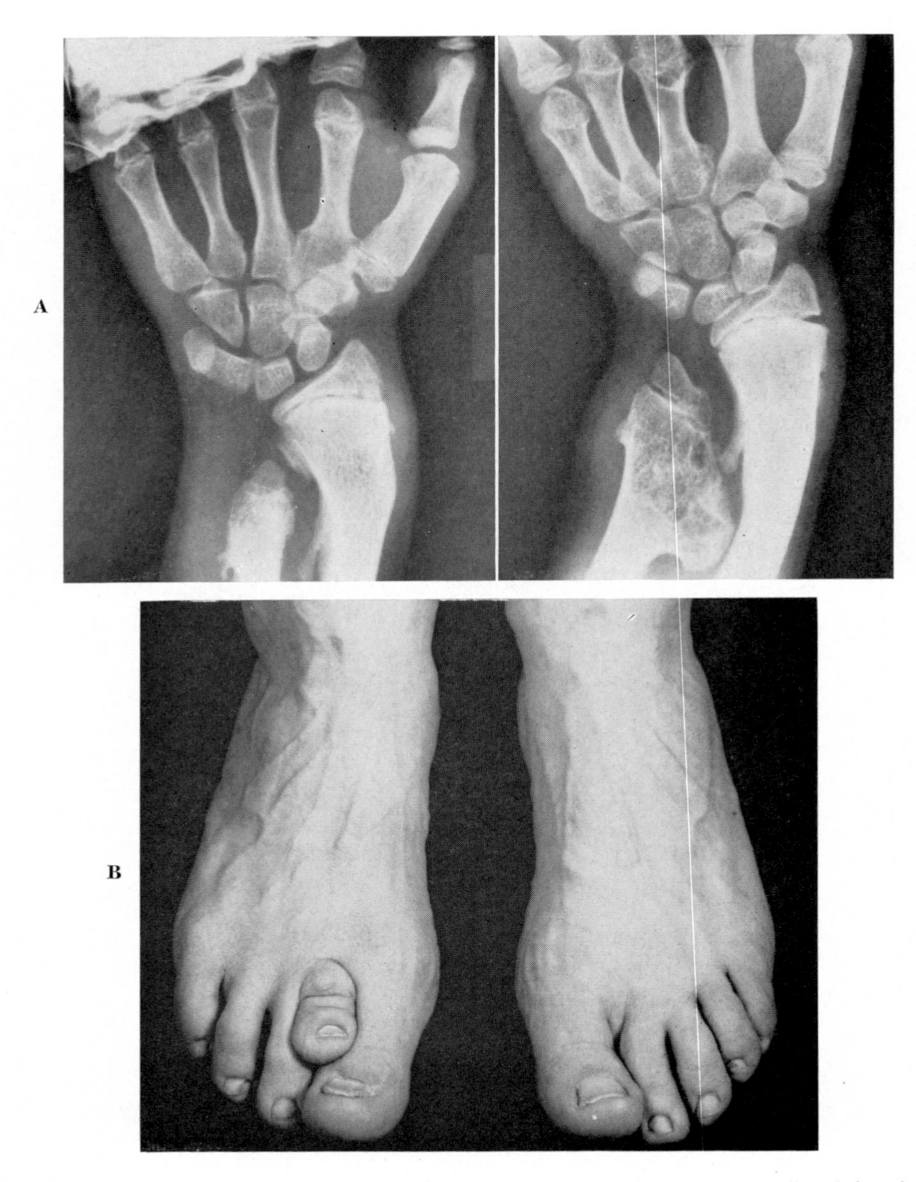

Fig. 10-30. Deformity of extremities from multiple exostoses. **A,** Madelung-like deformity of forearm. **B** and **C,** Short second metatarsal on right. **D,** Short fourth metacarpal.

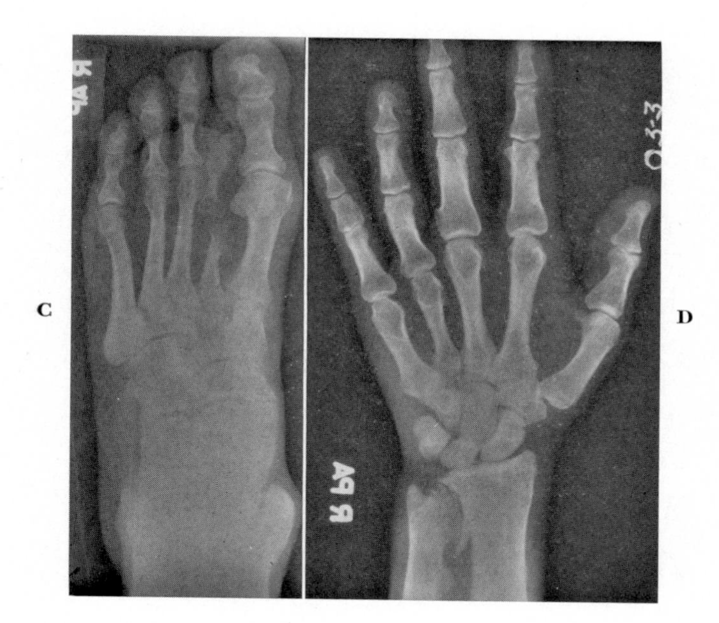

Fig. 10-30, cont'd. For legend see opposite page.

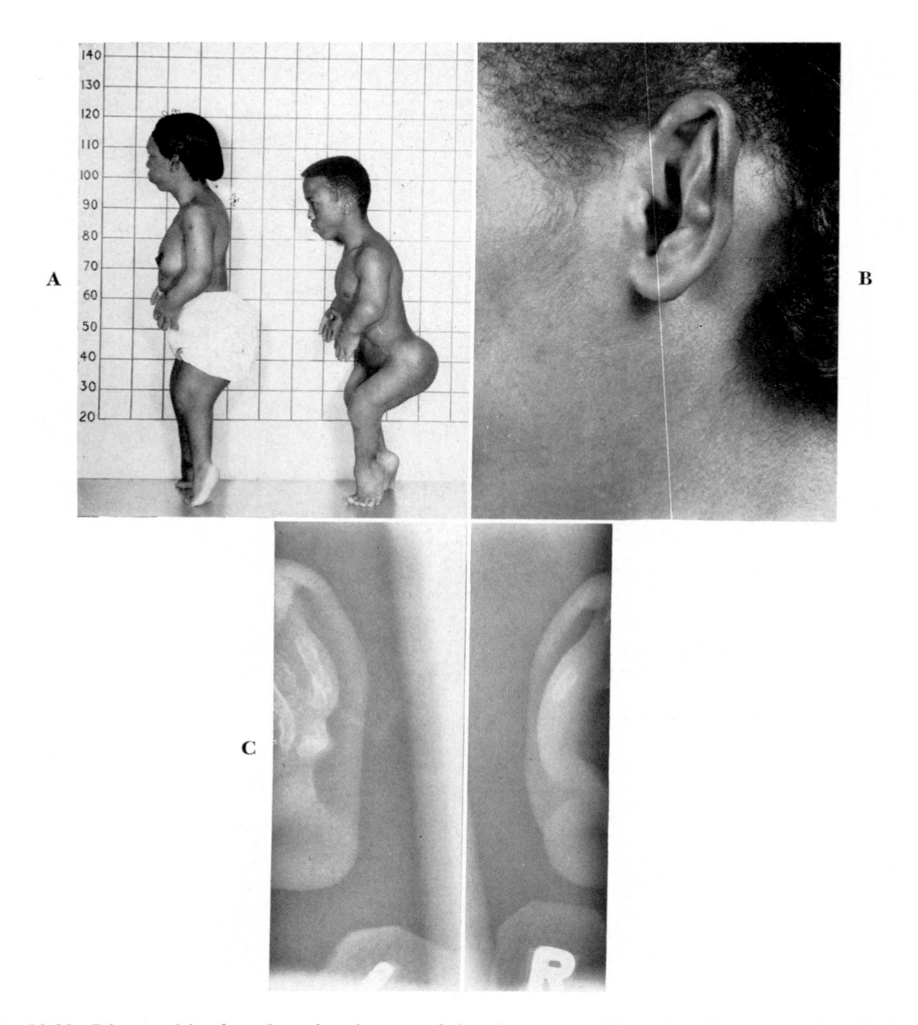

Fig. 10-31. Diastrophic dwarfism in sister and brother, ages 19 and 15, respectively. Clubbed hands and feet and marked dwarfism are shown in **A.** The ears are rigid and deformed, **B,** and show ossification of pinnal cartilages, **C.** The severe deformity of the hands, **D,** and feet, **E,** is demonstrated. The position of the thumb—"hitchhiker thumb"—is characteristic. Its metacarpal is very short. Ankylosis of the proximal interphalangeal joints in the second, third, and fourth fingers of both hands is also demonstrated. Because of the stiff fingers the patient's method of writing, **F,** is awkward. In **G** are demonstrated severe derangement of the hip, scoliosis, and precocious ossification of costal cartilages.

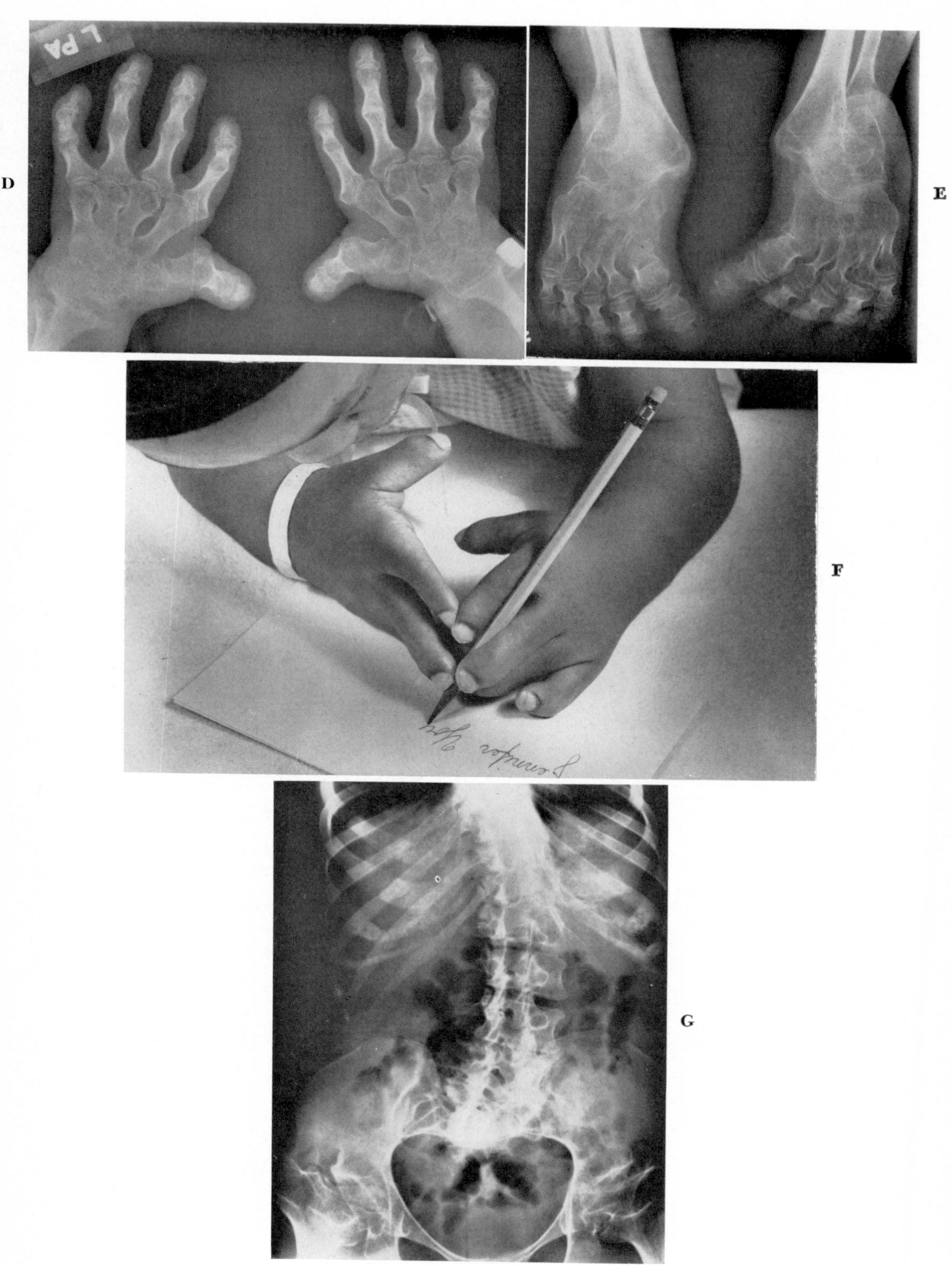

Fig. 10-31, cont'd. For legend see opposite page.

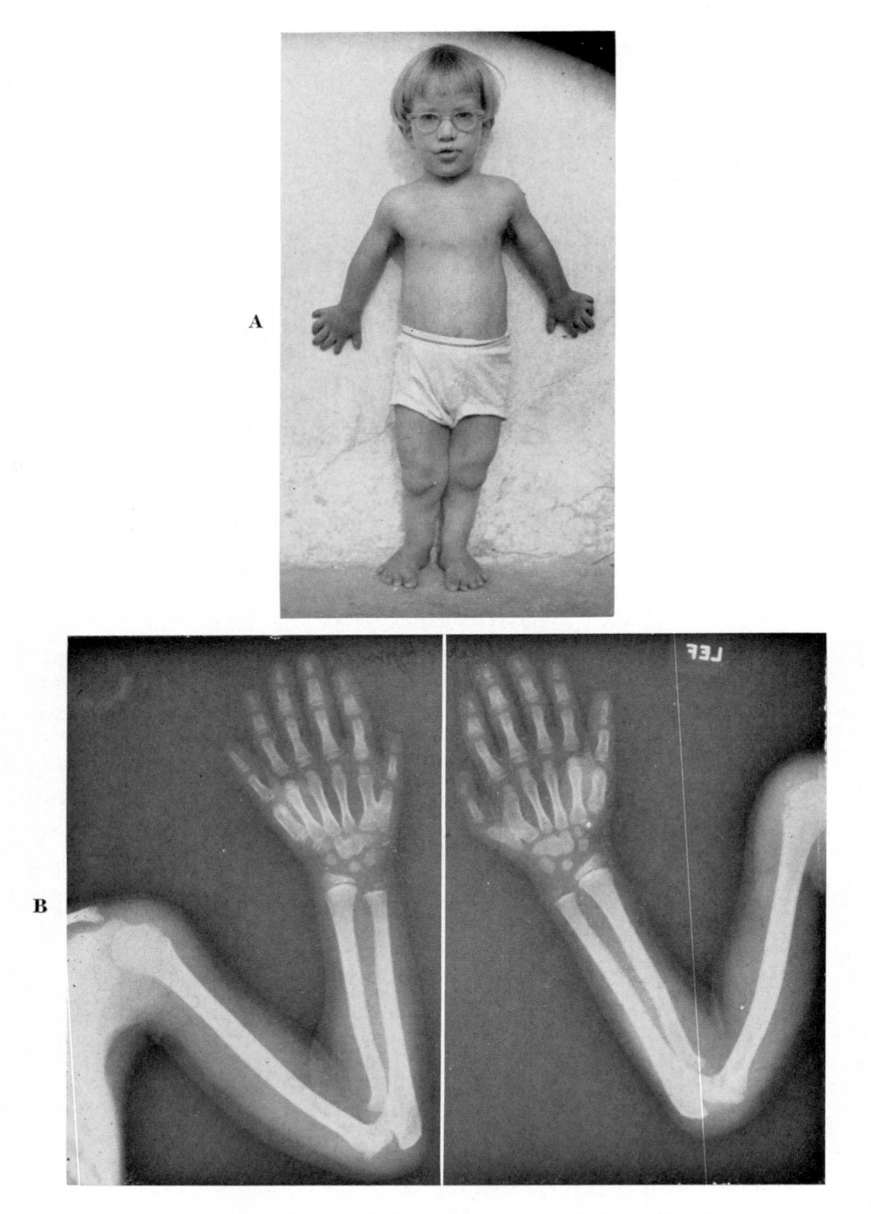

Fig. 10-32. Ellis-van Creveld syndrome. **A,** Boy, 5 years old. Polydactyly, knock-knees, and short extremities are demonstrated. **B,** Negro female, 9 years old. The appearance of the extra finger and the fusion of the hamate and capitate bones are characteristic. (From McKusick, V. A., and colleagues: Trans. Ass. Amer. Phys. **77**:154, 1964.)

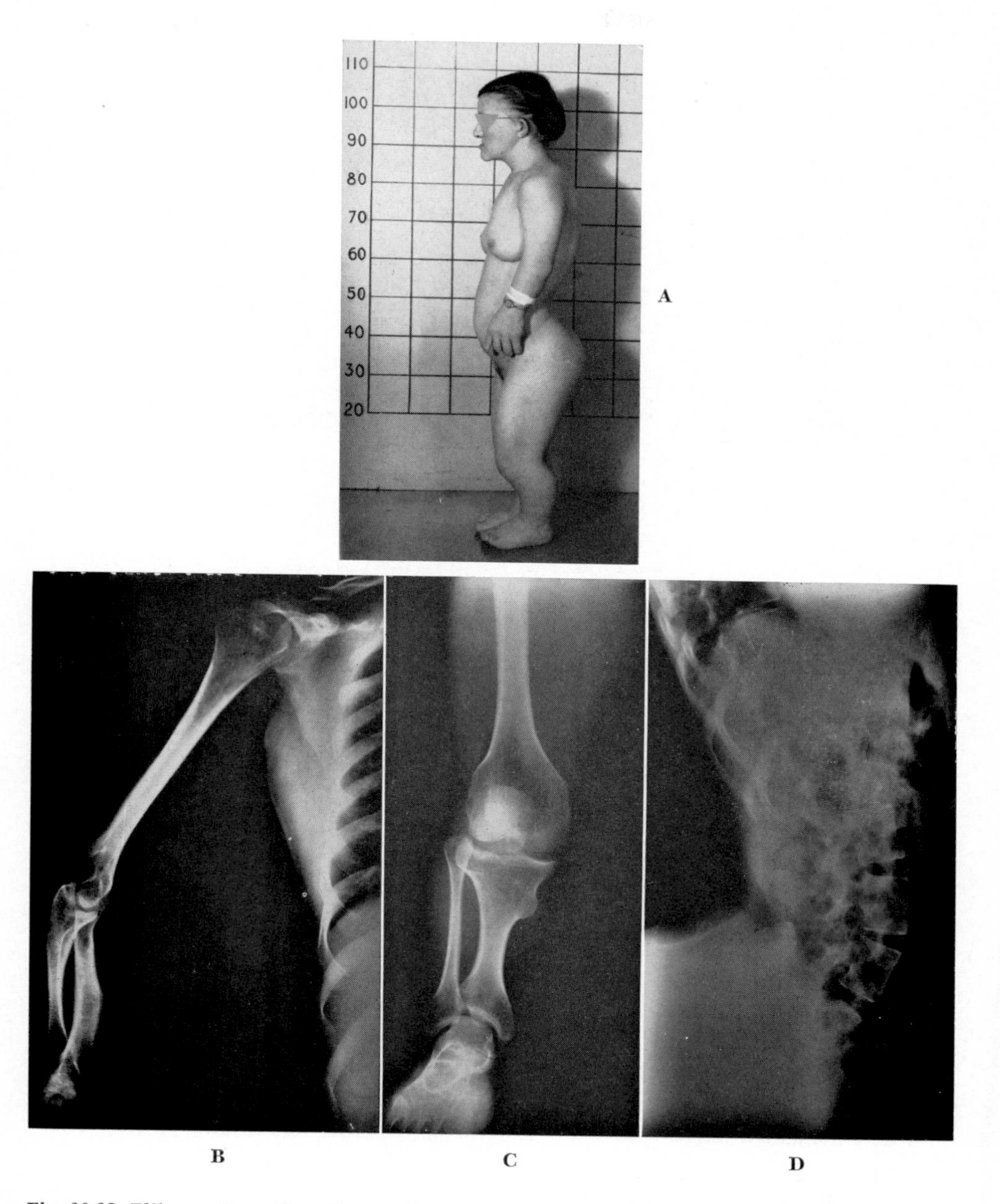

Fig. 10-33. Ellis-van Creveld syndrome. **A,** General appearance of 21-year-old female. The upper lip is retracted and sunken, in part due to early loss of teeth, in part due to "partial harelip." Signs of large atrial septal defect are present. The distal portion of the extremities is particularly short, **B** and **C.** Extreme spondylolisthesis is present, **D.** The fingernails are dystrophic, **E.** Extra fingers have been amputated.

Continued.

E

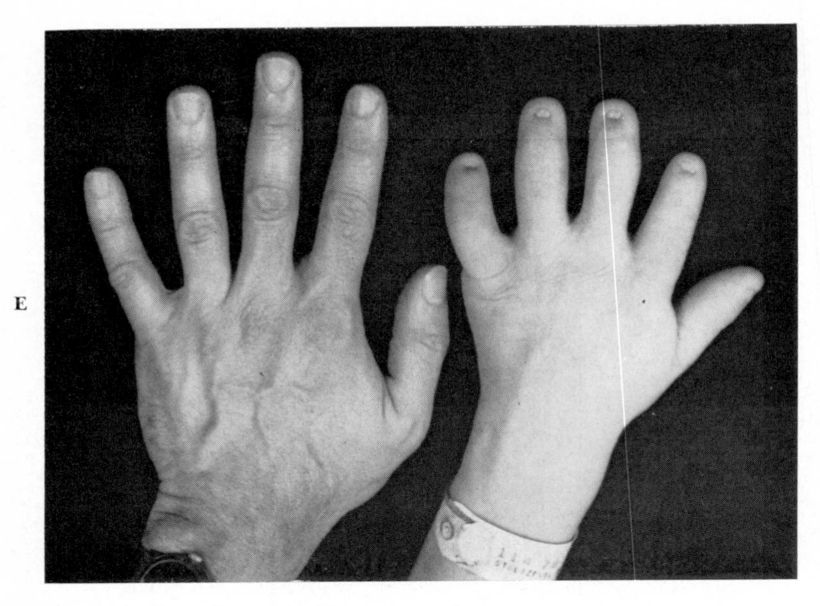

Fig. 10-33, cont'd. For legend see preceding page.

hands (e.g. short metacarpal) is frequent. The patients are usually of reduced stature. Cutaneous osteomata have been described as an associated feature.[237] Sarcomatous transformation is rather frequent.[222,264,297] Inheritance is autosomal dominant. Neurologic complications occur in some from pressure on the spinal cord or peripheral nerves.[271,322] The same disorder has been observed in horses.[295]

Diastrophic dwarfism, a recessive disorder, is manifested by clubbed feet and clubbed hands, severe dwarfism, scoliosis, and deformity of the pinnae.[268,283,328,330] Cleft palate occurs in some cases. Typically the proximal interphalangeal joints are fused. Calcification and even ossification of the pinnal cartilages and precocious calcification of costal cartilages are observed radiologically. Because of the bending of the spine and extremities, Lamy and Maroteaux,[268] who first delineated this entity, borrowed the term *diastrophic* from geology; diastrophism is that process of bending of the earth's crust by which mountains, continents, ocean basins, etc. are formed. Diastrophic dwarfism is autosomal recessive.

Hyperostosis corticalis generalisata, or van Buchem's disease,[334,341] is another osteosclerotic process involving the skull, mandible, clavicles, and ribs and accompanied by hyperplasia of the diaphyseal cortex of the long bones. The progessive changes probably begin during puberty and may lead to facial paralysis, optic atrophy, and perceptive deafness. Serum alkaline phosphatase is elevated. Inheritance is autosomal recessive.

The Ellis-van Creveld syndrome (chondroectodermal dysplasia) is manifested by dwarfism, polydactyly, dysplastic fingernails, and, in about half of cases, malformation of the heart, usually single atrium.[226,259] Cases have been observed in persons of many nationalities, including Caucasoids, Negroes, and Orientals. Many cases, about equalling the number reported in the literature, were observed[284,285] in a religious isolate, the Old Order Amish of Lancaster County, Pennsylvania. Inheritance is autosomal recessive.

Text continued on page 470.

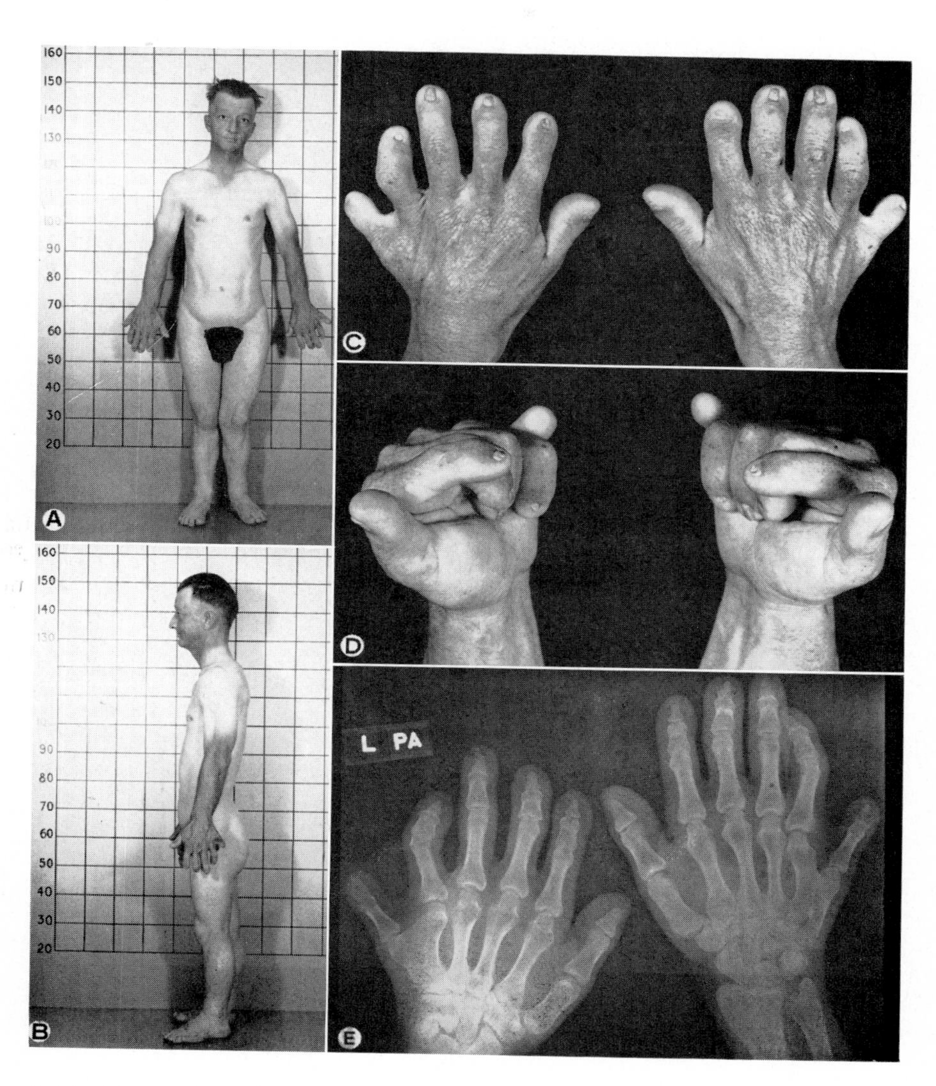

Fig. 10-34. Ellis-van Creveld syndrome in man now 45 years old. **A** and **B,** Note the particular shortening of the distal portion of the extremities. **C,** In the hands note the polydactyly, brachydactyly, and dysplastic fingernails. **D,** The patient cannot make a tight fist. The reason is shown in **E.** The proximal phalanges are long relative to the middle and distal phalanges. Note the partial fusion of the hamate and capitate bones of the wrist. (From McKusick, V. A., Egeland, J. A., Eldridge, R., and Krusen, D. E.: Bull. Hopkins Hosp. **115**:306, 1964.)

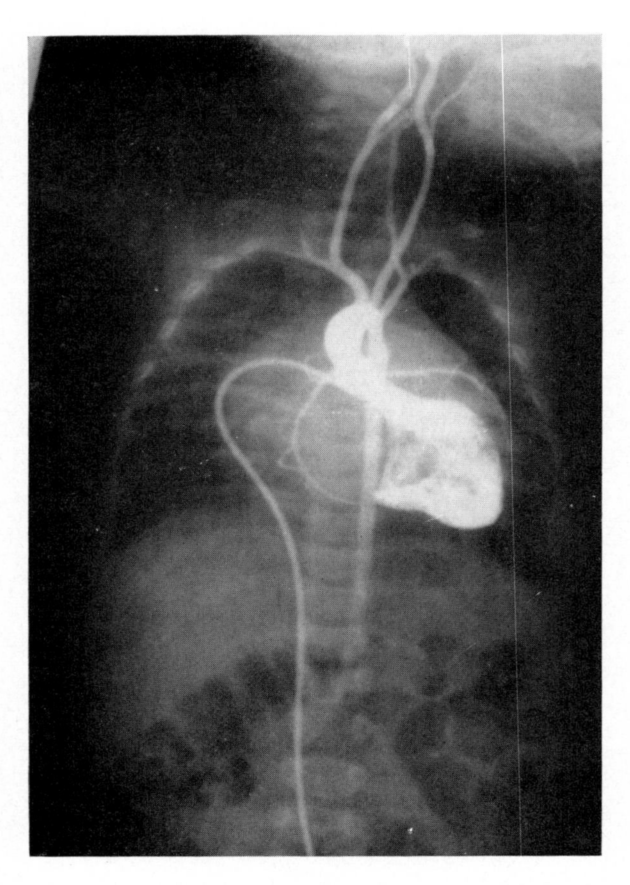

Fig. 10-35. Ellis-van Creveld syndrome with single atrium in 4-month-old infant (L. E., B47024). The catheter introduced via a leg vein has passed into the left ventricle from the single atrium. (From McKusick, V. A., Egeland, J. A., Eldridge, R., and Krusen, D. E.: Bull. Hopkins Hosp. **115**:306, 1964.)

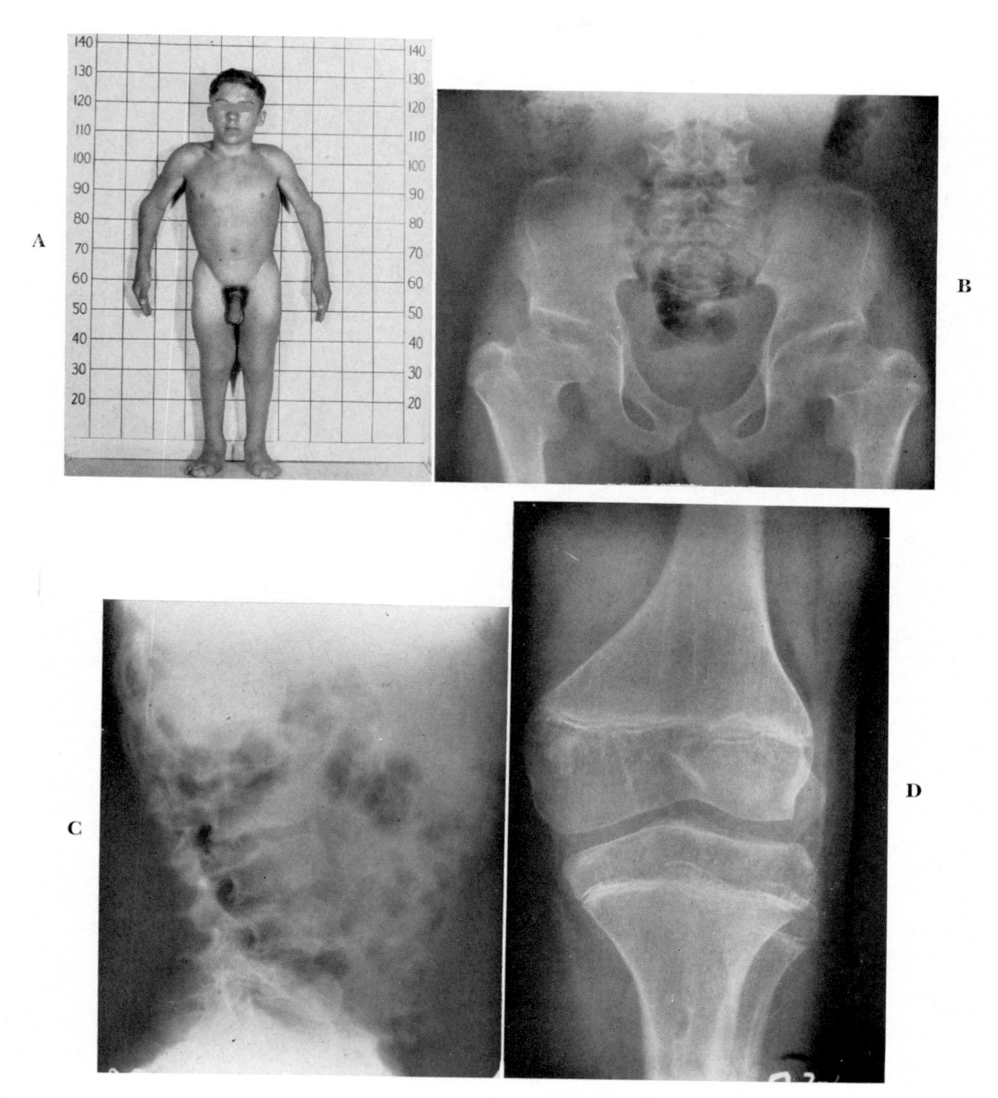

Fig. 10-36. Early cataract with skeletal disease. D. B. (764114), age 16 years at the time of these studies, **A,** has a form of spondyloepiphyseal dysplasia as demonstrated by the changes in the hips, **B,** lumbar spine, **C,** and knees, **D.** A mature cataract was removed at the age of 13 years. Detachment of the left retina was detected at that time. He is totally blind in the left eye and severely myopic in the right. No other members of the family are similarly affected, and the parents are apparently not related.

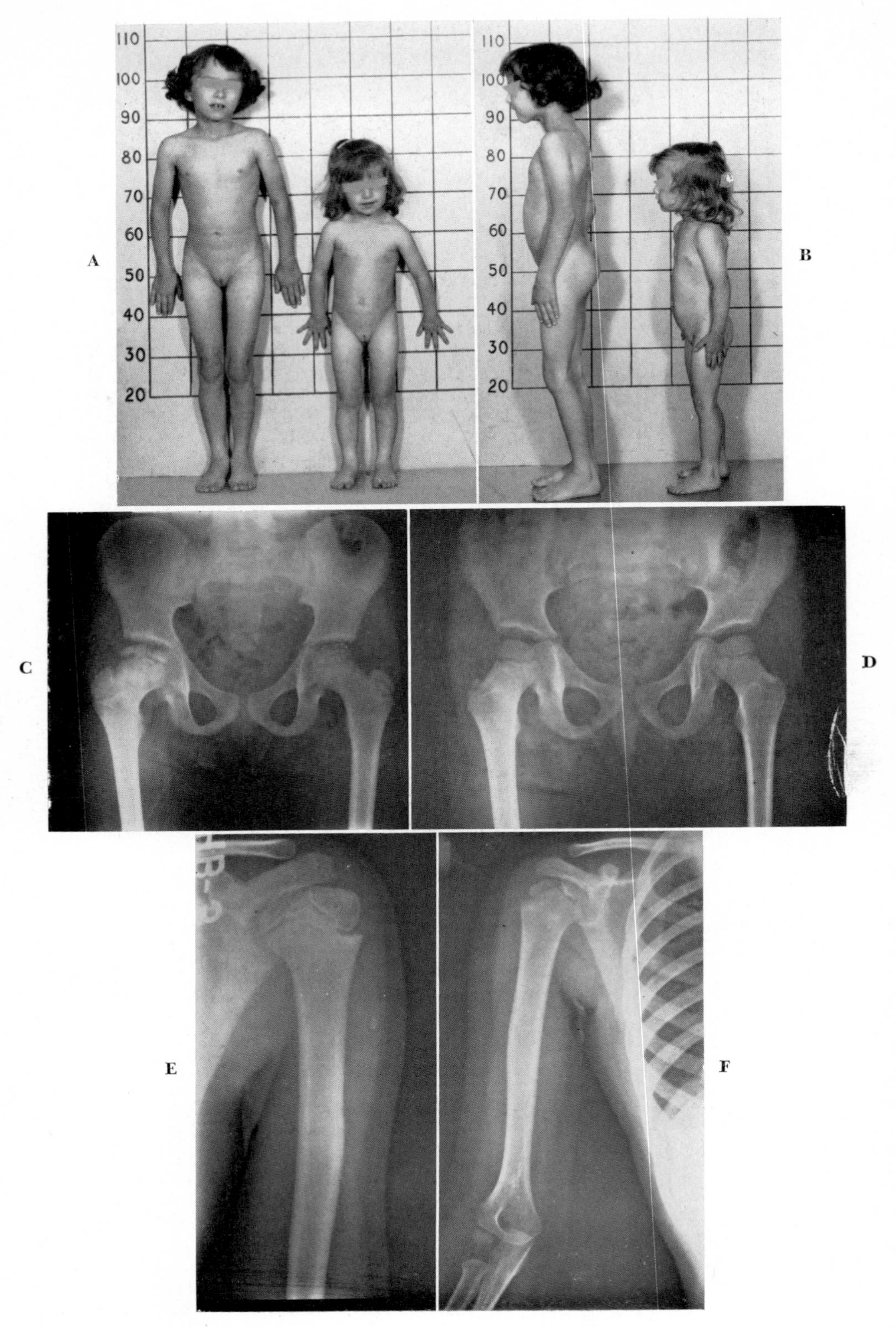

Fig. 10-37. For legend see opposite page.

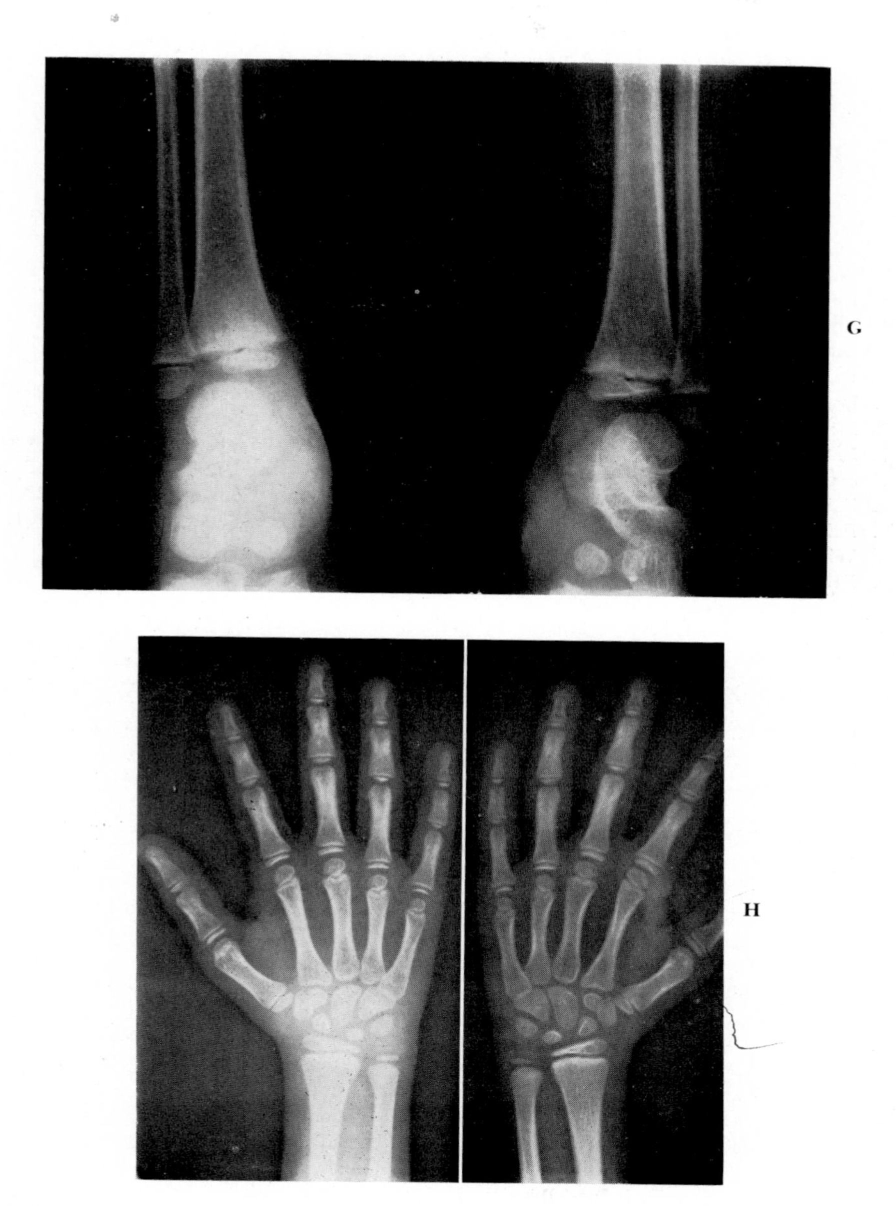

Fig. 10-37. Early cataract with epiphyseal disease. D. S. (1073527) and T. S. (1073528) are sisters, 8 and 4 years old in **A** and **B.** Each has had bilateral cataract extraction. Both have Legg-Perthes type of change in the femoral heads, **C** and **D,** bipartite proximal epiphysis of the humerus, **E** and **F,** and flattening of the distal tibial epiphyses, **G,** as well as those at the wrist and in the fingers, **H.** A third sister has also developed cataracts and epiphyseal disease by 3½ years of age.

Other very rare disorders

A few disorders of the osseous skeleton have been reported only very rarely, and their nosology and genetics are incomplete. This category includes peripheral dysostosis[320] and Léri's dyschondrostéose.[276] Bruland[225] pointed out that childhood rheumatism (Still's disease) may result in dwarfism suggesting chondrodystrophy ("pseudochondrodystrophia rheumatica"). See Figs. 10-36 and 10-37 for the association of epiphyseal disease with cataract, in two families.

REFERENCES

Fibrodysplasia ossificans progressiva (FOP)

1. Barker, L. F.: Medical clinics, Philadelphia, 1922, W. B. Saunders Co.
2. Bauer, K. H., and Bode, W.: Erbpathologie der Stützgewebe beim Menschen. Handbuch der Erbbiologie des Menschen, vol. 3, Berlin, 1940, Julius Springer, p. 105.
3. Bell, J.: On hereditary digital anomalies. Part I. On brachydactyly and symphalangism. The treasury of human inheritance, London, 1951, Cambridge University Press.
4. Brooks, W. D. W.: Calcinosis, Quart. J. Med. **3**:293, 1934.
5. Burton-Fanning, F. W., and Vaughan, A. L.: A case of myositis ossificans, Lancet **2**:849, 1901.
6. Drago, A.: Contributo allo studio della moisite ossificente progressive multipla, Pediatria **27**:715, 1919.
7. Eaton, W. L., Conkling, W. S., and Daeschner, C. W.: Early myositis ossificans progressiva occurring in homozygotic twins; a clinical and pathologic study, J. Pediat. **50**:591, 1957.
8. Fairbank, H. A. T.: Myositis ossificans progressiva, J. Bone Joint Surg. **32-B**:108, 1950.
9. Fairbank, H. A. T.: An atlas of general affections of the skeleton, Baltimore, 1951, The Williams & Wilkins Co.
10. Falls, H. F.: Skeletal system, including joints. In Sorsby, A.: Clinical genetics, St. Louis, 1953, The C. V. Mosby Co., chap. 14.
11. Fränkel, B.: Ein Fall von erblicher Deformität, Berl. Klin. Wschr. **8**:418, 1871.
12. Frejka, B.: Heterotopic ossification and myositis ossificans progressiva, J. Bone Joint Surg. **11**:157, 1929.
13. Freke, J.: Philos. Trans. Roy. Soc., London, 1740. Quoted by Ralph H. Major: Classic descriptions of disease, with biographical sketches of the authors, ed. 3, Springfield, Ill., 1945, Charles C Thomas, Publisher, p. 304.
14. Garrod, A. E.: The initial stage of myositis ossificans, St. Bartholomew's Hosp. Rep. **43**:43, 1907.
15. Gaster, A.: Discussion in meeting of West London Medico-Chirurgical Society, Oct. 7, 1904, West London Med. J. **10**:37, 1905.
16. Geschickter, C. F., and Maseritz, I. H.: Myositis ossificans, J. Bone Joint Surg. **20**:661, 1938.
17. Glimcher, M. J.: Specificity of the molecular structure of organic matrices in mineralization. In Sognnaes, R. F., editor: Calcification in biological systems, Washington, D. C., 1960, American Association Adv. Science, p. 421.
18. Greig, D. M.: Clinical observations of the surgical pathology of bone, Edinburgh, 1931, Oliver & Boyd, p. 170.
19. Griffith, G.: Progressive myositis ossificans; report of a case, Arch. Dis. Child. **24**:71, 1949.
20. Gruber, G. B.: Anmerkungen zur Frage der Weichteilverknöcherung, besonders der Myopathia osteoplastica, Virchows Arch. **260**:457, 1926.
21. Gutman, A. B., and Yü, T. F.: A further consideration of the effects of beryllium salts on in vitro calcification of cartilage. Metabolic interrelations, Trans. Josiah Macy Jr. Found. **3**:90, 1950.
22. Guyatt, B. L., Kay, H. D., and Branion, H. D.: Beryllium "rickets," J. Nutr. **6**:313, 1933.
23. Helferich, H.: Ein Fall von sogenannter Myositis ossificans progressiva, Aerztl. Intelligenz-Blatl. **26**:485, 1879.
24. Hirsch, F., and Löw-Beer, A.: Ueber einen Fall von Myositis ossificans progressiva, Med. Klin. **25**:1661, 1929.
25. Huggins, C. B.: The formation of bone under the influence of epithelium of the alimentary tract, Arch. Surg. **22**:377, 1931.
26. Hutchinson, J.: Reports of hospital practice, M. Times Gaz. **1**:March 31, 1860.

27. Klemper, F. W., Miller, J. M., and Hill, C. J.: The inhibition of alkaline phosphatase by beryllium, J. Biol. Chem. **180**:281, 1949.
28. Koontz, A. R.: Personal communication.
29. Koontz, A. R.: Myositis ossificans progressiva, Amer. J. Med. Sci. **174**:406, 1927.
30. Kubler, E.: Neue Gesichtspunkte bei der Beurteilung der Verlaufsformen der Myositis ossificans progressiva, Fortschr. Roentgenstr. **81**:354, 1954.
31. Lins, F. M., and Abath, G. M.: Doenca ossificante progressiva, Pediat. Prát. **30**:131, 1959.
32. Lockhart, J. D., and Burke, F. G.: Myositis ossificans progressiva. Report of a case treated with corticotropin (ACTH), Amer. J. Dis. Child. **87**:626, 1954.
33. Lutwak, L.: Myositis ossificans progressiva. Mineral, metabolic and radioactive calcium studies of the effects of hormones, Amer. J. Med. **37**:269, 1964.
34. Magruder, L. F.: Myositis ossificans progressiva. Case report and review of the literature, Amer. J. Roentgen. **15**:328, 1926.
35. Mair, W. F.: Myositis ossificans progressiva, Edinburgh Med. J. **39**:13, 69, 1932.
36. Mather, J. H.: Progressive myositis ossificans, Brit. J. Radiol. **4**:207, 1931.
37. Maudsley, R. H.: Case of myositis ossificans progressiva, Brit. Med. J. **1**:954, 1952.
38. Michelsohn, J.: Ein Fall von Myositis ossificans progressiva, Z. Orthop. Chir. **12**:424, 1904.
39. Neuman, W. F., and Neuman, M. W.: Chemical dynamics of bone mineral, Chicago, 1958, University of Chicago Press, p. 179.
40. Nutt, J. J.: Report of a case of myositis ossificans progressiva, with bibliography, J. Bone Joint Surg. **5**:344, 1923.
41. Pack, G. T., and Braund, R. R.: Development of sarcoma in myositis ossificans, J.A.M.A. **119**:776, 1942.
42. Paul, J. R.: A study of an unusual case of myositis ossificans, Arch. Surg. **10**:185, 1925.
43. Pol: "Brachydaktylie," "Klinodaktylie," Hyperphalangie und ihre Grundlagen. Form und Entstehung der meist unter dem Bild der Brachydaktylie auftretenden Varietäten, Anomalien und Missbildungen der Hand und des Fusses, Virchows Arch. **299**:388, 1921.
44. Riley, H. D., Jr., and Christie, A.: Myositis ossificans progressiva, Pediatrics **8**:753, 1951.
45. Rolleston, H. D.: Progressive myositis ossificans with references to other developmental dieases of the mesoblast, Clin. J. **17**:209, 1901.
46. Rosenstirn, J.: A contribution to the study of myositis ossificans progressiva, Ann. Surg. **68**:485, 591, 1918.
47. Ryan, K. J.: Myositis ossificans progressiva. Review of the literature with report of a case, J. Pediat. **27**:348, 1945.
48. Stickler, G. B., Belau, P. G., Farrell, F. J., Jones, J. D., Pugh, D. G., Steinberg, A. G., and Ward, L. E.: Hereditary progressive arthro-ophthalmopathy, Mayo Clin. Proc. **40**:433, 1965.
49. Stonham, C.: Myositis ossificans, Lancet **2**:1481, 1892.
50. Sympson, T.: Case of myositis ossificans, Brit. Med. J. **2**:1026, 1886.
51. Tutunjian, K. H., and Kegerreis, R.: Myositis ossificans progressiva with report of a case, J. Bone Joint Surg. **19**:503, 1937.
52. Van Creveld, S., and Soeters, J. M.: Progressive myositis ossificans, Amer. J. Dis. Child. **62**:1000, 1941.
53. Vastine, J. H., II, Vastine, M. F., and Arango, O.: Genetic influence on osseous development with particular reference to the deposition of calcium in the costal cartilages, Amer. J. Roentgen. **59**:213, 1948.
54. Vastine, J. H., II, Vastine, M. F., and Arango, O.: Myositis ossificans progressiva in homozygotic twins, Amer. J. Roentgen. **59**:204, 1948.
55. Viparelli, V.: La miosite ossificante progressiva, Ann. Neuropsichiat. Psicoanal. **9**:297, 1962.
56. Wheeler, C. E., Curtis, A. C., Cawley, E. P., Grekin, R. H., and Zheutlin, B.: Soft tissue calcification, with special reference to its occurrence in the "collagen diseases," Ann. Intern. Med. **36**:1050, 1952.
57. Wilkins, W. E., Reagan, E. M., and Carpenter, G. K.: Phosphatase studies on biopsy tissue in progressive myositis ossificans, Amer. J. Dis. Child. **49**:1219, 1935.

Osteopoikilosis

58. Albers-Schönberg, H.: Eine seltene bisher nicht bekannte Strukturanomalie des Skelettes, Fortschr. Roentgenstr. **23**:174, 1915.
59. Albronda, J.: Familiale osteopoikilie, Nederl. T. Geneesk. **100**:3533, 1956.
60. Bistolfi: Cited by Curth.[68]

61. Bloom, A. R.: Osteopoecilia, Amer. J. Surg. **22**:239, 1933.
62. Busch, K. F. B.: Familial disseminated osteosclerosis, Acta Radiol. Scand. **18**:693, 1937.
63. Buschke, A., and Ollendorff, H.: Ein Fall von Dermatofibrosis lenticularis disseminata und Osteopathia condensans disseminata, Derm. Wschr. **86**:257, 1928.
64. Cocchi, U.: In Schinz, H. R., Baensch, W. E., Friedl, E., and Uehlinger, E.: Roentgen-diagnostics (J. T. Case, editor of American edition), New York, 1951, Grune & Stratton, Inc., p. 744.
65. Copeman, W. S. C., editor: Textbook of rheumatic diseases, Edinburgh and London, 1955, E. & S. Livingston, Ltd., p. 307.
66. Coughlin, E. J., Jr., Guare, H. F., and Moskovitz, A. J.: Chondrodystrophia calcificans congenita: case report with autopsy, J. Bone Joint Surg. **32-A**:938, 1950.
67. Crespo, D. I.: Osteopoikilosis, A.I.R. **4**:71, 1961.
68. Curth, H. O.: Dermatofibrosis lenticularis disseminata and osteopoikilosis, Arch. Derm. Syph. **30**:552, 1934.
69. Curth, H. O.: Follicular atrophoderma and pseudopelade associated with chondrodystrophia calcificans congenita, J. Invest. Derm. **13**:233, 1949.
70. Erbsen, H.: Die Osteopoikilie (Osteopathia condensans disseminata), Ergebn. Med. Strahlenforsch. **7**:137, 1936.
71. Funstein, L., and Kotschiew, K.: Ueber die Osteopoikilie, Fortschr. Roentgenstr. **54**:595, 1936.
72. Green, A. E., Ellswood, W. H., and Collins, J. R.: Melorheostosis and osteopoikilosis; with a review of the literature, Amer. J. Roentgen. **87**:1096, 1962.
73. Hinson, A.: Familial osteopoikilosis, Amer. J. Surg. **45**:566, 1939.
74. Jeter, H., and McGehee, C. L.: Osteopoikilosis, J. Bone Joint Surg. **15**:990, 1933.
75. Koch, J. C.: The laws of bone architecture, Amer. J. Anat. **21**:177, 1917.
76. Luzsa, G.: Osteopoikilia familiaris, Orv. Hetil. **103**:1267, 1962.
77. Martinčić, N.: Osteopoikilie (spotted bones), Brit. J. Radiol. **25**:612, 1952.
78. Nichols, B. H., and Shiflett, E. L.: Osteopoikilosis. Report of an unusual case, Amer. J. Roentgen. **32**:52, 1934.
79. Osgood, E. C.: Polyostotic fibrous dysplasia and osteopathia condensans disseminata, Amer. J. Roentgen. **56**:174, 1946.
80. Reilly, W. A., and Smith, F. S.: Stippled epiphyses with congenital hypothyroidism (cretinoid epiphyseal dysgenesis), Amer. J. Roentgen. **40**:675, 1938.
81. Risseeuw, J.: Familiäre osteopoikilie, Nederl. T. Geneesk. **80**:3827, 1936.
82. Ritterhoff, R. J., and Oscherwitz, D.: Osteopoikilosis associated with bronchogenic carcinoma and adenocarcinoma of stomach, Amer. J. Roentgen. **48**:341; 1942.
83. Schmorl, G.: Anatomische Befunde bei einem Fall von Osteopoikilie, Fortschr. Roentgenstr. **44**:1, 1931.
84. Smith, A. D., and Waisman, M.: Connective tissue nevi: familial occurrence and association with osteopoikilosis, Arch. Derm. **81**:249, 1960.
85. Steenhuis, D. J.: About a special case of osteitis condensans disseminata, Acta Radiol. **5**:373, 1926.
86. Stieda, A.: Ueber umschriebene Knochenverdichtungen im Bereich der Substantia spongiosa im Röntgenbilde, Beitr. Klin. Chir. **45**:700, 1905.
87. Šváb, d'Vaclav: A propos de l'ostéopoecilie héréditaire, J. Radiol. Electr. **16**:405, 1932.
88. Traub, E.: Epiphyseal necrosis in pituitary gigantism, Arch. Dis. Child. **14**:203, 1939.
89. Von Bernuth, F.: Ueber Sklerodermie, Osteopoikilie und Kalkgicht im Kindesalter, Z. Kinderheilk. **54**:103, 1932.
90. Voorhoeve, N.: A hitherto undescribed picture of abnormality of the skeleton, Acta Radiol. **3**:407, 1924.
91. Wilcox, L. R.: Osteopoikilosis (disseminated condensing osteopathy), Amer. J. Roentgen. **27**:580, 1932.
92. Windholz, F.: Ueber familiäre Osteopoikilie und Dermatofibrosis lenticularis disseminata, Fortschr. Roentgenstr. **45**:566, 1932.

Léri's pleonosteosis

93. Cocchi, U.: Hereditary diseases with bone changes. In Schinz, H. R., Baensch, W. E., Friedl, E., and Uehlinger, E.: Roentgen-diagnostics (J. T. Case, editor of American edition), New York, 1951, Grune & Stratton, Inc., vol. 1, pp. 720 ff.

94. Cohen and de Herdt: Pléonostéose familiale, J. Neurol. Psychiat. **28**:395, 1928.
95. Copeman, W. S. S., editor: Textbook of the rheumatic diseases, Edinburgh and London, 1955, E. & S. Livingston, Ltd.
96. Feiguine, E., and Tikhodéeff, S.: Un cas rare d'osteopathie systematisée—un cas de pléonostéose en U. R. S. S., Arch. Méd. Enf. **35**:654, 1932.
97. Léri, A.: Une maladie congénitale et heréditaire de l'ossification: la pléonostéose familiale, Bull. Soc. Méd. Hôp. Paris **45**:1228, 1921.
98. Léri, A.: Dystrophie osseuse généralisée congénitale et heréditaire: la pléonostéose familiale, Presse Méd. **30**:13, 1922.
99. Léri, A.: Sur la pléonostéose familiale,. Bull. Soc. Méd. Hôp. Paris **48**:216, 1924.
100. Materna, A.: Zur Pathologie der Pléonosteose (Léri), Beitr. Path. Anat. **112**:112, 1952.
101. Neel, J. V., and Schull, W. J.: Human heredity, Chicago, 1954, University of Chicago Press, p. 309.
102. Rocher, H. L., and Pesme, P.: Un cas de pléonostéose (maladie de Léri) avec cornées opalescentes, J. Méd. Bordeaux **123**:121, 1946.
103. Rocher, H. L., and Roudil, G.: La pléonostéose (maladie de Léri), Bordeaux Chir. **4**:359, 1932.
104. Rothea, M.: La pléonostéose familiale (maladie d'André Léri), Theses, Paris and Nancy, No. 421.
105. Rouillard, J., and Barreau, P.: Un nouveau cas de pléonostéose heréditaire avec atteintes graves des grosses articulations, Bull. Soc. Méd. Hôp. Paris **51**:794, 1927.
106. Rukavina, J. G., Falls, H. F., Holt, J. F., and Block, W. G.: Léri's pleonosteosis. A study of a family with a review of the literature, J. Bone Joint Surg. **41-A**:397, 1959.
107. Watson-Jones, R.: Léri's pleonosteosis, carpal tunnel compression of the medial nerves and Morton's metatarsalgia, J. Bone Joint Surg. **31-B**:560, 1949.

Paget's disease

108. Albright, F., and Reifenstein, E. C., Jr.: The parathyroid glands and metabolic bone disease. Selected studies, Baltimore, 1948, The Williams & Wilkins Co., pp. 284-301.
109. Aschner, B. M., Hurst, L. A., and Roizin, L.: Genetic study of Paget's disease in monozygotic twin brothers, Acta Genet. Med. **1**:67, 1952.
110. Ashley-Montagu, M. F.: Paget's disease (osteitis deformans) and heredity, Amer. J. Hum. Genet. **1**:94, 1947.
111. Brunner, H.: Zur Pathologie der Ostitis deformans (Paget) des Schläfenbeins, Klin. Wschr. **2**:174, 1931.
112. Brunner, W.: Osteodystrophia deformans Paget unter besonderer Berücksichtigung unserer Erfahrungen der letzten 10 Jahre, Deutsch. Z. Chir. **52**:585, 1939.
113. Chauffard, A.: Discussion of paper by Gilles de la Tourette and Marinesco, Bull. Soc. Méd. Hôp. Paris **11** (ser.3):426, 1894.
114. Clegg, J. T.: Paget's disease with mental symptoms and choroiditis, Lancet **2**:128, 1937.
115. Cockayne, E. A.: Quoted by Rast and Weber.[148]
116. Crumpacker, E. L., and Lipscomb, P. R.: The familial incidence of Paget's disease of bone (osteitis deformans). Report of occurrence in three siblings, Med. Clin. N. Amer. **35**:1203, 1951.
117. Dandy, W. E.: Personal communication.
118. Dickson, D. D., Camp, J. D., and Ghormley, R. K.: Osteitis deformans (Paget's disease of bone), Radiology **44**:449, 1945.
119. Dubreuilh, W., and Laubie: Maladie osseuse de Paget chez deux frères, Bull. Soc. Franc. Derm. **3**:87, 1924.
120. Edholm, O. G., Howarth, S., and McMichael, J.: Heart failure and bone blood flow in osteitis deformans, Clin. Sci. **5**:249, 1945.
121. Faugeron, R.: Essai sur les rapports de la syphilis et de la maladie osseuse de Paget, Thèse de Paris, 1923.
122. Goldenberg, R. R.: The skeleton in Paget's disease, Bull. Hosp. Joint Dis. **12**:229, 1951.
123. Gutman, A. B., and Kasabach, H. H.: Paget's disease (osteitis deformans). Analysis of 116 Cases, Amer. J. Med. Sci. **191**:361, 1936.
124. Hanke, H.: Osteodystrophische Erkrankungen und ihre Begrenzung, Deutsch. Z. Chir. **245**:641, 1935.
125. Harrison, C. V., and Lennox, B.: Heart block in osteitis deformans, Brit. Heart J. **10**:167, 1948.

126. Higbee, W. S., and Ellis, A. G.: A case of osteitis deformans, J. Med. Res. **24**:43, 1911.
127. Hurwitz, S. H.: Osteitis deformans, Paget's disease: a report of six cases, Bull. Hopkins Hosp. **24**:263, 1913.
128. Hurwitz, S. H.: Osteitis deformans (Paget's disease), Bull Hopkins Hosp. **24**:266, 1913.
129. Irvine, R. E.: Familial Paget's disease with early onset, J. Bone Joint Surg. **35-B**:106, 1953.
130. John, E., and Strasser, U.: Zur Aetiologie, Klinik und Therapie der Ostitis fibrosa deformans (Paget), Deutsch. Z. Nervenheilk. **97**:81, 1927.
131. Kay, H. D., Simpson, S. L., and Riddock, G.: Osteitis deformans, Arch. Intern. Med. **53**:208, 1934.
132. Kilner, J.: Two cases of osteitis deformans in one family, Lancet **1**:221, 1904.
133. Koller, F.: Ueber die Heredität der Ostitis deformans Paget, Helv. Med. Acta **13**:389, 1946.
134. Laederich, L., Mamon, H., and Beuchesne, H.: Un cas de maladie osseuse de Paget avec cataracte de type endocrinien, Bull. Soc. Méd. Hôp. Paris **65**:529, 1938.
135. Lambert, R. K.: Paget's disease with angioid streaks of the retina, Arch. Ophthal. **22**:106, 1939.
136. Lunn, J. R.: Four cases of osteitis deformans, Trans. Clin. Soc. London **18**:272, 1885.
137. Martin, E.: Considérations sur la maladie de Paget, Helv. Med. Acta **14**:319, 1947.
138. Moehlig, R. C.: Paget's disease (osteitis deformans) and osteoporosis: similarity of the 2 conditions as shown by familial background and glucose tolerance studies, Surg. Gynec. Obstet. **62**:815, 1936.
139. Moehlig, R. C.: Osteitis deformans: familial constitutional hereditary background as etiological factors, J. Mich. Med. Soc. **51**:1004, 1027, 1952.
140. Monroe, R. T.: Diseases of old age, Cambridge, 1951, Harvard University Press, p. 304.
141. Morrison, W. H.: Osteitis deformans with angioid streaks. Report of a case, Arch. Ophthal. **26**:79, 1941.
142. Mozer, J. J.: Discussion of Koller.[133]
143. Murphy, W.: Osteitis deformans in a brother and sister, Med. J. Aust. **1**:507, 1950.
144. Narins, L., and Oppenheimer, G. D.: Calcification of vas deferens associated with Paget's disease of bone, J. Urol. **67**:2118, 1952.
145. Paget, J.: Remarks on osteitis deformans, Illust. Med. News **2**:181, 1889.
146. Parry, T. W.: A case of osteitis deformans in which fracture of a femur took place as the result of stooping, Brit. Med. J. **1**:879, 1912.
147. Pick: Osteitis deformans, Lancet **2**:1125, 1883.
148. Rast, H., and Weber, F. P.: Paget's bone disease in three sisters, Brit. Med. J. **1**:918, 1937.
149. Roberts, R. E., and Cohen, M. J.: Osteitis deformans (Paget's disease of bone), Proc. Roy. Soc. Med. **19**:13, 1936.
150. Rosenkrantz, J. A., Wolf, J., and Kaicher, J.: Paget's disease (osteitis deformans); review of 111 cases, Arch. Intern. Med. **90**:610, 1952.
151. Sabatini, G.: Ostitis fibrosa di Paget in due coppie di coniugi, Minerva Med. **39**:607, 1948.
152. Schmorl, G.: Ueber Ostitis deformans Paget, Virchows Arch. **283**:694, 1932.
153. Schwartz, L. A.: Paget's disease in 3 male siblings; clinical report, J. Mich. Med. Soc. **47**:1244, 1948.
154. Seligman, B., and Nathanson, L.: Metastatic calcification in the soft tissues of the legs in osteitis deformans, Ann. Intern. Med. **23**:82, 1945.
155. Smith, S. M.: A case of osteitis deformans in which the disease is present in father and son, Trans. Med. Soc. London **28**:224, 1904-1905.
156. Sornberger, C. F., and Smedel, M. I.: Mechanism and incidence of cardiovascular changes in Paget's disease; critical review of literature with case studies, Circulation **6**:711, 1952.
157. Stahl, B. F.: Osteitis deformans, Paget's disease, with reports of two cases and autopsy in one, Amer. J. Med. Sci. **143**:525, 1912.
158. Stein, I., Stein, R. O., and Beller, M. L.: Living bone in health and disease, Philadelphia, 1955, J. B. Lippincott Co.
159. Stemmermann, W.: Die Ostitis deformans Paget unter Berücksichtigung ihrer Vererbung, Ergebn. Inn. Med. **3** (n.s.):185, 1952.
160. Storsteen, K. A., and Jones, N. J.: Arteriography and vascular studies in Paget's disease of bone, J.A.M.A. **154**:472, 1954.
161. Terry, T. L.: Angioid streaks and osteitis deformans, Trans. Amer. Ophthal. Soc. **32**:555, 1934.

162. Van Bogaert, L.: Ueber eine hereditäre und familiäre Form der Pagetschen Ostitis deformans mit Chorioretinitis pigmentosa, Z. Ges. Neur. **147**:327, 1933.
163. Von der Heydt, R.: Osteitis deformans with pigmented corneal degeneration, Amer. J. Ophthal. **20**:1139, 1937.
164. Wells, H. G., and Holley, S. W.: Metastatic calcification in osteitis deformans, Arch. Path. **34**:435, 1942.
165. Wilton, A.: On the genesis of osteitis deformans (Paget), Acta Orthop. Scand. **24**:30, 1954.
166. Woodcock, C. W.: Transactions of the Cleveland Dermatological Society, Arch. Derm. Syph. **65**:623, 1952.

Other possible hereditary and generalized disorders of connective tissue

167. Bloom, D.: Heredity of keloids, New York J. Med. **56**:511, 1956.
168. Boatwright, H., Wheeler, C. E., and Cawley, E. P.: Werner's syndrome, Arch. Intern. Med. **90**:243, 1952.
169. Böhme, A.: Kasuistischer Beitrag zur Thiemannschen Epiphysenerkrankung, Z. Ges. Inn. Med. **18**:491, 1963.
170. Bunnell, S.: Surgery of the hand, Philadelphia, 1948, J. B. Lippincott Co.
171. Christiaens, L., Marchant-Alphant, A., and Fovet, A.: Emphysème congénital et cutis laxa, Presse Méd. **62**:1799, 1954.
172. Cockayne, E. A.: Inherited abnormalities of the skin and its appendages, London, 1933, Oxford University Press, p. 310.
173. Conway, H.: Dupuytren's contracture, Amer. J. Surg. **87**:161, 1954.
174. Craig, H. R.: Epidermolysis bullosa, Amer. J. Dis. Child. **39**:989, 1930.
175. Debré, R., Marie, J., and Seringe, P.: "Cutis laxa" avec dystrophie osseuse, Bull. Soc. Méd. Hôp. Paris **61**:1038, 1937.
176. Early, P. F.: Dupuytren's contracture, J. Bone Joint Surg. **44-B**:602, 1962.
177. Early, P. F.: Genetics of Dupuytren's contracture, Brit. Med. J. **1**:908, 1964.
178. Engman, M. F., and Mook, W. H.: A further contribution to the study of elastic tissue in epidermolysis bullosa, J. Cut. Dis. **28**:275, 1910; study of some cases of epidermolysis bullosa with remarks upon the congenital absence of elastic tissue, J. Cut. Dis. **24**:55, 1906.
179. Fittke, H.: Ueber eine ungewöhnliche Form "multipler Erbabartung" (Chalodermie und Dysostose), Z. Kinderheilk. **63**:510, 1942.
180. Garrod, A. E.: On an unusual form of nodule upon the joints of the fingers, St. Bartholomew's Hosp. Rep. **29**:157, 1893.
181. Garrod, A. E.: Concerning pads upon the finger joints and their clinical relationship, Brit. Med. J. **2**:8, 1904.
182. Ghormley, R. K.: A case of congenital osteosclerosis, Bull. Hopkins Hosp. **33**:404, 1922.
183. Haverkamp Begemann, N., and van Lookeren Campagne, A.: Homozygous form of Pelger-Huët's nuclear anomaly in man, Acta Haemat. **7**:295, 1952.
184. Hunt, A. C., and Ley, D. G.: General arterial calcification of infancy, Brit. Med. J. **1**:385, 1957.
185. Irvin, G. W., and Ward, P. B.: Werner's syndrome, with a report of two cases, Amer. J. Med. **15**:266, 1953.
186. Kanoky, J. P., and Sutton, R. L.: Epidermolysis bullosa congenita (epidermolysis bullosa hereditaria of Köbner), J.A.M.A. **54**:1137, 1910.
187. Klein, H.: Die Pelger-Anomalie der Leukocyten und die pathologische Anatomie des neugeborenen homozygoten Pelger-Kaninchens. Ein Beitrag zum Formenkries der fetelen Chondrodystrophie, Z. Menschl. Vererb. Konstitutionsl. **29**:551, 1949.
188. Kostia, J.: A Dupuytren contracture family, Ann. Chir. Gynaec. Fenniae **46**:351, 1957.
189. Lamb, J. H., and Halpert, B.: Epidermolysis bullosa of the newborn, Arch. Derm. Syph. **55**:369, 1947.
190. Ling, R. S. M.: The genetic factor in Dupuytren's disease, J. Bone Joint Surg. **45-B**:709, 1963.
191. Lund, M.: Dupuytren's contracture and epilepsy, Acta Psychiat. Neur. **16**:465, 1941.
192. Menten, M. L., and Felteman, G. H.: Coronary sclerosis in infancy. Report of three autopsied cases, two in siblings, Amer. J. Clin. Path. **18**:805, 1948.
193. Meyer, R. J.: The medical significance of lenticular opacities (cataract) before the age of fifty, with emphasis on their occurrence in systemic disorders, New Eng. J. Med. **252**:622, 665, 1955.

194. Murley, R. S.: Peyronie's disease, Brit. Med. J. **1**:908, 1964.
195. Nachtsheim, H.: Pelger anomaly in man and rabbit, J. Hered. **41**:131, 1950.
196. Perloff, J. K., and Phelps, E. T.: A review of Werner's syndrome, with a report of the second autopsied case, Amer. Intern. Med. **48**:1205, 1958.
197. Reed, R., Seville, R. H., and Tattersall, R. N.: Werner's syndrome, Brit. J. Derm. **65**:165, 1953.
198. Schourup, K.: Plastic induration of the penis, Acta Radiol. **26**:313, 1945.
199. Seegmiller, J. E., Laster, L., and Howell, R. R.: Biochemistry of uric acid and its relation to gout, New Eng. J. Med. **268**:712, 764, and 821, 1963.
200. Sestak, Z.: Ehlers-Danlos syndrome and cutis laxa: an account of families in the Oxford area, Ann. Hum. Genet. **25**:313, 1962.
201. Skoog, T.: Dupuytren's contraction with special reference to etiology and improved surgical treatment; its occurrence in epileptics; note on knucklepads, Acta Chir. Scand., supp. 138, 1948.
202. Smith, E. W., and Conley, C. L.: Genetic variants of sickle cell disease, Bull. Hopkins Hosp. **94**:289, 1954.
203. Smith, R. C., Winer, L. H., and Martel, S.: Werner's syndrome; report of two cases, Arch. Derm. **71**:197, 1955.
204. Teleky, L.: Dupuytren's contraction as occupational disease, J. Indust. Hyg. **21**:233, 1939.
205. Thannhauser, S. J.: Werner's syndrome (progeria of the adult) and Rothmund's syndrome; two types of closely related heredofamilial atrophic dermatoses with juvenile cataracts and endocrine features; a critical study with five new cases, Ann. Intern. Med. **23**:559, 1945.
206. Van der Sar, A.: The Pelger-Huët familial nuclear anomaly of the leucocytes, Amer. J. Clin. Path. **15**:544, 1944.
207. Wamoscher, Z., and Farhi, A.: Hereditary Legg-Calvé-Perthes disease, Amer. J. Dis. Child. **106**:97, 1963.
208. Weber, F. P.: A note on Dupuytren's contraction, camptodactylia and knuckle pads, Brit. J. Derm. Syph. **50**:26, 1938.
209. Weiss, R. S.: A case of epidermolysis bullosa, showing loss of elastic tissue in the apparently normal skin, J. Cut. Dis. **35**:26, 1917.
210. White, W. H.: On pads on the finger joints, Quart. J. Med. **1**:479, 1908.
211. Williams, A. L. (Melbourne): Personal communication, 1959.
212. Williams, A. L. (Melbourne): The pathology of cardiac failure in infancy, M.D. thesis, University of Melbourne, 1958.
213. Wyngaarden, J. B., and Jones, O. W.: The pathogenesis of gout, Med. Clin. N. Amer. **45**:241, 1961.

Genetic disorders of the osseous skeleton

214. Albers-Schönberg, H.: Eine bisher nicht beschriebene Allgemeinerkrankung des Skelettes im Röntgenbilde, Fortschr. Roentgenstr. **11**:261, 1907.
215. Alexander, W. G.: Report of a case of so-called "marble-bones" with a review of the literature and a translation of article, Amer. J. Roentgen. **10**:280, 1923.
216. Allansmith, M., and Senz, E.: Chondrodystrophia congenita punctata (Conradi's disease): review of literature and report of case with unusual features, Amer. J. Dis. Child. **100**:109, 1960.
217. Bakwin, H., and Krida, A.: Familial metaphyseal dysplasia, Amer. J. Dis. Child. **53**:1521, 1937.
218. Barrie, H., Carter, C., and Sutcliffe, J.: Multiple epiphyseal dysplasia, Brit. Med. J. **2**:133, 1958.
219. Bean, W. B.: Dyschondroplasia and hemangiomata (Maffucci's syndrome), Arch. Intern. Med. **95**:767, 1955.
220. Beisel, W. R., Austen, K. F., Rosen, H., and Herndon, E. G., Jr.: Metabolic observations in adult hypophosphatasia, Amer. J. Med. **29**:369, 1960.
221. Beisel, W. R., Benjamin, N., and Austen, K. F.: Absence of leucocyte alkaline phosphatase activity in hypophosphatasia, Blood **14**:975, 1959.
222. Bennett, G. E., and Berkheimer, G. A.: Malignant degeneration in a case of multiple benign exostoses: with a brief review of the literature, Surgery **10**:781, 1941.

223. Bethune, J. E., and Dent, C. E.: Hypophosphatasia in the adult, Amer. J. Med. **28:**615, 1960.
224. Brailsford, J. F.: Radiology of bones and joints, ed. 5, Baltimore, 1953, The Williams & Wilkins Co.
225. Bruland, H.: Pseudo-chrondrodystrophia rheumatica (rheumatic dwarfism): review and discussion of two cases, Acta Rheum. Scand. **6:**209, 1960.
226. Caffey, J.: Chondroectodermal dysplasia (Ellis-van Creveld disease), report of three cases, Amer. J Roentgen. **68:**875, 1952.
227. Caffey, J.: Pediatric x-ray diagnosis, ed. 4, Chicago, 1961, Year Book Medical Publishers, Inc.
228. Callender, G. R., Jr., and Miyakawa, G.: Osteopetrosis in adult; case report, J. Bone Joint Surg. **35-A:**204, 1953.
229. Carleton, A., Elkington, J. S. C., Greenfield, J. G., and Robb-Smith, A. H. T.: Maffucci's syndrome (dyschondroplasia with haemangiomata), Quart. J. Med. **11:**203, 1942.
230. Christensen, W. R., Lin, R. K., and Berghout, J.: Dysplasia epiphysalis multiplex, Amer. J. Roentgen. **74:**1059, 1955.
231. Cleveland, M., and Fielding, J. W.: Chondrodysplasia (Ollier's disease): report of a case with a thirty-eight year follow-up, J. Bone Joint Surg. **41-A:**1341, 1959.
232. Cohen, J.: Osteopetrosis; case report, autopsy findings and pathologic interpretation; failure of treatment with vitamin A, J. Bone Joint Surg. **33-A:**923, 1951.
233. Cowan, D. J.: Multiple epiphysial dysplasia, Brit. Med. J. **2:**1629, 1963.
234. Currarino, G., Neuhauser, E. B. D., Reyersback, G. C., and Sobel, E. H.: Hypophosphatasia, Amer. J. Roentgen. **78:**392, 1957.
235. Daeschner, C. W., Singleton, E B., Hill, L. L., and Dodge, W. F.: Metaphyseal dysostosis, J. Pediat. **57:**844, 1960.
236. Dent, C. E. (London): Personal communication, 1964.
237. Donaldson, E. M., and Summerly, R.: Primary osteoma cutis and diaphyseal aclasis, Acta Derm. **85:**261, 1962.
238. Elliott, K. A., Elliott, G. B., and Kindrachuk, W. H.: The "radial subluxation—fingernail defect—absent patella" syndrome: observations on its nature, Amer. J. Roentgen. **87:**1067, 1962.
239. Elsbach, L.: Bilateral hereditary micro-epiphysial dysplasia of the hips, J. Bone Joint Surg. **41-B:**514, 1959.
240. Engelmann, G.: Osteopathia hyperostotica sclerotisans multiplex infantilis, Fortschr. Roentgenstr. **39:**1101, 1929.
241. Epstein, J. A., and Malis, L. J.: Compression of spinal cord and cauda equina in achondroplastic drawfs, Neurology **5:**875, 1955.
242. Evans, R., and Caffey, J.: Metaphyseal dysostosis resembling vitamin D–refractory rickets, Amer. J. Dis. Child. **95:**640, 1958.
243. Fairbank, H. A. T.: An atlas of general affections of the skeleton, Edinburgh, 1951, E. & S. Livingstone, Ltd.
244. Ford, N., Silverman, F. N., and Kozlowski, K.: Spondylo-epiphyseal dysplasia (pseudo-achondroplasia type), Amer. J. Roentgen. **86:**462, 1961.
245. Forland, M.: Cleidocranial dysostosis; a review of the syndrome and report of a sporadic case with hereditary transmission, Amer. J. Med. **33:**792, 1962.
246. Fraser, D.: Hypophosphatasia, Amer. J. Med. **22:**730, 1957.
247. Freiberger, R. H.: Multiple epiphyseal dysplasia: a report of three cases, Radiology **70:**379, 1958.
248. Ghormley, R. K.: A case of congenital osteosclerosis, Bull. Hopkins Hosp. **33:**444, 1922.
249. Gram, P. B., Fleming, J. L., Frame, B., and Fine, G.: Metaphyseal chondrodysplasia of Jansen, J. Bone Joint Surg. **41-A:**951, 1959.
250. Herndon, C. N.: Cleidocranial dysostosis, Amer. J. Hum. Genet. **3:**314, 1951.
251. Hinkel, C. L., and Beiler, D. D.: Osteopetrosis in adults, Amer. J. Roentgen. **74:**46, 1955.
252. Hobaek, A.: Problems of hereditary chondrodysplasias, Oslo, 1961, Oslo University Press.
253. Hodgkinson, H. M.: Double patellae in multiple epiphysial dysplasia, J. Bone Joint Surg. **44-B:**569, 1962.
254. Iversen, J.: Cleidocranial dysostosis, Acta Obstet. Gynec. Scand. **41:**93, 1962.
255. Jacobsen, A. W.: Hereditary osteochondrodystrophia deformans: a family with 20 members affected in five generations, J.A.M.A. **113:**121, 1939.

256. Jaffe, H. L.: Hereditary multiple exostoses, Arch. Path. **36**:335, 1943.
257. Kalliala, E., and Taskinen, P. J.: Cleidocranial dysostosis. Report of six typical cases and one atypical case, Oral Surg. **15**:808, 1962.
258. Keith, Sir A.: The nature of the structural alteration in the disorder known as multiple exostoses, J. Anat. **54**:101, 1919-1920.
259. Keizer, D. R. R., and Schilder, J. H.: Ectodermal dysplasia, achondroplasia, and congenital morbus cordis, Amer. J. Dis. Child. **82**:345, 1951.
260. Kelley, C., and Lawlah, J. W.: Albers-Schönberg disease: a family survey, Radiology **47**:507, 1946.
261. Khoo, F. Y., Chang, P. Y., Lee, C. T., and Fan, K. S.: Multiple cartilaginous exostoses (hereditary deforming chondrodysplasia), Chinese Med. J. **66**:252, 1948.
262. Klein, A.: Zur Frage der Erblichkeit der Marmorknochenkrankheit, Fortschr. Roentgenstr. **76**:366, 1952.
263. Kneal, E., and Sante, L. R.: Osteopetrosis (marble bones); report of a case with special reference to early roentgenologic and pathologic findings, Amer. J. Dis. Child. **81**:693, 1951.
264. Knight, J. D. S.: Sarcomatous change in three brothers with diaphysial aclasis, Brit. Med. J. **1**:1013, 1960.
265. Komins, C.: Familial metaphyseal dysplasia (Pyle's disease), Brit. J. Radiol. **27**:670, 1954.
266. Krooth, R. S., Macklin, M. A. P., and Hilbish, T. F.: Diaphysial aclasis (multiple exostoses) on Guam, Amer. J. Hum. Genet. **13**:340, 1961.
267. Lamy, M., and Maroteaux, P.: Les chondrodystrophies génotypiques, L'Expansion Scientifique Française, Paris, 1960.
268. Lamy, M., and Maroteaux, P.: Le nanisme diastrophique, Presse Méd. **68**:1977, 1960.
269. Landauer, W.: Studies on the creeper fowl. XII. Size of body, organs and long bone of late homozygous creeper embryos, Storrs Agric. Exper. Station, University of Connecticut Bull. No. 232, 1939; also: Studies on fowl paralysis. III. A condition resembling osteopetrosis (marble bone) in the common fowl, Bull. No. 222, 1938.
270. Langer, L. O., Jr.: Spondyloepiphyseal dysplasia tarda. Hereditary chondrodysplasia with characteristic vertebral configuration in an adult, Radiology **82**:833, 1964.
271. Larson, N. E., Dodge, H. W., Rushton, J. B., and Dahlin, D. C.: Hereditary multiple exostoses with compression of the spinal cord, Proc. Mayo Clin. **32**:728, 1957.
272. Laubmann, W.: Ueber die Knochenstruktur bei Marmorknochenkrankheit, Virchows Arch. **296**:343, 1935.
273. Lavine, L. S., and Koven, M. T.: Engelmann's disease (progressive diaphyseal dysplasia), J. Pediat. **40**:235, 1952.
274. Leeds, N. E.: Epiphyseal dysplasia multiplex, Amer. J. Roentgen. **84**:506, 1960.
275. Lennan, E. A., Schechter, M. M., and Hornabrook, R. W.: Engelmann's disease. Report of a case with a review of the literature, J. Bone Joint Surg. **43-B**:273, 1961.
276. Léri, A., and Weill, J.: Une affection congenitale et symétrique du développement osseux: la dyschondrostéose, Bull. Soc. Méd. Hôp. Paris, **53**:1491, 1929.
277. Licht, J., and Jesiotr, M.: Chondroangiopathia calcarea seu punctata (chondrodystrophia calcificans congenita): an atypical, stationary form of the disease, Amer. J. Roentgen. **78**:492, 1957.
278. Lorey and Reye: Ueber Marmorknochenkrankheit, Fortschr. Roentgenstr. **30**:35, 1923.
279. McCance, R. A., Fairweather, D. V. I., Barrett, A. M., and Morrison, A. B.: Genetic, clinical, biochemical and pathologic features of hypophosphatasia, Quart. J. Med. **25**:523, 1956.
280. McCune, D. J., and Bradley, C.: Osteopetrosis (marble bones) in an infant. Review of the literature and report of a case, Amer. J. Dis. Child. **48**:949, 1934.
281. McKusick, V. A.: Frederick Parkes Weber—1863-1962, J.A.M.A. **183**:45, 1963.
282. McKusick, V. A., and colleagues: Medical Genetics 1963, J. Chronic Dis. **17**:1077, 1964.
283. McKusick, V. A., and Milch, R. A.: The clinical behavior of genetic disease: selected aspects, Clin. Orthop. **33**:22, 1964.
284. McKusick, V. A., Egeland, J. A., Eldridge, R., and Krusen, D. E.: Dwarfism in the Amish: I. The Ellis-van Creveld syndrome, Bull. Hopkins Hosp. **115**:306, 1964.
285. McKusick, V. A., Eldridge, R., Hostetler, J. A., and Egeland, J. A.: Dwarfism in the Amish, Trans. Ass. Amer. Physicians **77**:151, 1964.
286. McKusick, V. A., Eldridge, R., Hostetler, J. A., Ruangwit, U., and Egeland, J. A.: Dwarfism in the Amish. II. Cartilage-hair hypoplasia, Bull. Hopkins Hosp. **116**:285, 1965.

287. McPeak, C. N.: Osteopetrosis: report of eight cases occurring in three generations of one family, Amer. J. Roentgen. **37**:816, 1936.
288. Maroteaux, P., and Lamy, M.: Les formes pseudo-achondroplastiques des dysplasies spondylo-epiphysaires, Presse Méd. **67**:383, 1959.
289. Maroteaux, P., and Lamy, M.: La pycnodysostose, Presse Méd. **70**:999, 1962.
290. Maroteaux, P., and Lamy, M.: Achondroplasia in man and animals, Clin. Orthop. **33**:91, 1964.
290a. Maroteaux, P., and Lamy, M.: The malady of Toulouse-Lautrec, J.A.M.A. **191**:715, 1965.
291. Maudsley, R. H.: Dysplasia epiphysealis multiplex, J. Bone Joint Surg. **37-B**:228, 1955.
292. Mikity, V. G., and Jacobson, G.: Progressive diaphyseal dysplasia (Engelmann's disease), J. Bone Joint Surg. **40-A**:206, 1958.
293. Moldauer, M., Hanelin, J., and Bauer, W.: Familial precocious degenerative arthritis and the natural history of osteochondrodystrophy. In Blumenthal, Herman T., editor: Medical and clinical aspects of aging, New York, 1962, Columbia University Press, pp. 226-233.
294. Mørch, E. T.: Chondrodystrophic dwarfs in Denmark, Opera ex Domo Biol. Hered. Hum., Univ. Hafn., vol. 3, 1941.
295. Morgan, J. P., Carlson, W. D., and Adams, O. R.: Hereditary multiple exostosis in the horse, J. Amer. Vet. Med. Ass. **140**:1320, 1962.
296. Mori, P. A., and Holt, J. F.: Cranial manifestations of familial metaphyseal dysplasia, Radiology **66**:335, 1956.
297. Munro, R. S., and Goldring, J. S. R.: Chondrosarcoma of the ilium complicating hereditary multiple exostoses, Brit. J. Surg. **39**:73, 1951-52.
298. Pearce, L., and Brown, W. H.: Hereditary osteopetrosis in the rabbit, J. Exp. Med. **88**:579, 597, 1928.
299. Peterson, J. C.: Metaphyseal dysostosis; questionably a form of vitamin D–resistant rickets, J. Pediat. **60**:656, 1962.
300. Pirie, A. H.: The development of marble bone, Amer. J. Roentgen. **24**:147, 1930; Marble bones, Amer. J. Roentgen. **30**:618, 1933.
301. Plotz, M., and Chakales, H. J.: Osteopetrosis (Albers-Schönberg disease; marble bone disease), New York J. Med. **53**:445, 1953.
302. Potterfield, T. C., and Gonzalez, I.: Ollier's dyschondroplasia, J. Pediat. **33**:705, 1948.
303. Pyle, E.: A case of unusual bone development, J. Bone Joint Surg. **13**:874, 1931.
304. Raap, G.: Chondrodystrophia calcificans congenita, Amer. J. Roentgen. **49**:77, 1943.
305. Resnick, E.: Epiphyseal dysplasia punctata in a mother and identical male twins, J. Bone Joint Surg. **25**:461, 1943.
306. Rubin, P.: Dynamic classification of bone dysplasias, Chicago, 1964, Year Book Medical Publishers, Inc.
307. Sanderson, G. H., and Smith, F. S.: Chondrodysplasia (Ollier's disease), J. Bone Joint Surg. **20**:61, 1938.
308. Schlesinger, B., Luder, J., and Bodian, M.: Rickets with alkaline phosphatase deficiency: an osteoblastic dysplasia, Arch. Dis. Child. **30**:265, 1955.
309. Schoeder, G.: Osteo-onychodysplasia hereditaria (albuminurica). Literaturbericht und Einordnung einer Sippe in dieses Missbildungssyndrom, Z. Menschl. Vererb. Konstitutionsl. **36**:42, 1961.
310. Schreiber, F., and Rosenthal, H.: Paraplegia from ruptured lumbar discs in achondroplastic dwarfs, J. Neurosurg. **9**:648, 1952.
311. Schwarz, E.: Craniometaphyseal dysplasia, Amer. J. Roentgen. **84**:461, 1960.
312. Schwarz, E., and Fish, A.: Roentgenographic features of a new congenital dysplasia, Amer. J. Roentgen. **84**:511, 1960.
313. Seigman, E. L., and Kilby, W. L.: Osteopetrosis; report of a case and review of recent literature, Amer. J. Roentgen. **63**:865, 1950.
314. Senturia, H. R., and Senturia, B. D.: Congenital absence of patellae associated with arthrodysplasia of elbows and dystrophy of nails, Amer. J. Roentgen. **51**:352, 1944.
315. Shnitka, T. K., Asp, D. M., and Horner, R. N.: Congenital generalized fibromatosis, Cancer **11**:627, 1958.
316. Shuler, S. E.: Pycnodysostosis, Arch. Dis. Child. **38**:620, 1963.
317. Silverman, J. L.: Apparent dominant inheritance of hypophosphatasia, Arch. Intern. Med. **110**:191, 1962.

318. Simril, W. A., and Thurston, D.: Normal interpediculate space in spines of infants and children, Radiology **64:**340, 1955.
319. Singleton, E. B., Daeschner, C. W., and Teng, C. T.: Peripheral dysostosis, Amer. J. Roentgen. **84:**499, 1960.
320. Singleton, E. B., Thomas, J. R., Worthington, W. W., and Hild, J. R.: Progressive diaphyseal dysplasia (Engelmann's disease), Radiology **67:**233, 1956.
321. Sjölin, K. E.: Gargoylism, forme fruste, Acta Paediat. **40:**165, 1951.
322. Slepian, A., and Hamby, W. B.: Neurologic complications associated with hereditary deforming chondrodysplasia: review of the literature and a report on two cases occurring in the same family, J. Neurosurg. **8:**529, 1951.
323. Spahr, A., and Spahr-Hartmann, I.: Dysostose metaphysaire familiale. Étude de 4 cas dans une fratrie, Helv. Paediat. Acta **16:**836, 1961.
324. Spillane, J. D.: Three cases of achondroplasia with neurological complications, J. Neurol. Neurosurg. Psychiat. **15:**246, 1952.
325. Stephens, F. E.: An achondroplastic mutation and the nature of its inheritance, J. Hered. **34:**229, 1943.
326. Stickler, G. B., Maher, F. T., Hunt, J. C., Burke, E. C., and Rosevear, J. W.: Familial bone disease resembling rickets (hereditary metaphysial dysostosis), Pediatrics **29:**996, 1962.
327. Stocks, P., and Barrington, A.: Hereditary disorders of bone development. Treasury of human inheritance, vol. 3, part 1, diaphysial aclasia (multiple exostoses), multiple enchondromatosis, cleidocranial dysostosis, London, 1925, Cambridge University Press.
328. Stoner, C. N., Hayes, J. T., and Holt, J. F.: Diastrophic dwarfism, Amer. J. Roentgen **89:**914, 1963.
329. Stout, A. P.: Juvenile fibromatoses, Cancer **7:**953, 1954.
330. Taybi, H.: Diastrophic dwarfism, Radiology **80:**1, 1963.
331. Thompson, E. A., Walker, E. T., and Wiens, H. T.: Iliac horns, osseous manifestation of hereditary arthrodysplasia associated with dystrophy of fingernails, Radiology **53:**88, 1949.
332. Thomsen, G., and Guttadauro, M.: Cleidocranial dysostosis associated with osetosclerosis and bone fragility, Acta Radiol. **37:**559, 1952.
333. Tips, R. L., and Lynch, H. T.: Malignant congenital osteopetrosis resulting from a consanguineous marriage, Acta Paediat. **51:**585, 1962.
334. Van Buchem, F. S. P., Hadders, H. N., Hansen, J. F., and Woldring, M. G.: Hyperostosis corticalis generalisata: report of seven cases, Amer. J. Med. **33:**387, 1962.
335 Von Knorre, G.: Ueber die hereditare Arthro-osteo-onycho-dysplasie (Turner-Kieser-Syndrome), Z. Menschl. Vererb. Konstitutionsl. **36:**118, 1961.
336. Vogl, A.: The fate of the achondroplastic drawf (neurologic complications of achondroplasia), Exp. Med. Surg. **20:**108, 1962.
337. Vogl, A., and Osborne, R.: Lesions of the spinal cord (transverse myelopathy) in achondroplasia, Arch. Neurol. Psychiat. **61:**644, 1949.
338. Weinberg, H., Frankel, M., and Makin, M.: Familial epiphysial dysplasia of the lower limbs, J. Bone Joint Surg. **42-B:**313, 1960.
339. Wiedemann, H.-R.: Die grossen Konstitutions-Krankheiten des Skeletts, Stuttgart, 1960, Gustav Fischer Verlag.
340. Wildervanck, L. S.: Hereditary congenital abnormality of elbows, knees and nails in five generations, Acta Radiol. **33:**41, 1950.
341. Witkop, C. J., Jr.: Genetics and dentistry, Eugen. Quart. **5:**15, 1958. Also in Pruzansky, S., editor: Congenital anomalies of the face and associated structures, Springfield, Ill., 1961, Charles C Thomas, Publisher.
342. Zimmer, E. A.: Heinrich Albers-Schönberg, Schweiz. Med. Wschr. **95:**140, 1965.
343. Zwerg, H. G., and Laubmann, W.: Die Albers-Schönbergsche Marmorkrankheit, Ergebn. Med. Strahlenforsch. **7:**95, 1936.

11

The future in the study of heritable disorders of connective tissue

Identification of the primary gene-determined defect is the goal in all these disorders. In the last decade (p. 15) it has been demonstrated that the primary function of the gene is to specify the amino acid sequence of a protein, all of whose properties are reflections of this sequence, or primary structure. The gene-determined protein may be an enzyme, and mutation in the relevant gene may lead to an inborn error of metabolism. Among the heritable disorders of connective tissue, homocystinuria and alkaptonuria are well-established examples. Or the gene-product may be a nonenzymic protein such as collagen.

The search for portein abnormalities, enzymic or nonenzymic, in those heritable disorders of connective tissue whose defect at the molecular level remains obscure—and this description applies to most of them—will be the task of the next few decades. The mode of inheritance can, as has been emphasized several times, serve as a guide to the type of defect to be sought. Enzymatic defects are to be expected in pseudoxanthoma elasticum, the mucopolysaccharidoses, and other recessive disorders such as diastrophic dwarfism and cartilage-hair hypoplasia. A substitution in the amino acid sequence of collagen should be sought in dominant disorders such as the Ehlers-Danlos syndrome and osteogenesis imperfecta.

Rich opportunity for further study of heritable disorders of connective tissue at the clinical level also remains: separation of the entities that presently are thought to be one, i.e. demonstration of genetic heretogeneity; improvement in methods for recognizing mild affection; analysis of the factors, particularly the environmental ones, which are involved in the variability in clinical severity; further nosologic study of all these conditions, particularly the genetic disorders of the osseous skeleton; further exploration of surgical procedures for correcting the structural effects, such as the aortic aneurysm and the scoliosis of the Marfan syndrome.

12

General summary and conclusions

1. In general, the clinical picture of each of the heritable disorders of connective tissue is as specific and predictable as that of other clinical entities—for example, infectious diseases. There is, of course, a certain amount of variability in clinical expression, such as the physician learns to expect. The clinical manifestations of each syndrome were summarized in tabular form in Chapter 1.

2. The heritable disorders of connective tissue are not congenital malformations in the conventional sense. Certain congenital malformations do seem to occur with increased frequency in association with some of these disorders. It is proposed that during embryogenesis the connective tissue defect sets the stage favorable to the development of the particular malformations. See Chapter 3 on the Marfan syndrome for examples.

3. Pseudoxanthoma elasticum behaves like an abiotrophy, as does also the aortic involvement in the Marfan syndrome. The peculiarities of growth in the Marfan syndrome and the Hurler syndrome are apparently intimately related to the basic defect of connective tissue. Certain features of the Hurler syndrome (specifically those relating to the brain, liver, spleen, and cardiovascular system) partake of the characteristics of a thesaurosis, or "storage" disease. In osteogenesis imperfecta and in the Ehlers-Danlos syndrome there appears to be a defect in the formation of collagen. Homocystinuria and alkaptonuria are inborn errors of metabolism. Both are also generalized heritable disorders of connective tissue.

4. Many principles of heredity are illustrated by these disorders. Examples of dominant, recessive, and sex-linked inheritance are provided. Phenomena of expressivity and penetrance are displayed.

5. The recognition of the more easily detectable expressions of the basic defect of connective tissue provides clinical clues to the nature of internal disturbances that are less accessible for study. Most dramatic among the illustrations of this time-honored principle are the associations of ectopia lentis with aortic regurgitation in the Marfan syndrome and of angioid streaks of the fundus oculi and characteristic skin changes with massive gastrointestinal hemorrhage in pseudoxanthoma elasticum.

6. The intimate interrelationships of the several elements of connective tis-

sue are indicated by the difficulties in identifying the specific element of connective tissue that is defective in several of these syndromes.

7. The heritable disorders of connective tissue are ripe for major advances in identification of the fundamental molecular defect, involving either an enzymic or a nonenzymic protein. An enzyme defect can be expected in those conditions with recessive inheritance; a defect in a nonenzymic protein, e.g. collagen, should be sought in those disorders which have a dominant mode of inheritance.

8. The heritable disorders of connective tissue can be useful tools for the study of the normal biology of connective tissue. Further confirmation is provided for the principle enunciated by Sir Archibald Garrod: the clinical and other investigation of hereditary disorders will shed light on normal developmental and biochemical mechanisms.

Index

B

T